7. 27. 92

Techniques in Extracorporeal Circulation

Techniques in Extracorporeal Circulation

Third Edition

Edited by

Philip H. Kay

Consultant Cardiothoracic Surgeon
The General Infirmary at Leeds
Leeds
UK

BUTTERWORTH
HEINEMANN

Butterworth-Heinemann Ltd
Linacre House, Jordan Hill, Oxford OX2 8DP

PART OF REED INTERNATIONAL BOOKS

OXFORD LONDON BOSTON
MUNICH NEW DELHI SINGAPORE SYDNEY
TOKYO TORONTO WELLINGTON

First published 1976
Second edition 1981
Reprinted 1982
Third edition 1992

British Library Cataloguing in Publication Data
Kay, Philip H.
Techniques in Extracorporeal
Circulation–3Rev. ed
I. Title II. Kay, P. H.
617.4
ISBN 0 7506 1391 2

Library of Congress Cataloguing in Publication Data
Techniques in extracorporeal circulation/edited by
Philip H. Kay.–3rd ed.
p. cm.
Rev. ed. of: Current techniques in extracorporeal
circulation. 1976.
Includes bibliographical references and index.
ISBN 0 7506 1391 2
1. Blood–Circulation, Artificial. I. Kay, Philip H.
II. Current techniques in extracorporeal circulation.
[DNLM: 1. Extracorporeal Circulation–methods.
2. Heart Surgery. WG 168 T255]
RD598.35.A77T43 1992
617.4'1–dc20
DNLM/DLC
for Library of Congress 91-36525
CIP

Composition by Scribe Design, Gillingham, Kent
Printed and bound in Great Britain by
The Bath Press, Avon.

Contents

Publisher's Preface vii
Preface to Third Edition ix
Preface to Second Edition xi
Preface to First Edition xiii
List of Contributors xv

1 Historical aspects 1
S.A. Livesey and S.C. Lennox
2 Physiology and pathophysiology of extracorporeal circulation 8
Robert H. Bartlett and Ralph E. Delius
3 Design and principles of the extracorporeal circuit 33
L. Bigi, N. Ghelli, A. Menghini and I. Panzani
4 Membrane and bubble oxygenators 42
Marc E. Voorhees and Roger Elgas
5 Filtration in cardiopulmonary bypass 56
Linda Marshall
6 Priming fluids for cardiopulmonary bypass 72
Mahesh V. Shah
7 Anaesthetic techniques for cardiopulmonary bypass 78
J.W.W. Gothard
8 Intraoperative myocardial protection 88
Simon J.M. Ledingham
9 Postoperative management following cardiopulmonary bypass 138
Martin K.G. Boylan
10 Haematological aspects of extracorporeal circulation 144
Mano S. Raja and Alan F. Penny
11 The role of the complement system during cardiopulmonary bypass 156
R.S. Bonser and D. Vergani
12 Changes in renal function associated with cardiopulmonary bypass 178
F.D. Thompson
13 The neurological sequelae of cardiopulmonary bypass 183
Peter Smith
14 Microbiological aspects of heart, heart–lung and lung transplant patients 194
Roger Freeman and Frances Kate Gould
15 Blood conservation following cardiovascular surgery 205
Altagracia M. Chavez and Delos M. Cosgrove III
16 Pulsatile flow during cardiopulmonary bypass 211
David Bregman, Michael Kesselbrenner and Jeffrey B. Sack
17 Low flow and circulatory arrest 230
P.H. Kay
18 Intra-aortic balloon counterpulsation 236
Michael Kesselbrenner, Jeffrey B. Sack, Robert A. Saporito Jr and David Bregman
19 Ventricular assist devices 268
Timothy Locke and Christopher McGregor
20 Artificial hearts – present and future 282
W.J. Kolff and Jack Kolff
21 Heart and heart–lung transplantation 299
G. Fradet, J.P. Scott, T.R. Graham, R.L. Smyth, E. Solis and J. Wallwork
22 Extracorporeal respiratory support 309
John H. Dark
23 Future developments and potential applications of extracorporeal circulation in medicine and surgery 321
Hans Zwart
Index 331

Publisher's Preface

In the years which have elapsed since the publication of the second edition of Marian Ionescu's *Techniques in Extracorporeal Circulation* there have been many advances in technology and thought on the topic, and these are reflected in the contents of this new edition, edited by Philip Kay. Drawing on an international team of contributors, the book is an essential reference for cardiothoracic surgeons, anaesthetists, perfusionists and support staff.

Preface to Third Edition

The heart is a unique organ, simple in concept as a muscle pump, but complex in design and function. Heart failure, from whatever cause, remains the commonest cause of death in the western world.

It is now almost 100 years since von Reyn contravened the dictates of Billroth, risked 'loosing the esteme of his colleagues' and successfully operated on the heart. However cardiac surgery proceeded at a slow pace until the development of the extracorporeal circuit. Thereafter the understanding of the complex anatomy, biochemistry, pharmacology and physiology of the heart has enabled us to take great strides in the complex repair work that is now so common place in the operating room. Concomitantly, advances in rheology and material science have provided a wider safety margin and therefore expanded the number of patients able to benefit from cardiac surgery. It is these advances that form the basis of the third edition of *Techniques in Extracorporeal Circulation.*

The first edition of this book, edited by Mr M. Ionescu and Mr G. Wooller 16 years ago laid a solid foundation for the student of extracorporeal circulation. It was followed by a second edition five years later and after a further 11 years by this edition. Yet progress in this field is so fast that many of the new developments in this book were not even contemplated in the final 'future developments' chapter of the second edition and so I am sure will be the case for the fourth edition. Similarly much progress has been made during the three years it has taken to produce this book. Nevertheless, this edition, like the original, provides a firm basis for doctors, nurses, perfusionists and physicians assistants alike, all students of the extracorporeal circulation and its ever increasing number of applications.

I hope that it will stimulate its readers to continuing the pioneering interface between the lone surgeon and the increasingly complex machinery that surrounds him.

P.H. Kay

Preface to Second Edition

The preface to the first edition of this book was preceded by Michelangelo's humble remark 'ancora imparo'. Even for the contents of this small book on techniques in extracorporeal circulation it proved its timeless veracity as we 'continue to learn'.

The first edition however, despite many shortcomings, has fulfilled its role.

During the past few years the energetic clinical and research activities have led to many advances and have further broadened the concept of artificial circulation and oxygenation so that an increasing number of subspecialties are now attaining a certain contour.

In recent years, several areas of extracorporeal circulation have assumed increasing importance. The progress made in the field of ischaemic heart disease and the major impact of myocardial protection through cardioplegia are only two of the most obvious examples. Refinements in the construction and performance of bubble oxygenators and the introduction of disposable membrane oxygenating systems have changed the techniques of heart–lung bypass and broadened its scope.

Many pioneers in these fields have discovered and rediscovered noteworthy features of great clinical significance.

This second edition attempts to summarize the major technical problems and touches on some of the more theoretical aspects of extracorporeal circulation but does not necessarily provide final answers.

In an effort to keep abreast of the many advances which have occurred, a number of additional topics have been included in this present edition. Several new, outstanding contributors have participated, whilst the great majority of those chapters which appeared in the first edition have been updated or augmented.

Despite the awareness of discontinuity and reiteration, this second edition of *Techniques in Extracorporeal Circulation* retains the structure of most modern books by being comprised of a series of individual chapters.

I wish to express my enthusiasm for the privilege of editing this text and gratefully acknowledge the outstanding contributions of the authors who have joined in this endeavour.

I should like to thank Miss Wendy Lawrence for the complex and seemingly endless secretarial work.

My sincere appreciation is extended to Messrs Butterworths for their unfailing attention to detail and for the maintenance of the high standards for which they are known.

Marian I. Ionescu

Preface to First Edition

ancora imparo
Michelangelo Buonarotti

Extracorporeal circulation with an artificial heart-lung machine has established itself as the routine adjunct to intracardiac and vascular surgery. Since its introduction in 1953 this method has been progressively improved by development and simplification of the equipment and by better understanding of the body response to the alterations induced by the use of artificial perfusions.

The method, established in the experimental laboratory, has been perfected by clinical use. For many poorly understood aspects the method has continued to be investigated in the laboratory, where answers and solutions have been found for innumerable bewildering and knotty clinical problems.

A superficial look at today's methods would give the uninformed the general impression that no substantial progress has been made in the past ten years. For example, the same principle of bubble oxygenation used at the beginning of the open-heart surgery era is almost universally employed today. The same may be said for metallic prosthetic valves with a ball or disc occluder mechanism. The best method for 'myocardial preservation' during open-heart surgery is yet to be established and the Montagues of hypothermia still have to convince the Capulets of coronary perfusion of the veracity and superiority of their principle just as much as they had to ten years ago.

On closer examination, one realizes that during the past ten years an enormous wealth of data and knowledge has been accumulated and the application of this knowledge has made clinical perfusions incomparably better and safer. The results of cardiovascular surgery obtained today, whether in the newborn or the elderly, for great arteries or coronary arteries, in routine cases or in emergencies, when compared with the results obtained only ten years ago, are the best proof of progress and continuous improvement in extracorporeal circulation.

During the past few years many new and exciting principles and techniques based on extracorporeal circulation have been brought into clinical use. Deep hypothermia for heart surgery in the newborn, prolonged extracorporeal oxygenation-perfusion for pulmonary insufficiency and intra-aortic balloon pumping for circulatory assistance are some of the major achievements of the past decade.

The paucity of books devoted exclusively to extracorporeal circulation has prompted us to bring together in a single volume standard *current techniques in extracorporeal circulation* along with the more recent developments in this field. This is an attempt to answer some of the innumerable practical problems associated with the routine use of artificial circulation and oxygenation and to present some models of standardized techniques.

A major problem with such a book is to decide what to include and what to omit. We are aware that omissions have been made but we have aimed to keep the subject matter strictly circumscribed in the interest of text size and readability. The esoteric has been omitted on purpose and emphasis is placed on the current practical methodology.

Advances in modern surgical and perfusion techniques have been developed to such a degree that an entirely new spectrum of problems evolves with each new development. Such rapid changes and improvements will certainly call for another publication in the near future and this is another reason for limiting the size of this book.

Since this is a multi-authored book and the chapters are designed to be read separately, some reiteration has been inevitable, although an attempt was made to avoid repetition.

Major attention has been focused on the cardiovascular system, the lung, the renal function and haematological changes. Clearly the brain, liver, gut, muscle masses and reticuloendothelial system are of great importance in the body response to extracorporeal circulation but the measurement of their function in the cardiovascular patient is at the moment largely in the realm of the investigator. Although the principles and techniques described have become routine for practical purposes, they are by no means beyond challenge. As William Hazlitt put it 'when a thing ceases to be a subject of controversy, it ceases to be a subject of interest'.

The Editors join the contributors in hoping that this volume will be of interest to those active in the field of cardiovascular surgery.

We take great pleasure in expressing our thanks to Dr Frank Gerbode for kindly writing the Foreword of this work. We are grateful to Miss Nancy Evans for her continuous and enthusiastic help.

Completion of this book within a few months was promised, but it has taken almost two years and we appreciate the forbearance and continuous help of our publishers, Butterworth and Co. Ltd.

M.I. Ionescu

Contributors

RH Bartlett MD
Professor of General and Thoracic Surgery
The University of Michigan Medical Center
Ann Arbor
Michigan
USA

L Bigi PhD
Scientific Affairs Director
Dideco SpA
Italy

RS Bonser MRCP, FRCS
Consultant Cardiothoracic Surgeon
Queen Elizabeth Hospital
Birmingham, UK

MKG Boylan BA(Hons), MB, ChB, FFARCS
Consultant Anaesthetist
The General Infirmary at Leeds
Leeds, UK

D Bregman MD, FACS
Department of Surgery
St Joseph's Hospital and Medical Center
Paterson
New Jersey
USA

AM Chavez MD
Assistant Professor of Surgery
MetroHealth Medical Center
Cleveland
Ohio, USA

DM Cosgrove III MD
Thoracic and Cardiovascular Surgery
Cleveland Clinic Foundation
Cleveland
Ohio
USA

JH Dark FRCS
Consultant Cardiothoracic Surgeon
Freeman Hospital
Newcastle upon Tyne, UK

RE Delius MD
Instructor in Surgery
The University of Michigan Medical Center
Ann Arbor
Michigan, USA

R Elgas
Cobe Cardiovascular Inc
Arvada
Colorado, USA

G Fradet
Transplant Fellow
Papworth Hospital
Cambridgeshire, UK

R Freeman MB,ChB, FRCPath
Reader in Bacteriology
University of Newcastle upon Tyne, UK

N Ghelli MSCE
R & D Department
Dideco SpA
Italy

JWW Gothard FFARCS
Consultant Anaesthetist
Anaesthetic Department
The Royal Brompton National
Heart and Lung Hospital
London, UK

FK Gould MBBS, MRCPath
Consultant Microbiologist
Freeman Hospital
Newcastle upon Tyne, UK

TR Graham FRCS
Transplant Fellow
Papworth Hospital
Cambridgeshire, UK

PH Kay DM, FRCS
Consultant Cardiothoracic Surgeon
The General Infirmary at Leeds
Leeds, UK

M Kesselbrenner MD, FACC
Fair Lawn
New Jersey
USA

WJ Kolff MD, PhD
Kolff's Laboratory Department of Surgery
University of Utah
Salt Lake City
Utah
USA

SJM Ledingham MD, FRCS
National Heart and Lung Institute,
London, UK

SC Lennox FRCS
The Brompton Hospital
Fulham Road
London, UK

SA Livesey FRCS
Consultant Cardiothoracic Surgeon
Southampton General Hospital
Southampton, UK

TJ Locke MD, FRCS
Consultant Cardiothoracic Surgeon
Northern General Hospital
Leeds, UK

L Marshall BSc, PhD
School of Biological Sciences
University of Manchester
Manchester, UK

A Menghini
Cardiopulmonary Group Product Manager
Dideco SpA
Italy

CGA McGregor MB, FRCS
Director of Cardiothoracic Transplantation
The Mayo Clinic
Minnesota
USA

I Panzani PhD
R & D Director
Dideco SpA
Italy

AF Penny BSc, MSc
Principal Biochemist
Department of Biochemistry
Seacroft Hospital
Leeds, UK

MS Rajah MBBS, FRCP
Consultant Clinical Haematologist
Department of Haematology
Killingbeck Hospital
Leeds, UK

JP Scott
Transplant Fellow
Papworth Hospital
Cambridgeshire, UK

MV Shah FFARCS
Diplomate of the American Board of
Anesthesiologists; and
Consultant Anaesthetist
The General Infirmary at Leeds
Leeds, UK

P Smith MBBS, MRCP, FRCS
Consultant Cardiothoracic Surgeon
Hammersmith Hospital
London, UK

RL Smyth
Transplant Fellow
Papworth Hospital
Cambridgeshire, UK

E Solis
Transplant Fellow
Papworth Hospital
Cambridgeshire, UK

FD Thompson FRCP
Consultant Nephrologist
St Philips Hospital
London, UK

D Vergani MD
Senior Lecturer in Immunology
King's College Hospital
London, UK

ME Voorhees PhD
Engineering Manager
Cobe Cardiovascular Inc
Arvada
Colorado, USA

J Wallwork FRCS
Consultant Cardiac Surgeon
Papworth Hospital
Cambridgeshire, UK

H Zwart MD, FACS, FACC
Hans Zwart MD and Associates Inc
Ohio
USA

1

Historical aspects

S.A. Livesey and S.C. Lennox

The progress of cardiac surgery over the last four decades will have delighted and amazed the pioneers whose work is briefly described in this chapter. From operating on only the most parlous patients with end-stage congenital heart disease the specialty has developed into a routine service with a minimal morbidity and mortality; this owes much to the development of a safe, reliable and versatile method of maintaining the circulation using extracorporeal support.

The concept of external support of the circulation has been with us for nearly two centuries. At the end of the eighteenth century physiologists were aware that the function of certain organs – the nervous system and muscles – could be restored after death by perfusing these organs with blood. In the mid-nineteenth century Brown-Sequard (1858) used his own blood to perfuse an animal limb and was able to restore local reflexes.

The concept of artificial oxygenation developed a little later. After several workers had shown that blood could be 'arterialized' by bubbling oxygen through it, von Frey and Gruber (1885) developed the first 'heart–lung' machine in 1885. In this machine blood was allowed to form a film on the inside of a hollow metal cylinder where it was exposed to oxygen. Later that century in 1895 Jacobj used an isolated animal lung as an oxygenator.

From the mid-nineteenth century it was apparent that untreated blood could not be used to maintain artificial perfusion because it clotted, so it was rendered incoagulable by whipping (which results in defibrination) and then it flowed freely. It was not until the discovery of heparin by McLean in 1916 that perfusion science could begin to make significant advances.

The development of satisfactory pumps was more troublesome to early workers in the field than was the development of oxygenators. Rubber balloons and various camshaft mechanisms were initially used but it was the development of the Dale–Schuster valved pump and later the DeBakey roller pump that allowed this aspect of perfusion to develop. The controversy over pulsatile and non-pulsatile perfusion has long been present. Hamel (1888) and Jacobj (1890) were aware of the desirability of pulsatile flow and constructed several elaborate devices to achieve this.

Much of the early drive in the development of extracorporeal techniques came from physiologists but they were to a certain extent unaware of the adverse effects various materials had on blood and sterility did not feature in early experiments. Unrecognized sepsis may have accounted for some instances of circulatory failure that were at the time thought to be a direct consequence of perfusion *per se*.

Although many scientists were working on techniques of extracorporeal circulation throughout the world, the credit for their introduction into clinical practice should go to Kolff who pioneered haemodialysis using an artificial kidney (1944) and to Gibbon (1954) who successfully repaired an atrial septal defect in a young woman in 1953 with the circulation totally supported by an extracorporeal pump oxygenator system.

Methods of oxygenation

Many methods of artificial oxygenation of blood have been investigated over the last century starting from the direct injection of oxygen into the bloodstream, to the use of chemicals to generate oxygen, proceeding to the film oxygenators which were used in the heyday of cardiac surgery and finally to the modern bubble and membrane oxygenators in use today.

In an experiment in 1811 Nysten injected oxygen intravenously into dogs breathing pure nitrogen and was able to prolong their survival by several minutes but no longer. Similar experiments in the twentieth century (Bourne and Smith, 1927) showed that the amount of intravenous oxygen needed to raise the oxygen saturation significantly resulted in circulatory embarassment due to gaseous pulmonary emboli. The concept was later extended by Singh (1935, 1960) who used hyperbaric chambers to increase the solubility of the injected oxygen and used the technique clinically along with hypothermia to reduce the patient's oxygen requirements.

The administration of oxygen by the subcutaneous or intraperitoneal routes was found to be of no value in raising the blood oxygen tension (Bourne and Smith, 1927).

The concept of using chemicals to generate oxygen has also been investigated. The injection of hydrogen peroxide intravenously produced severe hypertension though the use of dilute solutions was tried clinically (Abeatici, 1959). Injecting a solution of sodium percarbonate which degrades to produce oxygen microbubbles was also tried but this too gave rise to gas emboli as did the injection of oxygenated saline. Haemoglobin is much easier to oxygenate in the free form than when held in intact red cells. Amberson (1949) used a solution of free haemoglobin in Ringer's lactate to replace an animal's entire circulating volume and the animals behaved normally for several hours. However the free haemoglobin is taken up by the reticuloendothelial system and is also excreted in the urine so death resulted from hypoxia in 36h.

A technique of 'pervascular oxygenation' was described at the turn of the century (Magnus, 1902). Isolated organs were perfused with moist oxygen and basic organ functions continued for a limited time. In 1959 Sabiston kept an isolated heart beating for up to 8h with this technique.

All of these experiments concerned themselves with artificial oxygenation and ignored the need for removal of carbon dioxide.

Cross-circulation

The idea of using a 'donor' to support the vital function of a recipient circulation was conceived in the late nineteenth century. Fredericq (1890) diverted the circulation via glass tubes from the carotid artery of one animal to the carotid artery of another and was able to maintain cerebral function.

Cross-circulation for total body perfusion utilized what became known as the 'azygos principle'. It had initially been thought that flows comparable to the resting cardiac output were necessary to maintain vital centres during cardiopulmonary bypass, but Andreasen and Watson (1952) showed that dogs survived after clamping the venae cavae for up to 40 min provided the azygos vein was left open. The cardiac output was considerably reduced (about 10 ml kg^{-1} min^{-1}). Using this observation Cohen and Lillehei (1954) found that atrial operations could be tolerated but if ventriculotomy was to be performed, higher flows were found necessary – in the region of 20–40 ml kg^{-1} min^{-1}. This ability of the body to tolerate such low flows allowed the development of cardiac surgery supported by cross-circulation. Using a dual pump (arterial and venous) and a venous reservoir, Lillehei reported the use of this technique to repair intracardiac defects in 32 patients in 1955.

At the same time as conventional methods of cardiopulmonary bypass were being developed, various workers used preoxygenated blood held in a reservoir which was then slowly transfused to the recipient. However large volumes of blood were needed and the circulation could only be supported for a short period of time (and at low flow rates) by this method.

The lung as an oxygenator

The lung remains the ideal oxygenator since it also removes carbon dioxide and does not cause blood damage. In 1895 Jacobj used an isolated lung to oxygenate blood in various organ perfusion experiments and this technique was later developed to the point where it could be used as the oxygenator for whole body perfusion in animal experiments. Rather than use an isolated lung, Potts *et al.* (1952) cannulated the pulmonary circulation *in situ* and used this with a mechanical pump to perform cardiac operations on animals.

Mustard (1955) and other workers used animal lungs as oxygenators during human cardiac surgery after meticulous washing. However the system was complicated and not superior to artificial oxygenators being developed at the same time.

Right heart bypass was the natural extension of the isolated lung technique. This was used by Dodrill *et al.* (1953) to support the circulation while the right ventricle was excluded; this allowed open surgery to the right ventricular outflow tract. Combined right and left heart bypass using the lungs as an oxygenator was the next logical step and was apparently simple. However cannulation was sometimes difficult and achieving a balanced flow in the two circuits was also a problem. The problem of imbalance was resolved by Ross (1959) by allowing one reservoir to drain into the other if imbalance in venous drainage from each half of the circulation became too great.

Reduction of body temperature to 30°C allowed up to 10 min cardiac arrest, enough time to correct simple intracardiac lesions. Cooling below this temperature is liable to cause irreversible ventricular fibrillation. Combining hypothermia with cardiopulmonary perfusion overcame this problem and gave several advantages. Since the oxygen requirements of the body are reduced, the blood flow could be reduced. This in turn reduces collateral flow and gives a drier operative fields. Better oxygenation and less blood damage are also important benefits.

In dogs Bigelow (1950) showed that as their temperature was reduced, their oxygen requirement was reduced in an almost linear fashion. Drew (1958) combined profound hypothermia with combined right and left heart bypass using the patient's own lungs as the oxygenator. The patient was cooled to 15°C using right and left bypass allowing a much longer period of circulatory arrest. He reported seven cases with two deaths in which the circulatory arrest was up to 45 min. This time allowed much more complex lesions to be repaired especially as the operation was on a still bloodless heart. This was an important contribution at that time.

Oxygenators

Efficient gas exchange requires the exposure of blood to 'gas' over a large surface area to allow rapid equilibration between the two. Three basic types have been developed; bubble, film and membrane oxygenators.

Bubble oxygenators

Although the concept of oxygenation of blood by a continuous stream of oxygen bubbles was proposed at the turn of the century its use was initially confined to the intravenous injection of oxygen which led to pulmonary embolism and death. The use of a reservoir, bubble traps and defoaming agents to produce an essentially bubble-free arterial stream allowed the successful clinical use of bubble oxygenation (Clark *et al.*, 1950). The DeWall bubble oxygenator (DeWall *et al.*, 1956) used this principle. Oxygen was bubbled through blood which then flowed through a chamber coated with an antifoam compound. It then passed through a helical bubble trap and was filtered before being pumped to the patient. This oxygenator was intended to be easily sterilized and re-used. Eventually a disposable plastic version was developed which although only capable of low flow rates was efficient for about an hour.

The Rygg–Kyvsgaard 'bag' (Rygg and Kyvsgaard, 1956) took the same idea further. It combined the bubbling and settling chambers along with a reservoir in the same plastic 'bag'. Polythene sponges coated with an antifoam agent were used for debubbling. Flows of $3\,l\,min^{-1}$ were delivered from the early designs and they remained relatively efficient for several hours.

The bubble concept is also used in 'foam' oxygenators but they differ from the above in that venous blood enters from the top of the oxygenator and flows over the large bubbles created by oxygen being bubbled in at the bottom. Arterialized blood then collects at the base of the oxygenator and is pumped to the patient.

Film oxygenators

The oxygenator developed by Gibbon which was used for the first successful open heart operations to be supported by a heart–lung machine was of this type. The principle is extremely simple. Blood is allowed to form a very thin film on a metal plate and is exposed to oxygen. This is not dissimilar to von Frey and Gruber's original concept of an oxygenator.

Gibbon's first oxygenator using the thin film principle utilized a vertical cylinder (Gibbon, 1937). The stream of venous blood was directed against the inner surface of the rapidly revolving vertical cylinder on to which it spreads in a thin film. This is then exposed to a mixture of 95% oxygen and 5% carbon dioxide at a gas flow of $5\,l\,min^{-1}$. Roller pumps were used on both arterial and venous sides of the oxygenator. There was no reservoir in the circuit but a membrane manometer was attached to a T-tube on the venous line: resting on this was a column of mercury which operated an electric switch. Whenever the venous return stopped because of the caval wall being sucked against the cannula the pressure in the manometer fell and the switch shut the pump off. As the level rose again the pump was similarly switched back on. Gibbon surrounded the blood tubing by a water bath to maintain a constant temperature during perfusion.

This system was capable of delivering $500\,ml\,min^{-1}$ of oxygenated blood which was enough for his early experiments using cats in which he occluded the pulmonary artery for up to 25 min and supported the circulation with this system. Some of his animals survived for over a year. Gibbon felt at this time (1937) that his apparatus would not be capable of supporting the entire circulation of a man but that it might be able to be used as an assist device for the failing heart or be used in patients with massive pulmonary embolism until embolectomy could be performed.

The early film oxygenators were inefficient because diffusion of gas is limited to the superficial layer of the blood film. The efficiency can be increased by causing mixing of the blood and gas to occur. Gibbon's group used a screen of wire mesh to cause turbulence at the blood–gas interface and this greatly increased the efficiency of the oxygenator.

At the Mayo Clinic Kirlin's group built an oxygenator of the Gibbon screen type. It consisted of fourteen wire mesh screens, each 30 × 45 cm enclosed in a lucite case. Blood flowed on to the screens through a series of 0.006 mm slots; the gas flow was 10 l min^{-1} of oxygen the carbon dioxide flow being automatically varied according to the pH of the arterial blood leaving the oxygenator.

The efficiency of the film oxygenator could also be increased by increasing the surface area of the blood film.

Bjork (1948) realized that as oxygenation was almost instantaneous, blood only needed to be exposed to oxygen for a short time and that by rapid exchange of blood films efficient oxygenation could be achieved in relatively small apparatus.

He developed a film oxygenator comprising a number of vertical plates mounted on a central axle – he used 40 plates 13 cm in diameter arranged in groups of four along the axle. Each group was separated by a baffle in the floor of the oxygenator – this caused blood to mix and further improved efficiency.

Membrane oxygenators

As in the 'natural' lung the blood/gas interface is separated by a semi-permeable membrane (the alveolar capillary membrane), so in the membrane oxygenator this is replaced by a synthetic membrane. Separating the two media across a membrane has the advantage that a defoaming process is not needed and consequently blood trauma is reduced and longer bypass runs facilitated.

In his early dialysis experiments using a cellophane membrane Kolff (1944) observed that the venous blood became red. Later attempts to use this model as an oxygenator (rather than for dialysis) showed it to be a rather inefficient machine for gas exchange and only capable of arterializing blood at low flow rates (Kolff and Balzer, 1955).

Clowes and Neville used a multi-layered Teflon membrane oxygenator for human perfusion in 1957. However these oxygenators were rather bulky (the Clowes model had a membrane area of $25m^2$) difficult to assemble and sterility was difficult to guarantee. Priming this large membrane lung was tedious and heat loss across it was marked.

It was an early hope that membrane oxygenation would allow the support of patients with acute reversible pulmonary insufficiency for days rather than hours and this was the main stimulus to further research.

The prevention of blood clotting proved to be a significant problem in the early membranes, probably because the surface area of foreign materials was very high, blood flow rather slow and inadequate doses of heparin were used.

Silicone proved to be the most permeable material to both oxygen and carbon dioxide and the early membranes were made by dip coating a nylon mesh in silicone rubber.

The membrane lung was introduced into clinical practice in the late 1960s. The Bramson model was one of the earliest: this consisted of fourteen 'cells' – each cell having a silicone rubber membrane across which diffusion occurred (Bramson *et al.*, 1965).

The use of tubular capillary membranes rather than flat membranes (with a welcome reduction in the size of the oxygenator) was first proposed by Bodell (Bodell, Head and Head, 1963). In this system gas can either flow in the capillaries with blood on the outside or vice versa. The latter method has been the most successful approach and has led to the development of very efficient hollow fibre membrane oxygenators.

Blood pumps

The development of efficient atraumatic blood pumping devices lagged behind advances being made in oxygenator technology. Many different types of pumping mechanism were used – centrifugal pumps, conical rollers, double rollers (like the DeBakey pump), Archimedian screw, worm screw, piston, diaphragm and ventricle type pumps.

In early experiments at the turn of the nineteenth century, Jacobj (1895) and other scientists used a rubber bladder compressed by a motor driven eccentric shaft. Diaphragm pumps using valved inlet and outlet ports were one of the simplest early pumping devices. Dale and Schuster (1928) are given credit for the development and use of this type of pump. It consisted of a water-filled chamber which was intermittently compressed by a plunger; this in turn compressed a blood-filled chamber and blood flow was directed in the appropriate direction by valves on the inlet and outlet ports. The main problem with this type of pump was its limited output, though Jongbloed (1949) used six such pumps in parallel to obtain flows in the range needed for total cardiopulmonary bypass.

The commonest type of pumping device seen on perfusion apparatus today is the roller pump. This is usually associated with DeBakey who in 1934 described this type of pump as an aid to rapid blood transfusion, though many other workers used similar pumps.

Roller pumps have the advantage of simplicity but the disadvantage of being relatively traumatic to blood because of the extreme shearing forces developed by the repeated compression of blood in relatively narrow bore tubing. The amount of blood trauma is directly related to the degree of 'occlusiveness' of the pump's rollers and by reducing the occluding pressure the degree of haemolysis can be reduced.

Conduct of bypass

In the early years of cardiopulmonary bypass there was considerable discussion as to whether venous blood should reach the pump-oxygenator as a result of gravity drainage or be assisted by a suction pump. Initially suction drainage was preferred as this presented a relatively constant flow of blood to the oxygenator (the film type of oxygenator in particular was much more efficient when presented with a constant flow of blood) but obstruction of the venous cannulae was a constant problem. Many elaborate devices to prevent venous occlusion by the caval walls such as automatic relays to stop the pump (Kantrowitz, Reiner and Abelson, 1950) and arteriovenous connections which could be opened to unblock the venous lines were used.

Direct gravity drainage into the oxygenator had the advantage that it was simple and required little priming volume. However constant flow was difficult to ensure and this reduced the efficiency of the oxygenator. The problem was solved by using gravity drainage into a reservoir – the level of which could be varied to improve drainage – which then fed the oxygenator (Paneth *et al*., 1957). A pump was sometimes used to transfer blood from the reservoir to the oxygenator.

Arterial cannulation was also the subject of much controversy in the developing specialty. The limit to arterial return became not the blood pumps but the size of the arterial cannula which in turn was controlled by the size of the vessel to be intubated. Small cannulae resulted in high flow velocities and more haemolysis (Senning, 1952), so metal cannulae were preferred to the plastics available at the time because the ratio of internal to external diameter was high and thus for any given flow, velocity could be reduced.

In animal experiments the femoral, carotid and subclavian arteries had all been used for arterial cannulation. The subclavian approach fell out of favour when median sternotomy became the incision of choice. Many surgeons were initially worried that the direction of flow in the aorta was important and that inflow from the distal half of the body would not generate sufficient pressure to perfuse the cerebral and coronary vessels but femoral cannulation soon became the standard approach – though Kirklin felt that the external iliac artery was a better choice because it could accommodate a larger cannula.

Special cannulae which could be used conveniently for direct aortic cannulation were developed though it was many years before this became the standard route.

In the early days of bypass surgery the heart–lung machine was primed with fresh heparinized blood. Often large amounts were used and this caused an enormous strain on the blood banks. Postoperative bleeding was common and accentuated this problem. Controversy surrounded the amount of heparin required during the perfusion and the amount of protamine needed to neutralize it. The use of haemodilution has greatly simplified open heart surgery.

Clinical use

Possibly the first attempt to use cardiopulmonary bypass in the clinical setting was in Minneapolis in 1951. Dennis *et al*., 1951 had developed a Gibbon type oxygenator in a series of experiments in dogs. The problems in development were immense. They were able to produce a dry operating field but after only 30 min of perfusion 50% of the serum proteins had been lost, the platelet count had fallen by two-thirds and there was a marked metabolic acidosis. Fatal gastrointestinal haemorrhage often occurred in their animals. It was not until they realized that the perfusion apparatus was contaminated by *Escherichia coli* and that this was responsible for their problems were they able to progress by sterilizing the equipment in 3% formaldehyde for 12h. The system then had to be rinsed with 30 litres of saline before use. The group eventually modified Gibbon's rotating cylinder and used slowly rotating screen discs on to which blood was laid in fine jets. The 38 cm discs rotated 54 times per minute and could raise the oxygen saturation of a pint of blood from 45% to 95%. By using several similar discs mounted together on a shaft (after the method described by Bjork) they were able to use the system to operate on an adult patient.

On 5 April 1951, Dr R.L. Varco operated on a patient with a preoperative diagnosis of Lutembacher's syndrome (secundum atrial septal defect,) ASD, with mitral stenosis) using this system. The patient had 'pulmonary oedema and such cardiac enlargement as to completely collapse the left lung'. Bypass was set up between bicaval stainless steel cannulae and the right subclavian artery. Unfortunately the return of blood to the right atrium via the Thebesian veins was 250 ml min^{-1} and the lesion proved to be an ostium primum defect. An attempt was made to close it directly with interrupted sutures. Large amounts of citrated bank blood had to be added to maintain the circulation and it was felt that this caused the subsequent heart failure. The patient could not be weaned from bypass.

The work of Dr J.H. Gibbon Jr and his wife in the laboratories at Massachusetts General Hospital and later at the Jefferson Medical School in Philadelphia in the development of an efficient oxygenator culminated in the first successful clinical use of cardiopulmonary bypass for total support of the circulation when he repaired an ASD in a young woman in 1953.

He subsequently operated on four more patients all of whom died and he became disillusioned with his technique but his example remains one of the most significant achievements in surgery. Kirklin had also been working experimentally with a similar type of oxygenator and soon started to use it clinically (Kirklin *et al.*, 1955). He reported the repair of intracardiac defects in eight patients in 1955 using a Gibbon type of pump-oxygenator. (Four of these patients died; one because of reopening of a ventricular septal defect after direct suture; one 2h postoperatively because of heart failure; one because of respiratory failure and one could not be weaned from bypass because of unrecognized hypovolaemia. This was the only death which he attributed directly to a complication of perfusion.)

Since then enormous progress has taken place as has been outlined in this chapter. However organ and tissue damage still remains an important problem of cardiopulmonary bypass. Haemostasis was often difficult to achieve and although this is much less common it can still be a problem especially in patients undergoing further operations. Research into blood coagulation, particularly platelet function and the role of the endothelium, may improve this situation. The use of Aprotinin may be beneficial. Brain damage appears to be common although only a small number have an obvious clinical deficit.

References

Abeatici, S., Laugeri, V. and DeNunno, T. (1959) Sulle possibilita di ossigenazione ematica attraverso membrane porose mediante soluzione di perossido di idrogeno. *Minerva Chirurgica*, **13**, 860–868.

Amberson, W.R., Jennings, J.J. and Rhode, C.M. (1949) Clinical experience with haemoglobin-saline solutions. *Journal of Applied Physiology*, **1**, 469–489.

Andreasen, A.T. and Watson, F. (1952) Experimental cardiovascular surgery. *British Journal of Surgery*, **39**, 548–551.

Bigelow, W.G., Callaghan, J.C., Hopps, J.A. (1950) General hypothermia for experimental intracardiac surgery; use of electrophrenic respirations, artificial pacemaker for cardiac stand still and radio-frequency rewarming in general hypothermia. *Annals of Surgery*. **132**, 531–539.

Bjork, V.O. (1948) Brain perfusion in dogs with artificially oxygenated blood. *Acta Chirurgica Scandinavica Supplementum*, **96**, 137.

Bodell, B.R., Head, J.M. and Head, L.R. (1963) A capillary membrane oxygenator. *Journal of Thoracic and Cardiovascular Surgery*, **46**, 639–650.

Bourne, G. and Smith, R.G. (1927) The value of intravenous and intraperitoneal administration of oxygen. *American Journal of Physiology*, **82**, 328–334.

Bramson, M.L., Osborn, J.J., Main, F.B., *et al.* (1965) A new disposable membrane oxygenator with integral heat exchange. *Journal of Thoracic and Cardiovascular Surgery*, **50**, 391–400.

Brown-Sequard, E. (1858) Recherches experimentales sur les propetes physiologique et les usage du sang rouge et du sang noir et leurs principaux elements gazeux, l'oxygene et l'acide carbonique. *Journal de Physiologie de l'Homme*, **1**.

Clark, L.C., Gollan, F. and Gupta, V.B. (1950) The oxygenation of blood by gas dispersion. *Science*, **III**, 85–87.

Clowes, G.H.A. and Neville, W.E. (1957) Further developments of a blood oxygenator dependent upon the diffusion of gases through plastic membranes. *Transactions of the American Society for Artificial Internal Organs*, **3**, 53–58.

Cohen, M. and Lillehei, C.W. (1954) A quantitive study of the azygos factor during vena caval occlusion in the dog. *Surgery, Gynecology and Obstetrics*, **98**, 225–232.

Dale, H.H. and Schuster, E.A. (1928) A double perfusion pump. *Journal of Physiology*, **64**, 356–364.

DeBakey, M.E. (1934) A simple continuous flow transfusion instrument. *New Orleans Medical and Surgical Journal*, **87**, 386–389.

Dennis, C., Spreng, D.S., Nelson, G.E., *et al.* (1951) Development of a pump-oxygenator to replace the heart and lungs: an apparatus applicable to human patients and an application to one case. *Annals of Surgery*, **134**, 709–721.

DeWall, R.A., Warden, H.E., Gott, V.L., *et al.* (1956) Total body perfusion for open cardiotomy using the bubble oxygenator. *Journal of Thoracic Surgery*, **32**, 591–603.

Dodrill, F.D., Hill, E., Gerish, R.A. and Johnson, A. (1953) Pulmonary valvuloplasty under direct vision using the mechanical heart for a complete bypass of the right heart in a patient with congenital pulmonary stenosis. *Journal of Thoracic Surgery*, **26**, 584–597.

Drew, D.M., O'Rourke, J. (1958) The future of throacoplasty in pulmonary tuberculosis. *British Journal of Tuberculosis*. **52**, 319–324.

Fredericq, L. (1890) Sur la circulation cephalique croisee ou echange du sang carotidien entre deux animaux. *Archives Biologie*, **10**, 127–130.

Gibbon, J.H. Jr. (1937) Artificial maintenance of circulation during experimental occlusion of pulmonary artery. *Archives of Surgery*, **34**, 1105–1131.

Gibbon, J.H. (1954) Application of a mechanical heart and lung apparatus to cardiac surgery. *Minnesota Medicine*, **37**, 171.

Gibbon, J.H. Jr. Application of a mechanical heart and lung apparatus to cardiac surgery. *Recent Advances in Cardiovascular Physiology and Surgery*, University of Minnesota, 107–113.

Hamel, G. (1888) Die Bedentung de Pulse fur den Blustrom. *Zeitschrift fur Biologie*, **25**, 474–495.

Jacobj, C. (1890) Apparat zur Durchblutung isolierter uberlebender Organe. *Archiv fur Experimentelle Pathologie und Pharmakologie*, **26**, 388–400.

Jacobj, C. (1895) Ein Beitrag zur Technik der kunstlichen Durchblutung uberlebender Organe. *Archiv fur Experimetelle Pathologie und Pharmakologie*, **31**, 330–348.

Jongbloed, J. (1949) The mechanical heart/lung system. *Surgery, Gynecology and Obstetrics*, **89**, 684–691.

Kantrowtiz, A., Reiner, S. and Abelson, D. (1950) An automatically controlled inexpensive pump-oxygenator. *Journal of Thoracic and Cardiovascular Surgery*, **38**, 586–593.

Kirklin, J.W., DuShane, J.W., Patrick, R.T., *et al.* (1955) Intracardiac surgery with the aid of a mechanical pump oxygenator system (Gibbon type): report of eight cases. *Proceedings of Staff Meetings of Mayo Clinic*, **30**, 201–207.

Kolff, W.J. and Balzer, R. (1955) The artificial coil lung. *Transactions of the American Society for Artificial Internal Organs*, **1**, 39–42.

Kolff, W.J. and Berk, H.T.J. (1944) Artificial kidney: dialyster with a great area. *Acta Medica Scandinavica*, **117**, 121–134.

Lillehei, C.W., Cohen, M., Warden, H.E. and Varco, L. (1955) The direct-vision intracardiac correction of congenital anomalies by controlled cross-circulation. *Surgery*, **38**, 11–29.

McLean, J. (1916) The thromboplastic action of cephalin. *American Journal of Physiology*, **41**, 250–257.

Magnus, R. (1902) Die Thatigkeit des uberlebenden Saugethierherzens bei Durchstromung mit Gasen. *Archiv fur Experimentelle Pathologie und Pharmakologie*, **47**, 200–208.

Mustard, W.T. (1955) Clinical and experimental experience with homologous and heterologous lung perfusion. *Transactions of the American Society for Artificial Internal Organs*, **1**, 94–95.

Nysten, P.H. (1911) *Recherche de Physiologie et de Chimie Pathologique, pour faire suite a celles de Bichat sur la Vie et la Mort*. JA Brosson: Paris.

Paneth, M., Sellers, R., Goitt, V.L., *et al.* (1957) Physiologic studies upon prolonged cardiopulmonary bypass with the pump oxygenator with particular reference to (1) acid-base balance, (2) syphon caval drainage. *Journal of Thoracic Surgery*, **34**, 570–579.

Potts, W.J., Riker, W.L., DeBord, R. and Andrews, C.E. (1952) Maintenance of life by homologous lungs and mechanical circulation. *Surgery*, **31**, 161–166.

Ross, D.N. (1959) The technique of veno-venous cooling and rewarming. *Guys Hospital Report*, **108**, 245–251.

Rygg, I.H. and Kyvsgaard, E. (1956) A disposable polyethylene oxygenator system applied in the heart/lung machine. *Acta Chirurgica Scandinavica*, **112**, 433–437.

Sabiston, D.C., Talbert, J.L., Riley, L.H. and Blalock, A. (1959) Maintenance of the heartbeat by perfusion of the coronary circulation with gaseous oxygen. *Annals of Surgery*, **150**, 361–370.

Senning, A. (1952) Ventricular fibrillation during extracorporeal circulation. *Acta Chirurgica Scandinavica Supplementum*, **171**, 1–79.

Singh, I. (1935) Intravenous injection with the animal under ordinary and increased atmospheric pressure. *Journal of Physiology*, **84**, 315–322.

Singh, I. (1960) Life without breathing. *Archives Internationales de Pharmacodynamie*, **129**, 239–243.

von Frey, M. and Gruber, M. (1885) Untersuchungen uber den Stoffweschel isolierter Organe. *Archiv fur Physiologie*, **9**, 519–532.

2

Physiology and pathophysiology of extracorporeal circulation

Robert H. Bartlett and Ralph E. Delius

The term 'physiology' was coined by the great Dutch physician Boerhaave to describe the study of interdependent organ function under normal conditions. Extracorporeal circulation (ECC) imposes several conditions which lead to a series of changes in normal organ function. The physiology of ECC, for the purposes of this discussion, refers to interdependent organ function during the conditions imposed by venoarterial cardiopulmonary bypass. Physiological function under these conditions differs considerably from normal physiology. The changes occurring with ECC are outlined in Table 2.1. The normal functions of blood flow, gas exchange, blood surface interface effects and reticuloendothelial function are the physiological functions that are replaced in total or in part by the extracorporeal device. Subsequent changes in neurological, renal, hepatic, and other functions are secondary to these substitutions. The mechanical and pharmacological factors which are inherent in the design of the device (and hence responsible for physiological changes) are also listed in Table 2.1.

Abnormal, deteriorating, or inadequate organ function associated with extracorporeal circulation is the pathophysiology of ECC. It is difficult, if not impossible, to separate the uniform and ubiquitous changes in organ function that are associated with ECC from specific organ damage or deteriorating function that can occur when a mechanical device is used to substitute for the heart and lungs. In addition, all clinical studies of ECC are conducted on patients with underlying intrinsic disease, usually in conjunction with a cardiac operation. Therefore, 'physiology' and 'pathophysiology' are defined from an abnormal baseline. While some aspects of ECC can be clearly identified as pathophysiology (gross air embolism for example), in the current state of the art other aspects cannot be separated from normal function of the apparatus (platelet aggregation for example). In this sense Table 2.1 represents both the physiology of ECC and the inherent pathophysiology.

Haemodynamics, blood volume and endocrine response to cardiopulmonary bypass

Physiological studies of prolonged normothermic extracorporeal circulation (ECMO) have shown that minimal changes in haemodynamic measurements and other physiological parameters are present (Figure 2.1). The only substantial deviations from normal physiology during ECMO are the anticoagulation required and the non-pulsatile flow imposed by the system. Hence, much of the 'normal' physiology of ECC is probably best defined in patients requiring venoarterial bypass for respiratory failure. In contrast, cardiopulmonary bypass during cardiac surgery superimposes several other conditions which can alter normal physiology, including haemodilution, hypothermia, and relative hypoperfusion. Figure 2.1 illustrates that during ECMO we can go from total bypass to normal cardiac function and back to total bypass without significant changes in oxygen kinetics or metabolic changes, while Figure 2.2 shows that several haemodynamic functions are altered during conventional bypass with haemodilution, hypothermia, and low flow. Hypotension is common after initiation of bypass and has been attributed to several factors. First of all, flow is usually initiated at 2.4 $l\,m^{-2}\,m^{-1}$, which is less than normal perfusion. Also, elevated histamine levels have been documented in the circuit prime and have been shown to be elevated

Table 2.1 The physiology and pharmacology of extracorporeal circulation compared with normal circulation and pulmonary function

Normal function	Physiologic changes with ECC	Mechanical factors	Pharmacological factors
	↓ Total flow negative venous P	Venous cannula size	Steroids
	↑ Adrenergic response		Adrenergic blockers
	↑ Renin-angiotensin	Arterial cannula site	
	Abnormal distribution		Diuretics
Blood flow	Non-pulsatile	Pump characteristics	
	Non-servo		Volume expanders
	↓ Tissue washout		
	↓ Oxygen delivery	Heat exchanger	Hypothermia
	Acidosis		buffers-tris HCO_3^-
	O_2-CO_2 exchange requires large blood volume	Oxygenator: Disc Bubble Membrane	
Gas exchange			Defoamer
	Microbubbles		
	Emboli and aggregates	Reservoirs, connectors, tubing	? Platelet-active drugs
	Stagnant zones		
Blood-endothelial interface	Anticoagulation	Surface coating	Heparin priming solutions
	↑ Fibrinolytic activity		
	↓ Platelet function	Coronary suction	
	Blood dilution		Haemodilution
Reticuloendothelial function			
	Tissue histiocytes loaded	Filters	
	Phagocytosis ↓		

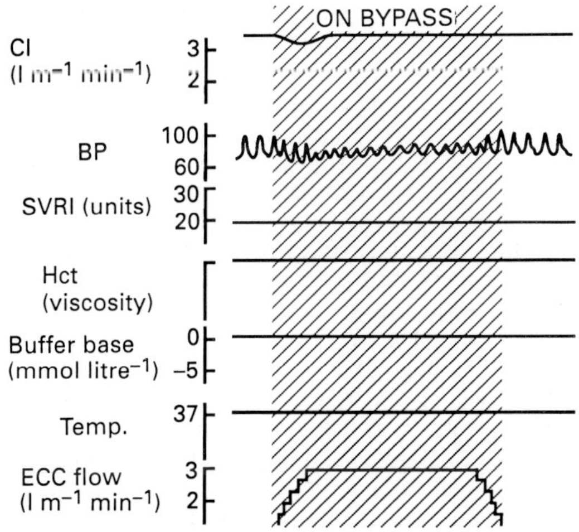

Figure 2.1 Typical haemodynamic changes during veno-arterial bypass in an infant on prolonged bypass (ECMO) with normal haematocrit, temperature, and flow. CI=cardiac index; BP=blood pressure; SVRI=systemic vascular resistance index; Hct=haematocrit; Temp.=temperature; ECC=Extracorporeal circulation.

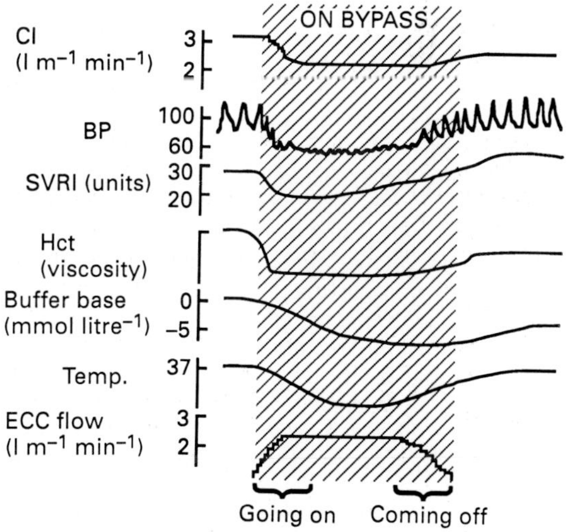

Figure 2.2 Typical haemodynamic changes during conventional venoarterial bypass with haemodilution, hypothermia, and low flow. CI=cardiac index; BP=blood pressure; SVRI=systemic vascular resistance index; Hct=haematocrit; Temp.=temperature; ECC=Extracorporeal circulation.

when ECC is initiated (Marath, Man and Taylor, 1987; Marath *et al.*, 1988). Hypotension due to vasodilation is a known response to histamine. Another factor that may contribute to hypotension is activation of the alternative complement pathways, with resultant formation of anaphylatoxins such as C3a (Chenoworth, 1986; Reigel *et al.*, 1988). Complement activation in turn has been associated with neutrophil activation and granule release (Cavarocchi *et al.*, 1986; Wachtfogel *et al.*, 1987), which may also adversely affect haemodynamics. A sudden decrease in systemic vascular resistance due to abrupt haemodilution, which affects blood viscosity, appears to be a significant cause of hypotension after initiation of ECC (Robicsek *et al.*, 1983).

If blood flow is held constant during perfusion, transfusion of blood and fluid will be necessary to maintain constant intravascular volume. While blood loss at the surgical site accounts for some of the loss of volume, other factors also appear to be involved. Several groups have demonstrated a significant increase in extracellular fluid following cardiopulmonary bypass (Breckenridge, Digerness and Kirklin, 1969; Cohn, Angell and Shumway, 1971). One mechanism for this may be related to the decreased plasma oncotic pressure which occurs as a result of haemodilution. However, an eventual increase in interstitial pressure and decrease in interstitial oncotic pressure leads to an equilibrium that appears to ultimately limit oedema formation (Rein, 1988). A primary increase in capillary permeability has been demonstrated by Smith *et al.*, 1987. The factors responsible for this increase in capillary permeability are uncertain, but activated neutrophils have been shown to increase capillary permeability (Henney *et al.*, 1971). This corresponds nicely with *in vitro* studies demonstrating disruption of the cytoskeleton in endothelial cells exposed to hydrogen peroxide, with resultant loss of cell shape (Hind *et al.*, 1988). Taken together, these studies suggest that activated neutrophils may injure endothelial cells and subsequently lead to an increase in microvascular permeability. Plasma volume loss may also result from diuresis induced by adding mannitol or a potent diuretic to the oxygenator priming solution. Venous return to the extracorporeal device is impaired if blood volume is not adequately replaced, which in turn results in a decreased arterial flow rate. Tissue perfusion is not optimal if this occurs and can lead to metabolic acidosis.

During operations requiring cardiopulmonary bypass there is a generalized increase in serum catecholamine levels in excess of that seen during operations not requiring ECC (Replogle *et al.*, 1962; Tan *et al.*, 1976; Fedderson, 1985). This release of catecholamines results from stimulation of both the carotid sinus and aortic baroreceptors (Harrison and Seton, 1973). These receptors appear to respond to low pulse amplitude which occurs during non-pulsatile perfusion (Stein and Perris, 1973), when total flow is decreased. Hypothermia also appears to be a major stimulus for catecholamine release and can adversely affect postoperative haemodynamics and increase oxygen consumption during rewarming. These adverse effects can be ameliorated by neuromuscular paralysis during the rewarming period (Zwischenberger *et al.*, 1987).

Vasopressin levels increase considerably during ECC, probably due to the decreased stimulation of baroreceptors that occurs during bypass (Fedderson *et al.*, 1985; Viinamaki, 1986). Renin secretion from the kidney is also increased in response to the decrease in mean arterial pressure and reduction of left arterial pressure, which in turn leads to angiotensin activation and subsequent aldosterone secretion (Kono *et al.*, 1983). The increase in catecholamines, vasopressin, and angiotensin II combine to increase arteriolar constriction, which returns the blood pressure toward normal.

If the total flow remains constant with the increase in pressure, blood is preferentially directed to organs which are more responsive to increased perfusion pressure and least dependent on arteriolar tone. This includes the two most important organs – the brain and the heart. At the same time blood flow is most decreased in organs such as skin and skeletal muscle, in which the vasculature is the least sensitive to increased perfusion pressure. The resulting redistribution of blood flow under these circumstances has been studied by several investigators (Lees *et al.*, 1970; Rudy, Heyman and Edmunds, 1970a and b). The results indicate that during cardiopulmonary bypass there is a redistribution of blood flow that is caused by factors other than the alterations in pulse pressure that occur when non-pulsatile perfusion is used. The factors include anaesthesia, peripheral emboli, amount of haemodilution, effects on blood elements, etc. This neuroendocrine response and redistribution phenomenon may be diminished by alpha-adrenergic blocking anaesthetic drugs, such as halothane, in which case the arterial pressure remains relatively low under conditions of constant flow. Adding to the blood volume causes an increase in perfusion pressure if flow is held constant. Occasionally the neuroendocrine sympathetic response will dominate the haemodynamics, creating the syndrome of hypertension at constant flow with poor organ perfusion which may be serious enough to require definitive alpha-adrenergic blockade (Maxwell *et al.*, 1958; Gomes and McGoon, 1969; Burack *et al.*, 1972; Mannucci, 1988; Lemiuz *et al.*, 1967).

These haemodynamic effects of ECC have been evaluated by Gazzaniga, Byrd and Gross (1970) and Gazzaniga *et al.* (1972), who utilized the method of skeletal muscle surface pH measurement to evaluate the perfusion metabolism relationship in that specific tissue. Since the arterial blood under conditions of anaesthesia or bypass is completely saturated with oxygen, decreasing muscle surface pH is a direct reflection of decreasing capillary flow. An initial decrease in muscle surface pH occurs with the induction of anaesthesia and its attendant minor myocardial depressant effects, demonstrating the sensitivity of the measurement. With the institution of cardiopulmonary bypass, muscle surface pH drops remarkably and then gradually continues to fall during the period of ECC, indicating inadequate tissue perfusion. The addition of blood volume results in an increase in arterial pressure at constant flow and minimizes decreased organ perfusion to some extent, leading to a low plateau of muscle surface pH rather than a continuing fall. Preloading with volume can further minimize the low flow. The addition of alpha-adrenergic blockade reverses or nearly eliminates the muscle surface acidosis, indicating the major role of alpha-adrenergic stimulation during ECC (Gazzaniga *et al.*, 1972). Venous pH, as a more general and less sensitive measure of organ perfusion, falls during bypass at a constant $P\text{CO}_2$. More specifically, a condition of metabolic acidosis can be detected by measurement of pH and $P\text{CO}_2$. Urine output usually falls during bypass, although the concomitant effects of antidiuretic endocrine stimuli and pharmacologically induced diuresis by mannitol or diuretics make observation of the urine output a questionable indicator of perfusion in a clinical situation. Similarly, Del Canale *et al.* (1988) have shown that hypothermic, low flow ECC leads to increased anaerobic metabolism in skeletal muscle, with a concurrent increase in lactate and decrease in phosphocreatine levels and intracellular pH. Fantini *et al.* (1987) have found that low flow hypothermic ECC leads to a decrease in skeletal muscle transmembrane potential and an increase in intracellular sodium and selective membrane permeability to sodium and potassium. These findings are similar to that found in haemorrhagic shock and supports the studies of Gazzaniga demonstrating inadequate tissue perfusion during ECC as usually performed for cardiac surgery.

Several other important endocrine changes occur in response to ECC. Atrial natriuretic factor (ANF) is a peptide hormone secreted by atrial cardiocytes in response to stretching of the atrial wall (Needleman and Greenwald, 1986). This hormone has a wide variety of actions, including an increase in glomerular filtration rate and pronounced natriuresis, inhibition of aldosterone secretion, attenuation of the vasopressin release which occurs in response to hypovolaemia, suppression of renin release, and direct relaxation of blood vessels, resulting in a decrease in systematic vascular resistance. Since ECC involves emptying of the atria for several hours it would be anticipated that ANF levels would decrease because the primary stimulus for ANF release, atrial stretch, would not be present. However, Dewar *et al.* (1988) surprisingly found a paradoxical increase in ANF during cardiopulmonary bypass and a decrease after termination of bypass. Furthermore, they found a lack of correlation between atrial filling pressure and ANF release in the early postoperative period. Two subsequent studies, however, did not show any significant change in ANF levels during ECC but found that ANF levels increased markedly early after bypass (Asari *et al.*, 1989; Schaff *et al.*, 1989). Although the clinical significance of these findings are uncertain, the perioperative changes in ANF release which are unique to operations performed during ECC may play a role in postoperative diuresis (Schaff *et al.*, 1989).

Several investigators have shown that ACTH and cortisol are elevated in response to ECC (Kono *et al.*, 1983; Pollack *et al.*, 1988). Cortisol secretion does not appear to be influenced by non-pulsatile flow. The secretion of cortisol and growth hormone during ECC contributes to the changes in glucose metabolism seen during cardiopulmonary bypass. A mild hyperglycaemia is seen during normothermic cardiopulmonary bypass which is due to increased gluconeogenesis and peripheral insulin resistance in response to the elevated levels of stress hormones (Kurtschan, Galletti and Hahn, 1986). Glucose levels are normal during hypothermic ECC, probably due to inhibition of hepatic gluconeogenesis during hypothermia. However, glucose levels rise during rewarming and glucose metabolism becomes similar to that seen during normothermic ECC (Kuntschen *et al.*, 1985).

Mechanical limitations to physiological cardiopulmonary bypass

Even with conditions of alpha-blockade and volume loading, can normal peripheral blood flow of $3.2\ \text{l m}^2$ min be achieved with an artificial device? Probably so, but at the expense of some loss of safety due to increased flow in the extracorporeal circuit. High arterial line pressure, more surface exposure per minute, increased cavitation, and possibly greater chance of aggregate embolism are present at high flow rates (Kirklin and Barratt-Boyes, 1986). With the current state of the art, bypass flow of $2.2\text{–}2.4\ \text{l m}^{-2}\ \text{min}^{-1}$ is generally considered a reasonable compromise (Replogle and Gross, 1961; Tarhan and Moffitt, 1971; Kirklin and Barratt-Boyes, 1986). The resulting moderate flow is well tolerated for the 1–2h required for most intracardiac operations and usually does not result in any permanent sequelae. Hence, flow levels of $2.4\ \text{l m}^{-2}\ \text{min}^{-1}$ have come to be considered the 'normal' physiology of extracorporeal circulation, although this is not necessarily the case.

Mechanical factors affecting bypass flow rates include the size and position of venous and arterial cannulae, the nature of the pump and type of oxygenator. The flow obtained in total bypass is a function of the blood volume and the diameter of the tubing used for the venous lines. Assuming that 100 cmH_2O of siphon suction is applied to the venous cannulae, the maximal possible flow increases linearly with tubing size until high flow rates are achieved (Peirce, 1969). Under conditions of inadequate venous return, whether due to low blood volume or low arterial perfusion with sequestration, the flow through the venous line is regulated by the collapsing of the vena cavae around the venous cannula. Under conditions of adequate venous return the bypass flow is limited by the size and length of the venous drainage lines. The resistance to flow is directly related to the length of tubing and inversely related to the fourth power of the radius of the tubing (Holloway *et al.*, 1988).

Theoretically, the size of the arterial cannula is not a major consideration during non-pulsatile flow. If $5\,l\,min^{-1}$ is pumped then $5\,l\,min^{-1}$ will flow through the arterial cannula. However, the flow rate will be maintained only at the expense of higher pressures and greater turbulence in the perfusion system. These factors may lead to haemolysis (Blacksheer, Dorman and Steinback, 1965) and also increases the risk of tubing separation or rupture. Arterial cannulae which are capable of providing adequate flow with a pressure gradient across the cannula of less than 100 mmHg and arterial line pressures of less than 250 mmHg have been recommended (Brodman *et al.*, 1985; Kirklin and Kirklin, 1990). Brodman *et al.* (1985) found that there is poor correlation between the pressure flow characteristics of arterial cannule and French designation, which is a measure of the outside diameter of the tip of the cannulae. Therefore, comparison of performance characteristics between similarly sized cannulae is difficult. Montoya, Merz and Bartlett (1990) have devised a numerical designation based on a Reynolds number friction factor correlation that can allow easy comparison of pressure flow characteristics between different cannulae.

Pulsatile flow during ECC has been a controversial subject for several decades. Since blood flow is normally pulsatile it would seem desirable to replicate this pulse contour with a mechanical device. There is universal agreement that the kidney perceives non-pulsatile flow as inadequate flow, resulting in renin release and antidiuresis. This phenomenon, first described over 35 years ago, has been found by several investigators (Many *et al.*, 1969; Goodman *et al.*, 1976). Nagaoka, Innami and Arai (1988) found lower levels of angiotensin II and aldosterone after pulsatile perfusion when compared with non-pulsatile perfusion, but did not find any advantages in regard to tissue metabolism. Olinger, Hutchinson and Borcheck (1983) and Matsuda *et al.* (1986) have found clinical benefits to pulsatile perfusion in patients with chronic renal insufficiency. Several groups have found clinical and experimental advantages to pulsatile perfusion, while others have not found any advantage to pulsatile perfusion (Dunn *et al.*, 1974; Harken *et al.*, 1980; Lindberg *et al.*, 1984; Tranmer *et al.*, 1986; Watanabe *et al.*, 1989). Hickey, Buckley and Philbin (1983) have suggested that the conflicting findings are due to various forms of pulsatile perfusion used by different groups which are not equivalent and make direct comparison between studies difficult. To this end a pulsatility index has been devised which allows quantification of pulsatile waveforms (Grossi *et al.*, 1985). However, the contradictions may also be resolved by careful examination of the experimental methods correlated with the classic studies of Harrison (Harrison *et al.*, 1970; Harrison and Seton, 1973).

Normally, blood flow is approximately 110 ml kg^{-1} body weight with a pulse amplitude of 20–40 mmHg (with some species variation). The studies that demonstrated acidosis and organ failure during non-pulsatile flow were conducted at flow rates ranging from 60 ml kg^{-1} to 100 ml kg^{-1}. Those investigators who found no difference between pulsatile and non-pulsatile flow used total perfusion rates between 130 ml kg^{-1} and 200 ml kg^{-1} (Rudy, Heyman and Edmunds, 1970a; Boucher, Rudy and Edmunds, 1974; Harken *et al.*, 1980). This relationship could have been predicted from the studies of Harrison (Harrison *et al.*, 1970; Harrison and Seton, 1973), which showed that adrenal catecholamine secretion is regulated in part by carotid sinus baroreceptors. Decreased pulse amplitude caused maximal catecholamine output when total flow was less than normal, but minimal catecholamine output during normal and above normal flow rates. From Harrison's findings, one might expect no difference between pulsatile perfusion and non-pulsatile perfusion at flow rates over 110 ml kg^{-1}. High vascular resistance and metabolic acidosis would occur during non-pulsatile perfusion only at flow rates of 80–110 ml kg^{-1} and would occur during both pulsatile and non-pulsatile perfusion at flow rates less than 70 ml kg^{-1} (Figure 2.3). This corresponds closely to the reports listed above.

The implications of these studies for total cardiopulmonary bypass in cardiac surgery are significant as total perfusion is usually carried out at flow rates of 70–100 ml kg^{-1}. At this abnormally low flow rate the adrenal catecholamine secretion is increased by the decreased pulse amplitude, hence pulsatile flow (Bregman, 1976) or alpha blockade should be used to ameliorate the systematic effects of the altered flow pattern. During partial

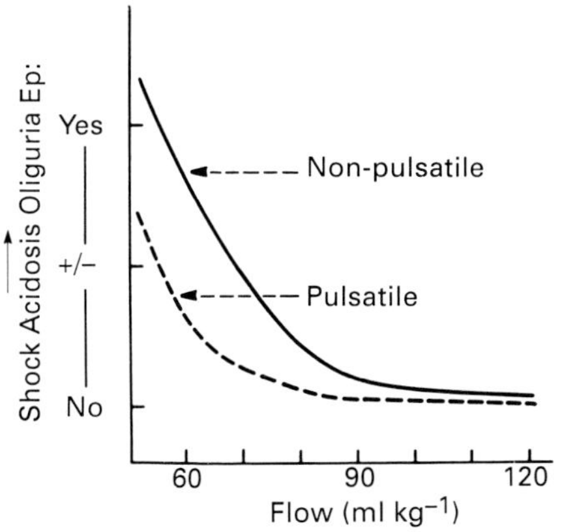

Figure 2.3 Low-flow syndrome related to total perfusion, with and without pulsation

pulmonary bypass for life support, total flow should be maintained as near normal as possible and should be regulated by whatever means necessary to assure a pulse amplitude of 15 mmHg or more.

Gas exchange and oxygen delivery

Gas exchange has proved to be the easiest problem of ECC. Flowing blood is exposed to oxygen either directly or through a gas permeable membrane. Oxygen diffuses into the blood plasma because of a gradient between high $P\text{O}_2$ in the gas phase and the low $P\text{O}_2$ in mixed venous blood. Oxygen then diffuses from the plasma through the red cell membrane to combine with unsaturated haemoglobin. The binding of oxygen to haemoglobin proceeds very rapidly and the limiting factor in oxygenation of flowing blood is the rate of oxygen diffusion through plasma (Bartlett, 1971). Hence, the thickness of the blood film between gas bubbles or surfaces, or between gas exchange membranes becomes the rate limiting factor. Carbon dioxide diffuses out of the flowing blood in the gas exchange device because of the gradient between the $P\text{CO}_2$ in mixed venous blood and the partial pressure of CO_2 in the ventilating gas. Although the gradient of CO_2 exchange is relatively low and can never be greater than the mixed venous $P\text{CO}_2$, the rate of diffusion through plasma is so rapid that CO_2 removal always proceeds more efficiently than oxygenation. Therefore, to avoid excess CO_2 removal with its attendant alkalosis, the gradient is diminished by adding CO_2 to the ventilating gas or by reducing the gas flow to the oxygenator.

Oxygenator performance

The performance characteristics of the gas exchange device must be thoroughly documented to plan the best extracorporeal circuit for any given patient. Since Co_2 removal is almost invariably greater than oxygenation, it is sufficient to describe the performance of gas exchange devices in terms of their oxygenating efficiency. The following factors must be known about the gas exchange device. How much oxygen can actually be supplied per minute? How much oxygen can be supplied under conditions of variable blood flow and variable mixed venous saturation? How much oxygen can be supplied at flow rates which are compatible with adequate perfusion for the patient in question (i.e. at least 2.4 l m^{-2} min^{-1})? What flow of ventilating gas is required? How much foreign surface is exposed to the flowing blood (this number is easy to derive for membrane oxygenators, but much more difficult for gas interface oxygenators)? What effects, if any, does the gas exchange device have on the components of flowing blood?

Many of these factors have been conveniently combined into a single expression of oxygenator performance defined as rated flow (Galletti, Richardson and Snider, 1972). The rated flow is the flow at which blood leaving the oxygenator is 95% saturated, under the conditions of mixed venous blood inflow. In other words, when venous blood (haemoglobin 15 g per 100 ml, $P\text{O}_2$ 40 mmHg, saturation 65%, O_2 content 15 ml per 100 ml) is pumped through a gas exchange device at 200 ml min^{-1}, the outflow blood will be 100% saturated ($P\text{O}_2$ 150 mmHg, O_2 content 20 ml per 100 ml). The amount of O_2 actually delivered by the device is determined by the flow rate and the arteriovenous (AV) difference. In this example the O_2 delivery is 5 ml per 100 ml blood × 100 ml min^{-1} = 5 ml O_2 delivery per minute. As blood flow through the device is increased, a point is reached at which the limiting factor is the thickness of the blood film and the rate at which O_2 diffuses through that particular film. When that point is exceeded, the outflow blood will exit at less than 100% saturation. The rated flow for a given device is that flow at which this limitation is reached. The rated O_2 delivery is the amount of O_2 that can be taken up by the blood at the rated flow. The upper limit of O_2 delivery is related to the flow and to the amount of unsaturated haemoglobin presented to the oxygenator per minute. If total bypass flow is decreased at a constant level of tissue oxygen consumption, venous saturation must decrease as more oxygen is extracted from the flowing blood. As long as this does not exceed the oxygenating capability of the gas exchange device, the oxygenator will compensate and function at a wider arteriovenous (AV) difference. Some of these variables are outlined in Figure 2.4, in which oxygen delivery per minute is related to the flow in litres per minute for different levels of venous saturation or arteriovenous difference. Notice that oxygen delivery is entirely depen-

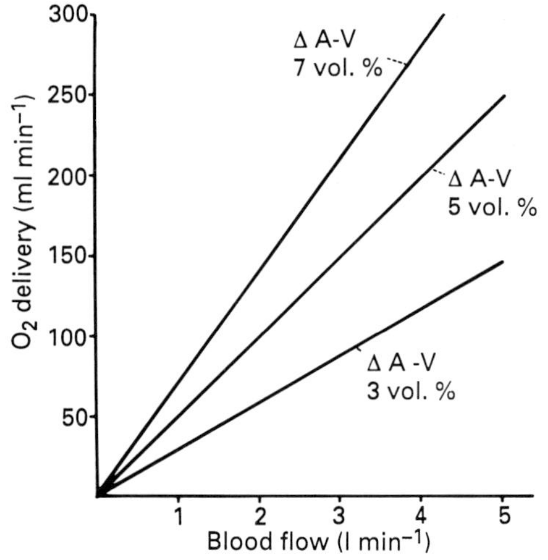

Figure 2.4 Oxygen delivery is directly related to blood flow and arteriovenous difference. The maximum oxygen that can be delivered for a given blood flow at a given venous saturation is shown here. This represents the maximum amount of oxygen delivery that could be accomplished by a gas exchange device under a given set of flow and inlet conditions

dent on flow. Decreasing flow severely decreases oxygen delivery, although fully saturated blood with a high Po_2 will be perfused into the arterial system.

Reports on oxygenation performance of gas exchange devices must include at least enough data to calculate inflow and outflow O_2 content and rated flow. In planning the components of an extracorporeal circuit the oxygen requirement of the patient at normothermia is calculated (150 ml min^{-1} m^{-2}). The blood flow which will deliver this amount of oxygen with an arteriovenous difference of 5 ml per 100 ml is calculated or determined from a graph (Figure 2.4). The cannulae, tubing and pump are chosen to provide the desired flow.

The concept of rated flow is demonstrated again in Figure 2.5 and the rated flow for several oxygenators is outlined in Figure 2.6. If a gas exchange device is operated at flow rates higher than its rated flow, desaturated blood will be perfused and the actual O_2 delivery per minute reaches a fairly level plateau regardless of flow rate.

Types of oxygenator

Assuming that the oxygenator will be used at appropriate flow rates below the rated flow, the choice of an oxygenator must be related to the ease of use and possible damage to blood components. Two basic types of gas exchange devices are used in extracorporeal circuits: a direct gas interface oxygenator in which O_2 is bubbled, filmed, or foamed directly through blood which is then defoamed or debubbled through some type of settling or filtering chamber, or a membrane oxygenator in which a gas exchange membrane is interposed between the gas phase and the blood phase. Older membrane membrane oxygenators used silicone 'rubber', while a new generation of membrane oxygenators utilize microporous materials such as polypropylene. These new oxygenators with either microporous hollow fibres or sheet membranes have much greater gas transfer capacities than membrane oxygenators used in the past (Bjork, Stenlieb and Davenport, 1985). Gas interface oxygenators have the advantage of simplicity, disposability and relatively low cost. Disadvantages include the possibility of gross or microscopic air embolism, relatively large priming volumes (although if the priming volume remains constant the exact volume is not important), variable reservoir level resulting in potential shifts in blood

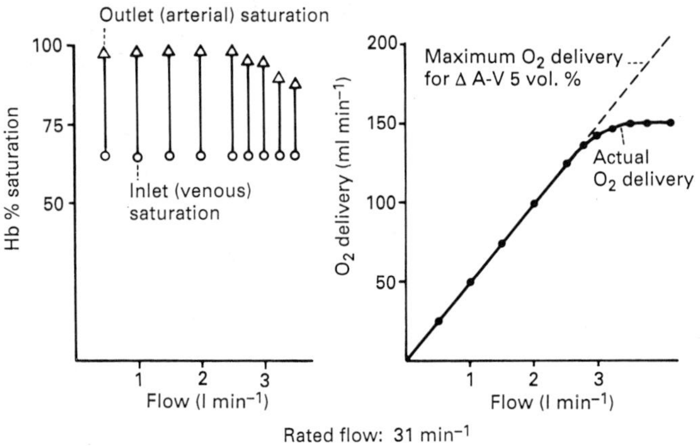

Figure 2.5 The concept of rated flow. A hypothetical gas exchange device has a maximum oxygen transfer capability of 150 ml min^{21} based on the surface area and blood flow characteristics. As long as the oxygen transport capability of flowing blood is less than 150 ml min^{-1}, fully saturated blood leaves the oxygenator. When the oxygen transport capability of flowing blood exceeds this amount, desaturated blood results. Under normal venous blood conditions this occurs at a flow rate of 3 l min^{-1}, the rated flow for this device. At flow rates in excess of 3 l min^{-1}, the outlet blood is desaturated, the arteriovenous difference is narrow, and the actual oxygen transferred reaches a plateau

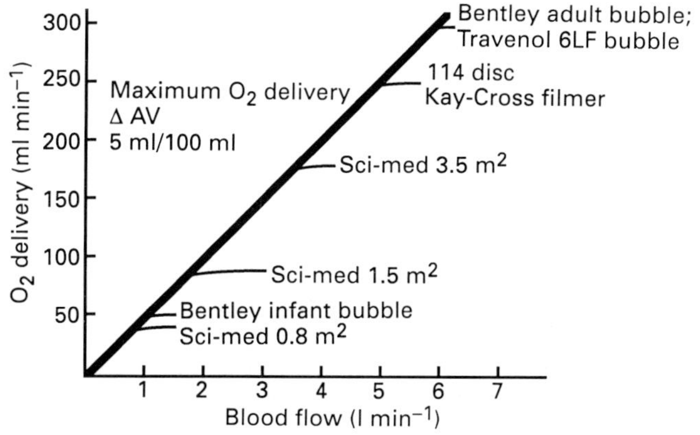

Figure 2.6 Rated flow under normal venous inlet conditions for a variety of commercial oxygenators. (Data based on publications cited in text or manufacturer's data sheet.) When modular units are used in parallel the rated flow becomes the sum of rated flows of all units in the circuit

volume between the intracorporeal and extracorporeal circuit and the effects of direct gas interface, including protein denaturation (Lee *et al.*, 1961; Dobell, 1965), increased haemolysis, platelet dysfunction, and thrombocytopenia (Van Oeveren *et al.*, 1985; Boonstra *et al.*, 1986). One group also found greater complement activation with bubble oxygenators (Cavarocchi *et al.*, 1986), although van Oeveren *et al.* (1985) were not able to demonstrate any difference in complement activation between membrane and bubble oxygenators. Membrane oxygenators have the advantage of eliminating blood–gas interface effects, ease of operation, less haemolysis, less platelet and neutrophil activation, better platelet preservation and less microemboli (Van Oeveren *et al.*, 1985; Boonstra *et al.*, 1986; Cavarocch *et al.*, 1986; Blauth *et al.*, 1990). The disadvantages of membrane oxygenators include expense, potential difficulty in eliminating all bubbles during priming, and moderately large, although constant, priming volumes in some instances.

Many of the published reports on pump or membrane oxygenator characteristics have included an open gas interface reservoir in the experimental design (Bernstein and Gleasor, 1967; Dutton and Edmunds, 1973). Data from these studies are applicable to ECC for cardiac surgery, as coronary suction, which has been to shown to injure platelets (Boonstra *et al.*, 1985), will always require some of the blood exposed to a direct gas interface. However, characterization of physiological changes of ECC or blood surface exposure should be done in experimental models which specifically exclude any gas interface to eliminate any variations caused by this factor.

Microporous membranes are made of non-wettable substances such as Teflon perforated with multiple small holes which permit gas transfer but preclude blood leakage because of surface tension effects. Oxygen and CO_2 transfer in a gas to gas test system are virtually unlimited with this type of membrane, but the plasma oxygen diffusion limitations still exist when blood is applied to the membrane. Hence, microporous membranes have oxygen transfer characteristics similar to other membrane oxygenators of similar flow design. Carbon dioxide transfer will be significantly better, however. The latter consideration is important only in oxygenators where mixing is intense (Bartlett *et al.*, 1974) and CO_2 transfer is the limiting design variable. Haemotologic studies indicate microporous membrane oxygenators cause less haemolysis and platelet dysfunction than bubble oxygenators (Van Oeveren *et al.*, 1985; Boonstra *et al.*, 1986; Calafiore *et al.*, 1987). Specific types of gas interface and membrane oxygenators and performance data are discussed in subsequent chapters in this book.

Oxygen delivery

An understanding of the relationship between oxygen delivery and consumption is necessary before the physiology of ECC can be fully appreciated. Systemic oxygen delivery during ECC is dependent on the flow supplied by the extracorporeal support device and the oxygen content of the blood, which in turn is affected by the haemoglobin content, degree of saturation, and factors which affect the haemoglobin–oxygen dissociation curve, such as temperature, $P\text{CO}_2$, level of 2, 3 diphosphoglycerate, etc. Oxygen consumption during ECC is normally influenced by factors such as body temperature and catecholamine release but may be modified by other circumstances such as sepsis. Normally, systemic oxygen delivery is five times systemic oxygen consumption. Measurement of mixed venous blood oxygen saturation provides a quick estimation of the relationship between oxygen delivery and consumption. If the arterial haemoglobin saturation is 100%, and 20% of the delivered oxygen is required for metabolic processes, then the saturation of the mixed venous blood will be approximately 80% (Zwischenberger *et al.*, 1986). If systemic oxygen delivery is reduced or if the systemic consumption of oxygen is increased, then the delivery:consumption ratio falls. For example, if the delivery:consumption ratio is 2:1 then one half of the oxygen supplied by the arterial blood is consumed. If the arterial saturation was 100% then the mixed venous saturation would be 50%. Hence, the measurement of mixed venous saturation provides a reasonably accurate approximation of the ratio between oxygen delivery and consumption. Organ function will be normal as long as the ratio between systemic oxygen delivery and consumption is 2.5 or greater. However, oxygen consumption will be impaired if the ratio is below this level. This can result in anaerobic metabolism, with resulting lactic acidosis and subsequent organ dysfunction and failure. These relationships are shown diagramatically in Figure 2.7. Point A represents normal physiological conditions. Point B represents the systemic oxygen delivery that occurs during low flow venoarterial bypass with haemodilution. This point is very close to the critical ratio at which anaerobic metabolism occurs. To compensate for this, oxygen consumption is decreased by lowering the metabolic rate through the use of hypothermia (point C). The segment between points D and C represents the margin of safety afforded by using flows that are in excess of that required by the hypothermic patient. This is reflected by an abnormally elevated mixed venous saturation, which demonstrates less systemic oxygen consumption at a given flow due to hypothermia. During rewarming the metabolic rate increases, so oxygen delivery must be increased to maintain the proper relationship between oxygen delivery and consumption.

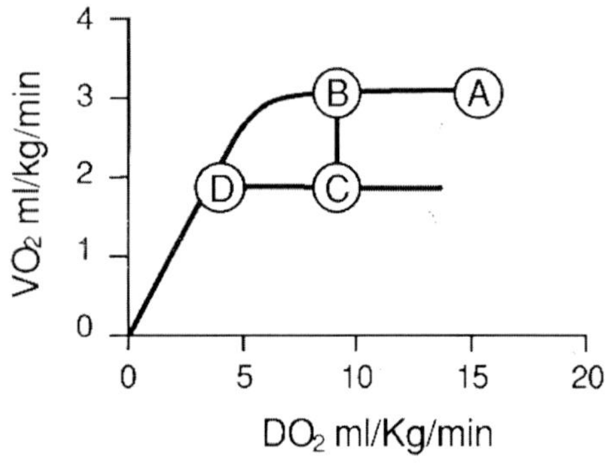

Figure 2.7 Relationship between oxygen consumption and oxygen delivery. See text for explanation

Blood surface interface effects

Normally, flowing blood is continuously exposed to endothelial cells. Fibrin formation probably takes place continuously on the endothelial surface balanced exactly by plasmin formation and concomitant fibrinolysis. Both of these reactions proceed at a slow and balanced rate so that the end effect is a slow but definitely measurable gradual conversion of fibrinogen to fibrin counterbalanced by an identical rate of fibrin degradation and elimination of fibrin degradation products. This delicate balance is abruptly upset by exposure of blood to collagen fibres underlying endothelial cells, tissue collagen, tissue thromboplastin, air, necrotic tissue or disrupted cells and to some extent foreign material in the bloodstream itself such as endotoxin. Under these circumstances the rate of conversion of fibrinogen to fibrin is greatly enhanced and proceeds to clotting at a much faster rate than fibrinolysis takes place. Concomitantly, platelet surfaces are altered, platelet adhesion and aggregation occurs and platelets release factors that further stimulate the formation of fibrin clot. This chain of events occurs during normal haemostasis. If any deficiencies occur in any of the factors required for coagulation. or if any of the steps are inhibited by a drug or lack of a catalyst such as calcium, or if platelet numbers or function are severely decreased, then haemostasis is severely disordered. The effects of ECC on the enzymes that constitute the coagulation system, as well as platelet function and physiology of the fibrinolytic system, have received a great deal of attention over the past 20 years.

Fibrin formation and lysis

During ECC the blood is exposed to a wide variety of surface textures and materials. During cardiac surgery, blood is aspirated from the field ('coronary' suction) and mixed with the perfusate. This aspirated blood may include tissue thromboplastin, clots, serum, gross particles of fat, muscle and bone, suture and other foreign material (Okies *et al.*, 1977). In addition, the extracorporeal circuit contains innumerable flat edges, right angle turns, stagnant zones, recirculating zones, jet zones and other flow characteristics not typically found in the normal circulatory system. All of these factors have the effect of stimulating platelet function, the coagulation cascade, and the fibrinolytic system. To date, heparin has been an absolutely indispensable drug in controlling these systems during ECC. At the current time heparin still plays a major role in the management of blood coagulation during ECC, but other drugs and devices as well as heparinless bypass systems are being studied intensively and may become commonplace in clinical practice in the near future (Whittlesey *et al.*, 1988; Bidstrup *et al.*, 1989; Von Segesser and Turina, 1989).

At the current time, the physiological changes associated with ECC must include those associated with heparinization as part of the normal baseline. To measure clotting accurately by any of the many tests which require a fibrin clot as an end point, the amount of heparin in the blood must be measured or estimated and inactivated with an appropriate agent. For intracardiac surgery it is desirable to maintain a prolonged clotting time with excessive amounts of heparin during the period of bypass. This requires at least 200 units kg^{-1} of patient weight and 200 units l^{-1} of blood in the priming solution. To provide an extra margin of safety most teams infuse 300 units kg^{-1} into the patient and 150 units kg^{-1} at 30 min intervals during the entire period of bypass. (Since heparin activity is measured by bioassay, activity is standardized in units of anticoagulant activity. Most heparin preparations are considered to contain 100 units mg^{-1}, although this may be technically incorrect.) Heparin carries a very strong negative charge and will become bonded to positive charges wherever they occur on glass or plastic surfaces; therefore, care must be taken when adding small amounts of heparin to fluids that are exposed to a large surface area.

Changes that occur in the coagulation system during prolonged ECC (24–48h) in a system without a direct gas interface are outlined in Figures 2.8 and 2.9. These studies are used as examples of extensive contact between blood and foreign surfaces. Changes during the first few hours are typical of those seen during cardiac surgery. In these studies partial (60–80%) venoarterial bypass was carried out in awake lambs and the heparin dose regulated at a low level. The initial drop in the levels of factors V and VIII after initiation of bypass are largely due to haemodilution. This has been corroborated in several clinical studies which have demonstrated that the drop in most clotting factors, as well as antithrombin III, plasminogen, and alpha-2-antiplasmin, correlates with the drop in haematocrit and is therefore due to haemodilution (Mammen *et al.*, 1985; Wolk *et al.*, 1985). One study has noted diminished factor VIII coagulant activity during bypass which does not correlate with the drop in haematocrit, suggesting consumption of this factor during ECC (Jones *et al.*, 1988). Desmopressin, a synthetic derivative of arginine-vasopressin, has been shown to increase the synthesis of von Willebrand factor and VIII:C (Mannucci, 1988). Administration of this agent to patients undergoing cardiac surgery has been shown to decrease blood loss (Salzman *et al.*, 1986). During prolonged bypass, a subsequent increase in fibrinogen and most other clotting factors is noted due to synthesis by the liver. The concentration of these proteins returns to

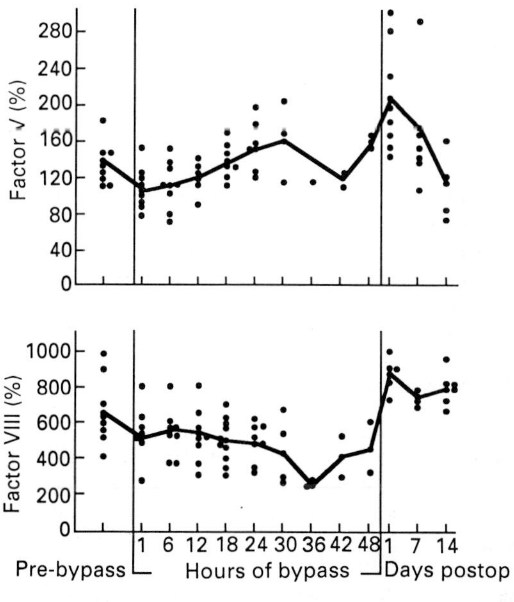

Figure 2.8 Changes in clotting factors during prolonged ECC in sheep. (Reproduced from Fong *et al.* (1974) by courtesy of *Transactions of the American Society for Artificial Internal Organs*)

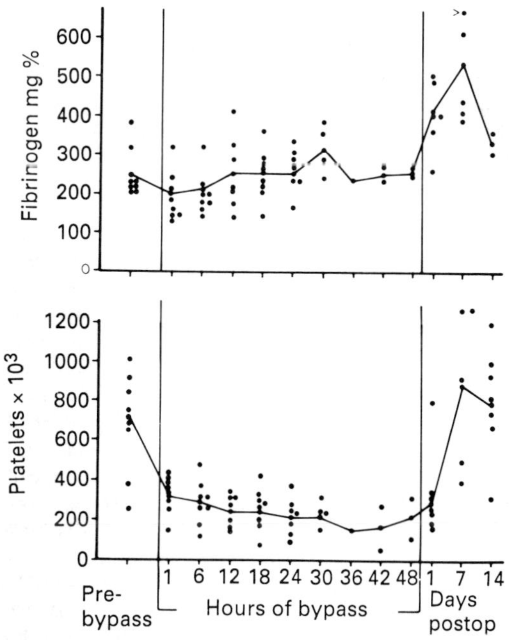

Figure 2.9 Changes in platelets and fibrinogen during prolonged ECC in sheep. (Reproduced from Fong *et al.* (1974) by courtesy of *Transactions of the American Society for Artificial Internal Organs*)

prebypass level within a period of hours and remains normal throughout the bypass period. However, during the 1–3h of ECC required for most intracardiac operations this compensation has not had time to proceed to completion and levels of most protein clotting factors are slightly decreased at the time bypass is discontinued and heparin is inactivated (Gans *et al.*, 1967). Clinical studies have also demonstrated a decrease in the levels of factors II and V as well as antithrombin III after termination of bypass (Mammen *et al.*, 1985; Wolk *et al.*, 1985).

Activation of circulating plasminogen to plasmin invariably occurs as fibrinogen is activated to fibrin; hence, any clot contains the enzymatic means for its own destruction. Evidence of active circulating plasmin can be detected whenever gross clotting is present. Tissue plasminogen activating factor, which is in part responsible for plasminogen activation, has been shown to be increased during ECC (Stibbe *et al.*, 1984). Numerous other factors are also responsible for plasmin activation, including proteases such as kallikrein. A correlation between protease activity and postoperative bleeding has been demonstrated (Hinshaw *et al.*, 1988). Aprotinin is a recently described protease inactivator that inhibits plasmin activation (Von Oeveren *et al.*, 1987). A recent European double blinded prospective clinical study with aprotinin demonstrated markedly less blood loss during cardiac surgery (Bidstrup *et al.*, 1989). Tranexamic acid, which binds to plasminogen and plasmin and blocks fibrinolysis, has also been shown to reduce postoperative blood loss (Horrow *et al.*, 1990). Agents such as aprotinin and tranexamic acid will likely gain wide acceptance in clinical practice in the future.

Platelet activity during extracorporeal circulation

Platelet physiology during ECC has been an area of intense interest over the past 15 years. It is of such importance that Chapter 10 of this book is devoted in large part to this subject. Studies have consistently shown that the concentration of platelets drops with the initiation of bypass and remains depressed as long as ECC continues. This has even been demonstrated in *in vitro* systems in which blood is circulated through a closed circuit (Addonizio and Colman, 1982). This suggests that interactions involving platelets and foreign surfaces are in large part responsible for the drop in platelet count during ECC. Fibrinogen is known to be absorbed to the circuit surface. Fibrinogen receptors on the surface of platelets appear to bind to the absorbed fibrinogen, resulting in adherence of platelets to the circuit surface as well as fragmentation of circulating platelets (Wenger *et al.*, 1989).

Other factors also appear to influence the adhesion of platelets to foreign surfaces, including surface texture, wettability, flow rates, and geometry of the blood flow through the circuit (Addonizio and Colman, 1982). Platelets also adhere to each other, forming aggregates. These platelet aggregates form microemboli and have been visualized in retinal vessels (Blauth *et al.*, 1990). The extent to which these microemboli cause damage and affect organ function is uncertain. Patients have been supported during prolonged ECC for periods of over 2 weeks without evidence of embolization, infarcts, or aggregates at autopsy. The platelet aggregates appear to disperse into individual platelet components in the microcirculation and reappear in the circulating blood (Hickey, Buckley and Philbin, 1983).

Platelet function also appears to be transiently affected by ECC (Harken, 1975; Tamari *et al.*, 1975). Platelet granule release occurs, suggesting some degree of activation. Platelets also become less sensitive to agonists such as ADP and epinephrine (Addonizio and Colman, 1982). These alterations in platelet function are probably significant and may contribute to bleeding complications related to ECC.

There has been considerable interest in the clinical use of agents which inhibit platelet activation during ECC. Prostaglandin E_1, dipyrimadole, prostacyclin (epoprostenol), and the stable prostacyclin analog iloprost have been used experimentally and clinically in an attempt to preserve platelet numbers and function during the postoperative period (Addonizio *et al.*, 1978; Fish *et al.*, 1986; Cottrell *et al.*, 1988; Teoh *et al.*, 1988). While potentially promising, a randomized, double blind clinical trial utilizing prostacyclin showed only minor clinical impact (Fish *et al.*, 1986). Use of this agent is also limited by hypotension, which is a significant side affect of this agent. An animal study with iloprost has demonstrated significant preservation of platelet number and function and suggests this agent may be clinically useful. Aprotinin, the serine protease inhibitor mentioned earlier, has not been shown to preserve platelet concentration but does appear to have beneficial effects on platelet function (Bidstrup *et al.*, 1989).

Haemodynamic and flow factors in relation to surface effects

Stagnant blood will clot even in undamaged surfaces lined with endothelium. Correspondingly, areas with very low flow in an extracorporeal circuit will form thrombus even when the patient is completely heparinized. Scientific validity was lent to this empirical observation by Spaeth *et al.* (1973) who demonstrated the formation of fibrin and platelet deposits on surfaces where flow was stagnant. It is equally important to avoid right-angled turns and eddy current areas in extracorporeal circuits. A 2 mm step-off between a connector and a piece of tubing in the bypass circuit would seem insignificant with 5–6 l min^{-1} of blood lavaging its surface. However, a stagnant area many microns in diameter will exist in the corner of such a junction where platelets and white cells may lie relatively still for long periods of time. Here, heparin may be metabolized and thrombus formation can occur. The fewer connections and access sites and the simpler the extracorporeal circuit, the less the problem of thrombus formation and direct embolization will be.

Use of filters

Since platelet aggregation may not be detrimental to microcirculation it appears unnecessary to attempt to filter out aggregates which form during a single pass through the extracorporeal circuit. The observation that significant amounts of material can be removed from the circulation by filters does not necessarily mean that filtration is clinically helpful (Gervin *et al.*, 1974). Aris *et al.* (1986) did not find any evidence that arterial line filters were beneficial in preventing subtle postoperative neuropsychiatric changes. The use of a 40 μm arterial line filter did not prevent microemboli from appearing in retinal vessels following cardiopulmonary bypass (Blauth *et al.*, 1988). In contrast to arterial line filtration, careful filtration of the coronary aspirate and of transfused blood is mandatory in order to filter out microaggregates that are glued together with fibrin, since these microaggregates will not break up when they arrive at a capillary bed. Total perfusion filtration may even be detrimental, as platelet aggregates will be removed from the circulation and may disaggregate more slowly in the prosthetic filter than in the spleen, liver, or lymph nodes. These filters can also contribute to complement activation. It should be noted, however, that filters serve as excellent microbubble traps and may be particularly useful when a bubble oxygenator is used (Padayachee *et al.*, 1988). It is doubtful that arterial line filtration is necessary if a membrane oxygenator and gas-free reservoir is used. Filters are not included in extracorporeal life support systems where ECC is used for days or weeks.

Interface effects on other formed elements

Damage to erythrocytes during ECC has largely been attributed to shear stresses (Kirklin and Barratt-Boyes, 1986). Most studies of this problem, however, have a blood–gas interface somewhere within the system. Bubble oxygenators cause a greater degree of haemolysis than membrane oxygenators (Clark and Mills, 1969). Coronary suction systems in particular appear to injure red blood cells (Kirklin and Barratt-Boyes, 1986). In contrast, experiments involving systems without a blood–gas interface demonstrate minimal haemolysis (Hill *et al.*, 1969; Bartlett and Gazzaniga *et al.*, 1978). Since ECC for cardiac surgery will usually involve a direct gas interface with coronary suction, the haemolysis which occurs after the red cells have been exposed to a gas interface will probably always be a part of ECC for cardiac surgery. Factors other than mechanical or shear stresses have also been implicated in ECC induced haemolysis. The deposition of terminal C5b-9 complement complexes on erythrocytes has been demonstrated during ECC. In this study, all red cell ghosts were found to have the terminal complement complex enbedded in the plasma membranes, while intact cells did not carry this complex. This suggests that complement activation may play a role in haemolysis (Salama *et al.*, 1988). Indeglia *et al.* (1967) studied red cell lysis under controlled conditions and found that haemolysis increased dramatically in lipaemic plasma and decreased with decreasing temperature in normal and lipaemic plasma. They concluded that the factors which predispose sensitized red cells to haemolysis are more chemical than mechanical, and pointed out the importance of avoiding lipaemic blood for transfusion or priming for ECC.

The effects of ECC on leucocyte kinetics, function and activation have been an area of intense interest during the past decade. Complement activation, largely through the alternative pathway, has been demonstrated in several studies (Kirklin *et al.*, 1983; Fosse, Mollnes and Ingvaldsen, 1987). Stimulation of the complement pathway can activate neutrophils, which release toxic oxygen species such as hydrogen peroxide as well as potentially damaging enzymes such as elastase (Hill *et al.*, 1972; Antonesen *et al.*, 1987; Wachtfagel *et al.*, 1987). Elevated levels of hydrogen peroxide have been demonstrated in patients during ECC (Cavarocchi *et al.*, 1986). Furthermore, increased levels of lipid peroxidation products have been found during cardiopulmonary bypass, suggesting significant oxidant activity (Royston *et al.*, 1986). Pulmonary leucocyte sequestration during ECC has been demonstrated and has been implicated as a possible cause of postoperative respiratory failure (Howard *et al.*, 1988; Utoh *et al.*, 1988). Neutrophil function during bypass will continue to be an active area of research during the next decade and interventions designed to limit the activation of neutrophils and to prevent damage from the oxidants released from these cells may come into clinical practice. Methylprednisolone and free radical scavengers such as superoxide dismutase have already been used in preliminary clinical studies (Tennenberg *et al.*, 1986).

Clinical significance of blood surface interface effects

Currently, coagulation during bypass is prevented with heparin, although many surface effects occur. The important clinical problem is returning to normal haemostasis and prevention of bleeding after ECC. First of all the heparin effect must be reversed. This is generally done by adding an appropriate does of protamine sulphate. Clots in the operative field are evidence of adequate heparin reversal. If the heparin effect persists more protamine is given and the measurements repeated. Reversal of heparin was studied by Jaberi, Bell and Benson (1973), who reported better heparin control with accelerated blood recalcification time, and more accurate protamine administration. These results were confirmed by Bull *et al.* (1975); Babka *et al.* (1977), and Friesen and Clement (1976). Activated clotting time (ACT) must be measured in whole blood (rather than plasma) because the heparin effect is inversely related to platelet count. We have found that kaolin-activated clotting (as in most commercial systems) is satisfactory when the platelet count is normal, but inadequate during thrombocytopenia. This may account for the erratic results reported by some (Arkin *et al.*, 1978). For measuring ACT during bypass, therefore, the reagent should contain fresh thromboplastins (Mullin *et al.*, 1976). Routine use of whole blood activated clotting time measurements when reversing heparin should be a routine aspect of ECC. Protamine is a moderate peripheral vasodilator and will cause hypotension when infused rapidly. It has a positive inotropic effect and peripheral flow appears to increase with protamine (Gourin, Strersand and Stuckey, 1970). Despite evidence of increased fibrinolytic activity and altered platelet function with ECC, postoperative bleeding that requires reoperation is almost always related to specific bleeding vessels (Gomes and McGoon, 1969). If the patient is allowed to bleed but transfused to the point of near total blood volume, then a coagulopathy associated with platelet-poor blood will be produced, requiring fresh platelet transfusion. The indication for reoperation should be precise and conservative (for example, cumulative chest drainage of 15% of the blood volume any time within the first 12h after bypass requires reoperation). When a significant coagulopathy occurs, it is associated with prolonged bypass with gas interface oxygenation, low platelet count, and multiple transfusions. The defect is largely due to platelet quantity and quality, and must be treated by fresh platelet concentrate or fresh blood. A recent study has suggested that one unit of fresh whole blood is more effective than platelet concentrates in improving haemostasis following cardiopulmonary bypass (Lavee, 1989).

Patients with platelet function defects before bypass will present severe bleeding problems after operation despite normal 'screening' tests of coagulation. These rare disorders are suggested by a history of bleeding with minor trauma and are detected by bleeding time or *in vitro* platelet function tests. Children with cyanotic heart disease appear to have abnormally functioning platelets which improve their function after correction of the cardiac defect (Ekert and Sheers, 1974). This platelet abnormality has been related to polycythaemia (Ware *et al.*, 1983). This may explain the propensity to bleeding which occurs after bypass in cyanotic heart disease (Kevy *et al.*, 1966).

After ECC, clotting factors and platelets return to normal or above normal levels (Fong *et al.*, 1974). In occasional cases where abnormal coagulation occurs 24h or more after bypass it is usually due to consumption coagulopathy associated with low cardiac output (Boyd *et al.*, 1972).

Organ function and damage during extracorporeal circulation

As noted in the previous section, total cardiopulmonary bypass, as usually carried out, invokes a moderate low-flow state. Changes in organ function which occur following ECC are those of 1–2h of relatively inadequate perfusion for metabolic demands, rather than specific effects of the bypass. Studies of prolonged near-total bypass in awake alert animals and patients without significant metabolic or functional sequelae substantiate this observation. The changes that do occur in heart, liver, lung, renal and cerebral function are discussed below.

Central nervous system

It has become clear that there is a significant incidence of neurological and neuropsychiatric symptoms after cardiopulmonary bypass. Shaw *et al.*, 1987 found that at the time of discharge 17% of patients had some degree of neurological disability and 38% had neuropsychiatric symptoms. Most of these findings were subtle. The occurrence of brain dysfunction is related to the duration of ECC, as shown by Lee *et al.* (1970) and Goy *et al.* (1984). The percentage of patients with central nervous system damage was 10% after 1h ECC, 25% after 2h, and 35% after 3h. Similar data was reported by Tufo, Ostfield and Shekelle (1970), Gilman, (1965), and Kornfeld *et al.* (1978). Most of this central nervous system damage is manifested as delirium or disorientation and the disturbance usually returns to normal in 1–4 weeks. Some follow-up studies of intellectual functioning showed return to preoperative levels (Frank *et al.*, 1972), but a recent study has shown that 25% of patients had a diminished IQ score 6 months after cardiopulmonary bypass compared with the preoperative score (Goy *et al.*, 1984). The reversible delirium syndrome, which is related to the duration of bypass with gas interface oxygenators and minimized by the use of membrane oxygenators, may be due to microbubble embolism. An earlier study by Carlson *et al.* (1973) reported results comparing bubble and membrane oxygenators combined with ultrasonic detection of microbubbles in the arterial circuit. A high correlation was found between bubble oxygenator use, microbubble embolism, and minor cerebral dysfunction following operation. Brain function by psychological testing was more nearly normal and returned to normal more quickly in the patients perfused with the membrane oxygenator, in whom no microbubbles were present in the arterial circuit. The use of a filter as a microbubble trap diminished particles and improved central nervous system (CNS) function with the bubble oxygenator. Blauth *et al.* (1988, 1990) recently studied cerebral microemboli by using fluorescein angiography to examine the retinal vessels. They were able to confirm the finding of Carlson *et al.* (1973) that membrane oxygenators produced less microemboli than bubble oxygenators. However, they found no benefit from the use of arterial filters in reducing the number of microemboli. These studies did not attempt to correlate postoperative cerebral function with the presence of microemboli. Aris *et al.* (1986) did not find arterial line filters useful in preventing neurologic and neuropsychiatric disturbances when a bubble oxygenator was used.

Cerebral effects of ECC can also be major and permanent. Brain damage that is not reversible is often lethal (Hicks *et al.*, 1973; Witoszka *et al.*, 1973) and may be detectable during operations by electroencephalography (EEG) (Witoszka *et al.*, 1973). It can be due to gross embolism of fat or other particles (Hicks *et al.*, 1973), or to hypotension during or after bypass in older patients, especially those with cerebrovascular disease (Tufo, Ostfield and Shekelle, 1970).

Neurologic sequelae after repair of congenital cardiac defects has also been documented (Ferry, 1987 and 1990). Acute symptoms in these patients include seizures, diminished level of consciousness, focal motor deficits, and movement disorders. Potential long term sequelae include language and learning disorders, mental retardation, seizures, and cerebral palsy. These have been attributed to embolization, hypoxia, decreased cerebral perfusion, and biochemical disturbances.

In summary, transient brain dysfunction is common and increases in incidence with the duration of bypass. It appears to be due to microbubble embolism and is most common with bubble oxygenators. Major brain damage is usually due to particulate embolism or hypotension superimposed on atherosclerosis. Scrupulous attention to cleaning the field before coronary suction and filtration of coronary suction will help to prevent particulate embolism. Maintenance of adequate perfusion pressure before and after ECC is recommended in patients with atherosclerosis.

Hepatic, renal, pulmonary and myocardial function

Liver damage is detectable by isoenzyme determination within minutes of the institution of bypass, but this is generally clinically insignificant. The incidence of hyperbilirubinaemia (>3 mg dl^{-1}) has been reported to be as high as 20–23% (Collins *et al.*, 1983; Chu *et al.*, 1984). When liver damage does occur it usually appears as cholestatic jaundice which regresses spontaneously. However, 'postpump jaundice' has been associated with a poor outcome, with a 25% mortality rate reported by Collins *et al.* (1983). The factors which contribute to postoperative jaundice, such as hypoxia and hypotension, are usually responsible for the high mortality seen in these patients rather than the liver injury *per se* (Chu *et al.*, 1984). When massive liver injury does occur after cardiopulmonary bypass it is almost invariably associated with a fatal outcome.

Gastrointestinal complications following ECC are rare, with clinical symptoms developing in 0.29–2% of patients (Reath, Maull and Wolfgang, 1983; Leitman *et al.*, 1987; Krasha *et al.*, 1988; Rosemurgy *et al.*, 1988). The most common gastrointestinal complications include bleeding, acute cholecystitis, intestinal ischaemia, and pancreatitis. These complications have been associated with mortality rates ranging from 24% to 59% (Reath, Maull and Wolfgang, 1983; Leitman *et al.*, 1987; Rosemurgy *et al.*, 1988). Risk factors include old age, valvar operations, decreased cardiac output, and prolonged bypass time. The incidence of hyperamylasaemia has been found to be 27–36%, but is usually not associated with clinical pancreatitis (Haas *et al.*, 1985; Svensson, Decker and Kinsley, 1985).

Renal failure of some degree occurring in 1–4% of patients on cardiopulmonary bypass has been reported by Norman, McDonald, and Sloan (1964), Heikkinen, Hargula and Merikallio (1985) and Baxter *et al.* (1985). This would be expected from the effects of renin and angiotensin on renal cortical flow related, at least in part, to the non-pulsatile contour. When renal failure does occur it is usually a manifestation of acute tubular necrosis and is reversible. If excessive haemolysis occurs through malfunction of a device or an excessively long perfusion period with a gas interface oxygenator, renal failure from haemoglobin casts may occur.

This may be minimized by alkanizing the urine during bypass with bicarbonate and inducing osmotic diuresis with mannitol. Mannitol has been found to be useful in maintaining renal plasma flow and glomerular filtration during and after cardiopulmonary bypass (Nishimura *et al.*, 1983). Benefits from mannitol administration during ECC have also been demonstrated in children (Rigden *et al.*, 1984). Acute renal failure has been associated with a high mortality rate (66–88%), probably from factors associated with renal failure (Abel *et al.*, 1976a and b; Baxter *et al.*, 1985; Heikkinen, Hargula and Merikallio, 1985).

Lung damage following heart–lung bypass used to be common enough to be described as 'pump lung'. Pulmonary insufficiency is now unusual following bypass of 2h or less but often occurs to some degree when perfusion is carried out for a longer period of time. This effect is probably not related to lung perfusion (Abel *et al.*, 1976a) or lack of perfusion (Shah-Mirany *et al.*, 1970) via the pulmonary artery or to primary increased pulmonary extravascular water (O'Connor *et al.*, 1971). The lung, more than any other organ, displays the effects of denatured proteins, cellular breakdown or microembolism. Any particulate material occurring in the blood before or after bypass will manifest itself as pulmonary damage. The decrease in pulmonary insufficiency over the past two decades is related to at least two important factors:

1. Prepackaged, sterile, single-use, easily primed circuits, which can be prepared immediately before instituting bypass rather than requiring long periods of recirculation and blood interface exposure prior to bypass.
2 A better understanding of pulmonary physiology and management after operation.

There is ample evidence that the well inflated alveolus is less susceptible to humoral damage than the collapsed alveolus (Bartlett *et al.*, 1972). The same principle holds true during ECC. Weedn, Coalson and Greenfield, 1970 demonstrated that lung dysfunction was least in a group of dogs managed with static inflation during ECC, rather than static deflation or conventional ventilation. The lungs should be managed by static inflation during ECC unless this interferes with cardiac exposure. As mentioned earlier in this chapter, complement and neutrophil activation occurs with cardiopulmonary bypass. In addition, sequestration of neutrophils in the lungs during ECC has been demonstrated (Utoh *et al.*, 1988). Neutrophil mediated pulmonary endothelial cell injury can lead to increased capillary permeability and may contribute to the adverse effects of ECC on pulmonary function (Kirklin and Barratt-Boyes, 1986; Hernandez *et al.*, 1987).

Cardiopulmonary bypass by itself does not affect myocardial function. Many changes occur in myocardial function after operation, related to the type of operation, the valve or cardiac chamber being repaired, or the constitution of the coronary perfusate during bypass. These considerations will be discussed in detail in subsequent chapters.

Reticuloendothelial function changes

Silva, Hoeksema and Fekety (1964) have reported an elegant study of phagocytosis and bacterial killing capacity of circulating leucocytes during ECC. Using the nitroblue–tetrazolium test for phagocytosis, they found significantly decreased phagocytic activity in the circulating white cells of 12 patients undergoing cardiopulmonary bypass. They postulated that these changes were due to derangements in oxidative metabolism of these circulating white cells and supported this hypothesis by demonstrating that the bactericidal activity was decreased in two of four patients in whom it was measured. This clinical study supported the laboratory work of Kusserow and Larrow (1968) in which decreased phagocytic activity during ECC in dogs was demonstrated. Decreased activity in fixed tissue phagocytes has been demonstrated by Subramanian, Lowman and Gans (1968). They conducted ECC and isolated liver perfusion in rats and demonstrated that the clearance of radioactive gold by Kupffer cells in the liver was significantly impaired with ECC. In a later study this same group demonstrated that blood which was recirculated *ex vivo* for 30 min caused the same effect when perfused through a rat liver. They concluded from these studies that the decreased reticuloendothelial function was due to mechanical or chemical effects of the extracorporeal circuit on blood rather than the effect on the liver itself. The reason for this impaired reticuloendothelial function of circulating and fixed phagocytes has not been identified, but these observations correlate very nicely with studies of platelet aggregation and uptake in reticuloendothelial organs. If circulating and fixed phagocytes become loaded with platelet aggregates or other microparticles and debris from coronary suction or the extracorporeal circuit, then the ability of these cells further to phagocytize radioactive gold or bacteria would be reduced. If this hypothesis is proven to be true, it affords further evidence that avoiding platelet aggregation by platelet active drugs or modification of the surface of the extracorporeal circuit may be important not only in haemostasis but in maintenance of normal reticuloendothelial function after ECC. It should be briefly pointed out however that the relationship of impaired reticuloendothelial function during cardiopulmonary bypass to significant clinical infection has yet to be demonstrated.

Metabolism and pharmacology related to extracorporeal circulation

Hypothermia

Aside from the moderate low-flow state imposed by most cardiopulmonary operations as mentioned earlier, there are no specific metabolic sequelae of extracorporeal circulation. One appropriate method to compensate for the moderate low flow is the use of moderate hypothermia which decreases oxygen requirement and carbon dioxide production so that the lower flow can be matched to specific metabolic requirements. The use of moderate hypothermia (to 30°C) is widely carried out, although the effects of skin and perhaps muscle ischaemia related to this cold temperature and the increased sympathetic effects may balance out any potential advantages. Moreover, shivering during rewarming has been associated with increased oxygen consumption (Chiara *et al.*, 1980; Zwischenberger *et al.*, 1986). Paralytic agents which prevent shivering have been shown to decrease oxygen consumption and improve haemodynamic stability during rewarming (Zwischenberger *et al.*, 1986). Another effect of hypothermia is that the blood viscosity increases as the temperature drops so that use of haemodilution to lower the haematocrit is required in order to decrease blood viscosity.

The major advantage of hypothermia is to allow a safety factor to the surgeon. Faced with excessive bleeding, the entire bypass circuit can be turned off safely and the brain protected by hypothermia for periods from 10 min at 30°C to 60 min at 4°C. Equally important is the possibility afforded by moderate hypothermia of cross-clamping the aorta, eliminating coronary perfusion and providing a dry field at 32°C. This can be carried out safely for 20–30 min, can be repeated at regular intervals if necessary, and extended longer with cardioplegic techniques. These techniques are discussed in detail by subsequent authors.

Haemodilution and priming

The priming volume of the circuit depends on the gas exchange device, the venous reservoir volume and the blood volume of the patient. It is feasible to avoid blood transfusion altogether at the expense of oxygen carrying capacity. A high haematocrit and excellent oxygen carrying capacity can be achieved with an all blood prime, but at the expense of increased viscosity, haemolysis and potential for transfusion reaction, hepatitis and other blood bourne diseases such as AIDS. These factors generally balance out at a bypass haemtocrit of 25–30% which generally requires 500–1000 ml of blood in the prime or to be infused during bypass. Blood should be less than 24h old to maintain adequate levels of active blood platelets; otherwise fresh components should be used. The remainder of the prime can be isotonic saline or a colloid solution. When non-blood prime is used the resultant 'exchange transfusion' and rapid haemodilution will result in equilibration of priming solution into the appropriate body fluid space, causing hypovolaemia as referred to earlier in this chapter. Saline or saline-like crystalloid solutions will equilibrate into the extracellular fluid, requiring volume supplement to return blood volume to normal. Prime with crystalloid solutions necessarily expands the total body water and the extracellular fluid compartments. Some studies have found no difference between crystalloid and colloid primes (Ohgrist, Settergren and Lundberg, 1981; Gallagher *et al.*, 1985), while others have found colloid preferable (Sade *et al.*, 1985). Colloid solutions containing albumin or hydroxyethyl starch appear to work equally well (Sade *et al.*, 1985; Lumb, 1987). One other potential prime solution that has received attention lately is Fluosol-DA, an oxygen carrying fluorocarbon solution. This solution has been found to be comparable to saline and blood as a priming solution in experimental studies (Rousou *et al.*, 1985; Stone *et al.*, 1986), but has not been widely studied clinically.

Several investigators have studied the effect of eliminating blood transfusion for the cardiac surgical patient altogether. The reasons for wishing to do this include cost, simplicity, saving vital blood bank stores, avoiding the possible effects of microembolism from platelet fibrin aggregates in stored blood as well as possible damage to lung and other organs from transfused white blood cells, and most importantly avoiding the risk of diseases transmitted through transfusion such as hepatitis and human immunodeficiency virus. Successful major open heart operations performed without the use of blood products have been described in adult and paediatric patients of the Jehovah Witness faith (Gombotz *et al.*, 1985; Hening, 1988). The use of blood salvage and autologous transfusion before and after ECC (Kaplan *et al.*, 1977; Schaff *et al.*, 1978) and reinfusion of washed cells from the used circuit (Moran *et al.*, 1978) are major advances that save blood bank resources.

Fluid and electrolyte changes

Fluid and electrolyte disorders following ECC for cardiac surgery are major clinical considerations. Sodium retention, expanded extracellular fluid (ECF) and decreased total body potassium are characteristic of the patient with some degree of cardiac failure preoperatively, particularly if the patient had been treated with diuretics. Inadequate postoperative myocardial function as a result of hypothermia, anoxia, or the cardiac lesion itself may cause similar problems. A sophisticated study of fluid compartment composition and electrolyte status was reported by Pacifico, Digerness and Kirklin (1970). They used moderate haemodilution and found a significant increase in extracellular fluid and exchangeable sodium with a significant decrease in total body potassium in response to ECC. The increased ECF would be expected from the equilibrium of a saline type of haemodilution priming solution, plus the effects of exposure of platelets, white cells and proteins to a gas interface, which might result in increased capillary permeability. The decreased total body potassium is explained on the basis of kaliuresis and anticipated maximal aldosterone response associated with maximum stress. Similar changes in blood potassium were reported by Dieter, Neville, and Pifarre (1969). Hypokalaemia is the only major electrolyte abnormality of significance and is important because of the potential of developing digitalis-induced dysrhythmias. Hypokalaemia should be avoided by including potassium chloride in the priming solution (Pacifico, Digerness and Kirklin, 1970; Henling *et al.*, 1985). Extensive studies on calcium (Pedersen and Juhl, 1983; Chambers *et al.*, 1984) and magnesium (Turnier *et al.*, 1972; Romero *et al.*, 1973) show that these cations decrease initially with dilution at the onset of bypass and remain somewhat low throughout the course of ECC. The normal feedback loop between parathyroid hormone and calcium does not appear to function normally during cardiopulmonary bypass (Chambers *et al.*, 1984). Therefore, levels must be maintained at normal by supplementing calcium at the end of ECC. Although it has been suggested that hypomagnesaemia may predispose to dyrhythmias in ECC patients (Turnier *et al.*, 1972), it appears that these minor variations in calcium and magnesium do not commonly cause significant clinical abnormalities.

Pathophysiology of extracorporeal circulation

It was noted in the introduction that pathophysiology of ECC refers to malfunction of this extracorporeal artificial organ. This may be due to a mechanical defect, failure of the system itself, or improper regulation of the device by the operator.

Mechanical failure should be avoided by a preventative maintenance programme of replacing elements of the bypass circuit at regular intervals. The use of single-use, disposable, pre-sterilized items for all blood contact has largely eliminated failures in this area. Careful attention to roller pump settings and continuous monitoring of flow and pressure in the arterial line during bypass will minimize complications. The pump team should rehearse rapid replacement of any part of the bypass circuit as well as drills to deal with man-made problems of air embolism, thrombosis in the oxygenator, aortic dissection, improper venous cannulation, etc. Attention to these details in avoiding pathophysiological function of the extracorporeal circuit will be discussed in other chapters in this book.

Components of the extracorporeal circuit must be absolutely clean, inert, sterile and non-toxic. Mechanical cleaning may not be adequate to remove all foreign proteins and pyrogens from reused portions of the circuit. Such a foreign protein was implicated as acting as a plasminogen activator and causing abnormal bleeding in open-heart patients in one study. Cleaning in 20% sodium hydroxide removed the offending material (Brooks and Bahnson, 1971). Prepackaged single-use components should be clean but may not be necessarily so. Systemic emboli of particles of Dacron and nylon thread, antifoam, or other materials may originate from components that are allegedly clean for single use. Some extracorporeal components may contain plasticizers or solvents which could leak out into the circulating blood during ECC. All plastic materials which are used for contact with human blood must meet United States Government standards for biomedical plastics. These standards involve injecting extracts of the material into animals and subcutaneous implantation of the material in animals. All medical plastics undergo this testing procedure. Designations such as 'medical grade' or 'implant tested' do not connote any specific standard or unique characteristic.

The fact that plastic raw materials have successfully undergone conventional United States Government testing does not mean that the finished product will be non-toxic. Adhesive used in construction, heat sealing, radiation or gas sterilization may alter the characteristics of the material or add new materials that are potentially damaging to the patient. A tragic experience with toxicity of ethylene oxide sterilization of an extracorporeal circuit resulting in a fatality and clearly identified later in dogs was reported by Stanley *et al.*, 1971.

This lethal toxicity associated with ethylene oxide has now been described from several sources; however, little is known of the interactions of drugs such as halothane, penthrane, nitrous oxide, narcotics, antibiotics and analgesics with prolonged exposure to various plastic surfaces. Clinical experience would indicate that minimal interaction takes place although we have all seen clear polyvinyl chloride tubing become turbid and white silicone tubing become yellow with prolonged blood exposure. The interrelationships of these type of plastics with blood components for long periods of time deserves further study.

Antifoam is coated on some part of all gas interface oxygenators. When present in excessive amounts or when incompletely adhered to the surface, particles of this material may break loose and embolize (Reed and Kittle, 1959). The plastic material itself can erode on the inside of the extracorporeal circuit. Polyvinyl chloride tubing in the roller pump usually deteriorates by cracking and breaking from the outer edge in; however, prolonged pumping with a roller pump on silicone rubber tubing results in crumbling away from the inside out (T. Hyans, personal communication).

If air is trapped in the extracorporeal circuit and suddenly enters the arterial perfusion line, systemic air embolism will result. The possibility of this occurring from the arterial line filters has been demonstrated by Wellons and Nolan (1973) who showed that air could be trapped in the arterial line filter. This problem was solved by ventilating the filter with carbon dioxide before priming. Carbon dioxide is much more soluble than oxygen or nitrogen in priming solution and bubbles can be completely removed in this fashion. The same procedure is helpful in priming membrane oxygenators. Prevention of air embolism from intracardiac chambers has been emphasized by many authors (Lawrence, McKay and Sherensky, 1971; Gomes *et al.*, 1973). Techniques to avoid air embolism from cardiac chambers while ECC is turned on and off for various manoeuvres are described in other chapters.

Finally, infection occurring as a result of contamination of the extracorporeal circuit is another form of pathophysiology associated with ECC. Blakemore *et al.* (1971) have shown that the extracorporeal circuit becomes contaminated from the coronary suction line although the ventilation gas fed to the oxygenator itself may be contaminated from the tubing or from nebulizing or humidification devices. Appropriate use of air filters wherever possible and meticulous attention to avoiding air contamination in the field of the coronary suction will help minimize this contamination. However, bloodstream contamination, particularly in the face of decreased phagocytic and bactericidal reticuloendothelial function, as mentioned previously, predispose the ECC patient to infection. The possibility of infection and contamination during ECC has prompted most surgeons to add prophylactic antibiotics to the perfusion system or to the patient during ECC, although their value is difficult to demonstrate (Benner, 1969; Conte *et al.*, 1972; Rosendorf, Daicoff and Baer, 1974).

Conclusions

Extracorporeal circulation involves the use of a prosthetic device totally to replace the function of the heart and lungs and partially replace the blood endothelial surface and reticuloendothelial system. Properly used, it allows the function of the other organs of the body to remain unchanged during the conduct of the procedure.

Moderate hypovolaemia due to haemodilution and hypotension usually accompany ECC, with systemic flow maintained at an adequate but barely normal level. Gas exchange is easily accomplished by any of a variety of devices. The major physiological alterations caused by ECC are related to prosthetic surface exposure, with resultant platelet aggregation and complement and neutrophil activation.

References

Abel, R.M., Buckley, M.J., Austen, W.G., *et al.* (1976a) Acute post-operative renal failure in cardiac surgical patients. *Journal of Surgical Research*, **20**, 341

Abel, R.M., Buckley, M.J., Austen, W.G., *et al.* (1976b) Aetiology, incidence, and prognosis of renal failure following cardiac operations. Results of a prospective analysis of 500 consecutive patients. *Journal of Thoracic and Cardiovascular Surgery*, **71**, 323

Addonizio, V.P. and Colman, R.W. (1982) Platelets and extracorporeal circulation. *Biomaterials*, **3**, 9

Addonizio, V.P., Strauss, J.F., Macarak, E.J., *et al.* (1978) Preservation of platelet number and function with prostaglandin E_1 during total cardiopulmonary bypass in rhesus monkeys. *Surgery*, **83**, 619

Antonesen, S., Brandslund, I., Clemensen, S., *et al.* (1987) Neutrophil lysosomal enzyme release and complement activation during cardiopulmonary bypass. *Scandinavian Journal of Thoracic and Cardiovascular Surgery*, **21** 47

Aris, A., Solanes, H., Camara, M.L., *et al.* (1986) Arterial line filtration during cardiopulmonary bypass. Neurologic, neuropsychologic, and hematologic studies. *Journal of Thoracic and Cardiovascular Surgery*, **91**, 526

Arkin, C.F., Shahsavari, M., Copeland, B.E. and Kim, A. (1978) Evaluation of the activated clotting time to control heparin and protamine dosage in open-heart surgery. *Journal of Thoracic and Cardiovascular Surgery*, **75**, 790

Asari, H., Kondo, H., Ishihara, A., *et al.* (1989) Extracorporeal circulation influence on plasma atrial natriuretic peptide concentration in cardiac surgery patients. *Chest*, **96**, 757

Babka, R., Colby, C., El-Etr, A. and Pifarré, R. (1977) Monitoring of intra-operative heparinization and blood loss following cardiopulmonary bypass surgery. *Journal of Thoracic and Cardiovascular Surgery*, **73**, 780

Bartlett, R.H., Drinker, P.A., Burns, N.E., *et al.* (1972) The toroidal membrane oxygenator: design, performance and bypass testing of a clinical model. *Transactions of the American Society for Artificial Internal Organs*, **18**, 369–373

Bartlett, R.H., Fong, S.W., Burns, N.E. and Gazziniga, A.E. (1974) Prolonged partial venoarterial bypass: physiologic, biochemical and hematologic responses. *Annals of Surgery*, **180**, 850

Bartlett, R.H. and Gazzaniga, A.B. (1978) Extracorporeal circulation for cardiopulmonary failure. *Current Problems in Surgery*, **15**, (5). Year Book Medical Publishers, Chicago

Bartlett, R.H. (1971) Posttraumatic pulmonary insufficiency. In: *Surgery Annual*. (eds) Cooper, P. and Nyhus, L.) Appleton-Century-Crofts, New York.

Baxter, P., Rigby, M.L., Jones, O.D., *et al.* (1985) Acute renal failure following cardiopulmonary bypass in children: Results of treatment. *International Journal of Cardiology*, **7**, 235

Benner, J.E. (1969) Metabolism of antibiotics during cardiopulmonary bypass for open-heart surgery. *American Society Microbiology*, **92**, 373

Bernstein, E.F. and Gleason, L.R. (1967) Facors influencing haemolysis with roller pumps. *Surgery*, **61**, 432

Bidstrup, B., Royston, D., Sapsford, R.N. and Taylor, K.M. (1989) Reduction in blood loss and blood use after cardiopulmonary bypass with high dose aprotinin (Trasylol). *Journal of Thoracic and Cardiovascular Surgery*, **97**, 364

Bjork, V.O., Sternlieb, J.J. and Davenport, C. (1985) From the spinning disc to the membrane oxygenator for open heart surgery. *Scandinavian Journal of Thoracic and Cardiovascular Surgery*, **19**, 207

Blacksheer, P.L., Dorman, F.D. and Steinback, J.H. (1965) Some mechanical effects that influence hemolysis. *Transactions of the American Society for Artificial Internal Organs*, **11**, 112

Blakemore, W.S., McGarrity, G.J., Thiurer, R.J., *et al.* (1971) Infection by air-borne bacteria with cardiopulmonary bypass. *Surgery*, **70**, 830

Blauth, C.I., Arnold, J.V., Schulenberg, W.E., *et al.* (1988) Cerebral microembolism during cardiopulmonary bypass. Retinal microvascular studies in vivo with fluorescein angiography. *Journal of Thoracic and Cardiovascular Surgery*, **95**, 668

Blauth, C.I., Smith, D.L., Arnold, J.V., *et al.* (1990) Influence of oxygenator type on the prevalence and extent of microembolic retinal ischemia during cardiopulmonary bypass. *Journal of Thoracic and Cardiovascular Surgery*, **99**, 61

Boonstra, P.W., Vermeulen, F.E., Leusink, J.A., *et al.* (1986) Hematological advantage of a membrane oxygenator over a bubble oxygenator in long perfusions. *Annals of Thoracic Surgery*, **41**, 297

Boonstra, P.W., van Imhoff, G.W., Eysman, L., *et al.* (1985) Reduced platelet activation and improved hemostasis after controlled cardiotomy suction during clinical membrane oxygenator perfusions. *Journal of Thoracic and Cardiovascular Surgery*, **89**, 900

Boucher, J.K., Rudy, L.W. and Edmunds, L.H. (1974) Organ blood flow during pulsatile cardiopulmonary bypass. *Journal of Applied Physiology*, **36**, 86

Boyd, A.D., Engelman, R.M., Beaudet, R.L and Lackner, H. (1972) Disseminated intravascular coagulation following extracorporeal circulation. *Journal of Thoracic and Cardiovascular Surgery*, **64**, 685.

Breckenridge, I.M., Digerness, S.B. and Kirklin, J.W. (1969) Validity of concept of increased extracellular fluid after open-heart surgery. *Surgical Forum*, **20**, 169

Bregman, D. (1976) Mechanical support of the failing heart. *Current Problems in Surgery*, **13**, (12). Year Book Medical Publishers, Chicago

Brodman, R., Siegel, H., Lesser, M. and Frater, R. (1985) A comparison of flow gradients across disposable arterial perfusion cannulas. *Annals of Thoracic Surgery*, **39**, 225

Brooks, D.H. and Bahnson, H.T. (1971) An outbreak of haemorrhage following cardiopulmonary bypass. Epidemiologic studies. *Journal of Thoracic and Cardiovascular Surgery*, **63**, 449

Bull, B.S., Korpman, R.A., Huse, W.M. and Briggs, D.B. (1975) Heparin therapy during extracorporeal circulation. Problems inherent in existing heparin protocols. *Journal of Thoracic and Cardiovascular Surgery*, **69**, 674

Burack, B., Marcus, D., Miyamoto, A., *et al.* (1972) Response of class IV patients to alpha blockade prior to open-heart surgery. *American Heart Journal*, **84**, 456

Calafiore, A.M., Glieca, F., Marchesani, F., *et al.* (1987) A comparative clinical assessment of a hollow fibre membrane oxygenator (Capiox II) and bubble oxygenator (Harvey 1500). *Journal of Cardiovascular Surgery*, **28**, 633

Carlson, R.G., Landé, A.J., Landis, B., *et al.* (1973) The Landé–Edwards membrane oxygenator during heart surgery. *Journal of Thoracic and Cardiovascular Surgery*, **66**, 894

Cavarocchi, N.C., England, M.D., Schaff, H.V., *et al.* (1986) Oxygen free radical generation during cardiopulmonary bypass: correlation with complement activation. *Circulation*, **74**, 111–130

Cavarocchi, N.C., Pluth, J.R., Schaff, H.V., *et al.* (1986) Complement activation during cardiopulmonary bypass. Comparison of bubble and membrane oxygenator. *Journal of Thoracic and Cardiovascular Surgery*, **91**, 252

Chambers, D.J., Karimzandi, N., Baimbridge, M.V., *et al.* (1984) Hormonal and electrolyte responses during and after open heart surgery. *Journal of Thoracic and Cardiovascular Surgery*, **32**, 358

Chenoworth, D.E. (1986) Anaphylatoxin formation in extracorporeal circuits. *Complement*, **3**, 152

Chiara, O., Giomarelli, P.P., Biagioli, B., *et al.* (1980) Hypermetabolic response after hypothermic cardiopulmonary bypass. *Critical Care Medicine*, **15**, 995

Chu, C.M., Chang, C.H., Liaw, Y.F. and Hsieh, M.J. (1984) Jaundice after open-heart surgery: A prospective study. *Thorax*, **39**, 52

Clark, R.E. and Mills, M. (1969) The infant temptrol oxygenator. *Journal of Thoracic and Cardiovascular Surgery*, **60**, 54

Cohn, L.H., Angell, W.W. and Shumway, N.E. (1971) Body fluid shifts after cardiopulmonary bypass. Effects of congestive heart failure and haemodilution. *Journal of Thoracic and Cardiovascular Surgery*, **62**, 423

Collins, J.D., Bassendine, M.F., Ferner, R., *et al.* (1983) Incidence and prognostic importance of jaundice after cardiopulmonary bypass surgery. *Lancet*, **i**, 1119

Conte, J.E., Jr, Cohen, S.N., Roe, B.B. and Elashoff, R.M. (1972) Antibiotic prophylaxis and cardiac surgery: a prospective double-blind comparison of single-dose versus multiple-dose regimens. *Annals of Internal Medicine*, **76**, 943

Cottrell, E.D., Kappa, J.R., Stenach, N., *et al.* (1988) Temporary inhibition of platelet function with iloprost (ZK36374) preserves canine platelets during extracorporeal membrane oxygenation. *Journal of Thoracic and Cardiovascular Surgery*, **96**, 535

Del Canale, S., Fiaccadori, E., Vezzani, A., *et al.* (1988) Cell metabolism response to cardiopulmonary bypass in patients undergoing aorto-coronary grafting. *Scandinavian Journal of Thoracic and Cardiovascular Surgery*, **22**, 159

Dewar, M.L., Walsh, G., Chiu, R.C.-J., *et al.* (1988) Atrial natriuretic factor: Response to cardiac operation. *Journal of Thoracic and Cardiovascular Surgery*, **96**, 266

Dieter, R.A., Neville, W.E. and Pifarré, R. (1969) Hypokalaemia following haemodilution cardiopulmonary bypass. *Annals of Surgery*, **171**, 17

Dobell, A.R.C., Mitri, M., Galva, R., *et al.* (1985) Biologic evaluation of blood after prolonged recirculation through film and membrane oxygenators. *Annals of Surgery*, **161**, 617

Dunn, J., Kirsch, M., Harness, J., *et al.* (1974) Haemodynamic, metabolic, and haematologic effects of pulsatile cardiopulmonary bypass. *Journal of Thoracic and Cardiovascular Surgery*, **68**, 138

Dutton, R.C. and Edmunds, L.H., Jr. (1973) Measurement of emboli in extracorporeal perfusion system. *Journal of Thoracic and Cardiovascular Surgery*, **65**, 523

Ekert, H. and Sheers, M. (1974) Preoperative and postoperative platelet function in cyanotic congenital heart disease. *Journal of Thoracic and Cardiovascular Surgery*, **68**, 184

Fantini, G.A., Zadeh, B.J., Chiao, J., *et al.* (1987) Effect of hypothermia on cellular membrane function during low-flow extracorporeal circulation. *Surgery*, **102**, 132

Fedderson, K., Aurell, M., Delin, K., *et al.* (1985) Effects of cardiopulmonary bypass and prostacyclin on plasma catecholamines, angiotensin II and arginine-vasopressin. *Acta Anaesthesiologica Scandinavica*, **29**, 224

Ferry, P.C. (1987) Neurologic sequelae of cardiac surgery in children. *American Journal of Diseases of Children*, **141**, 309

Ferry, P.C. (1990) Neurologic sequelae of open-heart surgery in children. *American Journal of Diseases in Children*, **144**, 369

Fish, K.J., Sarnquist, F.H., van Steenis, C., *et al.* (1986) A prospective randomized study of the effects of prostacyclin on platelets and blood loss during coronary bypass operations. *Journal of Thoracic and Cardiovascular Surgery*, **91**, 436

Fong, S.W., Burns, N.E., Williams, G., *et al.* (1974) Changes in coagulation and platelet function during prolonged extracorporeal circulation (ECC) in sheep and man. *Transactions of the American Society for Artificial Internal Organs*, **20**, 239

Fosse, E., Mollnes, T.E. and Ingvaldsen, B. (1987) Complement activation during major operations with or without cardiopulmonary bypass. *Journal of Thoracic and Cardiovascular Surgery*, **93**, 860

Frank, K.A., Heller, S.S., Kornfeld, D.S. and Malm, J.R. (1972) Long-term effects of open-heart surgery on intellectual functioning. *Journal of Thoracic and Cardiovascular Surgery*, **64**, 811

Friesen, R.H. and Clement, A.J. (1976) Individual responses to heparinization for extracorporeal circulation. *Journal of Thoracic and Cardiovascular Surgery*, **72**, 875

Gallagher, J.D., Moore, R.A., Kerns, D., *et al.* (1985) Effects of colloid or crystalloid administration on pulmonary extravascular water in the postoperative period after coronary artery bypass grafting. *Anesthesia and Analgesia*, **64**, 753

Galletti, P.M., Richardson, P.D. and Snider, M.T. (1972) A standardized method for defining the overall gas transfer performance of artificial lungs. *Transactions of the American Society for Artificial Internal Organs*, **18**, 359

Gans, H., Castaneda, A.R. and Subramanian, V.A. (1967) Problems in haemostasis during open-heart surgery. IX. Changes observed in the plasminogen-plasma system and their significance for therapy. *Annals of Surgery*, **166**, 980

Gazzaniga, A.B., Byrd, C.L. and Gross, R.E. (1970) The use of skeletal muscle surface hydrogen ion concentration to monitor peripheral perfusion: experimental and clinical results. *Surgical Forum*, **21**, 147

Gazzaniga, A.B., Byrd, C.L., Stewart, D.R. and Gross, R.E. (1972) Effects of dexamethasone and chlorpromazine on skeletal muscle surface hydrogen ion concentration during cardiopulmonary bypass. *Annals of Surgery*, **176**, 757

Gervin, A.S., McNeer, J.F., Wolfe, W.G., *et al.* (1974) Ultrapore haemofiltration during extracorporeal circulation. *Journal of Thoracic and Cardiovascular Surgery*, **67**, 237

Gilman, S. (1965) Cerebral disorders after open-heart operations. *New England Journal of Medicine*, **272**, 489

Gombotz, H., Metzler, H., Hiotakis, K. and Dacar, D. (1985) Open heart surgery in Jehovah's Witnesses. *Wiener Klinische Wochenschrift*, **97**, 525

Gomes, M.M.R. and McGoon, D.C. (1969) Bleeding patterns after open-heart surgery. *Journal of Thoracic and Cardiovascular Surgery*, **60**, 87

Gomes, O.M., Pereira, S.N., Castagna, R.C., *et al.*, (1973) The importance of the different sites of air injection in the tolerance of arterial air-embolism. *Journal of Thoracic and Cardiovascular Surgery*, **65**, 563

Goodman, T.A., Gerard, D.F., Bernstein, E.F. and Dilley, R.B. (1976) The effects of pulseless perfusion on the distribution of renal cortical blood flow and on renin release. *Surgery*, **80**, 31

Gourin, A., Streisand, R.L. and Stuckey, J.H. (1970) Total cardiopulmonary bypass, myocardial contractility, and the administration of protamine sulfate. *Journal of Thoracic and Cardiovascular Surgery*, **61**, 160

Goy, M., Schmitt, R., Sabatier, M. and Kreitmann, P. (1984) Effect of open heart surgery on intellectual efficiency. Prospective study apropos of 40 cases. *Archives des Maladies du Coeur et des Vaisseaux*, **77**, 167

Grossi, E.A., Connally, M.W., Krieger, K.H., *et al.* (1985) Quantification of pulsatile flow during cardiopulmonary bypass to permit direct comparison of the effectiveness of various types of 'pulsatile' and 'nonpulsatile' flow. *Surgery*, **98**, 547

Haas, G.S., Warshaw, A.L., Daggett, W.M. and Aretz, H.T. (1985) Acute pancreatitis after cardiopulmonary bypass. *American Journal of Surgery*, **149**, 508

Harken, L.A., Malpass, T.W., Branson, H.E., *et al.* (1980) Mechanism of abnormal bleeding in patients undergoing cardiopulmonary bypass: Acquired transient platelet dysfunction associated with selective alpha granule release. *Blood*, **56**, 824

Harken, A.H. (1975) The influence of pulsatile perfusion on oxygen uptake by the isolated canine hind limb. *Journal of Thoracic and Cardiovascular Surgery*, **70**, 237

Harrison, T.S. and Seton, J.F. (1973) An analysis of pulse frequency as an adrenergic excitant in pulsatile circulatory support. *Surgery*, **73**, 868

Harrison, T.S., Chawla, R.C., Seton, J.F. and Robinson, B.H. (1970) Carotid sinus origin of adrenergic responses compromising the effectiveness of artificial circulatory support. *Surgery*, **68**, 20

Heikkinen, L., Hargula, A. and Merikallio, E. (1985) Acute renal failure related to open heart surgery. *Annales Chirurgiae et Gynaecologiae*, **74**, 203

Hening, C.R. (1988) *Modern Cardiovascular Physiology*. Little, Brown and Company, Boston

Henling, C.E., Carmichael, M.J., Keats, A.S. and Cooley, D.A. (1985) Cardiac operation for congenital heart disease in children of Jehovah's Witnesses. *Journal of Thoracic and Cardiovascular Surgery*, **89**, 914

Henney, P.R., Riemenschneider, T.A., DeLand, E.C., Maloney, J.V., Jr. (1971) Prevention of hypokalaemic cardiac arrhythmias associated with cardiopulmonary bypass and haemodilution. *Surgical Forum*, **21**, 145

Hernandez, L.A., Grisham, M.B., Twohig, B. (1987) Role of neutrophils in ischemia-reperfusion induced microvascular injury. *American Journal of Physiology*, **253**, H699

Hickey, P.R., Buckley, M.J. and Philbin, D.M. (1983) Pulsatile and nonpulsatile cardiopulmonary bypass: review of a counterproductive controversy. *Annals of Thoracic Surgery*, **36**, 720

Hicks, R.E., Dutton, R.C., Ries, C.A., *et al.* (1973) Production and fate of platelet aggregate emboli during venovenous perfusion. *Surgical Forum*, **24**, 250

Hill, J.D., Aguilar, M.J., Baranco, A., Gerbode, F. (1969) Neuropathological manifestations of cardiac surgery. *Annals of Thoracic Surgery*, **7**, 409

Hill, J.D., DeLeval, M.R., Fallat, R.J., *et al.* (1972) Acute respiratory insufficiency: Treatment with prolonged extracorporeal oxygenation. *Journal of Thoracic and Cardiovascular Surgery*, **64**, 551

Hind, C.R., Griffin, J.F., Pack, S., *et al.* (1988) Effect of cardiopulmonary bypass on circulating concentrations of leucocyte elastase and free radical activity. *Cardiovascular Research*, **22**, 37

Hinshaw, D.B., Armstrong, B.C., Burger, J.M., *et al.* (1988) ATP and microfilaments in cellular oxidant injury. *American Journal of Pathology*, **132**, 479

Holloway, D.S., Summaria, L., Sandesara, J., *et al.* (1988) Decreased platelet number and function and increased fibrinolysis contribute to postoperative bleeding in cardiopulmonary bypass patients. *Thrombosis and Haemostasis*, **59**, 62

Horrow, J.C., Hlavacek, J., Strong, M.D., *et al.* (1990) Prophylactic tranexamic acid decreases bleeding after cardiac operations. *Journal of Thoracic and Cardiovascular Surgery*, **99**, 70

Howard, R.J., Crain, C., Franzini, D.A., *et al.* (1988) Effects of cardiopulmonary bypass on pulmonary leukostasis and complement activation. *Archives of Surgery*, **123**, 1496

Indeglia, R., Shea, M.A., Varco, R.L and Bernstein, E.F. (1967) Mechanical and biological considerations in erythrocyte damage. *Surgery*, **62**, 47

Jaberi, M., Bell, W.R. and Benson, D.W. (1973) Control of heparin therapy in open-heart surgery. *Journal of Thoracic and Cardiovascular Surgery*, **67**, 133

Jones, D.K., Luddington, R., Higenbottam, T.W., *et al.* (1988) Changes in factor VIII proteins after cardiopulmonary bypass in man suggests endothelial damage. *Thrombosis and Haemostasis*, **60**, 199

Kaplan, J.A., Cannarella, C., Jones, E.L., *et al.* (1977) Autologous blood transfusion during cardiac surgery. A re-evalaution of three methods. *Journal of Thoracic and Cardiovascular Surgery*, **74**, 4

Kevy, S.V., Glickman, R.M., Bernhard, W.F. (1966) The pathogenesis and control of the haemorrhagic defect in open-heart surgery. *Surgery, Gynecology and Obstetrics*, **126**, 313

Kirklin, J.W. and Barratt-Boyes, B.G. (1986) Hypothermia, circulatory arrest, and cardiopulmonary bypass. In *Cardiac Surgery*. Wiley, New York, pp. 30–74

Kirklin, J.K. and Kirklin, J.W. (1990) Cardiopulmonary bypass for cardiac surgery. In *Surgery of the Chest*, 5th edn (eds D.C. Sabiston and F.C. Spencer), WB Saunders Company, Philadelphia, pp. 1107–1122

Kirklin, J.K., Westaby, S., Blackstone, E.H., *et al.* (1983) Complement and the damaging effects of cardiopulmonary bypass. *Journal of Thoracic and Cardiovascular Surgery*, **86**, 845

Kono, K., Philbin, D.M., Coggins, C.H., *et al.* (1983) Adrenocortical hormone levels during cardiopulmonary bypass with and without pulsatile flow. *Journal of Thoracic and Cardiovascular Surgery*, **85**, 129

Kornfeld, D.S., Heller, S.S., Frank, K.A., *et al.* (1978) Delirium after coronary artery bypass surgery. *Journal of Thoracic and Cardiovascular Surgery*, **76**, 93

Krasha, M.J., Flancbaum, L., Trooskin, S.Z., *et al.* (1988) Gastrointestinal complications after cardiac surgery. *Surgery*, **104**, 773

Kuntschen, F.R., Galletti, P.M., Hahn, C., *et al.* (1985) Alterations of insulin and glucose metabolism during cardiopulmonary bypass under normothermia. *Journal of Thoracic and Cardiovascular Surgery*, **89**, 97

Kuntschen, F.R., Galletti, P.M. and Hahn, C. (1986) Glucose insulin interactions during cardiopulmonary bypass. Hypothermia versus normothermia. *Journal of Thoracic and Cardiovascular Surgery*, **91**, 451

Kusserow, B.K. and Larrow, R. (1968) Studies of leukocyte responses to prolonged blood pumping–effects upon phagocytic capability and total white cell count. *Transactions of the American Society for Artificial Internal Organs*, **14**, 261

Lavee, J., Martinowitz, U., Mohr, R., *et al.* (1989) The effect of transfusion of fresh whole blood versus platelet concentrates after cardiac operations. A scanning electron microscope study of platelet aggregation on extracellular matrix. *Journal of Thoracic and Cardiovascular Surgery*, **97**, 204

Lawrence, G.H., McKay, H.A. and Sherensky, R.T. (1971) Effective measures in the prevention of intraoperative aeroembolus. *Journal of Thoracic and Cardiovascular Surgery*, **62**, 731

Lee, W.H., Jr, Brady, M.P., Rowe, J.M., Miller, W.C., Jr. (1970) Effects of extracorporeal circulation upon behavior, personality, and brain function: Part II, Haemodynamic, metabolic and psychometric correlations. *Annals of Surgery*, **173**, 1013

Lee, W.H., Jr, Krumhaar, D., Fonkalsrud, E.W., *et al.* (1961) Denaturation of plasma proteins as a cause of morbidity and death after intracardiac operations. *Surgery*, **50**, 29

Lees, M.H., Herr, R.H., Hill, J.D., *et al.* (1970) Distribution of systemic blood flow of the rhesus monkey during cardiopulmonary bypass. *Journal of Thoracic and Cardiovascular Surgery*, **61**, 570

Leitman, I.M., Paull, D.E., Barie, P.S. (1987) Intra-abdominal complications of cardiopulmonary bypass operations. *Surgery Gynecology and Obstetrics*, **165**, 251

Lemieux, M., Tice, D.A., Reed, G.E. and Chauss, R.H. (1967) Chlorpromazine; adjunct to physiologic perfusion. *Journal of Thoracic and Cardiovascular Surgery*, **53**, 425

Lindberg, H., Svennevig, J.L., Lilleaasen, P., Vatne, K. (1984) Pulsatile vs. non-pulsatile flow during cardiopulmonary bypass. A comparison of early postoperative changes. *Scandinavian Journal of Thoracic and Cardiovascular Surgery*, **18**, 195

Lumb, P.D. (1987) A comparison between 25% albumin and 6% hydroxyethyl starch solutions on lung water accumulation during and immediately after cardiopulmonary bypass. *Annals of Surgery*, **206**, 210

Mammen, E.F., Koets, M.H., Washington, B.C., *et al.* (1985) Hemostasis changes during cardiopulmonary bypass surgery. *Seminars in Thrombosis and Hemostasis*, **11**, 281

Mannucci, P.M. (1988) Desmopressin: a nontransfusional form of treatment for congenital and acquired bleeding disorders. *Blood*, **72**, 1449

Many, M., Giron, F., Birtwell, W.C., *et al.* (1969) Effects of depulsation of renal blood flow upon renal function and renin secretion. *Surgery*, **66**, 242

Marath, A., Man, W., Taylor, K.M. (1988) Plasma histamine profiles in paediatric cardiopulmonary bypass. *Agents and Actions*, **23**, 339

Marath, A., Man, W., Taylor, K.M. (1987) Histamine release in paediatric cardiopulmonary bypass–a possible role in the capillary leak syndrome. *Agents and Actions*, **20**, 299

Matsuda, H., Hirose, H., Nakano, S., *et al.* (1986) Results of open heart surgery in patients with impaired renal function as creatinine clearance below 30 ml/min. The effects of pulsatile perfusion. *Journal of Cardiovascular Surgery*, **27**, 595

Maxwell, G.M., Rowe, C.G., Castillo, G., *et al.* (1958) Haemodynamic effects of chlorpromazine: including studies of cardiac work and coronary blood flow. *Anesthesiology*, **19**, 64

Montoya, J.P., Merz, S.I., Bartlett, R.H. (1990) A standardized system for describing flow/pressure relationships in vascular access devices. *Transactions of the American Society for Artificial Internal Organs*, **37**, 4–8

Moran, J.M., Babka, R., Silberman, S., *et al.* (1978) Immediate centrifugation of oxygenator contents after cardiopulmonary bypass. *Journal of Thoracic and Cardiovascular Surgery*, **76**, 510

Mullin, P., Lee, S., Burd, S., *et al.* (1976) A new device for the rapid automated determination of the activated clotting time for whole blood. *American Society of Extra-Corporeal Technology Proceedings*, pp. 6–8

Nagaoka, H., Innami, R. and Arai, H. (1988) Effects of pulsatile cardiopulmonary bypass on the renin–angiotensin–aldosterone system following open heart surgery. *Japanese Journal of Surgery*, **18**, 390

Needleman, P. and Greenwald, J.E. (1986) Atriopeptin: a cardiac hormone intimately involved in fluid, electrolyte, and blood pressure homeostasis. *New England Journal of Medicine*, **314**, 828

Nishimura, O., Tokutsu, S., Sakurai, T., *et al.* (1983) Effects of hypertonic mannitol on renal function in open heart surgery. *Japanese Heart Journal*, **24**, 245

Norman, J.C., McDonald, H.P. and Sloan, H. (1964) The early and aggressive treatment of acute renal failure following cardiopulmonary bypass with continuous peritoneal dialysis. *Surgery*, **56**, 240

O'Connor, N.E., Sheh, J.M., Bartlett, R.H., Gazzaniga, A.B. (1971) Changes in pulmonary extravascular water volume following mitral valve replacement. *Journal of Thoracic and Cardiovascular Surgery*, **61**, 342

Ohgrist, G., Settergren, G. and Lundberg, S. (1981)

Pulmonary oxygenation, central hemodynamics and glomerular filtration following cardiopulmonary bypass with colloid and non-colloid priming solution. *Scandinavian Journal of Thoracic and Cardiovascular Surgery*, **15**, 257

Okies, J.E., Goodnight, S.H., Kitchford, B., *et al*, (1977) Effect of infusion of cardiotomy suction blood during extracorporeal circulation for coronary artery bypass surgery. *Journal of Thoracic and Cardiovascular Surgery*, **74**, 440

Olinger, G.N., Hutchinson, L.D. and Bonchek, L.T. (1983) Pulsatile cardiopulmonary bypass for patients with renal insufficiency. *Thorax*, **38**, 543

Pacifico, A.D., Digerness, S. and Kirklin, J.W. (1970) Acute alterations of body composition after open intracardiac operations. *Circulation*, **41**, 331

Padayachee, T.S., Parsons, S., Theobold, R., *et al.* (1988) The effect of arterial filtration on reduction of gaseous microemboli in the middle cerebral artery during cardiopulmonary bypass. *Annals of Thoracic Surgery*, **45**, 647

Pedersen, K.O. and Juhl, O. (1983) Blood ionized calcium measurements during aortocoronary bypass graft operations. *Scandinavian Journal of Clinical and Laboratory Investigation. Supplement*, **165**, 107

Peirce, E.C. II. (1969) *Extracorporeal Circulation for Open-heart Surgery*. Thomas, Springfield

Pollack, E.M., Pollock, J.C., Jamieson, M.P., *et al.* (1988) Adrenocortical hormone concentrations in children during cardiopulmonary bypass with and without pulsatile flow. *British Journal of Anaesthesia*, **60**, 536

Reath, D.B., Maull, K.I. and Wolfgang, T.C. (1983) General surgical complications following cardiac surgery. *American Surgeon*, **49**, 11

Reed, W.A. and Kittle, C.F. (1959) Observations on toxicity and use of antifoam. *Archives of Surgery*, **78**, 220

Rein, K.A., Semb, G.K., Myhre, H.O., *et al.* (1988) Transcapillary fluid balance in subcutaneous tissue of patients undergoing aortocoronary bypass with extracorporeal circulation: *Scandinavian Journal of Thoracic Cardiovascular Surgery*, **22**, 267

Replogle, R.L. and Gross, R.E. (1961) Renal function during extracorporeal circulation. *Journal of Surgical Research*, **1**, 91

Replogle, R.L., Levy, M., DeWall, R.A. and Lillehei, R.C. (1962) Catecholamine and serotonin response to cardiopulmonary bypass. *Journal of Thoracic and Cardiovascular Surgery*, **44**, 638

Riegel, W., Spillner, G., Schlosser, V. and Horl, W.H. (1988) Plasma levels of main granulocyte components during cardiopulmonary bypass. *Journal of Thoracic and Cardiovascular Surgery*, **95**, 1014

Rigden, S.P., Dillon, M.J., Kind, P.R. (1984) The beneficial effect of mannitol on postoperative renal function in children undergoing cardiopulmonary bypass surgery. *Clinical Nephrology*, **21**, 148

Robicsek, F., Masters, T.N., Niesluchowski, W. (1983) Vasomotor activity during cardiopulmonary bypass. In *Pathophysiology and Techniques of Cardiopulmonary Bypass*, (ed. J. Utley), Williams and Wilkins, Baltimore, pp. 1–13

Romero, E.G., Castillo-Olivares, J.L., O'Connor, F. (1973) The importance of calcium and magnesium ions in serum and cerebrospinal fluid during cardiopulmonary bypass. *Journal of Thoracic and Cardiovascular Surgery*, **66**, 668

Rosemurgy, A.S., McAllister, E. and Karl, R.C. (1988) The acute surgical abdomen after cardiac surgery involving extracorporeal circulation. *Annals of Surgery*, **207**, 323

Rosendorf, L.L., Daicoff, G. and Baer, H. (1974) Sources of gram negative infection after open-heart surgery. *Journal of Thoracic Cardiovascular Surgery*, **67**, 195

Rousou, J.A., Engleman, R.A., Amisimowicz, L. and Dobbs, W.A. (1985) A comparison of blood and fluosol-DA for cardiopulmonary bypass. *Journal of Cardiovascular Surgery*, **26**, 447

Royston, D., Fleming, J.S., Desai, J.B., *et al.* (1986) Increased production of peroxidation products associated with cardiac operations. Evidence of free radical generation. *Journal of Thoracic and Cardiovascular Surgery*, **91**, 759

Rudy, L.W., Heyman, M.A. and Edmunds, L.H. (1970a) Distribution of systemic blood flow during total cardiopulmonary bypass in rhesus monkeys. *Surgical Forum*, **21**, 149

Rudy, L.W., Heymann, M.A. and Edmunds, L.H. (1970b) Distribution of systemic blood flow during cardiopulmonary bypass. *Journal of Applied Physiology*, **34**, 194

Sade, R.M., Stroud, M.R., Crawford, F.A., Jr, *et al.* (1985) A prospective randomized study of hydroxyethyl starch, albumin, and lactated Ringer's solution as a priming fluid for cardiopulmonary bypass. *Journal of Thoracic and Cardiovascular Surgery*, **89**, 713

Salama, A., Hugo, F., Heinrich, D., *et al.* (1988) Deposition of terminal C5b-9 complement complexes on erythrocytes and leukocytes during cardiopulmonary bypass. *New England Journal of Medicine*, **318**, 408

Salzman, E.W., Weinstein, M.J., Weinstraub, R.M., *et al.* (1986) Treatment with desmopressin acetate to reduce blood loss after cardiac surgery. A double-blind randomized trial. *New England Journal of Medicine*, **314**, 1402

Sanderson, J.M., Wright, G. and Simms, F.W. (1972) Brain damage in dogs immediately following pulsatile and nonpulsatile blood flows in extracorporeal circulation. *Thorax*, **27**, 275

Schaff, H.V., Hauer, J.M., Bell, W.R., *et al.* (1978) Autotransfusion of shed mediastinal blood after cardiac surgery–a prospective study. *Journal of Thoracic and Cardiovascular Surgery*, **75**, 632

Schaff, H.V., Mashburn, J.P., McCarthy, P.M., *et al.* (1989) Natriuresis during and after early cardiopulmonary bypass: relationship to atrial natriuretic factor, aldosterone, and antidiuretic hormone. *Journal of Thoracic and Cardiovascular Surgery*, **98**, 979

Shah-Mirany, J., Najafi, H., Serry, C., *et al.* (1970) Pathophysiological alterations in perfused and nonperfused lungs during cardiopulmonary bypass. *Annals of Thoracic Surgery*, **10**, 402

Shaw, P.J., Bates, D., Cartlidge, N.E., *et al.* (1987) Neurologic and neuropsychological morbidity following major surgery: comparison of coronary artery surgery and peripheral vascular surgery. *Stroke*, **18**, 700

Silva, J., Jr, Hoeksema, H. and Fekety, F.R. (1974) Transient defects in phagocytic functions during cardiopulmonary bypass. *Journal of Thoracic and Cardiovascular Surgery*, **67**, 175

Smith, E.E.J., Naftel, D.C., Blackstone, E.H. and Kirklin, J.W. (1987) Microvascular permeability after cardiopulmonary bypass. *Journal of Thoracic and Cardiovaascular Surgery*, **94**, 225

Spaeth, E.E., Roberts, G.W., Yadwadkar, S.R., *et al.* (1973) The influence of fluid shear on the kinetics of blood coagulation reactions. *Transactions of the American Society for Artificial Internal Organs*, **19**, 179

Stanley, P., Bertranou, E., Forest, F. and Langevin, L. (1971) Toxicity of ethylene oxide sterilization of polyvinyl chloride in open-heart surgery. *Journal of Thoracic and Cardiovascular Surgery*, **61**, 309

Stein, J.H. and Perris, T.F. (1973) The physiology of renin. *Archives of Internal Medicine*, **131**, 860

Stibbe, J., Kluft, C., Brommer, E.J., *et al.* (1984) Enhanced fibrinolytic activity during cardiopulmonary bypass in open-heart surgery in man is caused by extrinsic (tissue-type) plasminogen activator. *European Journal of Clinical Investigation*, **14**, 375

Stone, J.J., Piccione, W., Berrizbeitia, L.D., *et al.* (1986) Hemodynamic, metabolic, and morphological effects of cardiopulmonary bypass with a fluorocarbon primary solution. *Annals of Thoracic Surgery*, **41**, 419C

Subramanian, V., Lowman, J. and Gans, H. (1968) Effect of extracorporeal circulation on retoculoendothelial function. *Archives of Surgery*, **97**, 330

Svensson, L.G., Decker, G. and Kinsley, R.B. (1985) A prospective study of hyperamylasemia and pancreatitis after cardiopulmonary bypass. *Annals of Thoracic Surgery*, **39**, 409

Tamari, Y., Aledort, L., Puszkin, E., *et al.* (1975) Functional changes in platelets during extracorporeal circulation. *Annals of Thoracic Surgery*, **19**, 639

Tan, C.-K., Glisson, S.N. and El-Etr, A.A., Ramakrishnaiah, K.B. (1976) Levels of circulating norepinephrine and epinephrine before, during, and after cardiopulmonary bypass in man. *Journal of Thoracic and Cardiovascular Surgery*, **71**, 928

Tarhan, S. and Moffitt, E.A. (1971) Anaesthesia and supportive care during and after cardiac surgery. *Annals of Thoracic Surgery*, **11**, 64

Tennenberg, S.D., Bailey, W.W., Cotter, L.A., *et al.* (1985) The effects of methylprednisolone on complement-mediated neutrophil activation during cardiopulmonary bypass. *Surgery*, **100**, 134

Teoh, K.H., Christakis, G.T., Weisel, R.D., *et al.* (1988) Dipyridamole preserved platelets and reduced blood loss after cardiopulmonary bypass. *Journal of Thoracic and Cardiovascular Surgery*, **96**, 266

Tranmer, B.I., Gross, C.E., Kindt, G.W. and Adey, G.R. (1986) Pulsatile versus nonpulsatile flow in the treatment of acute cerebral ischemia. *Neurosurgery*, **19**, 724

Tufo, H.M., Ostfeld, A.M. and Shekelle, R. (1970) Central nervous system dysfunction following open-heart surgery. *JAMA*, **212**, 1333

Turnier, E., Osborn, J.J., Gerbode, F. and Popper, R.W. (1972) Magnesium and open-heart surgery. *Journal of Thoracic and Cardiovascular Surgery*, **64**, 694

Utoh, J., Yamamoto, T., Kambara, T., *et al.* (1988) Complement conversion and leukocyte kinetics in open heart surgery. *Japanese Journal of Surgery*, **18**, 259

van Oeveren, W., Jansen, N.J., Bidstrup, B.P., *et al.* (1987) Effects of aprotinin on hemostatic mechanisms during cardiopulmonary bypass. *Annals of Thoracic Surgery*, **44**, 640

van Oeveren, W., Kazatchkine, M.D., Descamps-Latscha, B., *et al.* (1985) Deleterious effects of cardiopulmonary bypass. A prospective study of bubble versus membrane oxygenation. *Journal of Thoracic and Cardiovascular Surgery*, **89**, 888

Viinamaki, O., Nuutinen, L., Hanhela, R., *et al.* (1986) Plasma vasopressin levels during and after cardiopulmonary bypass in man. *Medical Biology*, **64**, 289

von Segesser, L.K. and Turina, M. (1989) Cardiopulmonary bypass without systemic heparinization. *Journal of Thoracic and Cardiovascular Surgery*, **98**, 386

Wachtfogel, Y.T., Kucich, U., Greenplate, J., *et al.* (1987) Human neutrophil degranulation during extracorporeal circulation. *Blood*, **69**, 324

Ware, J.A., Reaves, W.H., Horak, J.K. and Solis, R.T. (1983) Detective platelet aggregation in patients undergoing surgical repair of anoxic congenital heart disease. *Annals of Thoracic Surgery*, **36**, 289

Watanabe, T., Orita, H., Kobayashi, M. and Washio, M. (1989) Brain tissue pH, oxygen tension, and carbon dioxide tension in profoundly hypothermic cardiopulmonary bypass. Comparative study of circulatory arrest, nonpulsatile low flow perfusion, and pulsatile low-flow perfusion. *Journal of Thoracic and Cardiovascular Surgery*, **97**, 396

Weedn, R.J., Coalson, J.J. and Greenfield, L.J. (1970) Effects of oxygen and ventilation on pulmonary mechanics and ultrastructure during cardiopulmonary bypass. *American Journal of Surgery*, **120**, 584

Wellons, H.A., Jr and Nolan, S.P. (1973) Prvention of air embolism due to trapped air in filters used in extracorporeal circuits. *Journal of Thoracic and Cardiovascular Surgery*, **65**, 476

Wenger, R.K., Lukasiewicz, H., Mikuta, B.S., *et al.* (1989) Loss of platelet fibrinogen receptors during clinical cardiopulmonary bypass. *Journal of Thoracic and Cardiovascular Surgery*, **97**, 235

Whittlesey, G.C., Kundu, S.K., Salley, S.O., *et al.* (1988) Is heparin necessary for extracorporeal circulation? *Transactions of the American Society for Artificial Internal Organs*, **34**, 823

Witoszka, M.M., Tamura, H., Indeglia, R., *et al.* (1973) Electroencephalographic changes and cerebral complications in open-heart surgery. *Journal of Thoracic and Cardiovascular Surgery*, **66**, 855

Wolk, L.A., Wilson, R.F., Burdick, M., *et al.* (1985) Changes in antithrombin, antiplasmin, and plasminogen during and after cardiopulmonary bypass. *American Surgeon*, **51**, 309

Zwischenberger, J.B., Cilley, R.E., Kirsh, M.M., *et al.* (1986) Does continuous monitoring of mixed venous oxygen saturation (SvO_2) accurately reflect oxygen delivery (DO_2) and oxygen consumption (vO_2) following coronary artery bypass grafting (CABG?). *Surgical Forum*, **37**, 66

Zwischenberger, J.B., Kirsch, M.M., Dechert, R.E. (1987) Suppression of shivering decreases oxygen consumption and improves hemodynamic stability during postoperative rewarming. *Annals of Thoracic Surgery*, **43**, 428

3

Design and principles of the extracorporeal circuit

L. Bigi, N. Ghelli, A. Menghini and I. Panzani

History of cardiopulmonary bypass

The first proposal of an 'artificial circulation' was put forward by Le Gallois in 1812 when he perfused rabbit brains through carotid arteries. Between 1848 and 1853 Brown Sequard obtained bright red oxygenated blood by shaking dark venous blood and demonstrated that such blood could serve as a perfusate to maintain electrical activity of the isolated brain specimen.

In 1882 Shroder assembled the first bubble oxygenator. Two years later von Frey and Gruber created the first membrane oxygenator. In 1900 Howell, Holt and McLean discovered the efficacy of heparin as an anticoagulant.

The true beginning of modern extracorporeal circulation occurred in 1953 when Gibbon performed the first open heart operation using a 45 min period of extracorporeal perfusion at the Massachusetts General Hospital. He realized that the key to extracorporeal circulation was the oxygenator and developed a disc oxygenating device with a 4 m^2. exchange surface. Since then the technology of extracorporeal circulation has rapidly evolved.

In 1955 Lillehei used the first bubble oxygenator. A year later Rygg developed a disposable bubble oxygenator, from which time development in extracorporeal circulation have aimed at achieving completely disposable products.

Components of the extracorporeal circuit

The extracorporeal system consists of a series of interconnected devices for the oxygenation and circulation of blood temporarily replacing the function of the heart and the lungs. The main components of the circuit are a pump (artificial heart), an oxygenator (artificial lungs), a cardiotomy reservoir, a heat exchanger, cannulae, filters and inter-connected tubings.

There are two fundamental circuits dependent on whether a membrane or bubble oxygenator is used (Figures 3.1 and 3.2).

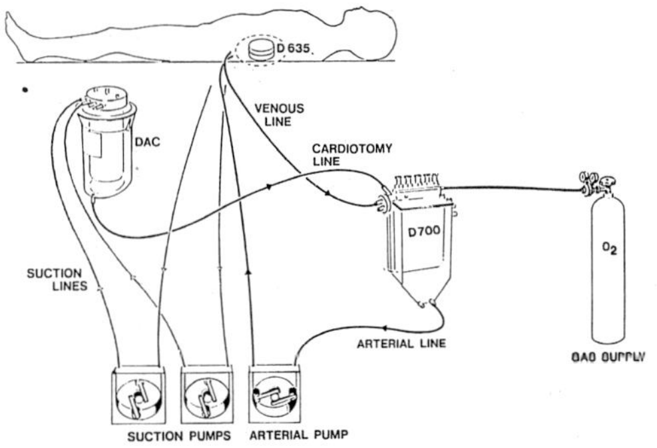

Figure 3.1

Bubble oxygenators

With the bubble oxygenator bubble formation allows direct contact between blood and gas with the exchange of oxygen and carbon dioxide occurring at the bubble surface.

A bubble oxygenator can be divided into four sections: oxygenating chamber, defoaming section, heat exchanger and venous reservoir.

The venous blood arrives at the oxygenating chamber from the venous reservoir by gravity drainage. In the Dideco Hi-Flex system bubbles are provided by ten precalibrated spargers. These are made of non-deformable materials and ensure the functional characteristics of the oxygenator and its gas exchange efficiency are maintained. The bubble size is predetermined. Too large bubbles would result in decreased efficiency of gas exchange. Alternatively tiny bubbles preclude adequate carbon dioxide exchange and present difficulties with defoaming leading to microemboli. In general terms bubbles of between 3 mm and 4 mm will provide acceptable oxygenation. The ratio of gas to blood flow is important as high gas flows lead to increased haemolysis.

A heat exchanger is generally integrated into all bubble oxygenators in the form of tubes or spirals. The special modular configuration of the Hi-Flex bubble oxygenator allows the operator to adjust the actual thermal exchange need according to the patient's size (Figure 3.3).

The defoaming section serves to remove bubbles from the blood via the surface which is coated with an antifoam compound. This can either be made of silicone or sponge coated with surfactants performing an antibubble action. A 120 μm filter removes particles of higher calibre.

The venous reservoir has a storage capacity of between 3.5 litres and 4.5 litres enabling the operation to meet the flow variation requirements. The reservoir must be of a highly transparent material permitting early detection of level variations. The geometric configuration is also important to allow laminar progress of the blood flow, eliminating vortices or turbulence which might provoke sources of microemboli.

Though bubble oxygenators are currently largely being superceded by membrane oxygenators they still have an important contribution in operations where the cardiopulmonary bypass time is less than 2 h duration.

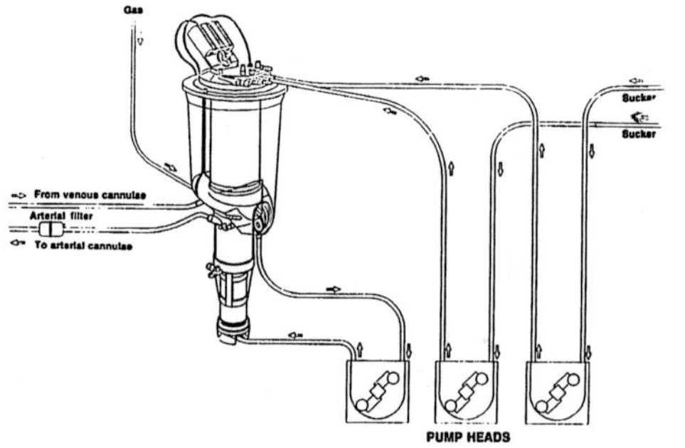

Figure 3.2

Membrane oxygenators

In the membrane oxygenators the oxygenating gas is separated from the blood by a permeable membrane. There is no direct contact between blood and gas. The membrane is normally made from either silicone rubber or polypropylene. The transmembrane pressure causes gas to diffuse from the high pressure area into the low pressure one. The rate of transfer depends on both the pressure gradient across the membrane and the permeability of the membrane.

The first membrane oxygenators had blood flowing inside polypropylene microporous capillaries with oxygenating gas flowing outside (Figure 3.4). In 1983 microporous hollow fibre oxygenators were developed in which the gas flowed inside the membrane with blood outside the capillary. This was a more efficient arrangement as there was less resistance in the oxygenating system. In addition there was less damage to the blood, the 'laying phenomenon' due to the viscosity of blood flowing inside capillaries was obviated and it was easier to defoam the blood during the priming phase.

The membrane oxygenator is superior to the bubble oxygenator with reduced trauma to the elementary constituents of the blood, no direct blood gas contact, independent control of Po_2 and Pco_2 low priming volumes, and high efficiency of gas and temperature exchange.

The challenge for most manufacturing companies has been to produce a membrane oxygenator that is simple to set up and use. Currently most models incorporate the cardiotomy filter, venous reservoir, oxygenator and heat exchanger (Figure 3.4).

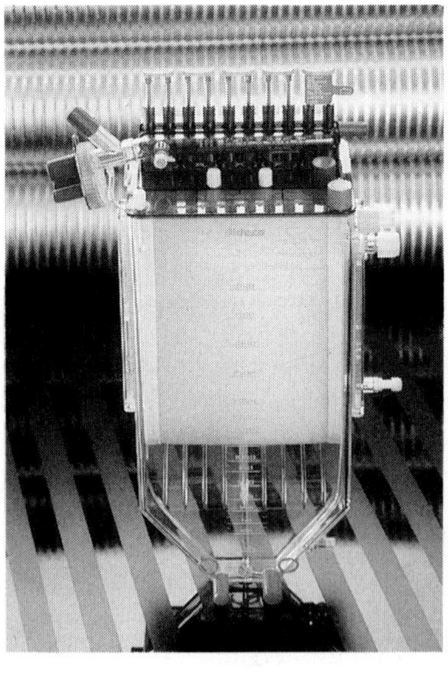

Figure 3.3

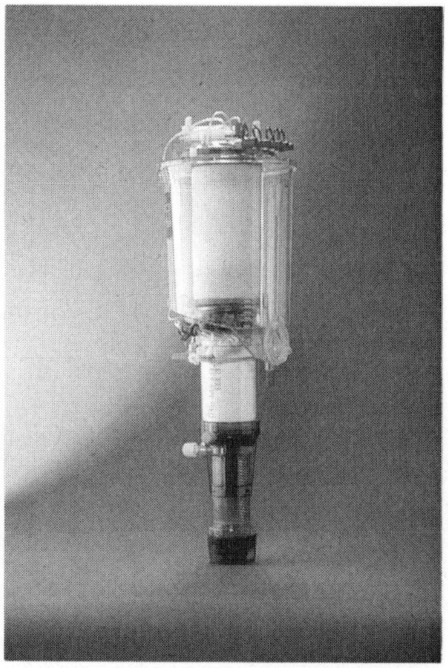

Figure 3.4

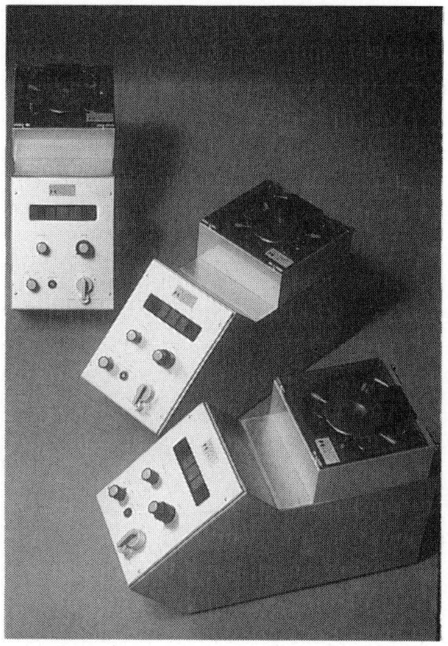

Figure 3.5

Pumps

While the oxygenator performs the tasks of the lungs during cardiopulmonary bypass the pump takes over the role of the heart. Its sole function is to provide an adequate flow of oxygenated blood to the patient's arterial circulation. The main technical requirements of the pumps are as follows:

1. Wide flow range (up to $7\,l\,min^{-1}$)
2. Low haemolytic effect
3. Minimum turbulence and blood stagnation
4. Simplicity and safety of use
5. Capacity for pulsatile flow
6. Cost effectiveness

There are two principle types of pumps available for use.

Roller pumps

At present the roller pump is the commonest type of pump used in the extracorporeal circuit (Figure 3.5). The pump comprises a semicircular stator and a rotor with twin rollers sited at 180° to each other. The blood tubing is compressed between the stator and the rotor. Thus blood never comes into direct contact with the rotor. The flow is unidirectional as one of the rollers keeps compressing the tube at all times. Roller pumps require routine adjustment to control the stroke volume of the blood displaced. A partially occlusive pump setting is preferable. Pump occlusivity is calibrated to allow a $1\,cm\,min^{-1}$ drop along a 1 metre high saline column created with three-eighths of an inch tubing ($2\,cm\,min^{-1}$ with a quarter inch tubing).

Pump function must be monitored carefully at all times throughout the bypass. A line restriction upstream would create an excessive vacuum leading to degassing of the blood and generation of a 'bubble train' inside the circuit. Conversely a line restriction downstream would lead to excessive pressure build-up and blow out of the line itself. Safety features include adequate pressure monitors and ultrasonic bubble sensors placed along the line.

Though roller pumps generate non-pulsatile perfusion it is possible to adapt the pump to generate pulsatile flow (Figure 3.6).

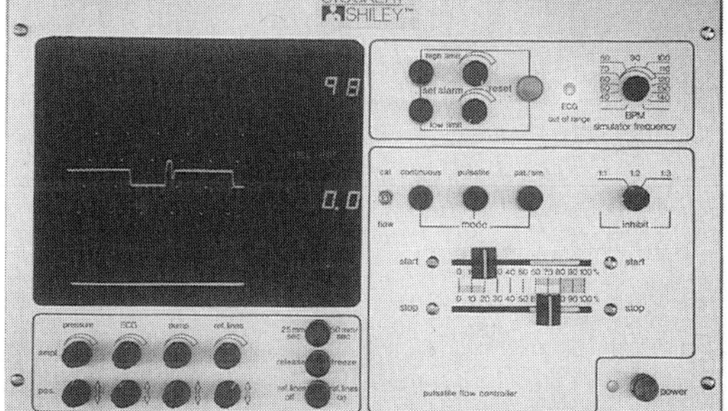

Figure 3.6

Centrifugal pumps

With the centrifugal pump blood is driven through a rotating impeller creating a centrifugal force which imparts kinetic energy to the blood. A magnetic linkage with the drive motor makes it possible hermetically to seal the entire pumping chamber which is disposable.

Figure 3.7 shows the Biomedicus pump in which the impeller is vaneless and includes three cones. Blood is propelled by the vortex generated by the spinning cones. The blood inlet is axial while the outlet is at the periphery of the outer chamber. The magnet is situated within the rotating elements. A rotary seal is placed around the shaft in order to prevent blood from entering the turning element.

The Sarns-3M disposable centrifugal pump (Figure 3.8) has two chambers. The drive force occurs in the upper chamber while the magnets are situated in the lower chamber. Blood is confined to

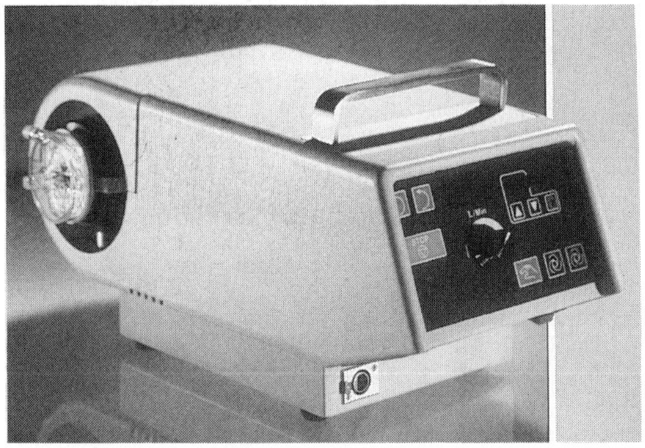

Figure 3.7

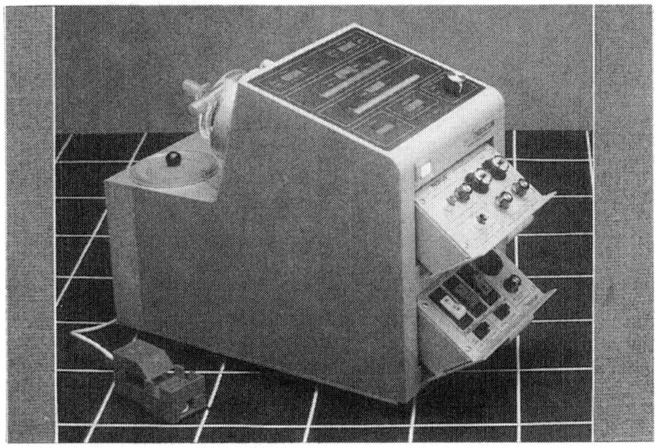

Figure 3.8

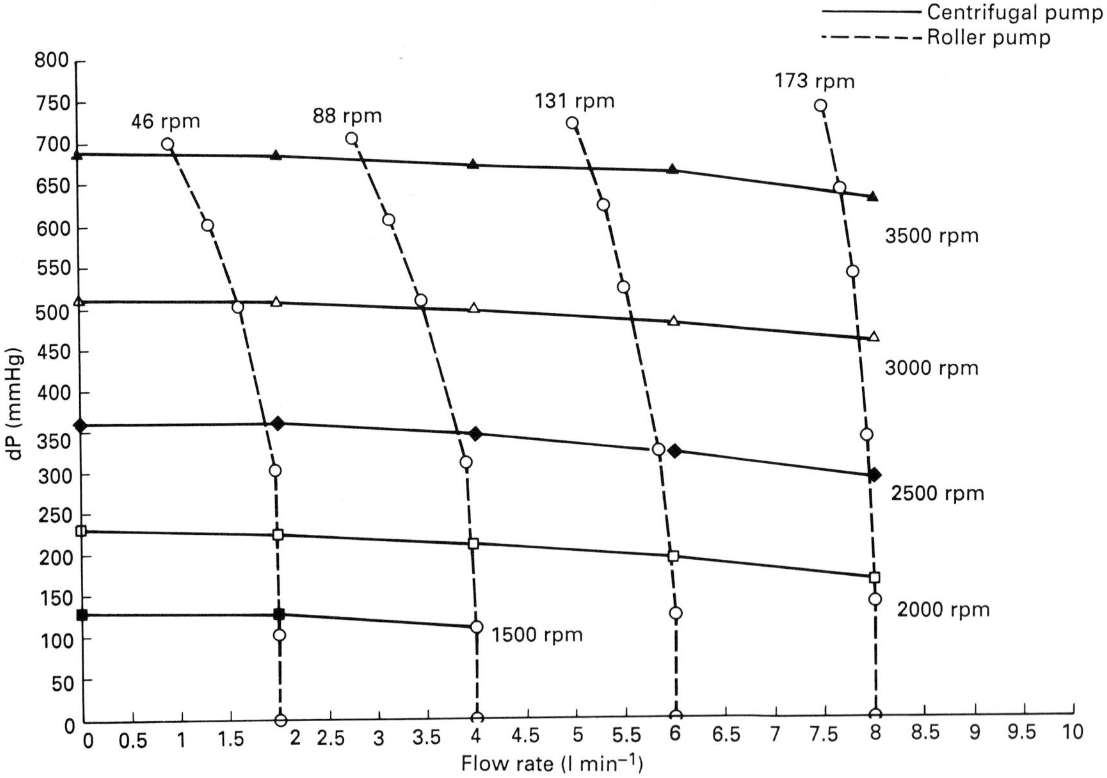

Figure 3.9

the first chamber by means of a rotary seal around the axle.

The centrifugal pumps are designed to minimize both haemolysis and clotting in the event of stagnation.

Centrifugal pumps are not occlusive and are therefore load sensitive, i.e. if the resistance to flow increases the blood flow decreases. This is easily seen in Figure 3.9 (Pressure Head versus Flow Rate).

During operation centrifugal pumps require strict flow control which is exerted by means of electromagnetic or ultrasonic flow metre probes placed along the line. This information enables pump speed adjustments to be made related to load variations.

Centrifugal pumps are extremely practical. They are compact, durable and easy to set up. They cause minimal haemolysis compared with roller pumps and have a second advantage in that if air enters the system the pump is no longer able to transmit kinetic energy to the blood, therefore stopping the fluid motion and minimizing the incidence of massive air embolism. However at present the relatively high cost of the disposable pump head precludes their routine use in cardiac centres.

Venous reservoir

The principal functions of the venous reservoir are to accumulate blood from the patient's venous system and to remove both air and microaggregates present in venous blood. Reservoirs may be either rigid or soft.

Rigid reservoir

This consists of reservoirs made of hard transparent materials with a defoaming layer and a filtering screen (100–200 μm). The reservoir capacity may range between 1 litre and 4.5 litres.

Soft reservoir

The 'bag' consists of soft PVC with a 100–200 μm filtering screen and a defoaming polyurethane layer. Bag capacity may range between 200 ml and 3000 ml.

The advantage of soft reservoirs is that they can be used as a closed system. As the reservoir empties the venous bag collapses preventing gaseous emboli.

Originally the rigid reservoir was used as an open system. In the event of sudden emptying of the reservoir there was no intrinsic safety mechanism against massive gaseous emboli. However more recently a silicone safety valve has been incorporated into the outlet of the rigid reservoir providing the same degree of safety offered by the closed system (Figure 3.10).

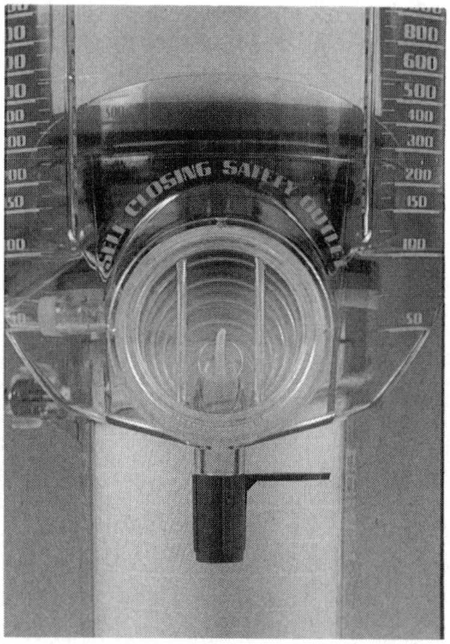

Figure 3.10

Cardiotomy reservoir

Blood from the cardiotomy suckers and vents is initially received into the cardiotomy reservoir. This serves as a storage area and also filters the large number of solid and gaseous microemboli. The rigid cardiotomy reservoir is normally made of polycarbonate. The defoamer is comprised of layers of open cell polyurethane foam or polyester screens. The screens incorporate a filter of between 20 μm and 40 μm.

The current trend is to combine both the cardiotomy reservoir and the venous reservoir with a filter positioned at the upper end of the cardiotomy reservoir.

Heat exchanger

During cardiopulmonary bypass the temperature of the perfusate may be adjusted to improve myocardial protection and optimize the operating conditions for the patient. The heat exchanger is composed of two chambers one containing blood the other water which are separated from each other by means of a surface allowing thermal exchange between the two fluids. The surface may be composed of anodized aluminium, stainless steel or plastic and be organized in one of the following configurations: spiral thin tube, tubes, spine tube, pleated sheet. The inlet and outlet of the two chambers in the heat exchangers are organized so that blood and water flow in the opposite directions. The heat exchanger performance factor may be calculated using the formula:

$$\text{Performance factor} = \frac{T_{B_o} - T_{B_i}}{T_{W_i} - T_{B_i}}$$

where:
T_{B_o} = Blood outlet temperature
T_{B_i} = Blood inlet temperature
T_{W_i} = Water inlet temperature

The performance factor varies considerably between various exchanger models depending on the materials used and their arrangement in the heat exchanger. Anodized aluminium has very good thermal conductivity but is biologically unsatisfactory. Stainless steel offers an excellent compromise. Plastic materials are characterized by very low thermal conductivity compared with metallic materials. The heat exchanger can be integrated into either the venous reservoir or the oxygenator. When the exchanger is in the venous reservoir it is of a spiralled or corrugated type with water flowing inside the tube and blood outside. Such systems have poor thermal performance, a high priming volume and cannot be used for ECMO. When the heat exchanger is integrated into the oxygenator a tube or pleated sheet is used. This arrangement has a much higher thermal performance, a low priming volume and can be used for ECMO.

The heat exchanger may also be used to adjust the temperature of blood cardioplegia solutions.

Tubing

Though most research has focused on the principle components of the extracorporeal circulation the tubing system remains a vital component. Several metres of tubing of different size and rigidity linked by multiple-way connectors form the pathway for draining venous blood from the right atrium to returning oxygenated blood to the aorta.

The most widely used tubing material is PVC. This offers appealing characteristics to the medical profession. It is preferably transparent, has low toxicity and good biocompatibility. It may be manufactured in different sizes and with a wide range of rigidity in large quantities at moderate cost. The main limitation of PVC is that its elasticity decreases with temperature thus causing potential problems under serious hypothermia. Furthermore the PVC has a limited shelf life due to migration of the plasticizer towards the surfaces.

Latex from natural rubber has good elastic characteristics and was originally used in the proximity of the pumps and rollers. However in the last few years synthetic elastomers (silicone rubber) have gradually replaced natural rubber. Though silicone has a good chemical inertia its resistance to abrasion is poor and during prolonged cardiopulmonary bypass particles may be released (Figure 3.11).

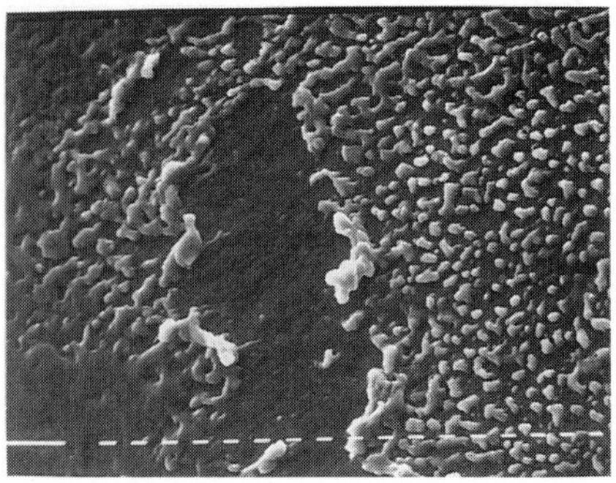

Figure 3.11

In general the tubing circuit is now made entirely of PVC connected with polycarbonate connectors.

Adequacy of perfusion

During cardiopulmonary bypass the main responsibility of the perfusion is to ensure that all the organs of the body supplied by the extracorporeal circuit are adequately perfused (see Tables 3.1–3.4). In order to achieve this the perfusionist continually monitors the following parameters:

1. Acid–based status (metabolic/respiratory)
2. Blood flow rate
3. Oxygen consumption rates (oxygen delivery/oxygen demand)
4. Vascular resistance (patient pressure)
5. Renal function
6. Coagulatory status

Table 3.1 Normal values: acid–base chemistry of whole blood

Arterial blood	
pH	7.38–7.45
$P\text{CO}_2$	35–40 mmHg
$P\text{O}_2$	95–100 mmHg
O_2SAT	94–100%
CO_2 content	19–24 mmol l^{-1}
B.E.	−2.5 to +2.5
Venous blood	
pH	7.35– 7.41
$P\text{CO}_2$	40–45 mmHg
CO_2 content	22–26 mmol l^{-1}
B.E.	−2.5 to +2.5

Table 3.2 Normal values: haematology

Activated clotting time*	Approx. 100–200 s (whole blood), (400 s during bypass).
Blood volume	Male: 69 ml kg^{-1} Female: 65 ml kg^{-1}
Fibrinogen	200–400 mg dl^{-1} (Plasma)
Haematocrit	Male: 40–54% Female: 38–47%
Haemoglobin	Male: 13.5–18 g dl^{-1} Female: 12.0–16 g dl^{-1}
Partial thromboplastin time	60–70 s
Platelet count	150 000–400 000 mm^{-3}
Plasma volume	Male: 39 ml kg^{-1} Female: 40 ml kg^{-1}
Prothombin time	12–14 s
Red cell count	Male: 4.6–6.2 × $10^{6\ mm^{-3}}$ Female 4.2–5.4 × $10^{6\ mm^{-3}}$
Viscosity	1.4–1.8 times water
White cell count	4500–11 000 mm^3

*Hemochron system.

Table 3.3 Normal values: chemistry of blood

Bicarbonate	21–28 mmol l^{-1} (plasma)
Calcium	4.5–5.3 mmol l^{-1} (serum)
Chloride	95–103 mmol l^{-1} (serum)
Cholesterol	150–200 mg dl^{-1} (serum)
Creatinine	Male: 0.2–0.6 mg dl^{-1} (serum) Female: 0.6–1.0 mg dl^{-1} (serum)
Glucose, fasting	70–110 mg dl^{-1} (serum)
Haemoglobin	Male: 13.5–18.0 g dl^{-1} (blood) Female: 12.0–16.0 g dl^{-1} (blood)
Plasma haemoglobin	0.5–5.0 mg dl^{-1} (serum or plasma)
Magnesium	1.5–2.5 mmol l^{-1} (serum)
Osmolality	280–295 mmol kg^{-1} (serum)
Potassium	3.8–5.0 mmol l^{-1} (plasma)
Sodium	136–142 mmol l^{-1} (plasma)
Triglycerides	10–200 mg dl^{-1} (serum)
Urea nitrogen	8–18 mg dl^{-1} (serum)

Table 3.4 Haemodynamic parameters

Parameter	*Definition*	*Normal values*
Cardiac output (CO) CO = HR × SV	Total blood flow rate ejected by the heart each minute	Adult: 4–8 l min^{-1}
Heart rate (HR)	Number of times the heart beats in one minute	Adult: 60–100 b.p.m.
Stroke volume (SV) SV = CO/HR	Volume of blood ejected by the heart with each beat	Adult: 60–130 ml per beat
Body surface area (BSA) BSA = 71.84 × $Wt^{0.425}$ × $Ht^{0.725}$ Wt = Weight (kg) Ht = Height (cm) BSA = Body surface area (m^2)	Surface area of the body according to Dubois formula	Varies with body size
Cardiac index (CI) CI = CO/BSA also CO = CI × BSA	Cardiac index is an adjustment of cardiac output for body size (BSA)	Adult 2.5–3.1 l $min^{-1}m^{-2}$
Blood flow rate (ml min^{-1})/Body Wt (kg) ml min^{-1} kg^{-1} = CO/WT	Total blood flow rate (CO) indexed to body weight	Range 40–100 ml $min^{-1}kg^{-1}$
Arterial blood pressure (BPA)	Blood pressure on arterial walls	Adult 130/70 mmHg
Central venous pressure (CVP)	Blood pressure within the central venous system (in or near the vena cavae)	4–10 mmHg Increases with cardiac failure

Acid–base status

The blood pH is maintained in the range 7.35–7.45. Within the body three mechanisms are present to maintain the acid-base equilibrium:

1. The buffer system is a rapidly acting system for the neutralization of excess acid. The principle ion is the bicarbonate ion with phosphate ions and negatively charged proteins also contributing.
2. The respiratory system adjusts the level of CO_2 removal by varying the ventilation of the lungs.
3. The kidneys excrete excess acid or alkaline. Though this is the most efficient system it is also the slowest.

Four kinds of acid-base disequilibrium are recognized:

1. Respiratory acidosis (raised $P\text{CO}_2$)
2. Respiratory alkalosis (low $P\text{CO}_2$)
3. Metabolic acidosis (excessive formation of H^+ ions)
4. Metabolic alkalosis (decreased formation of H^+ ions)

Blood pH and $P\text{CO}_2$ can be monitored in the extracorporeal circuit either by continuous in-line sampling or by isolated sampling at regular intervals for analysis on a distant blood gas machine. Membrane oxygenators are ideally suitable for adjusting $P\text{CO}_2$ as this can be performed independently of blood oxygenation (cf. bubble oxygenators).

Some difficulty arises with regard to the regulation of blood pH under conditions of hypothermia. There are two different theories of control:

1. The pH stat theory maintains pH at physiological value (7.4) independent of body temperature, imitating the behaviour of hibernating animals.
2. The alpha stat system adjusts to physiological value when corrected for normothermia, imitating the behaviour of poikilotherms.

Blood flow rate

During cardiopulmonary bypass the blood flow rate controlled by the pump is matched to the patient's metabolic demand. With hypothermic techniques the metabolic rate is reduced and therefore it is possible to reduce the overall pump flow rate. An extreme example of this is the use of circulatory arrest associated with profound hypothermia. This is fully detailed in Chapter 17.

Oxygen consumption rate

In addition to hypothermia the patient's total oxygen demand varies according to the level of type of anaesthesia used. Furthermore in the presence of an aortic cross clamp the coronary circulation is excluded.

Vascular resistance

The systemic vascular resistance (SVR) is defined by the general blood flow equation:

$$\text{SVR} = \frac{Pa - Pv}{\text{Co}} \times \frac{1}{n}$$

where:

Pa = mean arterial pressure
Pv = mean venous pressure
Co = cardiac output
n = blood viscosity

(Adult normal values = 900–1500 dyn × s/cm^{-5})

NB The above formula must be used with caution as blood is a non-Newtonian fluid, the blood circuit is a complex arrangement of distensible tubes and the blood viscosity is not a constant. The cardiac output is maintained as constant by the pump. However different values of systemic vascular resistance occur during total cardiopulmonary bypass and therefore will be an alteration in the pressure. In general the perfusion pressure should be maintained in the region of 60–80 mmHg during normothermia and as a minimum of 60 mmHg throughout the whole perfusion. Hypotension may be counted initially by an increase in the total flow rate. Alternatively vasopressor agents may be used. Hypertension should be treated with vasodilators.

Renal function

In addition to the acid–base status adequacy may be rapidly checked by assessing the urine output. A urine output of greater than 1 ml kg^{-1} min^{-1} suggests adequate tissue perfusion.

Coagulatory status

Before the commencement of extracorporeal circulation heparin is used to prevent coagulation in the circuit. Heparin is an acid electronegative mucopolysaccharide. Its primary action is to bind antithrombin III. During cardiopulmonary bypass the activated clotting time is monitored by the perfusionist. At the commencement of bypass 300 units kg^{-1} of heparin are given and the ACT maintained at greater than 400 sec. At the end of perfusion protamine is given to reverse the heparin. Protamine is a base and competes with the heparin antithrombin III complex.

Future developments

The continuous evolution of science and the appearance of new technologies allows us to foresee important conceptual and practical developments in the future. Substantial changes may be expected in the following areas:

1. *Materials.* The principle goal of the scientist working on surface treatments should be to provide completely biocompatible systems abolishing the need for anticoagulation.
2. *Pumping systems.* The combination of new technology and new material should provide an ideal pumping system which is non-occlusive, autocalibrating and pulsatile. The pump should be disposable and completely incorporated in the extracorporeal circuit.
3. *Oxygenating systems.* Further developments in technology and materials should provide more efficient and reliable oxygenating systems.
4. *Monitoring.* Advances in computer science will permit real time monitoring in an increased number of parameters including pH, $P\text{O}_2$, $P\text{CO}_2$, oxygen saturation, pressure, temperature, blood flow, haematocrit, coagulation status, electrolyte concentration, renal blood flow, cerebral blood flow, blood viscosity.
5. *Blood saving.* The serious problem of blood availability together with the efficacy of its use demands solution. This may take the form of either improved blood conservation or the use of blood substitutes.
6. *Circulatory assistance.* The development of ventricular assist devices has opened a whole field of technology to patients with end stage cardiac failure.
7. *Artificial heart.* This remains the ultimate goal of the bioengineer.

Conclusion

The translation of scientific and technological development into practical patient care continues to evolve at an exhilarating rate. Many basic items of the extracorporeal circuit will soon become obsolete to the benefit of mankind.

4

Membrane and bubble oxygenators

Marc E. Voorhees and Roger Elgas

The primary function of an extracorporeal blood oxygenator is to replace the respiratory function of the natural lung. In addition, the oxygenator as used in open heart surgery today, must store blood and provide a means to cool and warm the patient during cardiopulmonary bypass. Oxygenators also need to operate for as long as 6–8 h and with blood flow-rates as high as 6–7 $l\ min^{-1}$. These functions must be carried out without damaging blood proteins and formed elements.

Since the first clinical applications of extracorporeal blood oxygenators in the early 1950s, the technology has evolved significantly. The oxygenators of today are inexpensive, disposable, very efficient and much less traumatic than those early units. In the last few years, advances in membrane oxygenator technology have resulted in the design of devices with such high quality and performance that the forerunners are almost forgotten. This chapter will only highlight a few of the numerous milestones that have paved the way for the development of the current generation of oxygenators. Several excellent reviews on early oxygenators are available (Galletti and Brecher, 1962; Drinker, 1972; Galletti, 1976). This chapter also will focus on the specifics of gas transfer and blood trauma as they pertain to the design and evaluation of bubble and membrane oxygenators.

Historical milestones

LeGallois (1812) first suggested the concept of extracorporeal circulation to preserve life in an organ separated from the rest of the body by passing blood through it. The work of Brown-Séquard (1858) pointed out the necessity of oxygenating this blood. Both the bubble and film oxygenators can trace their beginning to the period of time shortly after this. The continuous oxygenation of blood by a stream of oxygen bubbles was devised by von Schröeder (1882) and von Frey and Gruber (1885) designed the film oxygenator where the blood was spread out so that a thin film was exposed to oxygen.

The film type of oxygenator was predominant for the next 70 years because of the impossibility of removing excess gas bubbles from the arterialized blood. Most of the pioneering works in the use of extracorporeal circulation as an aid to cardiac surgery was done with the film oxygenator (Gibbon, 1937; Björk, 1948; Dennis *et al.*, 1951; Gibbon, 1954; Cross *et al.*, 1956). Blood trauma was an early problem encountered with the film oxygenator, but the basic inefficiency of gas transfer remained a problem even after the blood handling problems were improved.

The key to the development of the bubble oxygenator was when Clark, Gollan and Gupta (1950) thought of using silicone compounds as defoaming agents. Arterialized blood was passed over or through surfaces coated with silicone polymers causing the bubbles to burst and resulting in a perfusate relatively free of bubbles. Blood trauma was still a challenge, but the gas transfer efficiency was significantly improved.

The development of the membrane oxygenator also began about the same time as the bubble oxygenator when Kolff and Berk (1944) observed that the dark venous blood entering their artificial kidney would brighten during its course through the cellophane dialysing tube. The membrane oxygenator held the promise of reduced blood trauma due to the elimination of the very large blood–gas interface present in the film and bubble oxygenators, but the inefficient gas transfer due to the membrane materials available to early developers (Kolff and Balzer, 1955; Clowes, Hopkins and Neville, 1956) limited its early clinical application.

The next advance in the evolution of the clinical oxygenators of today occurred in the late 1950s with the development of disposable bubble oxygenators constructed of plastic materials (DeWall *et al.*, 1956; Rygg and Kyvsgaard, 1956; Gott *et al.*, 1957). These designs greatly reduced the time and effort for cleaning and resterilization of the film oxygenators (Cooley *et al.*, 1958).

Bubble oxygenator development progressed little in the early 1960s. There were minor improvements and refinements, but the introduction of the Bentley Temptrol series of disposable bubble oxygenators in the late 1960s with its integral heat exchanger and efficient gas exchange (Kalke, Casteneda and Lillehei, 1969) was a major advance. It utilized clear polycarbonate plastic sheets in its construction and was a significant advance in both set-up and ease of use. With the advent of coronary artery bypass surgery in this same time period, the bubble oxygenator became the device of choice for routine bypass due to these characteristics. The next step in the evolution of the bubble oxygenator was the introduction of a high efficiency heat exchanger which supported the use of hypothermia during cardiopulmonary bypass. The Harvey disposable blood oxygenator accomplished this by locating the heat exchanger on the venous side of the oxygenator where the bubbles could be used to break up the thermal boundary layer (Page and Haller, 1974). Refinements in the gas exchange have resulted in lower gas to blood flow ratios, thus lowering the blood trauma, but the bubble oxygenators of today are essentially the same design as this generation. They are nearly all made from a clear polycarbon resin and use a venous heat exchanger.

The initial clinical applications of the membrane oxygenator in the late 1950s and early 1960s demonstrated its superiority over film and bubble oxygenators in terms of blood trauma and microemboli formation and encouraged further development of these devices. The recognition of the favourable gas permeability properties of silicone polymers and the introduction of these materials in the form of thin sheets and tubular capillaries by Dow Corning in the early 1960s was a key element in the evolution of the membrane oxygenator. The Bramson Lung (Bramson *et al.*, 1965) was the first commercially available membrane oxygenator and it was followed closely into the marketplace by the Landé–Edwards membrane oxygenator (Landé *et al.*, 1970). Both of these designs used silicone rubber sheets, but the complexity of their designs and problems with the leak due to pin holes and the fragile nature of the membrane limited their clinical acceptance for routine open heart surgery.

The decade of the 1960s saw a search for both stronger membranes and methods to enhance the gas transfer (Kolobow and Bowman, 1963; Pierce and Dibeluis, 1968). The use of tubular capillaries was first explored by Bodell *et al.* (1963) as a means of controlling the dimensions of the blood compartment and strengthening the membrane geometry. Capillary or hollow fibre membrane oxygenators at this time were mainly designed with the blood inside the tubes and the oxygen flushing the exterior surfaces (Wilson, Shepley and Llewellyn-Thomas, 1965; de Fillippi *et al.*, 1968; Dorson, Baker and Hull, 1968; Dutton *et al.*, 1971), but designs with the gas inside the fibre were also being investigated (Zingg, 1967).

The early 1970s was a time when industry made significant advances in the problems of large scale production, reliability and quality of membrane oxygenators. The development of microporous membrane materials was also a significant milestone in the development of membrane oxygenators which occurred at this time. The carbon dioxide transfer capability of these membranes was much higher than that of silicone rubber (Dantowitz and Borsanyi, 1969; Lautier *et al.*, 1969; Gille *et al.*, 1970). In fact, the gas transfer performance of the Travenol Modulung-Teflo membrane oxygenator approached that of bubble oxygenators (Esato and Eiseman, 1975).

The membrane oxygenators of the 1970s were able to provide low blood trauma and the gas transfer efficiency of bubble oxygenators, but the complexity of the priming procedures and ancillary equipment still limited their use to a maximum of 15–20% of the total open heart procedures performed. In 1982 the COBE CML membrane oxygenator was introduced. This oxygenator combined the integrated reservoir and heat exchanger of bubble oxygenators with the low blood trauma and high gas transfer efficiency of membrane oxygenators. Its introduction paved the way for today's generation of efficient, safe and easy to use membrane oxygenators which currently are used for over 60% of all open heart procedures. The day of the membrane oxygenator has clearly arrived.

Gas transfer in blood oxygenators

The physical processes which occur during respiration in the natural lung are convection, diffusion and chemical reaction. As blood flows through the alveolar capillaries, carbon dioxide diffuses from the blood across the alveolar membrane and into the alveolar space while oxygen diffuses from the alveolar space across the alveolar membrane and into the plasma and red cells. Diffusional resistances to the gas exchange process occur in the blood, the alveolar membrane and the alveolar air spaces. The natural lung is a remarkably efficient device in terms of respiratory gas exchange because of its large surface area (approximately 70 m^2) and small diffusional distances (approximately 10 μm). As a result, in the healthy lung arterial blood equilibrates with the alveolar gases for the full range of metabolic requirements and cardiac outputs.

The physical processes which occur during gas exchange in an artificial lung or blood oxygenator also are convection, diffusion and chemical reaction. Diffusional resistances to gas exchange in artificial lungs occur in the blood, the membrane (for membrane oxygenators), and the gas space. Diffusional distances are much greater than in the lung (100–500 μm) and the surface area of gas exchange is also considerably less than in the natural lung (less than 10 m^2). As a result, gas exchange is much less efficient and ventilating gases do not normally reach equilibrium with the blood stream. Thus, maintaining arterial blood gases at desired levels during cardiopulmonary bypass is not accomplished as readily as it is with the natural lung.

A comprehensive understanding of the gas exchange process has evolved over the last 25 years and many mathematical models exist which allow prediction of oxygenator performance and rational design of these devices (Spaeth, 1973; Colton, 1976; Eberhart, Dengle and Curtis, 1978). The most widely used approach in modelling gas exchange in blood oxygenators is to treat blood as a homogeneous fluid. This macroscopic model is justified for all blood oxygenators because the diffusional distances are much larger than individual red cell dimensions and concentration gradients are large.

The differential mass balance on an element of blood is based on Fick's first law of diffusion and takes the form:

$$\frac{DC_i}{Dt} = \nabla . \, D_i \, \nabla \, C_i + R_i$$

for a particular component i. The term on the left-hand side of the equation represents the rate of accumulation in a flowing element. The first term on the right-hand side of the equation represents the net rate of diffusion from the element and the second term on the right-hand side of the equation represents the net generation by reaction in the element. This differential balance is valid for both oxygen and carbon dioxide transfer in blood oxygenators.

Oxygen transfer in blood oxygenators

The majority of theories developed to predict oxygen transfer in blood oxygenators have treated blood as a continuum with the transferring species in local chemical equilibrium. All approaches of this type have assumed dissolved oxygen and oxyhaemoglobin to be the convected species with dissolved oxygen as the only important diffusing specie. This assumption is justified since the haemoglobin is confined physically to the interior of the red cell. In addition, facilitated diffusion is thought to be masked by the large oxygen partial pressure gradients present in oxygenators. The highly non-linear nature of the oxyhaemoglobin dissociation curve has necessitated numerical solutions to the convective-diffusive equation. As a result, solutions apply only for the particular set of parameters selected. Adequate summaries of the various theoretical models used to predict oxygen transfer can be found in a number of review articles (Spaeth, 1970; Spaeth, 1973; Colton, 1976; Dorson and Voorhees, 1976).

An alternative approach to the exact numerical solutions results from applying the advancing front theory of oxygen transfer. This theory was developed by investigators studying the transport of oxygen through blood films. Because of the large binding capacity the haemoglobin for oxygen and the very rapid oxygen–haemoglobin kinetics, these investigators postulated that two distinct zones existed in the blood film. These are a fully saturated region and an unsaturated region. Oxygen diffuses through the fully saturated region leading to a front where the unsaturated haemoglobin reacts with dissolved oxygen (Hill, 1929; Roughton, 1959; Marx *et al.*, 1960). The advancing front theory for artificial blood oxygenators is depicted in Figure 4.1. Application of the advancing front theory allows a unified approach for analysing oxygen transfer in both bubble and membrane oxygenators. Relevant parameters which results from these analyses are summarized in Table 4.1.

The advancing front theory for bubble oxygenators was first reported by Dindorf (Lightfoot, 1974).

Table 4.1 Variables for oxygen transfer in artificial lungs

C_{Hb}	=	Concentration of haemoglobin
S_A	=	Oxygen saturation of haemoglobin at oxygenator outlet
S_V	=	Oxygen saturation of haemoglobin at oxygenator inlet
P_g	=	Partial pressure of oxygen in gas phase
P_o	=	Partial pressure of oxygen in blood at oxygenator inlet
D_{o2}	=	Oxygen diffusivity in blood
α_{o2}	=	Oxygen solubility in blood
F	=	Gas flow rate
Q	=	Blood flow rate
a	=	Half-channel thickness
r_H	=	Hydraulic radius
N	=	Number of blood channels
L	=	Length of blood channel
W	=	Width of blood channel
A_s	=	Surface area

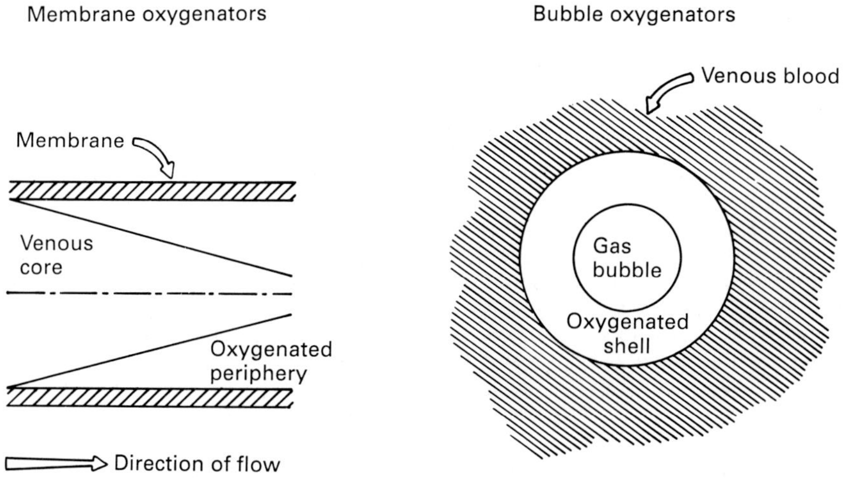

Figure 4.1 Advancing front theory as applied to blood oxygenators

A useful correlation for clinical bubble oxygenators was developed by Elgas and Van Way (1979). This correlation related a dimensionless contact time to the fractional oxygen saturation of haemoglobin (see Table 4.2). Oxygen transfer data obtained with one commercially available bubble oxygenator have been correlated and are shown in Figure 4.2. These data represent the full range of clinically relevant blood flow rates, gas flow rates, haemoglobin concentrations and venous saturations. Oxygen transfer for other bubble oxygenators have been successfully correlated by using this method (Elgas, unpublished data). The correlations demonstrate that the significant parameters which affect oxygen transfer in a bubble oxygenator being ventilated with pure oxygen are gas flow rate, blood flow rate and haemoglobin concentration.

Lightfoot (1968) derived the original advancing front equations for the hollow fibre membrane oxygenator with blood flow within the fibre lumen. The theory was extended by Elgas (1972) to include the effects of finite membrane resistance

Table 4.2 Correlating parameters for oxygen transfer in artificial lungs

Lung type	*Dimensionless length or contact time*
Bubble	$\dfrac{\alpha_{O_2}(P_g - P_o)F}{C_{b0}\,Q}$
Hollow fibre (blood flow outside fibres)	$\dfrac{\alpha_{O_2}(P_g - P_o)\,\pi\,NL\,D_{O_2}}{4\,C_{b0}\,Q}$
Hollow fibre (blood flow outside fibres)	$\dfrac{\alpha_{O_2}(P_g - P_o)\,A_s\,D_{O_2}}{16\,C_{b0}\,Q\,r_H}$
Flat plate	$\dfrac{\alpha_{O_2}(P_g - P_o)\,NLW\,D_{O_2}}{2\,C_{b0}\,Q_a}$

Where $C_{b0} = 1.34C_{Hb}\,(1 - S_v)$

Fractional saturation of haemoglobin $= \dfrac{S_A - S_V}{1 - S_V}$

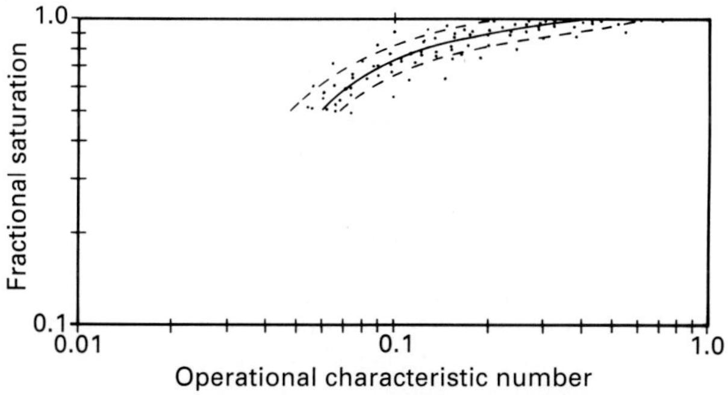

Figure 4.2 Correlation of oxygen transfer for a bubble oxygenator. The solid line represents the least squares fit to the data. The dashed lines represent one standard deviation from the least squares line

and by Dorson *et al.* (1971) to include the effects of dissolved oxygen in the saturated core. Dorson *et al.* (1971) presented data which validated the advancing front theory for single fibres. In the advancing front theory for hollow fibre membrane oxygenators the fractional oxygen saturation of haemoglobin is related to a dimensionless length as indicated in Table 4.2. Oxygen transfer data for two commercially available hollow fibre membrane oxygenators with blood flow inside the fibres are shown in Figure 4.3. Because of the high permeability of the microporous fibres used in these devices, membrane resistance to oxygen transfer is insignificant. The data fall below the dissolved correction prediction indicating the presence of blood or gas flow maldistribution.

Advancing front theory for oxygen transfer has recently been applied to hollow fibre membrane oxygenators with blood flow outside the fibres. Since the fibres are wound tightly in these devices, it was assumed that the blood flow path could be approximated by a series of parallel tubular channels. The effective diameter of these channels was determined from water pressure drop measurements. Data are presented in Figure 4.4 and this approach shows good agreement of data with the performance predicted by the advancing front theory. Again, the resistance to transfer of the microporous membrane was negligible.

Lightfoot (1968) also derived the original advancing front equations for the flat plate membrane oxygenator. The theory was later extended by Dorson and Voorhees (1974) to include the effects of wall resistance and dissolved oxygen in the saturated zone. In the advancing front theory for the flat plate membrane, the oxygenator saturation of haemoglobin is also related to a dimensionless length (see Table 4.2). Data from a commercially available flat plate membrane oxygenator are shown in Figure 4.5. The data lie above the performance predicted by the advancing front theory because of mixing in the blood channel resulting from a blood side screen.

A cardiopulmonary bypass simulator has been

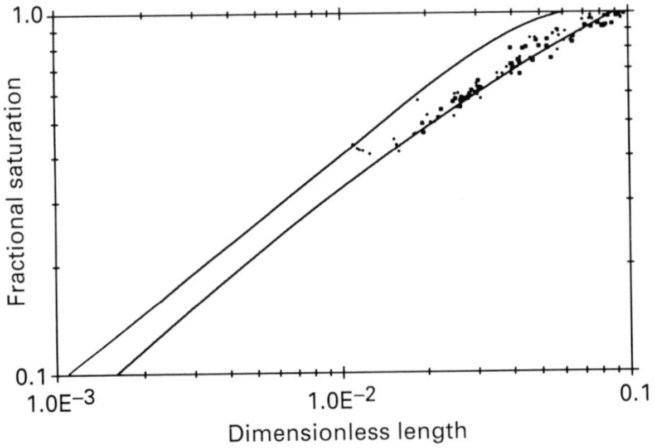

Figure 4.3 Correlation of oxygen transfer for two hollow fibre membrane oxygenators with blood flow inside the fibres. Surface areas are 5.4m² (■) and 3.3m² (·). The lower curve represents advancing front theory without the dissolved oxygen correction and the upper curve represents advancing front theory with the dissolved oxygen correction

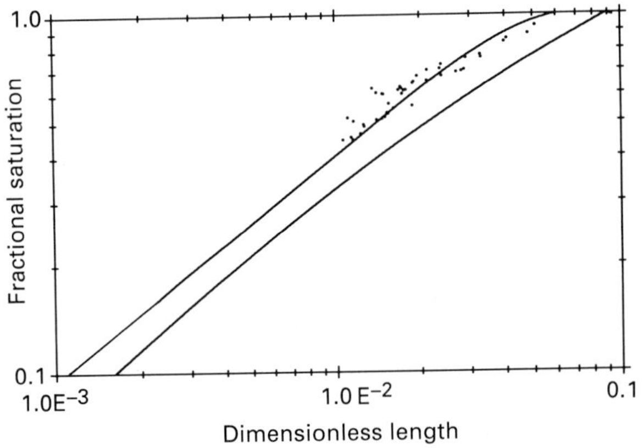

Figure 4.4 Correlation of oxygen transfer for a hollow fibre membrane oxygenator with blood flow outside of the fibres. The lower curve represents the advancing front theory without the dissolved oxygen correction and the upper curve represents the advancing front theory with the dissolved oxygen correction

developed which uses the oxygen transfer correlations presented above. This simulator allows the prediction of oxygen transfer under clinical situations and enables the effects of changing perfusion parameters to be determined. It differs from previously published models (Commin, Stecker and Dunelleroy, 1986; Leonard, 1988) in that it is a steady state model which requires the solution of only one non-linear algebraic equation. The value of such a model in understanding gas exchange in the clinical setting can be seen in the examples for the flat plate membrane oxygenator presented in Figures 4.6, 4.7 and 4.8. In Figures 4.6 and 4.7 patient oxygen consumption is 180 cm^3 min^{-1} which corresponds to a patient body surface area of 1.8 m^2, a basal oxygen consumption rate of 125 cm^3 min^{-1} m^{-2} (37°C), and a 20% reduction in oxygen consumption due to anaesthesia. The blood flow rate is 5 l min^{-1} (2.78 l min^{-1} m^{-2}), the haematocrit at 25%, the haemoglobin concentration at 8.3 g dl^{-1}, and the barometric pressure is 760 mmHg. The latter three values remain the same in Figure 4.8.

In Figure 4.6 the effect of gas phase oxygen concentration on arterial and venous oxygen saturation can be seen. Gas phase oxygen concentration is commonly controlled by using a respiratory blender. For reference purposes Po_2 = 100 mmHg at an oxygen saturation of 97.5% and Po_2 = 200 mmHg at an oxygen saturation of 99.2% (37°C with pH = 7.4, Pco_2 = 40 and P_{50} = 26.7 mmHg) (Severinghaus, 1979). With a gas phase oxygen concentration less than 80% the arterial oxygen saturation falls below 97.5%. In Figure 4.7 the effect of blood flow rate on arterial and venous saturation is seen. In this example the gas phase oxygen concentration has been set at 80%, and neglecting the potential effect of blood flow rate on oxygen consumption, both the arterial and venous oxygen saturations are seen to increase with increasing blood flow rate.

In the final example, Figure 4.8, the effect of patient oxygen consumption is seen, With an oxygen consumption rate of 125 cm^3 min^{-1} m^{-2} patient oxygen consumption would rarely exceed approximately 225 cm^3 min^{-1} even during the final

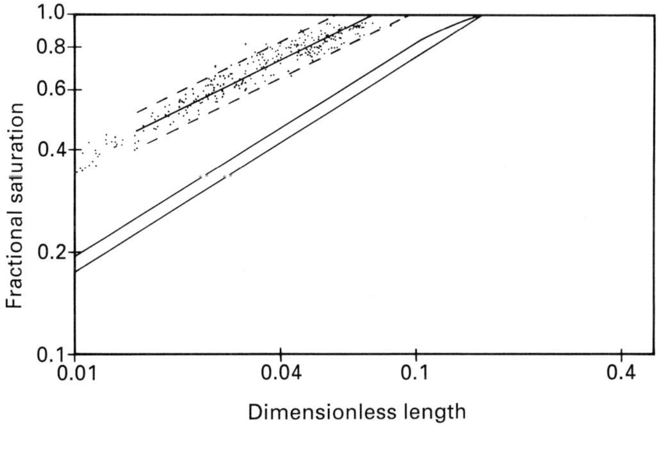

Figure 4.5 Correlation of oxygen transfer for a flat plate membrane oxygenator (n = 35). The lower two curves represent the advancing front theory with (*left*) and without (*right*) dissolved oxygen correction

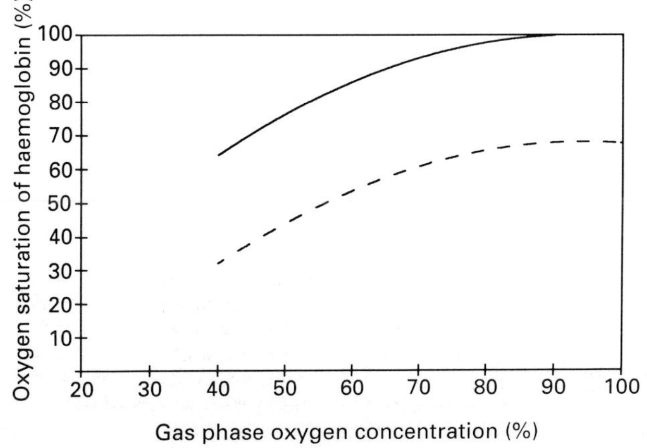

Figure 4.6 Effect of gas phase oxygen concentration on arterial and venous saturations for a flat plate membrane oxygenator. The solid line represents the arterial oxygen saturation and the dashed line represents the venous oxygen saturation. Blood flow rate is 5 l min^{-1}, haemoglobin concentration is 8.3 g dl^{-1} and patient oxygen consumption is 180 cm^3 min^{-1}. Atmospheric pressure is 760 mmHg

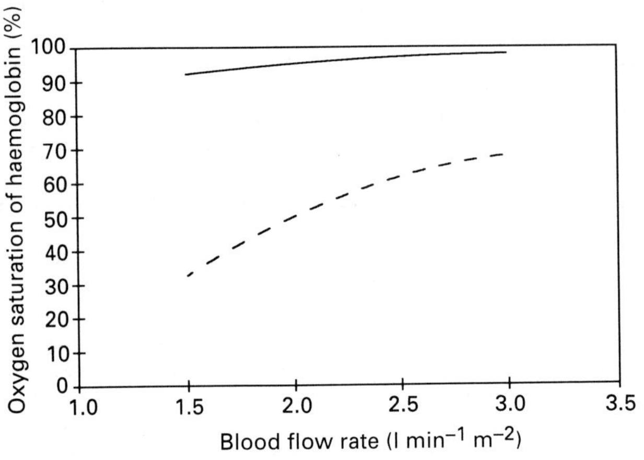

Figure 4.7 Effect of blood flow rate on arterial and venous oxygen saturations for a flat plate membrane oxygenator. The solid line represents the arterial oxygen saturation and the dashed line represents the venous oxygen saturation. Gas phase oxygen concentration is 80% of atmospheric pressure (sea level), haemoglobin concentration is 8.3 g dl^{-1}, and patient oxygen consumption is 180 cm^3 min^{-1}

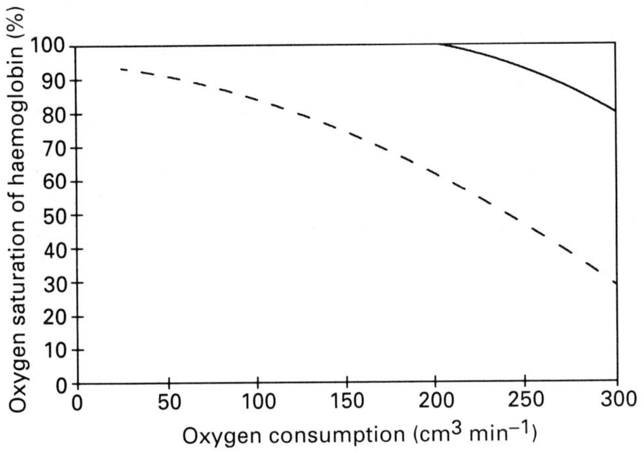

Figure 4.8 Effect of patient oxygen consumption on arterial and venous oxygen saturation for a flat plate membrane oxygenator. The solid line represents the arterial oxygen saturation and the dashed line represents the venous oxygen saturation. The blood flow rate is 5 l min^{-1}, the haemoglobin concentration is 8.3 g dl^{-1} and the gas phase oxygen concentration is 100% of atmospheric pressure (sea level)

stages of rewarming. However, unusual circumstances such as inadequate anaesthesia, shivering, patient temperature which is greater than 37°C, or a heavy, muscular patient might result in a total oxygen consumption greater than 225 cm^3 min^{-1} with resultant arterial oxygen saturations of less than 97.5%. Note that the oxygenator can deliver oxygen at rates of greater than 300 cm^3 min–1 but that the oxygen saturations are not optimal. Strategies available to the perfusionist to increase oxygen saturations include increasing blood flow rate as in Figure 4.7 or the addition of red cells (increasing haematocrit, results not presented).

These examples are based on mean values of gas exchange as shown in Figure 4.5. Due to the data scatter there is a statistical range for the predictions. However the value of the model is in the identification of trends and the relative sensitivity of oxygen saturation values to changes in perfusion parameters. Similar predictions of performance can be made with the other correlations presented above or for other oxygenators once the correlations have been developed.

Carbon dioxide transfer in blood oxygenators

Most theories developed to predict carbon dioxide transfer also have treated blood as a continuum with transferring species in local chemical equilibrium. Many early approaches assumed that dissolved carbon dioxide was the only important diffusing specie and neglected the contribution of bicarbonate ion (Colton, 1976). Later theories included the effect of bicarbonate ion (Benn, 1974; Voorhees, 1976; Mayes, Khoo and Gaylor, 1986). Due to the complexity of the carbon dioxide blood chemistries these theories again required numerical solution to the convective diffusive equation. A simplified approach to carbon dioxide transfer in flat plate and hollow fibre membrane oxygenators has been developed and successfully applied in estimating exchange for short blood residence times when appreciable membrane resistance to gas transfer exists (Voorhees, 1976). Theories have not been sufficiently developed for bubble oxygenation.

Application of carbon dioxide transfer theory to current clinical blood oxygenators further is complicated by the fact that gas phase carbon dioxide partial pressure varies significantly through these devices under all normal operating conditions. This situation occurs for bubble oxygenators since interfacial transfer resistance is negligible and gas flow rates are similar to blood flow rates. It occurs for membrane oxygenators with microporous membrane since membrane resistance to carbon dioxide transfer is negligible and gas flow rates are also similar to blood flow rates. As a consequence, empirical correlations of carbon dioxide transfer rates and gas to blood flow ratios have been the primary approach for examining carbon dioxide transfer in both bubble and membrane oxygenators. One such approach which is based on techniques used for analysis of heat exchange equipment has been particularly useful (Snider *et al.*, 1974). However, there is excess capacity for carbon dioxide in current bubble and membrane oxygenators and addition of carbon dioxide to the ventilating gas is necessary for some clinical protocols.

Blood damage in oxygenators

Contact of blood with oxygenator surfaces results in the immediate deposition of the plasma proteins fibrinogen, albumin, gammaglobulin and to a lesser extent the coagulation factors (US Department of Health and Human Services, Guidelines for Blood-Material Interactions, 1985). After initial protein absorption and conformation changes, platelets and leucocytes adhere to the surface. Platelets may become activated once they adhere to the surface thus resulting in recruitment of additional platelets and thrombus formation. The nature of protein layer initially deposited on the surface dictates the nature of subsequent events and is in turn dependent on surface composition and morphology. Circulation of blood through oxygenators also results in exposure of formed elements to shear stresses. Cell damage is a function of the shear stress level and exposure time. The shear stress/exposure time relationships have been established for red cells, platelets and white cells (Guidelines for Blood-Material Interactions, 1985), although the effect of multiple exposures to shear stress has not been elucidated. Sublethal damage to platelets and white cells occurs for shear stress of approximately 10 N m^{-1} and exposure times of 30 sec or greater which may be present in oxygenators. The blood–gas interface present in bubble-type oxygenators has been associated with increased blood trauma in the form of protein denaturation (Lee and Hairston, 1971) and cell lysis. Yang (1979) has shown that shearing forces due to bubble formation and collapse and not just the presence of the blood–gas interface is the mechanism responsible for cell lysis.

Analysis of blood damage in oxygenators is complicated by the multiplicity of materials and complexity of flow patterns. In an attempt to reduce variations inherent in *ex vivo* experiments, *in vitro* evaluation of different devices has been accomplished by using recirculating circuits containing different devices and utilizing a protocol similar to that recommended in the AAMI oxygenator standard (1982). Each circuit contains 2 litres of freshly collected bovine blood anticoagulated with heparin as the test fluid. Blood flow rate is 6 l min^{-1} and recirculation continues for 4.5h. Temperature is maintained at 37°C and blood gas values are controlled to $P\text{O}_2$ = 100–150 mmHg, $P\text{CO}_2$ = 35–45 mmHg, pH = 7.35–7.45, and base excess ± 5 mmol l^{-1}.

For a commercially available bubble oxygenator the data in Figure 4.9 demonstrate that haemolysis is a function of gas to blood flow ratio. Minimal haemolysis occurs when the gas to blood flow ratio equals zero. The haemolysis without gas flow in the bubble oxygenator circuit is the result of cell damage due to the roller pump and it is identical to haemolysis produced in membrane oxygenators utilizing a single roller pump. In Figure 4.10 the effect that gas flow has on platelet depletion is depicted. Significant platelet depletion occurs even without gas flow in the bubble oxygenator. This depletion is the result of foaming, and subsequent platelet activation, and adherence of platelets to surfaces which occurs as blood cascades from the gas exchange column through the defoamer. More rapid and complete damage occurs when gas is injected into the blood stream and platelets that remain in the circulating blood are activated and fragmented (Voorhees, Grover and Voorhees, 1990).

Platelet depletion is significantly reduced when membrane oxygenators are evaluated in this protocol although there are differences between devices. Figure 4.11 summarizes this data. Platelet depletion was more pronounced for a hollow fibre membrane oxygenator with blood flow inside the fibre lumen than for a hollow fibre membrane oxygenator with blood flow outside the fibre or a flat plate membrane oxygenator. This result is attributed to local shear damage which occurs in the manifolds of the hollow fibre membrane oxygenator with blood flow inside the fibre lumen. All oxygenators shown in Figure 4.11 were open reservoir systems with microporous membranes. When comparing open and closed reservoir systems for the same flat plate

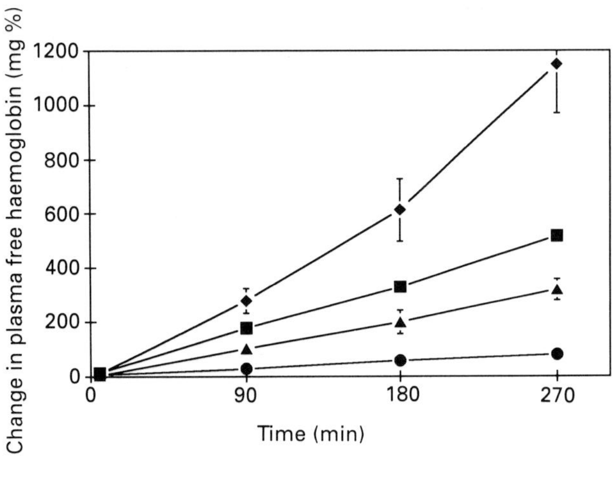

Figure 4.9 The effect of gas to blood flow ratio on haemolysis in a bubble oxygenator. Gas to blood flow ratio equals 0 (●, *n* = 4), 0.5 (▲, *n* = 2), 1.0 (■, *n* = 15) and 1.5 (◆, *n* = 2). Error bars represent one standard error of the mean

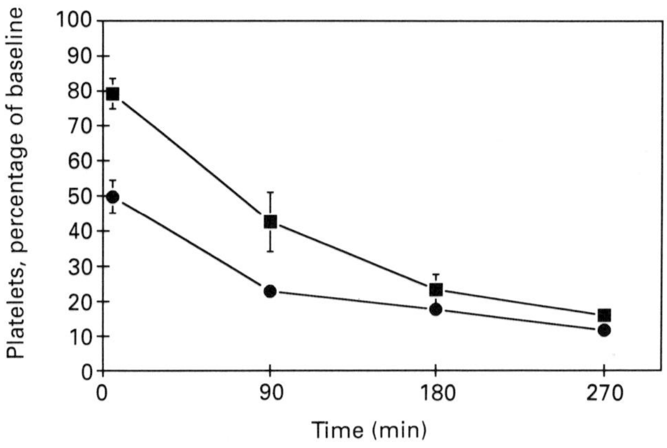

Figure 4.10 The effect of gas to blood flow ratio on platelet depletion in a bubble oxygenator. Gas to blood flow ratio equals 0 (●, *n* = 2) or 1.0 (■, *n* = 15). Error bars represent one standard error of the mean

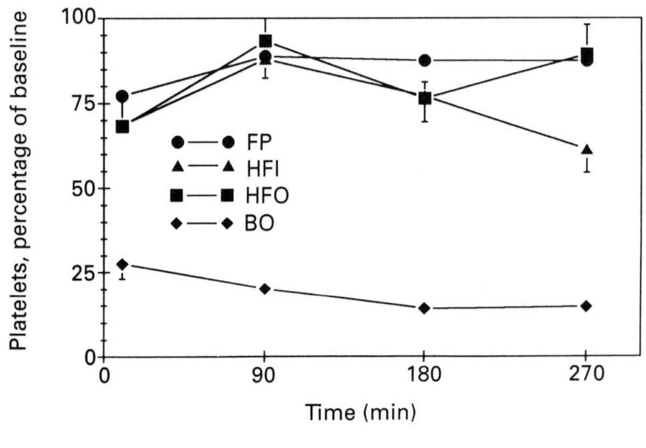

Figure 4.11 Platelet count as a function of time for membrane and bubble oxygenators. FP = flat plate membrane oxygenator (*n* = 12), HFO = hollow fibre membrane oxygenator with blood flow outside the fibres (*n* = 3), HFI = hollow fibre membrane oxygenator with blood flow inside the fibres (*n* = 3), BO = bubble oxygenator (*n* = 6, gas to blood flow ratio = 1.0). Error bars represent one standard error of the mean. (From Voorhees, C., Grover, R. and Voorhees, M., 1990 *Transactions of the American Society of Artificial Internal Organs*, **36**, by courtesy of the authors and publisher.)

membrane compartment, platelet depletion is statistically the same as shown in Table 4.3. In addition, membrane oxygenators having solid silicone rubber membranes have been associated with increased platelet depletion when compared with membrane oxygenators having microporous membranes (Lindsay *et al.*, 1976; Knight and Lyman, 1985).

A visual morphological scoring method has been described (Voorhees, Grover and Voorhees, 1990) that further quantitates damage to platelets that

Table 4.3 Effect of reservoir type on platelet depletion flat plate membrane oxygenator (platelets, percentage of baseline mean ± one standard deviation)

	Time (min)			
Reservoir type	5	90	180	270
Open *n* = 35	86 ± 12	73 ± 15	80 ± 12	77 ± 11
Closed *n* = 6	98 ± 9	75 ± 18	80 ± 6	78 ± 12

occurs during extracorporeal circulation with oxygenators. Briefly, this method assigns a numerical score to platelets based on their degree of damage as observed with phase microscopy. Normal discoid-shaped platelets receive a score of 4, spherical-shaped platelets receive a score of 2, platelets with dendrites or platelet fragments receive a score of 1 and large swollen platelets receive a score of 0. Data are normalized to baseline values and reported as a percentage termed the K-score. The K-score may by interpreted as follows: 1. 100% of baseline is a perfect K-score and indicates that no damage has occurred; 2. 90–100% of baseline indicates that slight damage has occurred; 3. 80–90% of baseline indicates that structural changes have occurred and damage is apparent; 4. 70–80% of baseline indicates increased fragmentation and dendrite formation with significant damage; 5. 70% and under of baseline indicates severe damage with altered platelet haemostatic function.

The K-score has been applied to *in vitro* evaluation of oxygenators using recirculating circuits as described above. The data are shown in Figure 4.12. In Figure 4.12a, K-score for a flat plate membrane oxygenator is compared with the K-score for a hollow fibre membrane oxygenator with blood flow outside the fibres. K-scores are statistically equivalent for all sample times. In Figure 4.12b the K-score for a flat plate membrane oxygenator is compared with the K-score for a hollow fibre membrane oxygenator with blood flow inside the fibre lumen. The K-score for the hollow fibre oxygenator is statistically lower than the K-score for the flat plate membrane oxygenator at 270 min. In Figure 4.12c the K-score for a flat plate membrane oxygenator is compared with the K-score for a bubble oxygenator (gas to blood flow ratio for the bubble oxygenator equal to 1.0). K-scores for the bubble oxygenator are statistically lower than the K-scored for the flat plate membrane oxygenator for all sample times.

For bubble oxygenation, the data presented indicate that damage to both red cells and platelets increases gas to blood flow ratios and duration of recirculation. Cellular damage is significantly greater for bubble oxygenation than for membrane oxygenation. For the flat plate membrane oxygenator, platelet depletion plateaus as circulating platelets reach an equilibrium with the oxygenator surfaces, while for the bubble oxygenator platelet depletion is rapid and continuous. For bubble

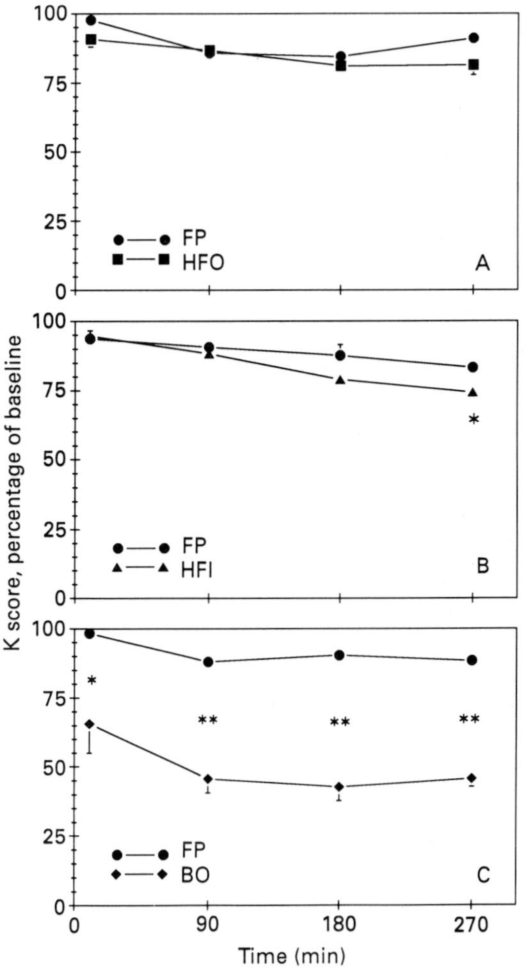

Figure 4.12 Platelet K-score for membrane and bubble oxygenators. FP = flat plate membrane oxygenator (*n* = 3 for all plots), HFO = hollow fibre membrane oxygenator with blood flow outside the fibres (*n* = 3), HFI = hollow fibre with blood flow inside the fibre (*n* = 3), and BO = bubble oxygenator (*n* = 3, gas to blood flow ratio = 1.0). Error bars represent one standard error of the mean and * $P < 0.05$, ** $P < 0.01$. (From Voorhees, C., Grover, R., Voorhees, M., 1990, *Transactions of the American Society for Artificial Internal Organs*, **36**, by courtesy of the authors and publisher)

oxygenation platelet function is significantly altered while for membrane oxygenation it is not. For some membrane oxygenators platelet consumption may be continuous due to the presence of high local shear stresses and platelet function may be reduced relative to other designs. In membrane oxygenators blood damage is not related to the gas exchange process as it is in bubble oxygenators.

Bovine blood has been chosen for *in vitro* testing because of availability and reduced risk of viral contamination. Adhesion of bovine platelets to polymeric materials has been shown to be similar to adhesion of human platelets to the same materials (Grabowski *et al.*, 1977; Park, Mosher and Cooper, 1986). Recirculation of human blood in *in vitro* circuits (Hennessy *et al.*, 1977; Addonizio *et al.*, 1979) and canine *ex vivo* experiments (Peterson, Dewanjee and Kaye, 1982) has resulted in similar reduction in platelet counts for both bubble and membrane oxygenators. Thus the use of the bovine model is reasonable for comparative evaluation of blood damage in blood oxygenators.

Extrapolation of *in vitro* data to the clinical setting is extremely difficult due to variations in blood flow rates, length of perfusion, temperature and the presence of anaesthetic agents or drugs that may alter platelet function. In addition, damaged cells and released constituents are cleared continuously and platelets may be sequestered as the result of hypothermia. Hope *et al.* (1981) have shown that activated platelets adhere to the defoamer of bubble oxygenators during bypass. Also, a significant source of blood damage during cardiopulmonary bypass is the cardiotomy suction/cardioplegia recovery system (Edmunds *et al.*, 1978; Wright and Sanderson, 1979; de Jong *et al.*, 1980). This system damages blood in the same manner as bubble oxygenation since air is entrained and then defoamed during the recovery of intracardiac blood. However, studies where cardiotomy suction and other perfusion variables are strictly controlled demonstrate haematological advantages of membrane oxygenators over bubble oxygenators (van den Dungen *et al.*, 1982; Pearson *et al.*, 1986).

Summary and conclusions

Oxygenator technology has evolved from the film oxygenators used in the first successful cardiopulmonary bypass procedures to bubble oxygenators used routinely in the 1970s. In the 1980s simple and easy to use membrane oxygenators replaced bubble oxygenators as the device of choice for the majority of routine cardiopulmonary bypass procedures.

The emergence of the membrane oxygenator in the 1980s was the result of a natural evolution of the technology. The superior blood handling characteristics of membrane oxygenators when compared with bubble oxygenators had been recognized even by the pioneers in the field. However, advances in membrane technology, gas transfer analysis, system design and large scale production were necessary in order for membrane oxygenators to be as widely used as they are today.

Additional refinements in membrane oxygenator design will occur in the 1990s and the popularity of these devices for routine cardiopulmonary bypass will continue to grow. Further improvements in membrane oxygenator blood handling characteristics will result as more biocompatible materials are used for fabrication. The ultimate benefits of membrane oxygenators will be realized as these materials are introduced and as the deleterious effects of cardiotomy suction are eliminated from the cardiopulmonary bypass circuit.

Acknowledgement

The authors would like to thank Toni Nugent for her assistance in preparation of the manuscript.

References

Addonizio, V.P., Strauss, J.F., Colman, R.W. and Edmunds, L.H. (1979) Effects of prostaglandin E_1 on platelet loss during in vivo and in vitro extracorporeal circulation with a bubble oxygenator. *Journal of Thoracic and Cardiovascular Surgery*, **77**, 119–126

Association for the Advancement of Medical Instrumentation (1982) *Standard for Blood/Gas Exchange Devices (Oxygenators) (Draft)*, AAMI, Washington, DC

Benn, J.A. (1974) Carbon dioxide transfer from weak acids and blood: the effect of carbonic anhydrase and oxygen uptake on carbon dioxide transfer in an oxygenator. PhD Dissertation, Massachusetts Institute of Technolgy, Boston, Massachusetts, USA

Bjork, V.O. (1948) Brain perfusions in dogs with artificially oxygenated blood. *Acta Chirurgia Scandinavica*, **96**, Suppl 137, 1–122

Bodell, B.R., Head, J.M., Head, L.R., *et al.* (1963) A capillary membrane oxygenator. *Journal of Thoracic and Cardiovascular Surgery*, **46**, 639–650

Bramson, M.L., Osbourne, J.J., Main, F.B., *et al.* (1965) A new disposable membrane oxygenator with integral heat exchange. *Journal of Thoracic and Cardiovascular Surgery*, **50**, 391–400

Brown-Sequard, E. (1858) Recherches experimentales sur les propriétés physiologiques et les usages du sang rouge et du sang noir et leurs principaux éléments gazeux, l'oxygéne et l'acide carbonique. *Journal Physiologie de l'Homme (Paris*, **1**, 95–122, 353–367, 729–735

Clark, L.C., Gollan, F. and Gupta, V.B. (1950) The oxygenation of blood by gas dispersion. *Science*, **111**, 85–87

Clowes, G.H.A., Hopkins, A.L. and Neville, W.E. (1956) An artificial lung dependent upon diffusion of oxygen and carbon dioxide through plastic membranes. *Journal of Thoracic Surgery*, **32**, 630–637

Colton, C.K. (1976) Fundamentals of gas transport in blood. In *Artificial Lungs for Respiratory Failure* (eds W.M. Zapol and J. Qvist), Academic Press, New York, pp. 3–41

Commin, P.L., Stucker, O. and Duvelleroy, M. (1986) Dynamic model of gas exchanges during cardiopulmonary bypass. *Life Support Systems*, **4**, Suppl 1, 23–33

Cooley, D.A., Belmonte, B.A., Latson, J.R. and Pierce, J.R. (1958) Bubble diffusion oxygenator for cardiopulmonary bypass. *Journal of Thoracic Surgery*, **35**, 131–134

Cross, F.S., Berne, K.M., Hirose, Y., *et al.* (1956) Evaluation of a rotating disc-type reservoir oxygenator. *Proceedings of the Society of Experimental Biology and Medicine*, **93**, 210–214

Dantowitz, P. and Borsanyi, A. (1969) Blood oxygenator with preformed, membrane lined capillary channels. In *Artificial Heart Program Proceedings, June 9–13* (ed. R. Hegyeli), Government Printing Office, Washington DC, pp. 339–346

de Filippi, R.P., Tompkins, F.C., Porter, J.H., *et al.* (1968) The capillary membrane blood oxygenator: in vitro and in vivo gas exchange measurement. *Transactions of the American Society for Artificial Internal Organs*, **14**, 236–241

de Jong, J.C.F., ten Duis, H.J., Smit Sibinga, C.T. and Wildervuur, C.R.H. (1980) Hematologic aspects of cardiotomy suction in cardiac operations. *Journal of Thoracic and Cardiovascular Surgery*, **79**, 227–236

Dennis, C., Spreng, D.S., Nelson, G.E., *et al.* (1951) Development of a pump oxygenator to replace the heart and lungs; an apparatus applicable to human patients and application to one case. *Annals of Surgery*, **134**, 709–721

DeWall, R.A., Warden, H.E., Read, R.C., *et al.* (1956) A simple, expandable, artificial oxygenator for open-heart surgery. *Surgical Clinics of North America*, **36**, 1025–1034

Dorson, W.J., Baker, E. and Hull, H. (1968) A shell and tube oxygenator. *Transactions of the American Society for Artificial Internal Organs*, **14**, 242–249

Dorson, W.J., Larson, K.G., Elgas, R.J. and Voorhees, M.E. (1971) Oxygen transfer to blood: data and theory. *Transactions of the American Society for Artificial Internal Organs*, **17**, 309–316

Dorson, W.J. and Voorhees, M.E. (1974) Limiting models for the transfer of CO_2 and O_2 in membrane oxygenators. *Transactions for the American Society for Artificial Internal Organs*, **20**, 219–228

Dorson, W.J. and Voorhees, M.E. (1976) Analysis of oxygen and carbon dioxide transfer in membrane lungs. In *Artificial Lungs for Respiratory Failure* (eds W.M. Zapol and J. Qvist), Academic Press, New York, pp. 43–68

Drinker, P.A. (1972) Progress in membrane oxygenator design. *Anesthesiology*, **37**, 242–260

Dutton, R.C., Mather, F.W., Walher, S.N., *et al.* (1971) Development and evaluation of a new hollow-fibre membrane oxygenator. *Transactions of the American Society for Artificial Internal Organs*, **17**, 331–336

Eberhart, R.C., Dengle, S.K. and Curtis, R.M. (1978) Mathematical and experimental methods for design and evaluation of membrane oxygenators. *Artificial Organs*, **2**, 19–34

Edmunds, L.H., Saxena, N.C., Hillyer, P. and Wilson, T.J. (1978) Relationship between platelet count and cardiotomy suction return. *Annals of Thoracic Surgery*, **25**, 306–310

Elgas, R.J. (1972) An analysis of recirculation in tubular membrane oxygenators. MS Thesis, Arizona State University, Tempe, Arizona, USA

Elgas, R. and Van Way, C.W. (1979) Dimensional analysis of oxygen transfer by bubble oxygenators. In *Proceedings of the 32nd Annual Conference on Engineering in Medicine and Biology* (Denver, Colorado 1979), Alliance for Engineering in Medicine and Biology, Washington DC

Esato, K. and B. Eiseman (1975) Experimental evaluation of Gore-tex membrane oxygenator. *Journal of Thoracic and Cardiovascular Surgery*, **69**, 690–697

Galletti, P.M. (1976) Membrane oxygenation: an overview. In *Artificial Organs* (eds R.M. Kenedi, J.M. Courtney, J.D.S. Gaylor and T. Gelchrist), University Park Press, Baltimore, pp. 11–19

Galletti, P.M. and Brecher, G.A. (1962) *Heart Lung Bypass*. Grune and Stratton, New York

Gibbon, J.H. (1937) Artificial maintenance of circulation during experimental occlusion of pulmonary artery. *Archives of Surgery*, **34**, 1105–1131

Gibbon, J.H. (1954) Application of a mechanical heart and lung apparatus to cardiac surgery. *Minnesota Medicine*, **37**, 171–180

Gille, J.P., Trudell, L., Snider, M.T., *et al.* (1970) Capability of the microporous membrane-lined, capillary oxygenator in hypercapnic dogs. *Transactions of the American Society for Artificial Internal Organs*, **16**, 365–374

Gott, V.L., DeWall, R.A., Paneth, M., *et al.* (1957) A self-contained disposable oxygenator of plastic sheet for intracardiac surgery. *Thorax*, **12**, 1–9

Grabowski, E.F., Didisheim, P., Lewis, J.C., *et al.* (1977) Platelet adhesion to foreign surfaces under controlled conditions of whole blood flow: human vs. rabbit, dog, calf, sheep, pig macaque, and baboon. *Transactions of the American Society for Artificial Internal Organs*, **23**, 141–151

Hennessy, V.L., Hicks, R.E., Niewarowski, S., *et al.* (1977) Function of human platelets during extracorporeal circulation. *American Journal of Physiology*, **232**, H622–H628

Hill, A.V. (1929) The diffusion of oxygen and lactic acid through tissues. *Proceedings of the Royal Society, London (Biology)*, **104**, 39–96

Hope, A.F., Heynes, A. duP., Löher, M.G., *et al.* (1981) Kinetics and sites of sequestration of indium 111-

labeled platelets during cardiopulmonary bypass. *Journal of Thoracic and Cardiovascular Surgery*, **81**, 880–886

Kalke, B.R., Casteneda, A. and Lillehei, C.W. (1969) A clinical evaluation of the new Temptrol (Bentley) disposable blood oxygenator. *Journal of Thoracic and Cardiovascular Surgery*, **57**, 679–687

Knight, P.M. and Lyman, D.J. (1985) Evaluation of the thrombogenicity of selected microporous membranes. *Artificial Organs*, **9**, 28–36

Kolff, W.J. and Balzer, R.R. (1955) Artificial coil lung. *Transactions of the American Society for Artificial Internal Organs*, **1**, 39–42

Kolff, W.J. and Berk, H.T.J. (1944) Artificial kidney: dialyzer with great area. *Acta Medica Scandinavica*, **117**, 121–134

Kolobow, T. and Bowman, R.L. (1963) Construction and evaluation of an alveolar membrane artificial heart-lung. *Transactions of the American Society for Artificial Internal Organs*, **9**, 238–243

Landé, A.J., Edwards, L., Block, J.H., *et al.* (1970) Prolonged cardiopulmonary support with a practical membrane oxygenator. *Transactions of the American Society for Artificial Internal Organs*, **16**, 352–356

Lautier, A., Rey, P., Bizot, J., *et al.* (1969) Comparison of gaseous transfer through synthetic membranes for oxygenators. *Transactions of the American Society for Artificial Internal Organs*, **15**, 144–150

LeGallois, J.J.C. (1812) *Expériences sur le Principe de la Vie*. D'Hautel, Paris

Lee, W.H. and Hariston, P. (1971) Structural effects on blood proteins at the gas-blood interface. *Federation Proceedings*, **30**, 1615–1622

Leonard, R.J. (1988) A total heart/lung bypass simulator. *Transactions of the American Society for Artificial Internal Organs*, **34**, 739–742

Lightfoot, E.N. (1968) Low-order approximations for membrane blood oxygenators. *American Institute of Chemical Engineering Journal*, **14**, 669–670

Lightfoot, E.N. (1974) *Transport Phenomena and Living Systems*, John Wiley and Sons, New York, pp. 319–324

Lindsay, R.M., Friesen, M., Cooper, J., *et al.* (1976) Platelet-foreign surface interactions with oxygenator membranes. In *Artificial Organs* (eds R.M. Kenedi, J.M. Courtney, J.D.S. Gaylor and T. Gilchrist), University Park Press, Baltimore, pp. 248–262

Marx, T.I., Snyder, W.E., St. John, A.D. and Moeller, C.E. (1960) Diffusion of oxygen into a film of whole blood. *Journal of Applied Physiology*, **15**, 1123–1129

Mayes, P.J.D., Khoo, G.T. and Gaylor, J.D.S. (1986) Modelling of CO_2 removal in membrane lungs. *Life Support Systems*, **4**, Suppl 1, 37–47

Page, P.A. and Haller, J.A. (1974) Clinical evaluation of the new Harvey H-200 disposable blood oxygenator. *Journal of Thoracic and Cardiovascular Surgery*, **67**, 213–220

Park, K., Mosher, D.F. and Cooper, S.L. (1986) Acute surface-induced thrombosis in the canine ex vivo model: importance of protein composition of the initial monolayer and platelet activation. *Journal of Biomedical Materials Research*, **20**, 589–612

Pearson, D.T., McArdle, B., Polslad, S.J. and Murray, A. (1986) A clinical comparison of the performance characteristics of one membrane and five bubble oxygenators: hemocompatibility studies. *Perfusion*, **1**, 81–96

Peterson, K.A., Dewanjee, M.K. and Kaye, M.P. (1982) Fate of indium 111-labeled platelets during cardiopulmonary bypass performed with membrane and bubble oxygenators. *Journal of Thoracic and Cardiovascular Surgery*, **84**, 39–43

Pierce, E.C. and Dibeluis, N.R. (1968) The membrane lung: studies with a new high permeability co-polymer membrane. *Transactions of the American Society for Artificial Internal Organs*, **14**, 220–226

Roughton, F.J.W. (1959) Transport of oxygen and carbon dioxide. In *Handbook of Physiology Respiration*, Washington DC, American Physiological Society, Section 3, **1**, pp. 767–825

Rygg, I.H. and Kyvsgaard, E. (1956) A disposable oxygenator system applied in a heart lung machine. *Acta Chirurgica Scandinavica*, **112**, 443–447

Severinghaus, J.W. (1979) Simple, accurate equations for human blood O_2 dissociation computations. *Journal of Applied Physiology*, **46**, 599–602

Snider, M.T., Richardson, P.D., Friedman, L.I. and Galletti, P.M. (1974) Carbon dioxide transfer rate in artificial lungs. *Journal of Applied Physiology*, **36**, 233–239

Spaeth, E.E. (1970) The oxygenation of blood in artificial devices. In *Blood Oxygenation*, (ed. D. Hershey), Plenum, New York, pp. 276–305

Spaeth, E.E. (1973) Blood oxygenation in extracorporeal devices: theoretical considerations. *CRC Critical Reviews in Bioengineering*, **1**, 383–416

U.S. Department of Health and Human Services (1985) *Guidelines for Blood-Material Interactions*, National Institutes of Health, Washington DC

van den Dungen, J.J.A.M., Karliczek, G.F., Brenken, V., *et al.* (1982) Clinical study of blood trauma during perfusion with membrane and bubble oxygenators. *Journal of Thoracic and Cardiovascular Surgery*, **83**, 108–116

von Frey, M. and Gruber, M. (1885) Untersuchungen über den stoffwechsel isolirter organe. *Virchow's Archiv für Physiologie*, **9**, 519–532

von Schröeder, W. (1882) Über die bildungsstätte des harnstoffs. *Archiv für Experimentelle Pathologie und Pharmakologie*, **15**, 364–402

Voorhees, M.E. (1976) Mutual transfer of carbon dioxide and oxygen to and from blood flowing in macrochannel devices. PhD Dissertation, Arizona State University, Tempe, Arizona, USA

Voorhees, C., Grover, R. and Voorhees, M. (1990) Evaluation of platelet damage in extracorporeal circuits using a visual platelet morphology method. *Transactions of the American Society for Internal Organs*, **36**, 664–667

Wilson, R., Shepley, D.J. and Lewellyn-Thomas, E. (1965) A membrane oxygenator with low priming volume for extracorporeal circulation. *Canadian Journal of Surgery*, **8**, 309–311

Wright, G. and Sanderson, J.M. (1979) Cellular aggregation and trauma in cardiotomy suction systems. *Thorax*, **34**, 621–628

Yang, W.J. (1979) Blood gas interactions and physiological implications. In *Advances in Cardiovascular Physics*, Vol. 3 (eds D.N. Ghista, E. Van Vollenbhoven, W.J. Yang and H. Raul), S. Karger, New York, pp. 45–99

Zingg, W. (1967) Membrane oxygenator for infants. *Transactions of the American Society for Artificial Internal Organs*, **13**, 334–337

5

Filtration in cardiopulmonary bypass

Linda Marshall

Filtration in cardiopulmonary bypass has undoubtedly increased over recent years. This is probably as a result of both greater awareness of clinical benefit to the patient i.e. the removal of microemboli, and as an important adjunct to perfusion safety. Gourlay (1988) has suggested arterial line filters to be the single most important safety item in the extracorporeal circuit utilized for open heart procedures and, more recently, filters have been advocated routinely whenever the surgeon or perfusionist wishes to minimize damage to the patient's central nervous system (Treasure, 1989).

It is the aim of this chapter to review the clinical relevance of filtration as well as to explain and clarify the mechanisms of filtration related to function. The term filtration in this context is used, essentially, to describe disposable filters placed into the extracorporeal circuit or an ancillary circuit during the bypass procedure. Haemofiltration to reduce fluid volumes, which has special relevance in cardiopulmonary bypass involving renal patients, is a quite different application and will not be discussed herein. However, the topic has been comprehensively reviewed by Wheeldon and Bethune (1986).

Filtration applications in cardiopulmonary bypass include removal of contaminants from blood in the arterial, cardiotomy, reperfusion and transfusion lines as well as clear fluid filtration during cardioplegia, circuit priming and introduction of intravenous (iv) fluids. A further application which appears to be generally accepted, though often overlooked, is the filtration of the oxygenator gas line. An additional gas line, if in use, is the patient's ventilation circuit which can also be included as a potential source of contamination and, therefore, as a candidate for filtration. For each of these applications the criteria for filtration are different although all share a requirement for clinical efficacy, low pressure drops, good flow characteristics, and suitability for use with other equipment.

The removal of potentially harmful particulate and gas emboli from blood must be attained without harming the viable cells being returned to the patient. Similarly the filtration must not initiate any adverse activation of biological systems e.g. the complement cascade.

Clear fluid filtration is more straight forward as cellular integrity is no longer an issue. In this instance we are usually dealing with non-biological fluids and can, therefore, achieve both the removal of microemboli and micro-organisms with the correct choice of filter.

Gas filtration works on different principles from liquid filtration but, as with clear fluid filtration, it can provide protection from particulates and micro-organisms. A key consideration for gas filtration is to ensure that the medium itself does not 'wet out' with moisture as this can compromise filtration efficiency by allowing the passage of contaminants through a liquid channel.

Thus, in the design and selection of a filter for a particular application general principles can be followed and these can then be supplemented by the user's individual needs.

Mechanisms of filtration and filter function

Liquid filtration

Blood filtration

The average erythrocyte is 5–7 μm in diameter while platelets are approximately 1–2 μm in size.

Any filtration of blood must allow the passage of these cells without hindrance. Historically two filtration methods were developed – *depth* and *screen* filtration. The removal ratings assigned to the filters varied between 10 μm and 40 μm and arose from work that had already been undertaken on the removal of microaggregates from stored blood (Swank, 1961). Both types of filter are able to remove particulate debris and microbubbles but do so by different mechanisms.

Depth, or adsorption, filters usually consist of packed fibres (e.g. Dacron wool) although filters made of porous plastic foam have also been available. The mechanism of filtration is one of impaction and subsequent adsorption of any particles on to the filter media (see Figure 5.1). As a consequence of the consistency of the filter material they do not have a defined 'pore' size i.e. impaction/adsorption is a statistical phenomenon and the diameter of channels within the filter medium can vary widely. However, the efficiency of the filter increases as the flow path through the filter becomes longer or narrower, hence, the synonym 'depth' for adsorption filters. Efficiency is maximized if the blood passes through a greater bulk of material – this provides both a larger number of tortuous pathways through which fluids must pass and a larger wetted surface for particle adsorption. As the blood flows into the filter very large particles will be retained on the initial surface while smaller particles will be carried by the liquid flow further down into the medium. As the blood passes through the internal structure of the filter the flow direction alters, at this point contaminant particles entrained in the fluid will resist the directional change and carry on in a straight line to impact on any wetted surface in its path. This impaction is related to the inertial mass of the particle. Once impacted on a filter fibre the particle will be held by adsorptive forces.

Screen filters consist of woven polymer threads (generally polyester) which create a material of defined 'pore' size; they work by direct interception (physical retention) of particles larger than the defined pore size. Thus, particle removal in screen filters is an absolute function of pore size (see Figure 5.1). Unlike depth filters there is very little involvement of adsorptive mechanisms although it is possible that particles smaller than the pore size may adhere to the filter material to a minor extent. If the screen is properly constructed, so as not to distort under pressure, all particles larger than the pore will be retained on the filter surface throughout the period of use. Screen filters do not require 'depth' to maximize efficiency but increased capacity can be achieved by enlarging the surface area available for blood to pass through – in practice this is usually done by pleating the screen filter, along with screen supports, to gain a large surface area in a minimal volume. Screen filtration provides efficient particle removal in combination with a very short 'contact time' between the blood and foreign surface.

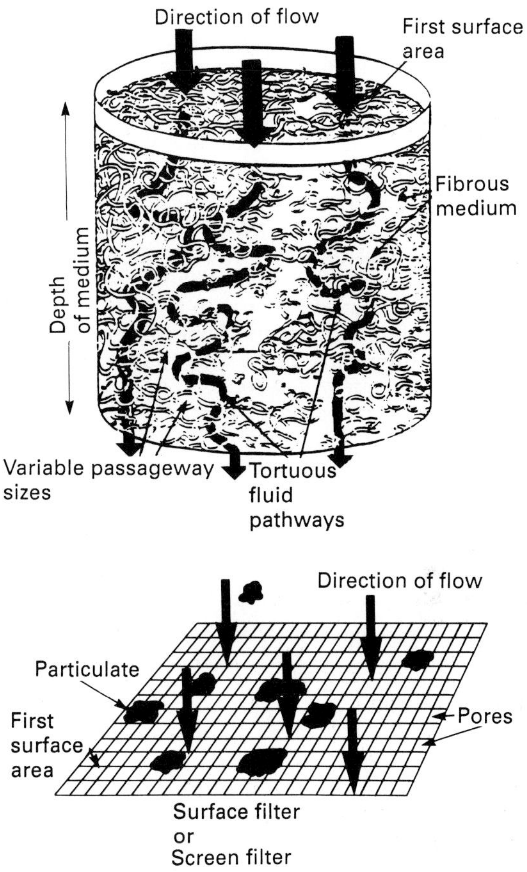

Figure 5.1 Schematic diagrams of mechanisms of blood filtration, (a) depth filtration and (b) screen filtration

Clear fluid filtration

Clear fluids (crystalloids and colloids) do not contain cellular components and, therefore, filtration of these fluids can be taken to a much lower level i.e. the removal of submicronic particles and micro-organisms. The packed fibres of depth filters or woven strands of screen filters cannot achieve this degree of filtration and so other technology must be employed – namely *membrane* filtration. Filter membranes are formed, rigid structures are produced rather like paper but to very particular standards. Although 'paper-like' to the human eye they do have relative depth to a bacterium. A typical bacterial-removal rated membrane (i.e.

0.2 μm) will have a thickness approximately 250 times the diameter of a bacterium. Membrane filters do not have absolute 'pore' size but are given a rating appropriate to the general distribution of channel size within the medium. The major filtration mechanism is direct interception but adsorption combined with charge interactions may be responsible for retention of particles smaller than the filter rating (Figure 5.2). This latter removal capability will be dependent on the surface properties of the filter material. As the channels within a 0.2 μm filter membrane are much smaller than those in a typical blood screen filter (20–40 μm) the resistance to flow must be considered. If a unit area of filter medium has 20 0.2 μm 'pores' the total flow, as compared with another unit area with 20 40 μm 'pores', will be very much smaller. The relationship between filter pore size and resistance to flow can be described by Poiseuille's equation:

$$Q = \frac{\Delta P \pi d^4}{128 \eta L}$$

where Q = flow, ΔP = pressure difference across the membrane, d = diameter of the pore, η = coefficient of viscosity and L = length of pore. Thus, if the pore size is increased from 1 unit to 2 units, the flow will be increased by a factor of 16. However the total cross sectional area available for liquid flow (open area) in a typical 0.2 μm rated nylon membrane can be as high as 85%. This fact, combined with a pleating technology for the filter membrane, allows manufacturers to provide a very large surface area filter, with low resistance, for bacterial and particulate removal in high flow applications e.g. cardioplegia and the prebypass prime.

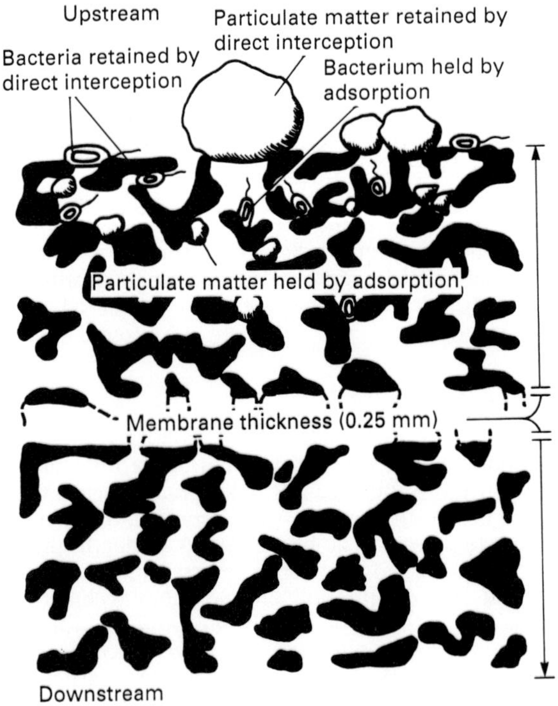

Figure 5.2 Schematic diagram of mechanisms of membrane filtration

Gas filtration

Some commercially available filters for breathing systems employ electrostatic interactions as a means of retaining particles. Most, however, perform the task by physical methods of interception and adsorption of which there are three basic mechanisms (see Figure 5.3):

1. direct interception
2. inertial impaction
3. diffusional interception

The extent to which each of these mechanisms is employed will depend on the contaminant being filtered, the structure of the filter material and the parameters of gas flow. Pore sizes are not usually given for gas filters as mechanisms (2) and (3) operate with particles that can be considerably smaller than the channels through the filter medium. Normally a percentage efficiency will be quoted for bacterial removal under particular conditions. For this reason it is important to consult the specifications of the manufacturer when discussing gas filtration. Mechanism (1) is akin to the direct interception previously described with screen filters. Large particles e.g. dust and scale debris are unlikely to pass the surface of the filter. Smaller particles e.g. bacteria are usually able to pass into the media but have sufficient inertial mass to impact upon the filter fibres when the gas flow moves around the internal structure of the filter. In this instance mechanism (2) can be likened to impaction/adsorption filtration in depth filters.

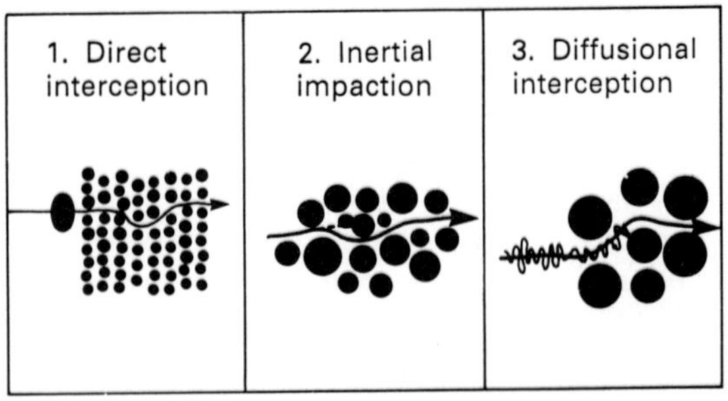

Figure 5.3 Schematic diagram of the three mechanisms of gas filtration

Diffusional interception (3) can occur with very small particles e.g. viruses. At a size of approximately 0.01 μm they are one hundred times smaller than a typical bacterium. In normal room air such small particles would have Brownian motion – a constantly varying direction. Under a directional gas flow the particles tend to assume an oscillating path which results in the particle offering a much greater apparent diameter to the medium. On entry to the filter medium they will also be intercepted upon the surface and retained by Van der Waal's forces.

If moisture comes into contact with a filter medium that is 'wettable' then a liquid channel can form which will prevent the normal gas filtration mechanisms occurring; contaminants may pass through the filter under these circumstances. Such an event results in a drop in efficiency and the resistance to gas flow is also likely to rise sharply. For this reason many gas line filters may be made of hydrophobic (water-hating) material. Liquid will not enter the medium but instead lies on the surface. Resistance to flow will only start to be affected if a considerable proportion of the filter surface becomes occluded; however, even in this event filter efficiency is not compromised.

A more detailed examination of the physics of gas and liquid filtration is provided by Suttle (1969).

Bubble removal in liquid filtration

Liquid filters are not only able to retain particulate microemboli but are also most effective at removing bubbles once they have been 'wetted' (primed) as long as a critical pressure, the bubble point pressure (BPP), is not exceeded. The BPP is the pressure required to push a bubble through the filter and is directly related to the pore size. The relationship can be described by the following equation, derived from the original quotation of Young and LaPlace describing capillarity:

$$P = \frac{4\ \gamma \cos \theta}{D}$$

where P = bubble point pressure (BPP), γ = surface tension (dependent on the liquid used), $\cos \theta$ = wetting angle (dependent on the filter material in combination with liquid used and is always less than 90° in a wettable material) and D = diameter of the filter pore. In essence the differential pressure across the membrane acts on the circular area of the bubble where it deforms at the pore, while in opposition, surface tension acts to try and keep the bubble spherical and the adsorptive forces of liquid (across the pore) resist dewetting. It is only when the pressure 'pushing' the bubble overwhelms the forces keeping it spherical that the bubble will pass through the pore (see Figure 5.4). It can be seen that the BPP is inversely proportional to the pore diameter; as the pore size diminishes, the pressure required to force a bubble through will increase. For example the BPP for a 40 μm polyester screen is typically around 37 mmHg (4.9 kPa) whereas the BPP for a 0.2 μm nylon membrane is approximately 26.90 mmHg (356.2 kPa). The removal of bubbles by filtration applies to bubbles greater than the filter pore size (this is equivalent to the largest channel in a depth filter) and will operate unless the BPP is exceeded. It should be stressed that the later scenario is highly unlikely to occur in clinical practice with a standard screen filter (Berman and Marin, 1986; Spielberg and Matkovich, 1986). A BPP of 35 mmHg may appear low if compared with typical circuit pressures, however, the BPP is the differential pressure that occurs on either side of the filter screen itself. At a flow of 5 l min^{-1} the pressure

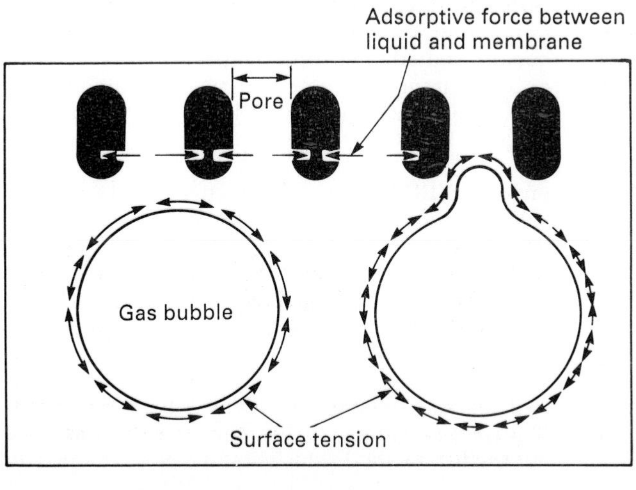

Figure 5.4 The forces of adsorption and surface tension when a gas bubble approaches a wetted filter screen or membrane

difference between the inlet and outlet of a standard 40 μm filter is 30 mmHg while the pressure difference across the actual screen is only a few mmHg (Berman and Marin, 1986).

Air venting

To enhance bubble removal capability manufacturers have incorporated vent ports and other design features into their filters which allow air to escape more readily. If air were to enter a filter and build up, the area for liquid filtration would be reduced (the air would be 'blocking' a proportion of the filter medium), and a substantial rise in pressure could then occur across the filter if flow is maintained. In these circumstances there is a potential for exceeding the BPP and so, in time, air would traverse the filter. This build up of pressure can be delayed or avoided if any entrained air is rapidly vented out of the filter so as to maintain the area available for liquid filtration.

Vent lines

The most obvious first step to vent air is to ensure that a vent port is present on the upstream side of the filter housing. Bubbles are naturally buoyant and so will rise and coalesce in the upper portion of the housing, where they can exit from the vent port. The port is attached to a vent line connected to a low pressure portion of the circuit e.g. the oxygenator. Venting to the cardiotomy reservoir is sometimes suggested but this may increase blood–foreign surface contact and the possibility of retrograde flow if the drain line becomes occluded (Berkowitz, 1980; Labinger *et al.*, 1981). The potential for pressure build up then becomes a balance between the amount of air entering the filter versus the ability of that air to escape along the vent line. This 'escape route' is reliant on several factors, firstly the patency of the vent line (for instance additional use for arterial blood sampling or pressure monitoring) and secondly the inherent resistance of the vent line. The resistance to flow through a channel is related to its length and diameter, as previously discussed. An ideal vent line is a piece of tubing with the largest possible diameter and shortest length. This may not only prove inconvenient from a practical viewpoint but would result in too great a degree of blood recirculation. A vent line flow of greater than 10% would be a good safety system but with a considerable loss of returned arterial blood, a flow of less than 2% would probably compromise the safety aspect too greatly.

A maximum one metre length of tubing with minimum diameter of 2.5 mm, using large bore stop cocks, will provide a fair compromise with reasonable venting capacity and tolerable recirculation losses (4–6%).

Automatic venting mechanisms

Many manufacturers have improved housing designs to encourage the passage of bubbles to the vent port; the air venting capability of several commercially available filters with varying designs has been studied by Gourlay, Gibbons and Taylor (1988). Nevertheless the venting may still be hampered by the need for a patent vent line. A further improvement has been the development of automatically vented filters – a system which relies on the use of a hydrophobic membrane at the apex of the filter, a permanently 'open' vent, rather than a vent line. An upstream housing design serves to separate microbubbles from a circular blood flow by centripetal force which are then vented through a hydrophobic membrane. A coalescer ring, before the filter, can be used to trap smaller bubbles with less buoyancy which would otherwise be carried along in the blood flow. This technology has increased the gas venting capabilities of conventional screen filters, particularly with respect to massive air removal (Spielberg and Matkovich, 1986; Gourlay *et al.*, 1987a; Gourlay and Taylor, 1988).

Filter 'wettability', surface tension and priming

Although patient protection and clinical safety efficacy are paramount in the development of any useful piece of equipment, ease of use is also of key importance. Clear, rigid, plastic housings are now available so that inside of filters can be viewed easily and, more recently, housing treatments and coatings have been applied to facilitate filter priming. If the 'wettability' of the internal surface(s) of a filter is increased the priming liquid will spread on the surface more easily and air will be expelled more rapidly. One way to increase 'wettability' is by attaching heparin to the filter cartridge via the surfactant benzalkonium chloride (also referred to as the biothyl complex). Studies have indicated that heparin-coated filters offer no particular advantages or disadvantages in respect of biocompatibility (Hill *et al.*, 1985; Justison *et al.*, 1986) but do prime more quickly. Though offering this advantage, a study by Palanzo (1988) has suggested that the bubble point pressure (BPP) may be affected adversely. The study suggested that release of the surfactant lowered the surface tension of the blood or priming fluid passing through the filters. With reference to the section on bubble removal (p. 59) it will be noted that as the surface tension decreases so too will the BPP and indeed potential variation in the surface tension of blood has been studied in patients with relation to bubble filtration (Butler, Kurusz and Conti, 1986). There is, however, an alternative method which has been developed to enhance priming. This involves a physical process that can modify surfaces without the use of any additional organic compounds or surfactants. The resultant surface modification increases the wettability of the filter and Palanzo's study found that filters produced in this way had an increased BPP.

Applications of filtration in relation to clinical need and safety

Blood filtration

Arterial and cardiotomy line filtration

At a relatively early stage in the history of cardiopulmonary bypass a number of investigators noted the presence of microemboli in the extracorporeal circuit and deleterious effects on the patients as a consequence of entry of these microemboli into their circulation. Jenevien and Weiss (1964) observed platelet emboli in the myocardium and renal glomeruli of patients dying within 4 postoperative days. These emboli were very similar to those identified in earlier studies on stored blood (Swank, 1961) as might be expected given the widespread use of blood primes at that time. Although the study of Jenevien and Weiss noted damage from microemboli in the heart and kidneys, potential cerebral damage became a focus of attention and an elevated incidence of neurological dysfunction was observed in early studies (Patterson and Kessler, 1969; Lee *et al.*, 1971). Tufo, Ostfeld and Shekelle (1970) noted that 43% of survivors following open-heart surgery displayed behavioural abnormalities preceded by focal neurological damage, and nine out of the ten patients who died were found to have small multiple lesions throughout the brain. It is important to remember that the body's own filter, the lung, is unavailable for cleansing of returned arterial blood to the patient. This was clearly demonstrated in a comparison of venovenous and venoarterial bypass in a dog model–considerable system organ damage was seen in the group undergoing venoarterial bypass whereas emboli were confined to the lung in the venovenous bypass group (Allardyce, Yoshida and Ashmore, 1966). It became apparent that there was a considerable variety of particulate debris that could be generated in the cardiotomy and arterial lines. The most logical target for primary filtration would appear to be the cardiotomy line due to the debris that could arise from the surgical site. Particulate debris identified in the cardiotomy line includes: fibrin clots, bone chips, calcium emboli, fat emboli, tissue fragments, other materials from the operating site, protein precipitates (arising at gas–liquid interfaces), platelet aggregates and microaggregates (consisting of leucocytes, platelets and fibrin) from stored blood. Early studies incorporating a cardiotomy line filter confirmed the effectiveness of debris removal in relation to patient mortality (Hill *et al.*, 1970; Osborn *et al.*, 1970). Connel *et al.* (1973) observed extensive occlusion of the lung vasculature in biopsies of patients who underwent open-heart surgery. The removal of particulate debris by filtration of the cardiotomy line reduced the extent of degenerative lesions, but interestingly, further protection was afforded by additional filtration of the arterial line and blood prime. It appeared, therefore, that cardiotomy line filtration was required but that it should be augmented by additional filtration in the arterial line for the maximum patient benefit. A filtration element is now generally incorporated as an integral part of the cardiotomy reservoir and so the need for separate blood filters in the cardiotomy line is usually unnecessary. There is still variation in the cardiotomy filters themselves and manufacturing debris may be present (Swanney, 1986). Although their sources are not as diverse as those from cardiotomy suction it is still evident that many particulate emboli can arise solely in the arterial line e.g. platelet and cellular aggregates (see Figure 5.5), protein precipitates, spallated plastic, other material from the oxygenator and tubing circuit, fibrin clots and thrombus in a centrifugal pump has also been noted (Bell-Thompson, Manero and Tyras, 1987).

The importance of arterial line filtration also became more widely recognized when it was realized that gas microemboli could be readily generated in the arterial line and they too were potentially harmful. Patterson and Kessler (1969) could not distinguish gas and particulate emboli with the Doppler technique used in their experimental circuit, but they did see an increase in signal frequency when gas flow increased, oxygenator blood volume decreased or the oxygenator was agitated. This was indicative of microbubble formation. Other ways in which gas microemboli may arise are: decreased solubility of gas (oxygen is less soluble than carbon dioxide), degassing due to increase in temperature or a negative pressure zone (e.g. inadvertent tubing clamp proximal to the pump head), incomplete defoaming, reservoir vortexing and runaway pump head. Bubble traps have been employed to try and overcome the problem of microbubbles but they are only useful at removing bubbles of about 200 μm and above. Arterial line filters were known to be effective bubble removers from bubble point pressure studies and so could perform a dual purpose – removal of both particulate and gaseous microemboli.

The evolution of bubbles within a circuit employing a bubble oxygenator is well accepted, however the problem is often considered to be avoided with the use of membrane oxygenators. Undoubtedly

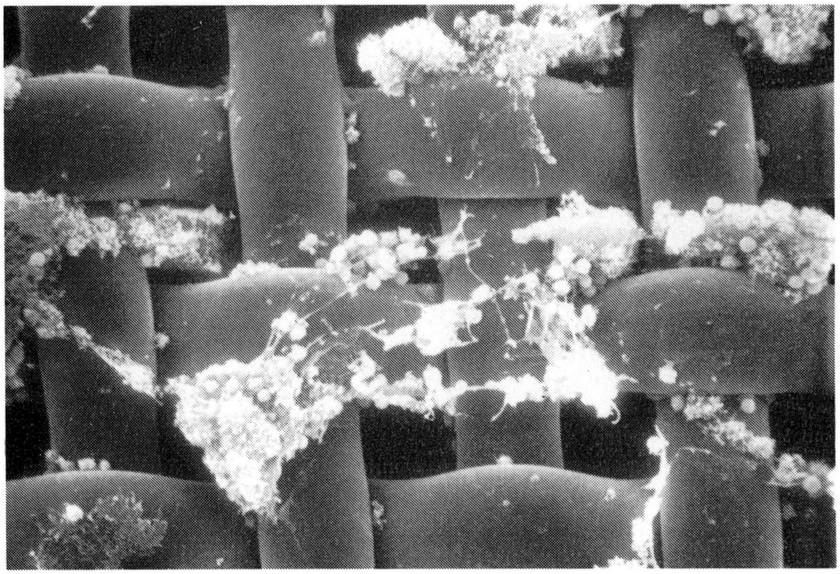

Figure 5.5 SEM of upstream surface of a 40 μm screen arterial line filter showing retained cellular debris

membrane oxygenators do not generate bubbles to the same extent as bubble oxygenators but gas emboli are still present in the circuit during use. Pearson *et al.* (1986) noted that gas microbubbles still arise as a result of entrainment of venous line air, cardiotomy suction, or injection of fluids and drugs into the oxygenator. In a recent clinical comparison of a bubble and membrane oxygenator the authors, though finding in favour of the membrane oxygenator, still recommend the use of a 40 μm arterial line filter (Smith, 1989).

Although air accidents have decreased significantly in the last decade they still remain the third most common cause of morbidity or mortality (Kurusz and Wheeldon, 1988). The clinical literature has noted that the use of a torpedo head exchanger and 40 μm screen filter delayed the passage of gas and added reaction time in a particular case of runaway pump head (Kurusz *et al.*, 1979).

Neurological dysfunction following open heart surgery is a recognized problem even with modern day equipment and surgical techniques. A study of 312 patients undergoing elective coronary artery bypass surgery found that 61% exhibited neurological complications; resolution of the order appeared in 4% of patients during their stay in hospital. No arterial line filters were used in this study although both bubble and membrane oxygenators were employed. The authors suggest micro- and macroembolizations, due to air and particles, as one of the possible aetiological mechanisms (Shaw *et al.*, 1985). It is interesting to note that in neurophysical studies the decline in patients' cognitive function has continued to 1 year (Newman *et al.*, 1989) and 5 year follow-ups (Willner *et al.*, 1983). The extent and assessment of neurological dysfunction and neuropsychological morbidity following bypass surgery has been discussed in further detail by several authors (Anon, 1989; Newman, 1989; Pearson, 1989; Shaw, 1989).

Specific attention has been paid to the aspect of micro- and macroembolization by assessing the use of filters in the bypass circuits – the outcome of these studies is summarized in Table 5.1.

The studies are mostly favourable but it must be remembered that all filters are not the same – removal of particulate debris must always be balanced against the trauma to viable components of the blood. Since filters were initially developed, it is the screen filters which have gained the most widespread acceptance to the point where depth filters are rarely used. Depth filters, although effective at removing particles, have been associated with increased haemolysis, decreased platelet counts and loss of bubble retaining capabilities due to 'channelling' in the medium. (Buley and Lumley, 1975; Cullen and Ferara, 1975; Krebber *et al.*, 1982). Certain screen filters too have proved to have no effect or even be detrimental in studies but they are all associated with filters made of nylon (associated with complement activation in heparinized blood) and/or a pore size of less than 40 μm (Bergdahl and Bjork, 1980; Chenoworth *et al.*, 1981; Yellon, Vernick and Golub, 1981; Willner *et al.*, 1983; Aris *et al.*, 1986). Polyester screen filters of 40 μm gauge

Table 5.1 Studies comparing filtered and non-filtered arterial line blood

Author	*Year*	*Patient groups and test method*	*Filter type*	*Findings*
Branthwaite	1975	Comparison of neurological damage pre and post use of cardiotomy and arterial filters and vasopressor agents.	40 μm polyester	Pre-use 19.2% incidence of neurological damage Post-use 7.4% incidence of neurological damage
Aberg and Kihlgren	1977	Patients with prophylactic protective measures including arterial line filters (1974–76) compared with earlier study group (1972–74) with psychometric tests.	40 μm polyester	Prophylactic measure undertaken in later groups resulted in decrease in cerebral complications from 14.5% to 3% in 1976
Taylor *et al.*	1980	Cardiopulmonary bypass undertaken on dogs and levels of brain specific creatine phosphokinase (CPK) assessed in cerebrospinal fluid in filter and non filter groups.	40 μm polyester	CPK is a marker for brain damage. Elevated levels of CPK arose in non-filter group which persisted postop. CPK elevation significantly reduced in filter group and returned to pre-op values within 24 h.
Willner *et al.*	1983	Psychometric testing (CLAT test) of patient groups with two different filters. Comparison with study 5 years previous (non-filter) and long term incidence of impairment.	Filter A – 40 μm polyester Filter B – 25 μm nylon	Filter A – 5% impairment. Filter B – 24% impairment. Non-filter – 14% impairment – 5 year follow-up of non-filter group showed that 94% patients had same incidence of impairment as postop
Pugsley	1989	Assessment of microembolic events in patients middle cerebral artery during bypass using transcranial Doppler. Filter and non-filter group.	40 μm polyester	Microembolic events: Filter group 0–10 per 30 min. Non-filter group 30–768 per 30 min ($P < 0.001$).
Treasure	1989	Patients in above study assessed pre and post operatively with 10 neuropsychological tests to check cognitive function and mood also assessed.	40 μm polyester	Neuropsychological tests: Filter / Non-filter Better 15/20 / 5/20 Unchanged 2/20 / 6/20 Worse 3/20 / 9/20 Beck depression score unchanged or better 18/20 / 11/20 Worse 2/20 / 9/20

have proved safe in use with insignificant haemolysis and platelet depletion (Patterson and Twichell, 1971; Guidon *et al.*, 1976; Taylor, 1986 Gourlay *et al.*, 1987b).

Other situations where extracorporeal circulation is undertaken may also be considered for filtration applications, especially where particulate or gaseous microemboli might be produced e.g. ECMO (Gerstmann and Cornish, 1987) and liver perfusion (Myers, 1987).

A further consideration for the future of arterial line filtration (and also, perhaps, in the perfusion of donated organs for transplant) is the possibility of removing potentially damaging leucocytes in the extracorporeal circuit. There is now a growing body of evidence implicating leucocytes in lung and myocardial reperfusion injury particularly related to the release of free radicals and other vasoactive mediators. (Engler, 1987; Hall *et al.*, 1987; Weiss, 1989). Removal of leucocytes in stored blood and platelets by filtration can now be achieved to very high degrees of efficiency and pilot studies utilizing adapted forms of this technology have revealed promising possibilities for the future with reference to preventing reperfusion injury (Bando *et al.*, 1989; Breda *et al.*, 1989).

Filtration of stored blood

A study of American perfusionists by Kurusz (1986) indicated that 94% of perfusionists filter stored blood using a microaggregate filter or a filtered cardiotomy reservoir. Stored blood is known to contain microaggregates (emboli consisting of non-viable platelets, leucocytes and fibrin strands). Following transfusion these microaggregates can result in pulmonary dysfunction if they block capillary arterioles in sufficient numbers while prior filtration significantly decreases the problem (Reul, Beall and Greenberg, 1974). They have also been implicated in posttransfusion thrombocytopenia (Bareford *et al.*, 1987) and fibronectin depletion (Snyder *et al.*, 1980). Again filtration has been shown to ameliorate these effects in both instances. Pourrat *et al.* (1985) demonstrated increased fibronectin depletion in bypass as compared with non-bypass surgery. Arterial line filtration was not used and the authors proposed that this supplementary decrease in fibronectin was due to particulates of various origin entering the blood during bypass. Thus, the combined onslaught of microaggregates and circuit particulates may cause a notable effect of plasma fibronectin levels in cardiac surgery. A further topic of particular interest in cardiac and transplant surgery is the transmission of cytomegalovirus (CMV). Adler, Baggett and McVoy (1985) found that reactivation of latent virus was the most common reason for CMV infection in adult cardiac patients although direct transmission from donor blood is also possible. Another case report cited impaired immune responses in a patient following an aortic value replacement due to acute CMV infection. This individual was CMV negative preoperatively but received 13 units of whole blood during surgery (Gould *et al.*, 1987). CMV resides in leucocytes and can be transmitted directly or reactivated in a patient's own cells by interaction with donor leucocytes. Removal of leucocytes by filtration can reduce or abolish the risk via either pathway and this has been shown to be effective in a variety of patients (Verdonck *et al.*, 1987; Murphy *et al.*, 1988; Gilbert *et al.*, 1989). In addition, transfusion of stored blood is known to have a variety of immunosuppresive effects (George and Morello, 1986) and most notable is the poor prognosis for patients receiving preoperative transfusion during solid tumour surgery (Blumberg *et al.*, 1985; Parrot *et al.*, 1987). The role of filters in microaggregate and leucocyte removal in stored blood has far reaching considerations in respect of the above effects being both simple, quick and non-invasive (Lloyd and Marshall, 1986; Marshall, 1989).

Filtration of autotransfused blood

Autotransfusion is a growing trend in cardiac surgery. The advantages of the technique are obvious – it eliminates possible immunological reactions or blood borne infectious agents and also results in less blood wastage and, therefore, does not deplete blood bank supplies. If autotransfusion is undertaken via a hand held suction device the blood should be filtered before transfusion to the patient as the potential for harmful debris is very similar to that previously described in the cardiotomy suction line. Alternatively if the blood is collected and stored in the cardiotomy reservoir there is still a need for additional transfusion filtration. A cardiotomy reservoir will remove operating site debris and the mediastinal blood will pass to the reservoir compartment. When mediastinal blood is shed and passes through the pericardium defibrination occurs and so no additional anticoagulant is added to stop blood clotting in the reservoir. However, the physical process of defibrination is rate dependent and in certain individuals the process may not be completed before collection and, therefore, the blood will still have the potential to clot or form aggregates. If the blood is left to rest (postcardiotomy filter) for any length of time it is then conceivable that particulate material may be directly transfused to the patient. Subsequent filtration at the time of transfusion has identified cellular aggregates in autotransfused blood which, without filtration, would have passed to the transfused patient (Fox and Wilkins, personal communication, 1989).

Clear fluid filtration

Cardioplegia and prebypass fluid filtration

The 1950s heralded the first awareness of the potentially harmful systemic effects of particulate debris in crystalline intravenous solutions and later other studies confirmed the problem (Jacques and Mariscal, 1951; Garvan and Gunner, 1971). The types of particles identified in intravenous therapy solutions included: glass and rubber fragments, lacquer flakes, cellulose, starch, talc, cotton fibres, metallic particles and plasticizers (Draft and Graf, 1974). Vast numbers of particles have also been identified in small volume additives – unlike large volume parenterals these small volume additives do not have to comply to any particulate limits in the UK. It is pertinent to note, however, that many of the particles seen in the additives appear to arise during storage (Backhouse *et al.*, 1987). A truly particle free solution or additive is probably impossible to achieve at this time, however stringent the manufacturers are, without the use of filtration at the time of use.

The significance of particles in clear fluids became relevant to cardiopulmonary bypass when clear fluid primes replaced blood primes and crystalloid cardioplegia gained popularity. It was quickly identified that the action of the pump head upon tubing could cause another type of particulate to arise – spallated plastic. Particles may also be released from various components of the circuit (see Figure 5.6). Particle counts are high as 175 000 after 120 min were seen with both PVC and Silastic tubing (Hubbard *et al.*, 1975). Another study noted that thousands of particles were produced in just a few minutes (Kemna and Docherty, 1979). Filters were suggested as a means of preventing the particles entering the patient and they were developed with a pore size of 3–8 μm. This size range was

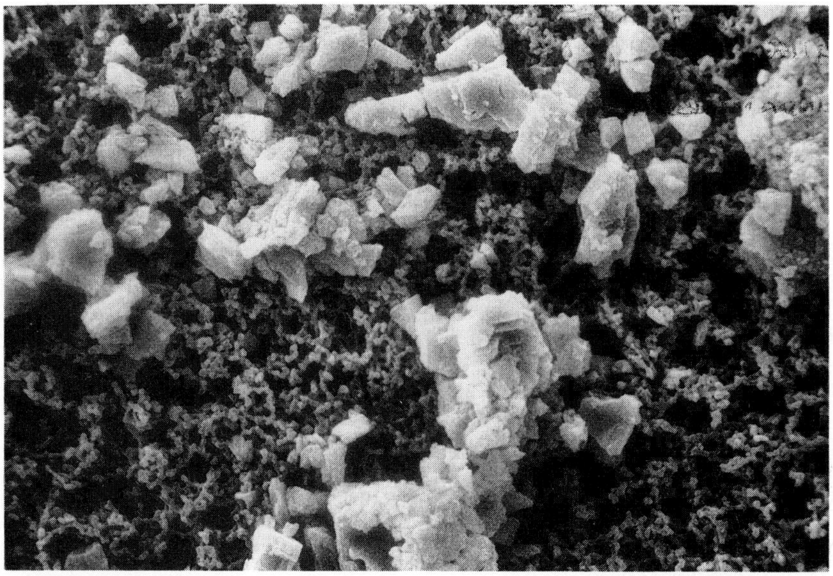

Figure 5.6 SEM of contaminants on a 0.8 μm analysis membrane filter after flushing membrane oxygenator

seen as being able to remove the large majority of particles while ensuring the resistance flow was not too great (Brooks *et al.*, 1979). Unfortunately, further studies indicated that most (greater than 90%) of the particles found in the clear fluids used in prebypass and cardioplegia were less than 5 μm in size (Gaillard *et al.*, 1984; Robinson, Braimbridge and Hearse, 1984). Further work was needed to discover whether a submicronic filter was viable in the cardioplegia and prebypass applications. A submicronic filter would not only remove a far more meaningful number of particles but would also provide bacteriological protection. Brooks (1980) found that a 0.45 μm filter was suitable as a prebypass filter, allowing adequate flow rates and he recommended a recirculation time of at least 15 min to remove the majority (85%) of loosened particles.

This finding has been supported by other studies i.e. most particles are released within the first 15 min or so of bypass and a submicronic filter removes a far greater proportion of particles than a 5 μm filter (Ueda, 1988). Although Brooks used a 0.45 μm rated filter in his study this rating has now been superseded by a 0.2 μm rating for full bacterial retention.

The potentially harmful effects of the particles inherent in clear solutions and arising from equipment use are well documented in i.v. therapy (Marshall and Lloyd, 1987) and there are now an increasing number of studies relating to bypass surgery and associated techniques which discuss the clinical significance in these areas (Kurusz *et al.*, 1980; Leong, 1982; Uretsky *et al.*, 1987). Orenstein *et al.* (1982) observed microemboli in the organ beds of patients who died following bypass surgery. The particles appeared to be mainly silicone antifoam but spallated PVC was also present. Post mortems of patients who have undergone haemodialysis have also identified silicone in the liver of 22 of 31 case studies. Further work noted particles in the liver in all post-mortem examinations as well as the marrow, lungs and lymph nodes in some cases (Leong, 1982; Leong, Disney and Gore, 1982; Leong and Gore, 1983). Studies on the isolated rat heart model with commonly used cardioplegia solutions, which all conformed to British Pharmacopeia particle standards, found that infusion of the fluid led to a mean reduction in coronary flow of 55.7%. This effect was abolished if the cardioplegia solution was filtered with a submicronic filter (0.8 μm).

In addition, when the rat hearts received unfiltered multi-dose cardioplegia they essentially failed to recover. In an identical set of experiments with 0.8 μm filtered solution the hearts recovered approximately 90% of their preischaemic function (Robinson, Braimbridge and Hearse, 1984). Further work by the same group demonstrated that the particles did not seem to cause direct vascular occlusion but acted by several non-specified mechanisms. The effects of the particles could also be overcome by the vasoactive drugs procaine, nifedipine and adenosine triphosphate (ATP) (Hearse *et al.*, 1985).

Particles are the main clinical concern in clear fluid filtration but the additional protection afforded by a 0.2 μm bacterial retentive rated filter cannot be overlooked. Reports of in-use contamination of i.v. fluids range between 5% and 30% (Denyer, 1982) but it is unlikely that contamination in the cardiac theatre would occur to the same extent. However, a report of five deaths following the administration of unfiltered cardioplegia solution inadvertently contaminated with *Enterobacter cloacae* reinforces the safety aspect of filtration (Hughes *et al.*, 1986). Incidences of bacterial contamination have not been widely reported but recent studies from a Danish group have highlighted another consideration – the presence of endotoxins in the extracorporeal circuit. Andersen *et al.* (1987) found a significant incidence of endotoxins in the circuit, pulmonary artery, and cardiotomy suction lines during bypass. Positive test results for the presence of endotoxins were seen with cardioplegic fluids, prebypass fluids, blood transfusions and ice for cooling. A subsequent study on the potential for tissue damage in patients with endotoxaemia noted that the endotoxin found in the patient's blood was derived from the priming fluids, the gut or both (Kharazmi *et al.*, 1989). Filtration (0.2 μm) capable of removing particles, bacteria and bacterially-associated endotoxins is already available (Baumgartner *et al.*, 1986; Marshall and Lloyd, 1987). This technology may prove beneficial with reference to the above findings.

It is relevant to point out that particles from drug additives administered during bypass, i.e. during blood circulation will not be trapped by a 40 μm arterial line filter. Such additives can be introduced via small 0.2 μm syringe filters to overcome this problem. The major portion of particles arising from the circuit and spallation can be effectively removed during approximately 15 min recirculation time before the removal of the prebypass filter before going on bypass.

Gas filtration

Oxygenator gas line filtration

It is a general belief that medical gases are both clean and dry but studies of medical grade compressed air have shown that this is not always the case. Bjerring and Oberg (1986) sampled compressed medical air from pipeline outlets in intensive care units and operating rooms. Of the samples 81% were found to be contaminated. Pathogens and normal skin flora were identified along with condensed water and oil droplets which allow bacterial proliferation. The authors pointed out that though medical gases must comply with chemical standards there are no recommendations with regard to bacterial contamination. They further suggest that 'until sterile air can be supplied we also recommend filters in ventilators and all other equipment driven by or requiring medical air'.

Another study found *Penicillum* spp. in the compressed air plant of a hospital and it was noted that *Aspergillus* spores are another likely contaminant. These authors also recommend filtration of compressed air (Warren *et al.*, 1986).

As well as protection against possible microbial contamination, a suitable gas line filter can help reduce the potential for mechanical damage to the oxygenator. Sharp particles of debris and scale are sometimes released from pipelines – these may cause blockage of an oxygen diffuser in a bubble oxygenator or pierce the membrane oxygenator. A 0.2 μm rated filter is both microbial and particulate retentive. It is also important that the filter is hydrophobic to ensure that liquid droplets do not traverse the filter; this would cause an increase in resistance and provide a channel for bacteria to cross.

Respiratory circuit filtration

As with the gas line there is a potential for intrinsic microbial contamination of anaesthetic gases. There is also potential for cross contamination of the anaesthetic machine, dependent on cleaning regimes and equipment use, which can lead to pneumonias and other infections (Daschner *et al.*, 1981; Nielsen *et al.*, 1980; Marc *et al.*, 1987). Studies in cardiac surgery and general surgery indicate that the ideal is to provide a completely clean circuit for each patient but this may prove expensive and difficult to undertake (Albrecht and Dryden, 1974; Deverill and Dutt, 1980). However, the use of an individual filter barrier to contamination (airborne bacteria and viruses along with contaminated liquid secretions) for each patient can prove clinically beneficial and cost effective (Gallagher, Strangeways and Allt-Graham, 1987; Nunn, 1988). Heat and moisture exchanging filters are now available which can provide both humidification and filtration to the individual patients but their properties vary (Bethune *et al.*, 1989).

Filter products available

This section has been compiled to give the reader an overview of currently available filters for extracorporeal perfusion. It is limited to the filters for arterial line, cardiotomy lines and prebypass priming fluid. Information on the other filtration applications discussed herein is readily available from manufacturers. Tables 5.2, 5.3 and 5.4 attempt to summarize key features of filters produced by a variety of manufacturers.

Table 5.2 Arterial line filters currently available from various manufacturers

Manufacturer	*Filter type*	*Pore size(S)*	*Filter material*	*Priming volume*	*Filter variants available*
Bard	Screen	33 μm	Polyester	195 ml	Adult, heparin coated easy prime
Bentley	Screen	25 μm and 40 μm	Polyester	220 ml and 115 ml	Adult, paediatric, heparin coated easy prime
Delta	Screen	37 μm	Nylon	250 ml and 120 ml	Adult, paediatric
Dideco	Screen	20 μm and 40 μm	Polyester	195 ml and 100 ml	Adult, paediatric
Gish	Screen	25 μm and	Polyester	195 ml	Adult
Johnson and Johnson	Screen	40 μm	Polyester	255 ml	Adult, heparin coated easy prime
Pall	Screen	40 μm	Polyester	220 ml, 200 ml, 110 ml, 35 ml	Adult, self venting, paediatric, surface modified easy prime
Polystan	Screen	40 μm	Nylon	220 ml	Adult
Shiley	Screen	40 μm and 20 μm	Nylon	215 ml	Adult
Sorin	Screen	25 μm and 40 μm	Polyester	200 ml	Adult
Swank	Depth	13 μm	Dacron wool	300 ml and 240 ml	Adult arterial and cardiotomy

Table 5.3 Prebypass filters currently available from various manufacturers

Manufacturer	*Pore size*	*Filter material*
Bard	5 μm	NA
Bentley	5 μm	German V5000T
Cobe	5 μm	NA
Delta	5 μm	NA
Dideco	5 μm	NA
Gish	5 μm	NA
Pall	0.5 μm	Nylon

NA = Not available from literature or UK company/distributor

Table 5.4 Cardioplegia filters currently available from various manufacturers

Manufacturer	*Pore size*	*Filter material*
Bentley	0.8 μm	Acryl copolymer with non-woven nylon and polyester PTFE hydrophobic vent
Cobe	0.2 μm	Nylon
Pall	0.2 μm	Nylon

Discussion

Filters are not an absolute requirement for successful cardiopulmonary bypass. They are, however, essential for the removal of undesirable gaseous and particulate microemboli arising from the circuit itself and in the introduction of additional fluids and gases. When properly utilized in an extracorporeal circuit these filters prevent microemboli entering the patient's circulation (see Figure 5.7). If filtration is not undertaken the microemboli can give rise to potentially harmful consequences, namely systemic lesions, neurologic dysfunction and neuropsychological impairment. Additionally, the air retentive/air venting properties of arterial line filters provide an extra margin of safety for the cardiac team in the event of accidental air entrainment, while bacterially retentive clear fluid and gas filters are an important barrier to inadvertent microbial contamination.

As with all technological developments the advantages of the technology must be balanced against any practical or economic factors. Controversy continues in the debate as to the necessity of filtration in cardiopulmonary bypass but they are relatively inexpensive and undoubtedly optimise the quality of all fluids and gases entering the patient. There is now a comprehensive body of knowledge to suggest that any disadvantages are far outweighed by numerous advantages.

Acknowledgements

I am grateful to Sarah Proctor for preparation of the manuscript.

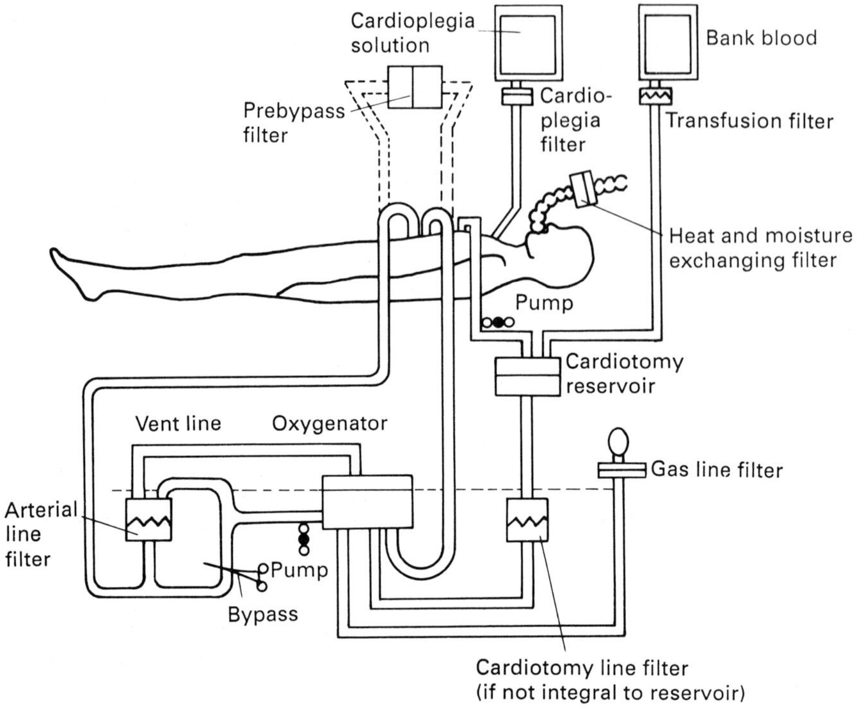

Figure 5.7 Applications of filtration in cardiopulmonary bypass surgery

References

Aberg, T. and Kihlgren, M. (1977) Cerebral protection during open heart surgery. *Thorax*, **32**, 525–533

Adler, S.P., Baggett, J. and McVoy, M. (1985) Transfusion associated cytomegalovirus infections in seropositive cardiac surgery patients. *Lancet*, **ii**, 743–746

Albrecht, W.H. and Dryden, G.E. (1974) Five year experience with the development of an individually clean anaesthesia system. *Anaesthesia and Analgesia*, **53**, 24–28

Allardyce, D.B., Yoshida, S.H. and Ashmore, P.G. (1966) The importance of microembolism in the pathogenesis of organ dysfunction caused by prolonged use of the pump oxygenator. Presented at *46th Annual Meeting of the American Association for Thoracic Surgery* (Vancouver, May 16–17, 1966)

Andersen, L.W., Baek, L., Degri, H., *et al.* (1987) Presence of circulating endotoxins during cardiac operations. *Journal of Thoracic and Cardiovascular Surgery*, **93**, 115–119

Anon (1989) Brain damage and open heart surgery. (Editorial). *Lancet*, **i**, 364–366

Aris, A., Solanes, H., Camara, M.L., *et al.* (1986) Arterial line filtration during cardiopulmonary bypass. *Journal of Thoracic and Cardiovascular Surgery*, **91**, 526–533

Backhouse, C.M., Ball, P.R., Booth, S., *et al.* (1987) Particulate contaminants of intravenous medications and infusions. *Journal of Pharmacy and Pharmacology*, **39**, 241–245

Bando, K., Pillai, R., Cameron, D.E., *et al.* (1989) Leukocyte depletion ameliorates free radical mediated lung injury following cardiopulmonary bypass. Presented at *The American Association for Thoracic Surgery, 69th Annual Meeting* (May 8–10th, 1989)

Bareford, D., Chandler, S., Hawker, R., *et al.* (1987) Splenic platelet sequestration following routine blood transfusion is reduced by filtered/washed blood products. *British Journal of Haematology*, **67**, 177–180

Baumgartner, T.G., Schmidt, G.L., Thakker, K.M., *et al.* (1986) In-line intravenous filters. *American Journal of Hospital Pharmacy*, **43**, 681–684

Bell-Thompson, J., Mongero, L. and Tyras, D.H. (1987) Thrombus formation in a Biomedicus centrifugal pump during cardiopulmonary bypass. *Perfusion*, **2**, 57–59

Bergdahl, L. and Bjork, V.O. (1980) The effect of a nylon mesh blood filter in the arterial line during extracorporeal circulation. *Scandinavian Journal of Thoracic and Cardiovascular Surgery*, **14**, 263–366

Berkowitz, D.A. (1980) Inspection and preventative maintenance of cardiopulmonary perfusion equipment and an overview of problems. *Journal of Extra Corporeal Technology*, **12**, 68–70

Berman, L. and Marin, F. (1986) Micropore filtration during cardiopulmonary bypass. In *Cardiopulmonary Bypass. Principles and Management* (ed. K.M. Taylor), Chapman and Hall, London, pp. 355–374

Bethune, D.W., Kerr, L., Ghosh, S., *et al.* (1989) Evaluation of four heat and moisture exchangers incorporating bacterial filters. Presented at *European Association of Cardiothoracic Anaesthesiologists, 4th Annual Meeting* (Uppsala, June 14–16th, 1989)

Bjerring, P. and Oberg, B. (1986) Bacterial contamination of compressed air for medical use. *Anaesthesia*, **41**, 148–150

Blumberg, N., Agarwal, M.M. and Chuang, C. (1985) Relation between recurrence of cancer of the colon and blood transfusion. *British Medical Journal*, **290**, 1037–1039

Branthwaite, M.A. (1975) Prevention of neurological damage during open heart surgery. *Thorax*, **30**, 258–261

Breda, M.A., Drinkwater, D.C., Laks, H., *et al.* (1989) Prevention of repurfusion injury in the neonatal heart with leukocyte depleted blood. *Journal of Thoracic and Cardiovascular Surgery*, **97**, 654–665

Brooks, J.D. (1980) Scientific investigation: use of the Gelman 0.45 μm mini capsule filter as a prebypass filter in the extracorporeal circuit. *Journal of Extra Corporeal Technology*, **5**, 103–106

Brooks, J.D., Beauchamp, R.A., Magrath, R.A. and Clark, R.E. (1979) Efficacy of particulate removal by a prebypass filter with different oxygenation systems. *Journal of Extra Corporeal Technology*, **11**, 175–182

Buley, R. and Lumley, J. (1975) Some observations of blood microfilters. *Annals of the Royal College of Surgeons of England*, **27**, 262–267

Butler, B.D., Kurusz, M. and Conti, V.R. (1986) Postbypass plasma surface tension and its role in bubble filtration. *Perfusion*, **1**, 187–191

Chenoweth, D.E., Cooper, S.W., Hugli, A.E., *et al.* (1981) Complement activation during cardiopulmonary bypass. *New England Journal of Medicine*, **304**, 497–502

Connell, R.S., Page, U.S., Bartley, T.D., *et al.* (1973) The effect on pulmonary ultrastructure of dacron wool filtration during cardiopulmonary bypass. *Annals of Thoracic Surgery*, **15**, 217–229

Cullen, D.J. and Ferrara, L.C. (1975) Fine screen filtration of pressurized whole blood, packed cells and fresh frozen erythrocytes. *Anaesthesiology*, **47**, 578–581

Daschner, F.D., Frey, P., Wolff, G., *et al.* (1982) Nosocomical infections in intensive care wards: a multi centre prospective study. *Intensive Care Medicine*, **8**, 5–9

Denyer, S.P. (1982) In-use contamination in intravenous therapy–the scale of the problem. In *Infusions and Infections? The Hazards of In-use Contamination in Intravenous Therapy* (ed P.F. D'Arcy), The Medicine Publishing Foundation, Oxford, pp. 1–15

Deverill, C.E. and Dutt, K.K. (1980) Methods of decontamination of anaesthetic equipment: daily sessional exchange of circuits. *Journal of Hospital Infection*, **1**, 165–170

Draft, R.G. and Graf, J. (1974) Identifying particle contaminants. *Bulletin of the Parenteral Drug Association*, **28**, 35–50

Engler, R. (1987) Granulocytes and oxidative injury in myocardial ischemia and reperfusion. *Federation Proceedings*, **46**, 2395–2396

Gaillard, D., Barthelemy, R., Bouilhac, M., *et al.* (1984) Particulate contamination of priming solutions and their manipulation. Presented at *CECEC* (Paris, June, 1984)

Gallagher, J., Strangeways, J.E.M. and Allt-Graham, J. (1987) Contamination control in long term ventilation. *Anaesthesia*, **42**, 476–481

Garvan, J.M. and Gunner, B.W. (1971) Particulate contamination of intravenous fluids. *British Journal of Clinical Practice*, **25**, 119–121

George, M.D. and Morello, P.J. (1986) Immunologic effects of blood transfusion upon renal transplantation, tumour operations and bacterial infections. *American Journal of Surgery*, **152**, 329–337

Gerstmann, D.R. and Cornish, J.D. (1987) A modified circuit and priming procedure for neonatal ECMO. *Perfusion*, **2**, 171–176

Gilbert, G.L., Hayes, K., Hudson, I.L. and James, J. (1989) Prevention of transfusion acquired cytomegalovirus infections in infants by blood filtration to remove leucocytes. *Lancet*, June 3, 1228–1231

Gould, F.K., Graham, T.R., Freeman, R. and Holden, M.P. (1987) Cytomegalovirus as a cause of immunosuppression following aortic value replacement. *Perfusion*, **2**, 181–183

Gourlay, T. (1988) The role of arterial line filters in perfusion safety. *Perfusion*, **3**, 195–204

Gourlay, T., Gibbons, M., Fleming, J. and Taylor, K.M. (1987a) Performance characteristics of a new arterial line filter. *Perfusion*, **2**, 19–26

Gourlay, T., Gibbons, M., Fleming, J. and Taylor, K.M. (1987b) Evaluation of a range of arterial line filters: Part I. *Perfusion*, **2**, 297–302

Gourlay, T., Gibbons, M. and Taylor, K.M. (1988) Evaluation of a range of arterial line filters. Part II. *Perfusion*, **3**, 29–35

Hall, T.S., Breda, M.A., Baumgartner, W.A., *et al.* (1987) The role of leucocyte depletion in reducing injury to the lung after hypothermic ischaemia. *Current Surgery*, **44**, 137–139

Hearse, D.J., Erol, C., Robinson, L.A., *et al.* (1985) Particle induced coronary vasconstriction during cardioplegic infusion. *Journal of Thoracic and Cardiovascular Surgery*, **89**, 428–438

Hill, A.G., Groom, R.G., Kurusz, M., *et al.* (1985) Arterial filtration: heparin bonded or unbonded: a comparison. *Proceedings of the American Academy of Cardiovascular Perfusion*, **6**, 132–139

Hill, J.D., Osborn, J.J., Swank, R.L., *et al.* (1970) Experience using a new dacron wool filter during extracorporeal circulation. *Archives of Surgery*, **101**, 649–652

Hubbard, L.C., Kletschka, H.D., Olsen, D.A., *et al.* (1975) Spallation using roller pumps and its clinical implications. *AMSECT Proceedings*, 27–31

Hughes, C.F., Grant, A.F., Leckie, B.D. and Baird, D.K. (1986) Cardioplegic solution: a contamination crisis. *Journal of Thoracic and Cardiovascular Surgery*, **91**, 296–302

Jacques, W.F. and Mariscal, G.G. (1951) A study of the incidence of cotton emboli. *Bulletin of Internal Association of Medical Museums*, **32**, 63

Jenevien, E.P. and Weiss, D.L. (1964) Platelet microemboli associated with massive blood transfusion. *American Journal of Pathology*, **45**, 313–325

Jutison, G.A., McCloskey, D.B., Riley, J.B. and Hurdle, M.B. (1986) A comparison of a heparin coated and a non-coated ECC arterial line blood filter. *Journal of Extra Corporeal Technology*, **18**, 55–60

Kamna, G.D. and Docherty, J.P. (1979) Why filter the cardiopulmonary circuit prebypass? *Journal of Extra Corporeal Technology*, **11**, 119–130

Kharazmi, A., Andersen, L.W., Baek, L., *et al.* (1989) Endotoxemia and enhanced generation of oxygen radicals by neutrophils from patients undergoing cardiopulmonary bypass. *Journal of Thoracic and Cardiovascular Surgery*, **98**, 381–385

Krebber, H.J., Lutz, G., Polonious, M.J. and Rodewald, G. (1982) Microembolization due to micro bubbles released from the oxygenator. In *Psychopathological and Neurological Dysfunction Following Open Heart Surgery* (eds R. Becker, J. Katz, M.J. Polonious and H. Speidel), Springer-Verlag, Berlin, pp. 352–361

Kurusz, M., Shaffer, C.W., Christman, E.W. and Tyers, G.F.O. (1979) Runaway pump head: a new cause of gas embolism during cardiopulmonary bypass. *Journal of Thoracic and Cardiovascular Surgery*, **77**, 792–795

Kurusz, M., Christman, E.W., Williams, E.H. and Tyers, G.F.O. (1980) Roller pump induced tubing wear: another argument in favour of arterial line filtration. *Journal of Extra Corporeal Technology*, **12**, 49–59

Kurusz, M. and Wheeldon, D.R. (1988) Perfusion safety. *Perfusion*, **3**, 97–112

Labinger, M.D., Applegate, B.J., Gabrhel, W.F., *et al.* (1981) A new idea for venting arterial line filters. *Journal of Extracorporeal Technology*, **5**, 247–248

Lee, W.H., Brady, M.P., Rowe, J.M. and Miller, W.C. (1971) Effects of extracorporeal circulation upon behaviour, personality and brain function. *Annals of Surgery*, **173**, 1013–1023

Leong, A.S-Y (1982) Particulate contamination in intravenous therapy and extracorporeal systems. *Medical Journal of Australia*, **2**, 309–310

Leong, A.S-Y. and Gore, D.W. (1983) Pathological findings in silicone spallation *in vitro* studies. *Pathology*, **15**, 189–192

Leong, A.S-Y., Disney, A.P.S. and Gore, D.W. (1982) Spallation and migration of silicone from blood pump tubing in patients on haemodialysis. *New England Journal of Medicine*, **306**, 135–140

Lloyd, G.M. and Marshall, L. (1986) Blood microaggregates: their role in transfusion reactions. *Intensive Care World*, **3**, 119–122

Marc, B., Guillou, C., Toubon, P., *et al.* (1987) Contamination of anaesthetic breathing machines related to the delay between two sterilisations. Presented at *1st International Conference of the Hospital Infection Society* (London, 31st August–4th September, 1987)

Marshall, L. (1988) Filtration in cardiopulmonary bypass: present and future. *Perfusion*, **3**, 135–147

Marshall, L. and Lloyd, G.M. (1987) Intravenous fluid filtration. *Care of the Critically Ill*, **3**, 10–17

Murphy, M.F., Grant, P.C.A., Hardiman, A.E., *et al.* (1988) Use of leucocyte poor blood components to prevent primary cytomegalovirus. *British Journal of Haematology*, **70**, 253–255

Myers, G.J. (1987) Perfusion applications during liver transplantation. *Perfusion*, **2**, 51–56

Newman, S. (1989) The incidence and nature of neuropsychological morbidity following cardiac surgery. *Perfusion*, **4**, 93–100

Nielsen, H., Jacobsen, J.B., Stokke, D.B., *et al.* (1980) Cross-infection from contamination anaesthetic equipment. *Anaesthesia*, **35**, 703–708

Nunn, S. (1988) Cost benefit of heat and moisture exchanging filter use in anaesthesia and intensive care. Presented at *Seminars at 9 Bedford Square, Association of Anaesthetists* (London, November 23rd, 1988)

Orenstein, J.M., Sato, N., Aaron, B., *et al.* (1982) Microemboli observed in deaths following cardiopulmonary bypass surgery: silicone antifoam agents and polyvinyl chloride tubing as sources of emboli. *Human Pathology*, **13**, 1082–1090

Osborn, J.J., Swank, R.L., Hill, J.D., *et al.* (1970) Clinical use of dacron wool filter during perfusion for cardiac surgery. *Journal of Thoracic and Cardiovascular Surgery*, **60**, 575–581

Palanzo, D. (1988) Does decreasing the surface tension on an arterial line filter affect its bubble point? Presented at the *Annual Seminar on Cardiovascular Perfusion of the American Academy of Perfusion* (New Orleans, September 26th, 1988). To be published in Annual Proceedings, Volume 9.

Parrott, N.R., Lennard, W.J., Taylor, R.M.R., *et al.* (1986) Effect of perio-operative blood transfusion on recurrence of colorectal cancer. *British Journal of Surgery*, **73**, 970–973

Patterson, R.H. and Kessler, J. (1969) Microemboli during cardiopulmonary bypass detected by ultrasound. *Surgery*, **129**, 505–510

Patterson, R.H. and Twichell, J.B. (1971) Disposable filter for microemboli. *Journal of the American Medical Association*, **215**, 76–80

Pearson, D.T. (1989) Assessing cerebral damage. *Perfusion*, **4**, 101–103

Pearson, D.T., Holden, M.P., Poslad, S.J., *et al.* (1986) A clinical evaluation of one membrane and five bubble oxygenators: gas transfer and gaseous microemboli production. *Perfusion*, **1**, 15–26

Pourrat, E., Sie, P.M., Desrez, X., *et al.* (1985) Changes in plasma fibronectin levels after cardiac and pulmonary surgery: role of cardiopulmonary bypass. *Scandinavian Journal of Cardiovascular Surgery*, **19**, 63–67

Pugsley, W. (1989) The use of Doppler ultrasound in the assessment of microemboli during cardiac surgery. *Perfusion*, **4**, 115–122

Reul, G., Beall, A.C. and Greenburg, S.D. (1974) Protection of the pulmonary vasculature by fine screen filtration. *Chest*, **66**, 4–9

Robinson, L.A., Braimbridge, M.V. and Hearse, D.J. (1984) The potential hazard of particulate contamination of cardioplegic solutions. *Journal of Thoracic and Cardiovascular Surgery*, **1**, 48–58

Shaw, P.J. (1989) The incidence and nature of neurological morbidity following cardiac surgery: a review. *Perfusion*, **4**, 83–91

Shaw, P.J., Bates, D., Cartlidge, N.E.F., *et al.* (1985) Early neurological complications of coronary artery bypass surgery. *British Medical Journal*, **291**, 1384–1387

Smith, P.L.C. (1989) Interventions to reduce cerebral injury during cardiac surgery–introduction and the effect of oxygenator type. *Perfusion*, **4**, 139–145

Snyder, E.L., Mosher, D.F., Hezzey, A., *et al.* (1980) Effect of blood transfusion on plasma fibronectin. *Anaesthesiology*, **53**, 5191

Speilberg, R. and Matkovich, V.J. (1986) Gas microemboli–detection, quantitation and elimination. *Chemical Engineering Communications*, **47**, 175–183

Suttle, H.K., *et al.* (1969) *Process Engineering Technique Evaluation. Filtration*, Morgan-Grampian, London

Swank, R.L (1961) Alteration of blood on storage: measurement of adhesiveness of 'aging' platelets and leucocytes and their removal by filtration. *New England Journal of Medicine*, **265**, 728–732

Swanney, P. (1986) A comparative study of five filtered cardiotomy reservoirs. *Journal of Extra Corporeal Technology*, **18**, 7–11

Taylor, K.M. (1986) Pathophysiology of brain damage during open heart surgery. *Texas Heart Institute Journal*, **13**, 91–96

Taylor, K.M., Devlin, B.J., Mittra, S.M. (1980) Assessment of cerebral damage during open heart surgery. A new experimental model. *Scandinavian Journal of Thoracic and Cardiovascular Surgery*, **14**, 197–203

Treasure, T. (1989) Interventions to reduce cerebral injury during cardiac surgery–the effect of arterial line filtration. *Perfusion*, **4**, 147–152

Tufo, H.M., Ostfeld, A.M. and Shekelle, R. (1970) Central nervous system dysfunction following open heart surgery. *Journal of the American Medical Association*, **212**, 1333–1340

Udea, M., Kondo, Y., Fuse, K.I., *et al.* (1987) Study of particle contamination in the extracorporeal circuit using an in-line particle counter. Presented at *The Convention of Artificial Organs* (Japan, November 4th, 1987)

Verdonck, L.F., de Graan-Hentzen, Y.C.E., Dekker, A.W., Mudde, G.C. and de Gast, G.C. (1987) Cytomegalovirus seronegative platelets and leucocyte poor red blood cells from random donors can prevent primary cytomegalovirus infection after bone marrow transplantation. *Bone Marrow Transplantation*, **2**, 73–78

Warren, R.E., Newsom, S.W.B., Matthews, J.A. and Arrowsmith, L.W.M. (1986) Medical grade compressed air. *Lancet*, June 21st, 1438

Weiss, S.J. (1989) Tissue destruction by neutrophils. *New England Journal of Medicine*, **320**, 365–374

Wheeldon, D.R. and Bethune, D.W. (1986) Blood conservation during CPB–autologous transfusion, cell saving and haemofiltration. In *Cardiopulmonary Bypass. Principles and Management* (ed. K.M. Taylor), Chapman and Hall, London, pp. 289–311

Willner, A.E., Caramante, L.L., Garvey, J.W., *et al.* (1983) The relationship between arterial filtration during open heart surgery and mental abstraction ability. *Proceedings of the American Academy of Cardiovascular Perfusion*, **4**, 56–65

Yellon, R.F., Vernick, S. and Golub, A.H. (1981) Complement activation by blood microfilters. *Transfusion*, **21**, 61

6

Priming fluids for cardiopulmonary bypass

Mahesh V. Shah

History

Fresh heparinized blood was used to prime heart–lung machines during the early days of cardiopulmonary bypass. The film oxygenators then used required large priming volumes (3–5 l), so extracorporeal circulation was in effect an exchange transfusion between the patient and the priming solution. Difficulties in obtaining adequate supplies of fresh donor blood soon forced clinicians to use blood preserved with an anticoagulant solution of acid-citrate-dextrose (Zuhdi *et al.*, 1960) despite the fears that this may provoke citrate toxication. Trihydroxymethylaminomethane (THAM) was added to the banked blood to buffer the fixed acidosis of the priming solution and to prevent further acidosis from developing during cardiopulmonary bypass (Malm *et al.*, 1963). Crystalloid solutions were suspected of causing pulmonary oedema and were barely used (Trede, 1969).

Perfusing patients with homologous blood posed problems. During the early bypass period there was a fall in arterial pressure and systemic venous return, and plasma migrated unpredictably from the intravascular compartment (Dow *et al.*, 1960). There was pooling of blood in the splanchnic circulation with subsequent hepatic congestion and portal hypertension (Dow, 1959). Metabolic acidosis also developed accompanied by coagulopathy, pulmonary congestion and renal failure. Postoperative pulmonary congestion and hypoxia (perfusion lung) were caused by obstruction of the pulmonary vascular bed with platelet aggregates (McNamara *et al.*, 1972) and immunologically triggered opening of pulmonary shunts (Melrose *et al.*, 1965). Gadboys, Slonim and Litwak (1962) described this combination of sequelae as the 'homologous blood syndrome' and postulated that it was precipitated by incompatibility reactions not only between donor and recipient but also between the individual pooled donor elements. There was also a risk of viral hepatitis of between 0.16% and 6% even after screening donors for the presence of Australia antigen (Doenicke, Grote and Lorenz, 1977). The above mentioned problems with blood prompted the search for alternative priming solutions.

Panico and Neptune in 1959 designed a pump oxygenator in which a saline prime was layered on top of the patient's blood, thus reducing the quantity of blood needed for perfusion. The concept of haemodilution prompted experimental and clinical studies at various centres. The large volume oxygenators used in those days prevented the use of total non-haemic primes to preserve the oxygen carrying capacity of the fluid.

Initial successful use of dextrose 5% in water was described by Zuhdi's group (1961) and by Cooley, Beall and Alexander (1961). Long *et al.* (1961) used low molecular weight dextran (LMWD) to prevent sludging of blood and to improve microcirculation, both alone and in various combinations with electrolyte and albumin solutions. They noted improved urine outputs and a reduction in haemolysis. Coagulation was not a problem provided the dose of LMWD did not exceed 20 ml kg^{-1} of body weight. On the contrary Hepps *et al.* (1963) found that with LMWD postoperative bleeding increased even though coagulation profiles were normal.

Modern oxygenators require only 1.5–2 l of prime, therefore there has been a significant reduction in the use of blood during cardiopulmonary bypass. Some authors have advocated primes of only electrolyte solutions (Lilleaason, Frøysaker and Stokke, 1978) while others recommend crystalloid-colloid mixtures (Sade *et al.*, 1985; McGrath, Gonzalez-Lavin and Neary, 1989).

Table 6.1 Priming fluids used in 30 National Health Service cardiothoracic units

Fluids	*Number of centres*
Hartmann's solution	15
Dextrose 5% and Hartmann's solution	2
Hartmann's solution and mannitol	4
Hartmann's solution and urea linked gelatin	6
Hartmann's solution, succinylated gelatin and mannitol	1
Plasmolyte 148 and urea linked gelatin	1
Plasmolyte 148 and hydroxyethyl starch	1

No obvious problems have been noted despite the diverse range of solutions used.

The results of a survey of priming fluids used in 30 National Health Service cardiothoracic units are shown in Table 6.1.

Principles of haemodilution

Regardless of the priming fluid selected the solution should be able adequately to oxygenate the body tissue during bypass and also be able to clear tissue metabolites. This depends upon:

1. an adequate oxygen carrying capacity of the fluid
2. the pattern of blood flow to the tissues.

Oxygen transport

The optimum haematocrit of normothermic blood is about 30% (Kessler and Messmer, 1975; Messmer, 1987). The need for blood transfusion to maintain this figure has recently been questioned since the discovery of the human immunodeficiency virus (Carson *et al.*, 1988). Induced hypothermia during cardiopulmonary bypass protects against further haemodilution because the oxygen consumption is reduced to 50% of normal at 30°C and 20% at 20°C (Gott *et al.*, 1962). This reduction in oxygen consumption also protects against the reduced oxygen availability to the tissues due to the shift to the left of the oxyhaemoglobin dissociation curve caused by hypothermia. Also, more oxygen is dissolved in plasma at lower temperatures.

Experimental attempts have been made to prime bypass machines with solutions of low haematocrit, with the help of liquids capable of transporting oxygen. Oxygen dissolves readily in fluorocarbon emulsions, which are inert, but the early experimental use of these solutions has not developed to the stage of clinical usage (Englemann *et al.*, 1981; Hoshino *et al.*, 1982). The temporary use of fluorocarbons during cardiopulmonary bypass causes retention of the fluorocarbon by the reticuloendothelial system and haemolysis in some animals. Stroma free haemoglobin solutions have also not yet developed to the stage where they can be used clinically. The small molecular size of stroma free haemoglobin means that they have rapid transcapillary leakage and renal clearance. Furthermore tissue oxygen availability is impaired because they have a greater oxygen affinity than intracorpuscular haemoglobin (Messmer *et al.*, 1978).

Tissue perfusion

Tissue perfusion depends upon the blood flow and vascular resistance:

$$\text{Perfusion pressure} = \text{blood flow} \times \text{vascular resistance}$$

Clowes (1972) has shown that at perfusion flow rates of less than 21 m^{-2} min^{-1}, oxygen consumption falls and base deficit increases during normothermic cardiopulmonary bypass.

The systemic vascular resistance depends upon arteriolar dilatation and viscosity. Arteriolar dilatation may occur at the commencement of bypass because of an alteration in baroreceptor perception as blood flow changes from a pulsatile to a non-pulsatile mode (Dunn *et al.*, 1974) and also due to a dilution of circulating catecholamines (Balasaraswathi *et al.*, 1980).

The viscosity of blood varies with its haematocrit. With crystalloid primes, the blood pressure falls significantly at the commencement of bypass because of a sudden reduction of viscosity as a result of haemodilution (Gordon *et al.*, 1975). Subsequently the fluid viscosity increases as the body temperature is decreased. Thus during bypass with high flow rates and moderate hypothermia adequate tissue oxygenation will be maintained with a haematocrit down to 20% (Kessler and Messmer, 1975).

Crystalloid solutions

Dextrose 5 mg/100 ml in water

Zuhdi's group (1961) first used low volume primes of 5% dextrose in water and perfused at low flow rates to minimize mechanical damage to erythrocytes. Cooley, Beall and Grondin (1962) and Paton and Rosenkrantz (1965) noted excellent intraoperative and postoperative diuresis when they used 5% dextrose, 20 ml kg^{-1} of body weight, with a bubble oxygenator. Patients were mentally alert after surgery and pulmonary congestion was not a problem.

Dextrose 5% is a cheap, slightly hypotonic, slightly acidotic solution (pH 4.0). When dextrose is metabolized the dilution effect of the water on the plasma bicarbonate may cause systemic metabolic acidosis (Ing *et al.*, 1977), hyponatraemia and hypokalaemia. The hypotonicity was also felt to be the cause of increased haemolysis (Paton and Rosenkrantz, 1965). Varying amounts of fluid shift out of the intravascular space and additional fluid has to be added during bypass.

Serum glucose and insulin levels are raised during non-pulsatile perfusion, even with non-glucose primes (Hewitt *et al.*, 1972). The addition of glucose can lead to very high blood glucose concentrations and may lead to hyperosmotic, hyperglycaemic, non-ketotic coma in diabetic patients (Mills *et al.*, 1973). Glucose included in cardioplegic solutions can have a damaging effect on the heart as a result of osmotic and metabolic effect (Hearse *et al.*, 1978). However dextrose, potassium and insulin may be beneficial to the ischaemic heart (Brachfield, 1973; Kones, 1975).

Balanced crystalloid solutions

Balanced crystalloid solutions were introduced so that the ion concentration of the perfusate and the patient's plasma were similar. Roe *et al.* (1964) used a small prime of a balanced electrolyte solution together with LMWD with a disposable oxygenator. Serum electrolytes were remarkably stable and metabolic acidosis was not a problem. Red cell damage was reduced and there were minimal postoperative pulmonary or renal problems. Neville *et al.* (1967) used buffered Ringer's lactate as a complete prime for a large volume disc oxygenator with similar good results.

Ringer's lactate primes have tended to cause fluid retention (Neville *et al.*, 1966; Sade *et al.*, 1985) which can be treated with fluid restriction and diuretics. Hypokalaemia has been observed with Ringer's lactate primes (Dieter *et al.*, 1970). The hypokalaemia occurs because in the renal tubules potassium is excreted in exchange for sodium. Hypokalaemia also occurs because of previous diuretic therapy (Lockey *et al.*, 1966), hyperglycaemia (Barnard *et al.*, 1959) and changes in phosphate metabolism (Vasko, DeWall and Riley, 1973). Administration of large volumes of normal saline may cause hyperchloraemic acidosis.

Plasmolyte 148 is the other balanced electrolyte solution in the UK. Compared with Ringer's lactate it has magnesium 1.5 mmol l^{-1} and has acetate and gluconate instead of lactate as sources for bicarbonate.

Mannitol

Mannitol is an inert, undissociated, six-carbon polyhydric alcohol which has long been used as an osmotic diuretic. It is also a free radical scavenger. The osmotic pressure of mannitol depends upon the strength of the solution. It is rapidly excreted by the kidneys, 80% of a 100 g dose appearing in the urine in 3h. Its addition to the prime has been noted to reduce haemolysis and the incidence of renal failure (Porter *et al.*, 1967).

Colloid solutions

Only 25–30% of crystalloid solutions administered to patients are distributed in the intravascular compartment (Shoemaker, 1976). The sole use of crystalloid solutions for cardiopulmonary bypass causes extravascular fluid shifts and weight gain (Neville *et al.*, 1966; Sade *et al.*, 1985). Additional fluid has to be added during the procedure and at the termination of bypass it is necessary to re-infuse the patient with a large portion of the diluted prime (Edie, Haubert and Malm, 1981). Greater somatic and pulmonary fluid accumulation has been observed in patients when only lactated Ringer's solution was used as the prime, compared with when colloids were added to it (Sade *et al.*, 1985). Positive fluid balance during bypass is associated with an increase in extravascular lung water accompanied by a deterioration of pulmonary gas exchange (Boldt *et al.*, 1986). Various colloid solutions have therefore been used in the priming fluid.

Albumin

Human albumin solutions are prepared from pooled human plasma, by cold ethanol fractionation. The solution is sterilized by filtration and then heated for 20h at 59.5°C to inactivate contaminating viruses. The oncotic pressure of the albumin solutions depends upon the albumin content. The plasma half-life is 15h.

Several authors have described the addition of albumin to the prime with good clinical results (Long *et al.*, 1961; Deihl, Lester and Cosgrove, 1982; Kirklin, Lell and Kouchoukos, 1984). Albumin also prevents red cell crenation in patients undergoing extracorporeal circulation (Kamada *et al.*, 1988). However the relative cost of albumin solutions has prompted the use of alternative colloid solutions.

Dextrans

Dextrans are high molecular weight polysaccharides linked predominantly in the a 1:6 glucosidic configurations. They are biosynthesized by the action of *Leuconostoc mesenteroides* on sucrose (Mishler, 1984). The two most commonly used preparations are dextran 40 and dextran 70 available in either 0.9% saline or 5% glucose. Dextran 40 has a greater oncotic and blood volume expanding effect immediately after infusion but because of its relative short half-life of 2.5h, the blood volume expanding effect is lost by 6h. Dextran 40 may cause oliguria and so it should be avoided in patients with impending renal failure (Matheson and Robertson, 1966). The beneficial effect of improved haemodynamics may last 24h or longer with dextran 70 because it has a longer half-life of approximately 25h.

Doses of dextran up to 1.5 g kg^{-1} of body weight induce no measurable changes in the clotting mechanism but the bleeding time is prolonged. Higher doses impair clotting by preventing platelet aggregation (Hassig and Stampfli, 1969) and by the facilitation of fibrinolysis by plasmin.

The incidence of anaphylactic reactions to dextran can be reduced with the preadministration of dextran 1, a monovalent haptid which binds presensitized antibodies (Renck *et al.*, 1983).

Dextrans prevent the sludging of red cells and have been used successfully as priming fluids for cardiopulmonary bypass (Drake *et al.*, 1961; Long *et al.*, 1961; McGrath *et al.*, 1989).

Gelatins

Gelatins are prepared by hydrolysis of bovine collagen. They have an average molecular weight of 35 000 and therefore are rapidly excreted in the urine, thus limiting their oncotic effect. There are two types of gelatin solutions, the urea-linked gelatin and the succinylated gelatin (modified fluid gelatin). Urea-linked gelatin has a higher calcium content so it should not be mixed with citrated blood because clots may form. This is not a problem with heparinized blood (personal observation). Urea-linked gelatins have been used effectively during cardiopulmonary bypass (Moyes, 1974; Merikallio, 1976). Both urea-linked and succinylated gelatins have been used extensively in our institution without any untoward effects.

Hydroxyethyl starch

Hydroxyethyl starch (HES) is a synthetic polymer manufactured by hydrolysing a waxy species of either maize or sorghum. Molecules of various sizes can be made and may contain variable numbers of substituted hydroxyethyl groups. Numerous studies have demonstrated the safety of high molecular weight HES which has an average molecular weight of 450 000 available as a 6% solution (Lee, Rubin and Huggins, 1975; Mishler *et al.*, 1975; Palanzo *et al.*, 1982; Saunders, Carlisle and Bick, 1983).

When HES containing primes were compared with lactated Ringer's solution or albumin, platelet counts were significantly decreased initially following bypass. However there were no significant differences in postoperative blood loss (Saunders, Carlisle and Bick, 1983; Sade *et al.*, 1985). It is recommended that the volume of HES administered should not exceed 20 ml kg^{-1} of body weight.

The lower molecular weight HES has an average molecular weight of 264 000 with a half-life of 2.5h. Studies describing its use in priming fluids have not yet appeared.

Anaphylactic reactions may occur after the infusion of any of the colloid solutions. Serious reactions occur in less than 1:5000 infusions. Ring and Messmer (1977) found the incidence of serious reactions to be 0.004% with plasma protein fractions, 0.006% with HES, 0.008% with dextran and 0.038% with gelatins. In contrast, Waldhausen, Keser and Harguardt (1988) in a report on 54 cases on anaphylaxis from a variety of causes, found that treatment with synthetic colloids produced marginally better results than albumin.

References

Balasaraswathi, K., Gilsson, S.N., El-Etr, A.A. and Azad, C. (1980) Effect of priming volume on serum catecholamines during cardiopulmonary bypass. *Canadian Anaesthetic Society Journal*, **27**, 135–139

Barnard, C.N., DeWall, R.A., Vasco, R.L. and Lillihei, C.W. (1959) Pre and postoperative care of patients undergoing open heart surgery. *Diseases of the Chest*, **35**, 194–211

Boldt, J., von Bormann, B., Kling, D., *et al.* (1986) The influence of extracorporeal circulation on extravascular lung water in coronary surgery patients. *Journal of Thoracic and Cardiovascular Surgery*, **34**, 110–115

Brachfeld, N. (1973) The glucose-insulin-potassium (GIK) regimen in the treatment of myocardial ischaemia. *Circulation*, **49**, 459–462

Carson, J.L., Poses, R.M., Spence, R.K. and Bonavita, G. (1988) Severity of anaemia and postoperative mortality and morbidity. *Lancet*, **i**, 727–729

Clowes, G.H.A. Jr. (1972) The physiologic basis of cardiac surgery. In *Cardiac Surgery*, 2nd edn, (ed. J.C. Norman), Appleton-Century-Crofts, New York, pp. 13–66

Cooley, D.A., Beall, A.C. Jr. and Alexander, J.K. (1961) Acute massive pulmonary embolism: successful surgical treatment using temporary cardiopulmonary bypass. *Journal of the American Medical Association*, **177**, 283–286

Cooley, D.A., Beall, A.C. Jr. and Grondin, P. (1962) Open-heart operations with disposable oxygenators, 5% dextrose prime and normothermia. *Surgery*, **52**, 713–719

Deihl, J.T., Lester III, J.L. and Cosgrove, D.M. (1982) Clinical comparison of hetastarch and albumin in postoperative cardiac patients. *Annals of Thoracic Surgery*, **34**, 674–679

Deiter, R.A. Jr., Neville, W.E. and Pifarre, R. (1970) Serum electrolyte changes after cardiopulmonary bypass with Ringer's lactate solution used for hemodilution. *Journal of Thoracic and Cardiovascular Surgery*, **59**, 169–177

Doenicke, A., Grote, B. and Lorenz, W. (1977) Blood and blood substitutes. *British Journal of Anaesthesia*, **49**, 681–688

Dow, J.W. (1959) The shock state in heart-lung bypass in dogs. *Transactions of the American Society for Artificial Internal Organs*, **5**, 689

Dow, J.W., Dickson III, J.F., Hamer, N.A. and Gadboys, H.L. (1960) Anaphylactoid shock due to homologous blood exchange in the dog. *Journal of Thoracic and Cardiovascular Surgery*, **39**, 449–456

Drake, C.T., Macalalad, F. and Lewis, F.J. (1961) The effect of low molecular weight dextran upon the blood flow during extracorporeal circulation. *Journal of Thoracic and Cardiovascular Surgery*, **42**, 735–742

Dunn, J., Kirsch, M.M., Harness, J., *et al.* (1974) Hemodynamic, metabolic and hematologic effects of pulsatile cardiopulmonary bypass. *Journal of Thoracic and Cardiovascular Surgery*, **68**, 138–147

Edie, R.N., Haubert, S.M. and Malm, J.R. (1981) The use of haemodilution and a non-haemic prime for cardiopulmonary bypass. In *Techniques in Extracorporeal Circulation*, 2nd edn, (ed. M.I. Ionescu) Butterworths, London, pp. 179–198

Englemann, R.M., Rousou, J.H. and Dobbs, W.A. (1981) Fluosol DA, an artificial blood for total cardiopulmonary bypass. *Annals of Thoracic Surgery*, **32**, 528–535

Gadboys, H.L., Slonim, R. and Litwak, R.S. (1962) Homologous blood syndrome: 1 Preliminary observations on its relationship to clinical cardiopulmonary bypass. *Annals of Surgery*, **156**, 793–804

Gordon, R.J., Ravin, M., Rawitscher, R.E. and Daicoff, G.R. (1975) Changes in arterial pressure, viscosity and resistance during cardiopulmonary bypass. *Journal of Thoracic and Cardiovascular Surgery*, **69**, 552–561

Gott, V.L., Bartlett, M., Long, D.M., *et al.* (1962) Myocardial energy substrates in the dog heart during potassium and hypothermic arrest. *Journal of Applied Physiology*, **17**, 815–819

Hassig, A. and Stampfli, K. (1969) Plasma substitutes, past and present. In *Modified Gelatins as Plasma Substitutes. Bibliotheca Haematologica*, **33**, 1–7

Hearse, D.J., Stewart, D.A. and Braimbridge, M.V. (1978) Myocardial protection during ischemic cardiac arrest. Possible deleterious effects of glucose and mannitol in coronary infusates. *Journal of Thoracic and Cardiovascular Surgery*, **76**, 16–23

Hepps, S.A., Roe, B.R., Wright, R.R. and Gardner, R.E. (1963) Amelioration of the pulmonary postperfusion syndrome with hemodilution and low molecular weight dextran. *Surgery*, **54**, 32–43

Hewitt, R.L., Woo, R.D., Ryan, J.R. and Drapanas, T. (1972) Plasma insulin and glucose relationships during cardiopulmonary bypass. *Surgery*, **71**, 905–912

Hoshino, S., Iwaya, F., Igari, T., *et al.* (1982) Extracorporeal circulation with perflurochemicals (Fluosol-DA). *Journal of Cardiovascular Surgery*, **23**, 463–469

Ing, T.S., Wu, C., Rosenberg, J.C., *et al.* (1977) Cerebrospinal fluid changes in experimental cardiopulmonary bypass using hemodilution with glucose water. *Neurology*, **27**, 85–89

Kamada, T., McMillan, D.E., Sternlieb, J.J., *et al.* (1988) Albumin prevents erythrocyte crenation in patients undergoing extracorporeal circulation. *Scandinavian Journal of Thoracic and Cardiovascular Surgery*, **22**, 155–158

Kessler, M. and Messmer, K. (1975) Tissue oxygenation during hemodilution. In *International Hemodilution. Bibliotheca Haematologica*, **41**, 16–33

Kirklin, J.K., Lell, W.A. and Kouchoukos, N.T. (1984) Hydroxyethyl starch versus albumin for colloid infusion following cardiopulmonary bypass in patients undergoing myocardial revascularization. *Annals of Thoracic Surgery*, **37**, 40–46

Kones, R.J. (1975) Glucose, insulin and potassium therapy for heart disease. History of GIK therapy. *New York State Journal of Medicine*, **75**, 1463–1492

Lee, W.H., Rubin, J.W. and Huggins, M.P. (1975) Clinical evaluation of priming solutions for pump oxygenator perfusion. *Annals of Thoracic Surgery*, **19**, 529–536

Lilleaason, P., Froysaker, T. and Stokke, O. (1978) Cardiac surgery in extreme haemodilution without donor blood, blood products or artificial macromolecules. *Scandinavian Journal of Thoracic and Cardiovascular Surgery*, **12**, 249–251

Lockey, E., Ross, D.N., Longmore, D.B. and Sturridge, M.F. (1966) Potassium and open-heart surgery. *Lancet*, **i**, 671–675

Long, D.M., Sanchez, L., Vasco, R.L. and Lillehei, C.W. (1961) The use of low molecular weight dextran and serum albumin as plasma expanders in extracorporeal circulation. *Surgery*, **50**, 12–28

McGrath, L.B., Gonzalez-Lavin, L. and Neary, M.J. (1989) Comparison of dextran 40 with albumin and Ringer's lactate as components of perfusion prime for cardiopulmonary bypass in patients undergoing myocardial revascularization. *Perfusion*, **4**, 41–49

McNamara, J.J., Burran, E.L., Larson, E., *et al.* (1972) Effect of debris in stored blood on pulmonary microvasculature. *Annals of Thoracic Surgery*, **14**, 133–139

Malm, J.R., Sullivan, S.F., Patterson, R.W., *et al.* (1963) The use of ACD blood titrated with THAM in extracorporeal circulation. *Transactions of the American Society for Artificial Internal Organs*, **9**, 216–219

Matheson, N.A. and Robertson, J.W. (1966) Effects of dextran 40 on postoperative haemodynamics. *Lancet*, **ii**, 251–253

Melrose, D.G., Nahas, R., Alvarez, D., *et al.* (1965) Postoperative hypoxia after extracorporeal circulation: a possible graft against host reaction. *Experimentia*, **21**, 47–50

Merikallio, E. (1976) Haemodilution in cardiopulmonary bypass using a gelatin derivative for priming. *Annals of Chirurgy and Gynaecology*, **65**, 138–144

Messmer, K. (1987) Acceptable haematocrit levels in surgical patients. *World Journal of Surgery*, **6**, 41–46

Messmer, K., Jesch, F., Schaff, J., *et al.* (1978) Oxygen supply by stroma-free haemoglobin. *Progress in Clinical and Biological Research*, **19**, 175–190

Mills, N.L., Baudet, R.L., Isom, D.W. and Spencer, F.C. (1973) Hyperglycaemia during cardiopulmonary bypass. *Annals of Surgery*, **177**, 203–205

Mishler, J.M. (1984) Synthetic plasma volume expanders–their pharmacology, safety and clinical efficacy. *Clinics in Haematology*, **13**, 75–92

Mishler, J.M., Nicora, R.W., Yoshitake, T., *et al.* (1975) Hemodilution with hydroxyethyl starch during cardiopulmonary bypass: Review of a multi-institutional study. *Journal of Extra Corporeal Technology*, **7**, 140–149

Moyes, D.G. (1974) Haemodilution with a plasma expander as priming solution in cardiopulmonary bypass. *South African Medical Journal*, **48**, 1615–1616

Neville, W.E., Colby, C., Peacock, H. and Kronkowski, T.C. (1967) Superiority of buffered Ringer's lactate to heparinized blood as total prime for the large volume disc oxygenator. *Annals of Surgery*, **165**, 206–216

Neville, W.E., Thomason, R.D. and Hirsch, D.M. (1966) Postperfusion hypervolaemia after hemodilution cardiopulmonary bypass. *Archives of Surgery*, **93**, 715–723

Palanzo, D.A., Grant, C.P., Parr, V.S., *et al.* (1982) Hetastarch as a prime for cardiopulmonary bypass. *Annals of Thoracic Surgery*, **34**, 680–683

Panico, F.G. and Neptune, W.B. (1959) A mechanism to eliminate donor blood prime from the pump oxygenator. *Surgical Forum*, **10**, 605–609

Paton, B.C. and Rosenkrantz, J. (1965) Non-hemic priming fluids for extracorporeal circulation. *Diseases of the Chest*, **48**, 311–318

Porter, G.A., Starr, A., Kimsey, J. and Lenertz, H. (1967) Mannitol haemodilution-perfusion: the kinetics of mannitol distribution and excretion during cardiopulmonary bypass. *Journal of Surgical Research*, **7**, 447–456

Renck, H., Lungstrom, K.G., Rosberg, B., *et al.* (1983) Prevention of dextran-induced anaphylactic reactions by hapten inhibition II. *Acta Chirurgica Scandinavica*, **149**, 349–353

Ring, J. and Messmer, K. (1977) Incidence and severity of anaphylactoid reactions to colloid volume substitutes. *Lancet*, **i**, 466–469

Roe, B.B., Swenson, E.E., Hepps, S.A. and Bruns, D.L. (1964) Total body perfusion in cardiac operations with perfusate of balanced electrolyte and low molecular weight dextran. *Archives of Surgery*, **88**, 128–134

Sade, R.M., Stroud, M.R., Crawford, F.A., *et al.* (1985) A prospective randomized study of hydroxyethyl starch, albumin and lactated Ringer's solution as priming fluid for cardiopulmonary bypass. *Journal of Thoracic and Cardiovascular Surgery*, **89**, 713–722

Saunders, C.R., Carlisle, L. and Bick, R.L. (1983) Hydroxyethyl starch versus albumin in cardiopulmonary bypass prime solutions. *Annals of Thoracic Surgery*, **36**, 532–539

Shoemaker, W.C. (1976) Comparison of the relative effectiveness of whole blood transfusions and various types of fluid therapy in resuscitation. *Critical Care Medicine*, **4**, 71–78

Trede, M. (1969) Experimental investigations into the behaviour of coagulation and renal function during high dilution perfusions with glucose, Haemaccel and Rheomacrodex. In *Modified Gelatine as Plasma Substitutes. Bibliotheca Haematologica*, **33**, 553–568

Vasko, K.A., DeWall, R.A. and Riley, A.M. (1973) Hypokalaemia: physiological abnormalities during cardiopulmonary bypass. *Annals of Thoracic Surgery*, **15** 347–353

Waldhausen, E., Keser, G. and Harguardt, B. (1988) Colloids anaphylaxis and the heart. *Lancet*, **ii**, 220

Zuhdi, N., McMollough, B., Carey, J. and Greer, A. (1960) The use of citrated banked blood for open heart surgery. *Anesthesiology*, **21**, 496–501

Zuhdi, N., McMollough, B., Carey, J., *et al.* (1961) Hypothermic perfusion for open-heart surgical procedures: a report on the use of a heart–lung machine primed with 5% dextrose in water inducing hemodilution. *Journal of the International College of Surgeons*, **35**, 319–326

7

Anaesthetic techniques for cardiopulmonary bypass

J.W.W. Gothard

The anaesthetist plays a major role in patient management during cardiac surgery. Anaesthesia is only one component of this role which includes manipulation of the circulation, control of ventilation and supervision of cardiopulmonary bypass. Ideally this supportive role of the anaesthetist should allow the surgeon to operate in optimal conditions and with no, or minimal, disturbance from outside the operative area. This is essential if good surgical results are to be achieved and maintained.

One chapter on cardiac anaesthesia cannot possibly cover the whole of the subject in detail. The principles of anaesthesia for cardiopulmonary bypass will therefore be outlined and, where appropriate, matters which remain controversial or are topical will be discussed in more detail.

Preoperative assessment

It is essential that cardiac surgical patients are seen and assessed by an anaesthetist preoperatively. Patients presenting for cardiac surgery either routinely or as an emergency have usually been fully investigated by the time an anaesthetist is involved in their management but points of specific anaesthetic interest may have been overlooked. Will endotracheal intubation be difficult, for example? Is there a likelihood of oesophageal reflux? Have there been anaesthetic problems in the past? These are just a few of the questions that need to be answered.

A full medical history and physical examination should be available from the case notes. These findings can be augmented by further questioning or clinical examination if this is indicated.

The anaesthetist should familiarize himself with the cardiac diagnosis and any relevant investigations that have been carried out such as cardiac catheterization, echocardiography, Doppler measurements and so on. Particular note should be made of factors that are likely to increase the risk of surgery or change anaesthetic management. In patients scheduled for coronary artery bypass known risk factors include left main stem coronary disease, congestive heart failure, a reduced ejection fraction, an increased left ventricular end-diastolic pressure, increasing age and female gender. Emergency coronary artery surgery is also associated with a higher mortality than an elective procedure.

Patients with valvular heart disease may be in an older age group but they also present risk factors relating to the natural history and pathophysiology of their disease. Myocardial failure is a late complication of both aortic incompetence and stenosis, for example, but is a particularly worrying feature with a purely regurgitant valve. In addition, patients with aortic stenosis do not tolerate a tachycardia or atrial fibrillation well because of the increased contribution of atrial systole to left ventricular diastolic volume in this disease. Severe pulmonary hypertension is an obvious risk factor in long standing mitral stenosis which may necessitate prolonged postoperative ventilation because of the associated decrease in lung compliance and increased work of breathing. In pure chronic mitral regurgitation, however, symptoms of pulmonary congestion are a worrying feature because the compliant left atrium usually accommodates the regurgitant blood from the left ventricle until late in the disease. Cardiac symptomatology can be assessed on the basis of the rather broad, but nevertheless helpful, New York Heart Association Classification (Table 7.1).

Following familiarization with the cardiac diagnosis a systematic review is made of the patient's general medical status, again concentrating on those

Table 7.1 The New York Heart Association Classification

Class 1	Heart disease, no symptoms
Class 2	Comfortable at rest, symptoms with ordinary activity
Class 3	Comfortable at rest Symptoms with minimal activity
Class 4	Symptoms at rest

points which will influence management during anaesthesia and cardiopulmonary bypass. The presence of carotid artery stenosis, for example, may require further investigation or treatment before cardiac surgery and will certainly influence management during cardiopulmonary bypass (see Chapter 13). Treatment schedules for other conditions such as diabetes may have to be modified before, and during, the surgical period. Routine laboratory investigations will include a full blood count, clotting screen, liver and renal function tests, blood grouping, blood crossmatch and a hepatitis screen. Cardiac enzyme levels should be requested in those patients who have had recent episodes of prolonged chest pain and other categories of patient may require specific tests such as sickle cell screening, drug levels, and so on. A recent chest radiograph and electrocardiogram should be available. Finally, all drug therapy and allergies are noted.

The majority of cardioactive drugs are continued up to and including the morning of surgery. It is particularly important to continue antianginal therapy in the form of β-adrenergic blockade, oral and transdermal nitrates and calcium channel blocking agents in order to minimize the risk of further ischaemia in the perioperative period. Theoretical problems of anaesthetic drug interactions and myocardial depression with these agents have not been realized in practice (Streisand and Wong, 1988). Antiarrhythmic drugs should, similarly, not be discontinued in the majority of cases before cardiac surgery. It has been a tradition to discontinue digoxin for 48h prior to operation but this seems unnecessary if the serum level is within the therapeutic range, particularly as serum potassium levels can now be readily measured in whole blood analysers situated in the operating theatre and intensive care unit.

Patients taking the antiplatelet drugs aspirin and dipyridamole should, ideally, discontinue these 7–10 days before surgery because there is a higher incidence of significant postoperative bleeding in their presence. The optimum management of patients taking coumarin-type anticoagulants is more difficult to define. Although these drugs are generally withdrawn a day or two before surgery, few surgeons insist on a normal prothrombin time preoperatively, preferring to operate when the prothrombin time is approximately twice control values. Rapid correction of the prothrombin time preoperatively with vitamin K and fresh frozen plasma may increase the risk of thrombosis in certain patients, particularly those with a history of embolic disease or those with a prosthetic valve *in situ*. If surgery is undertaken in the presence of a raised prothrombin time haemostasis must be meticulous and clotting factors should be administered on the basis of controlled laboratory tests.

Patients taking H_2 antagonists should continue this therapy, intravenously if necessary, throughout the perioperative period. Cardiac surgery is a stressful procedure and anticoagulation is often employed in the postoperative period so there is an increased risk of gastric erosion and bleeding.

Premedication

A sympathetic explanation of the proposed operation and the sequence of events in the perioperative period will allay many of the anxieties of the patient awaiting cardiac surgery. The majority of patients will still benefit from premedication, however.

The choice of premedicant drugs is rarely important. Many anaesthetists, and an increasing number of patients, prefer oral premedication. The benzodiazepine group of drugs is useful in this context but the longer acting agents should be avoided if an early resumption of spontaneous respiration is planned in the postoperative period. Many anaesthetists prefer to prescribe a morphine based opiate (usually papaveretum in the UK) combined with hyoscine and given intramuscularly 1.5–2h preoperatively. The main drawback of this combination is its tendency to cause a dry oropharynx.

Patients scheduled for routine coronary artery surgery are likely to tolerate relatively heavy premedication, although the need for this has lessened somewhat now that antianginal therapy is continued to control tachycardia and ischaemia in the preoperative period. Drug dosages must obviously be curtailed in elderly patients and it is wise to omit atropine from premedication for patients with valvular heart disease who will not tolerate a tachycardia. Occasionally patients presenting for emergency surgery have such a low cardiac output that it is preferable to withhold any preoperative sedation until adequate monitoring has been established (see below) either in the anaesthetic room or the operating theatre.

Choice of anaesthetic technique

In recent years there has been a wealth of information published on techniques of anaesthesia for cardiac surgery and the effect of anaesthetic agents on the myocardium and cardiovascular system. The majority of the work reported concerns the ischaemic heart. It is difficult to put in perspective the many reports of *in vitro* experimentation and studies in various animal species and man, although there has been much comment (Merin, Lowenstein and Gelman, 1986; Becker, 1987; Mangano, 1989) and several excellent reviews relating to these aspects of cardiac anaesthesia (Moffitt and Sethna, 1986; Reiz, 1988; Prys-Roberts, 1988; Streisand and Wong, 1988). In the following sections of this chapter management of anaesthesia for cardiopulmonary bypass is discussed from a practical standpoint in what remains a rapidly changing and controversial field.

Induction of anaesthesia

Anaesthesia for cardiac surgery in adults is invariably induced intravenously. The drugs used for induction of anaesthesia will depend to some extent on what agents are to be used for maintenance (see below). For example, if a high-dose opiate technique is to be employed then fentanyl can be given slowly to provide a satisfactory depth of anaesthesia without significant depression of the myocardium. The addition of nitrous oxide to a high dose opiate regime can, however, cause profound myocardial depression.

A more common approach to induction is to administer a moderate dose of opiate (fentanyl 10 $\mu g\ kg^{-1}$; alfentanil 50–100 $\mu g\ kg^{-1}$; sufentanil 10–15 $\mu g\ kg^{-1}$) before a minimal dose of thiopentone, etomidate or propofol. This technique provides a smooth induction and minimizes the drop in arterial blood pressure largely caused by a combination of myocardial depression and decrease in systemic vascular resistance when these agents are used alone in larger doses. Etomidate, which has minimal effects on the cardiovascular system in normal subjects, does tend to drop arterial pressure in patients with cardiac disease although to a lesser extent than other agents. This agent is therefore useful when coronary perfusion pressure is particularly critical in patients with mainstem disease of the left coronary artery and aortic valve stenosis. Etomidate must however be used with care in the elderly. Larsen *et al.* (1988) for example, in a study on geriatric patients demonstrated a pronounced drop in arterial pressure not only with propofol which was predictable, but also with etomidate.

Alternative techniques to those described above include the use of intravenous benzodiazepines and ketamine. Cardiovascular stability is well maintained when diazepam is used alone and therefore this drug can be used for sedation while invasive monitoring is established under local anaesthesia. The substantial rise in arterial pressure associated with the use of ketamine is undesirable before the majority of cardiac procedures and the drug is little used.

After induction of anaesthesia endotracheal intubation is carried out following the administration of a non-depolarizing muscle relaxant, intermittent positive pressure ventilation [IPPV] can then be commenced. Pancuronium (0.12–0.15 mg kg^{-1}) is widely used to provide muscle relaxation for cardiac surgery. This drug tends to cause a tachycardia and an elevation of arterial blood pressure, features which were considered an advantage when the drug was first introduced before the expansion of cardiac surgery for coronary artery disease. Thomson and Putnins (1985) showed that the use of pancuronium combined with high-dose fentanyl in patients undergoing surgery for ischaemic heart disease may cause significant elevations in heart rate and electrocardiographic (ECG) evidence of ischaemia. Significant tachycardia, however, is less likely in patients taking adequate doses of β-adrenergic blocking agents up to the time of surgery. In addition, O'Connor *et al.* (1989) using an anaesthetic technique of fentanyl combined with enflurane have recently demonstrated a low incidence of ischaemia in patients undergoing coronary artery surgery when either pancuronium or vecuronium was used as the muscle relaxant. Vecuronium does not influence heart rate or arterial pressure in fit patients undergoing general anaesthesia (Wierda *et al.*, 1989) and in the study of O'Connor *et al.* (1989) significant tachycardia (more than 90 beats per minute) was much more frequent in patients receiving pancuronium. This tachycardia was treated with propranolol and there was no significant difference in the incidence of ischaemia between the two groups. It would seem reasonable to continue to use the longer acting drug, pancuronium, to produce muscular paralysis for cardiac surgery on present evidence, provided its cardiovascular side effects are controlled. Vecuronium should be considered, however, for patients prone to tachy-dysrhythmias and those undergoing short procedures.

Maintenance of anaesthesia

Anaesthesia not only provides complete analgesia and lack of awareness for the patient but also a means of promoting cardiovascular stability during the operative period. In the case of coronary artery disease systemic pressures are kept in a low-normal range, taking account of the preoperative blood pressure, and avoiding both tachycardia and ischaemia. Anaesthetic agents alone, however, can rarely provide complete haemodynamic control so that additional drug therapy with β-adrenergic blockade and a variety of vasoactive drugs is necessary (see Cardiovascular management before cardiopulmonary bypass, p. 83).

An adequate depth of anaesthesia can be maintained with intravenous opiates, an inhalational agent or a combination of the two. Nitrous oxide should be used with care in patients with poor myocardial function because of its cardiodepressant effects which are more marked in combination with narcotics. Moffitt and Sethna (1986) have suggested that nitrous oxide should be avoided completely in patients with coronary artery disease because it 'involves an insidious risk of myocardial ischaemia not always identified by the ECG'. Many centres now use an air/oxygen mixture as the inspired gas and add to this a volatile inhalational agent as required.

Morphine was originally used as the drug of choice for a high dose opiate technique but this has largely been superseded by the shorter-acting synthetic opiod fentanyl. Fentanyl has been used as a sole anaesthetic agent for cardiac surgery in doses as high as 50–100 μg kg^{-1}. Even at the higher dose levels, however, fentanyl does not dependably abolish autonomic stimulation and the decrease in circulating fentanyl levels at the onset of bypass is greater than can be attributed to dilution alone, probably because of uptake by the oxygenator (Rosen *et al.*, 1988). The majority of anaesthetists therefore now use fentanyl in more moderate doses (10–30 μg kg^{-1}), in combination with a suitable inhalational agent, and take further measures to prevent awareness during the bypass period.

The cardiovascular effects of the available inhalational agents enflurane, halothane and isoflurane are summarized in Table 7.2. Isoflurane was initially heralded as the ideal cardiac anaesthetic agent because it preserved cardiac output with a reduced peripheral resistance and did not significantly depress myocardial contractility. More recent studies carried out in animal (Buffington *et al.*, 1987; Cason *et al.*, 1987; Priebe and Foex, 1987; Sill *et al.*, 1987; Conzen *et al.*, 1989) and man (Reiz and Ostman, 1985; Moffitt and Sethna, 1986) has focused attention on the coronary vasodilator effect of isoflurane. This can in certain circumstances cause a deleterious redistribution of coronary blood flow increasing flow to healthy areas of myocardium by diverting it from potentially ischaemic areas supplied by diseased coronary arteries–the so-called 'coronary steal' effect. The clinical implications of the animal work on isoflurane were the subject of an interesting editorial (Becker, 1987) entitled 'Is isoflurane dangerous for the patient with coronary artery disease?'. Becker advocated that isoflurane should be avoided in patients with coronary artery disease, particularly those with multivessel disease and left ventricular failure who are at increased risk of subendocardial ischaemia.

The prevalence of patients prone to coronary steal has since been investigated by Buffington *et al.* (1988). In a retrospective study based on the Coronary Artery Surgery Study (CASS) this group estimated that 23% of the 16249 patients had 'steal-prone' coronary anatomy.

Despite the evidence discussed above more recent work tends to suggest that the choice of anaesthetic agent does not significantly affect the outcome of coronary artery surgery (Slogoff and Keats, 1989; Tuman *et al.*, 1989a), although editorial comment on this issue has remained cautious (Mangano, 1989). Anaesthetists continue to use isoflurane for cardiac patients but in relatively low dosage combined with a background of opiod anaesthesia/analgesia. Isoflurane is less likely to sensitize the myocardium to catecholamines and is therefore useful in the presence of significant cardiac arrhythmias. It is also the volatile agent of choice if there is the possibility of halogen-induced hepatitis after repeat exposure to anaesthetic agents.

The controversy surrounding the use of isoflurane has somewhat overshadowed interest in the other two agents, halothane and enflurane. The classic work of Moffitt and Sethna (1986) has shown that the combination of an opiod such as fentanyl with a halothane or enflurane as the potent inhalational anaesthetic agent provides near ideal anaesthesia for the cardiac patient with good ventricular function. In their studies both agents caused controlled myocardial depression but myocardial oxygen consumption was also reduced to an even greater degree so that myocardial oxygen supply was not compromised and myocardial ischaemia was not a feature of their use. Halothane and enflurane therefore remain a sensible choice of anaesthetic agent for cardiac surgery provided the well known side effects of halothane are taken into consideration.

Table 7.2 The cardiovascular effects of the inhalational anaesthetic agents

	Heart rate	*Peripheral vascular resistance*	*Mean arterial pressure*	*Myocardial function/contractility*	*Cardiac output*
Enflurane	Increased	Decreased	Decreased	Decreased	Decreased
Halothane	Unchanged	Decreased	Decreased	Decreased	Decreased
Isoflurane	Increased	Decreased	Decreased	Maintained or slightly decreased	Maintained

See test for effects on myocardial oxygen consumption and coronary blood flow.

Monitoring

Monitoring techniques for cardiopulmonary bypass now differ little from unit to unit. Before anaesthesia a four lead electrocardiogram (ECG) plus V5 chest lead is attached to the patient and monitored. A radial artery cannula is then inserted percutaneously under local anaesthetic and the arterial wave form is displayed. In high risk cases it may be prudent to insert central venous monitoring lines and a pulmonary artery catheter (PAC) under local anaesthetic at this stage, but for routine cases this can be done following the induction of anaesthesia via a peripheral intravenous line. The preferred route for central venous cannulation is the right internal jugular vein (English *et al.*, 1969) because, unlike the left internal jugular vein, recordings will not be affected if the innominate vein is stretched when the chest is opened. Separate cannulae can be inserted into the internal jugular to provide routes for monitoring pressures, transfusion of fluid and the administration of vasoactive drugs. If there is any difficulty locating the internal jugular vein it is safer to use a Seldinger technique and if it is considered that several infusion sites may be required it is preferable to use a triple-lumen venous catheter plus one other large-bore catheter (or PAC sheath) for rapid transfusion.

In addition to the monitoring detailed above oxygen saturation and end-tidal carbon dioxide levels should be monitored from the start of the procedure. Central temperature probes (nasopharyngeal and/or rectal) and a urinary catheter can be inserted after induction of anaesthesia. Intra-oesophageal echocardiography remains an expensive research tool. Finally, many units now monitor cerebral function in a variety of ways although this is by no means established as routine clinical practice and is often used as part of a research programme. There remains a significant incidence of cerebral damage following cardiopulmonary bypass, however, so that cerebral function monitoring is likely to become more widespread. This topic is discussed in detail in Chapter 13–Neurological sequelae of cardiopulmonary bypass.

One area of controversy remains in relation to monitoring of the cardiac patient and that relates to the routine use of pulmonary artery catheters (PACs). PA catheterization allows measurement of pulmonary artery pressure, pulmonary artery capillary wedge pressure (which in most circumstances relates to left atrial pressure) and, in the more specialized forms of the catheter, permits measurement of thermodilution cardiac output and continuous mixed venous oxygen saturation. A variety of haemodynamic indices can then be calculated from this data and that taken from less complex measurements of systolic/diastolic blood pressure and central venous pressure. In patients with ventricular failure the measurement of both right and left heart filling pressures can be invaluable, but at operation left-sided pressures can be measured using a left atrial line or, more simply, with a fine needle temporarily inserted into the left atrium and connected to a pressure transducer. Much information can also be ascertained by observing the contraction and the filling state of the right and left heart and the pulmonary artery without recourse to invasive PA monitoring and its attendant risks (see Table 7.3). Several centres have now reported excellent surgical results without the universal utilization of PACs (Bashein and Ivey, 1987) or with no use of them at all in patients undergoing routine coronary artery surgery (Liban and Davies, 1986).

Table 7.3 Complications of pulmonary artery catheterization

Infection
Thrombosis or embolism
Pneumothorax
Rhythm disturbances
Pulmonary haemorrhage
Pulmonary artery disruption
Knotting of catheter
Vascular damage during insertion

Inserting PACs in all patients undergoing cardiac surgery is a practice advocated by certain North American centres whereas in the UK very few centres have, in the past, placed PACs either in the routine or high risk cardiac case. This divergence of opinion has become much less over recent years as American centres have become more aware of the complications and costs of routine PAC placement and UK anaesthetists have become more aware of their value in managing the high risk case. A recent paper by Tuman *et al.* (1989b) gives some credence to this change in attitude. These authors prospectively investigated the occurrence of complications and outcome of cardiac surgery in 1094 consecutive patients monitored, irrespective of cardiac risk, with either elective PACs (537 patients) or central venous pressure monitoring (557 patients). No significant difference in any of the outcome variables was noted between any groups of patients with similar risk factors. A group of 39 patients monitored initially with central venous pressure only were thought to require PAC monitoring during the study because of the occurrence of major haemodynamic events. Late utilization of PAC monitoring in this group did not affect outcome variables when compared with a similar group of patients monitored with PACs from the outset.

On the basis of these findings it seems reasonable to confine pulmonary artery catheterization to patients in a high risk category, particularly those with poor left ventricular function. An alternative approach is to place an introducer sheath for the PAC into the internal jugular vein at induction of anaesthesia. A PAC can then be easily introduced, when required, during the procedure or at a later stage in the intensive care unit.

Cardiovascular management before cardiopulmonary bypass

As discussed above in the section on maintenance of anaesthesia haemodynamic control cannot be achieved solely with the use of anaesthetic agents. In the case of coronary artery surgery systemic pressures are kept in a low-normal range avoiding tachycardia and ischaemia. Anaesthesia can be deepened at particularly stimulating times such as endotracheal intubation, skin incision and sternotomy but this is often insufficient to eliminate hypertension or tachycardia in those patients with good ventricular function. β-Adrenergic blocking agents can be used intravenously to control tachycardia unless they are contraindicated because of myocardial failure, asthma, potential heart-block or a drug interaction. As a general rule those patients already taking β-adrenergic blockers can be given increments intravenously at operation. If patients have angina but are not on these drugs preoperatively it may merely mean they are intolerant to minor side effects, but could indicate that they were witheld or withdrawn because of more serious side effects. In the face of intractable hypertension at operation β-adrenergic blockade can be given in combination with α-blockade as the drug labetalol. This is given intravenously either as a bolus injection (10–20 mg) or as a continuous infusion.

Apart from β-blocking agents, vasodilator drugs are the main agents used to treat hypertension in the perioperative period although there is increasing interest in the use of calcium-channel blocking agents by the intravenous route. Before bypass vasodilators with a short duration of action are chosen because this is a period of cardiovascular instability, when hypertension may quickly change to hypotension as the heart is manipulated or the venous return is impeded as the pericardium is lifted to improve access to the heart. Intravenous nitroglycerin is a useful drug at this stage. Although a venodilator it is usually sufficient to control blood pressure in the majority of patients when given as a bolus (50 μg initially, quickly increasing the dose if tolerated) or as an infusion. Nitroglycerin has a short duration of action and has the great benefit of producing coronary vasodilatation without a 'steal effect'. If venodilatation does not lower systemic pressure sufficiently α-blockade can be used in the form of phentolamine by bolus injection (1–5 mg) or sodium nitroprusside by continuous infusion. Hydralazine is an alternative drug which acts almost exclusively on arteriolar smooth muscle. It can be given intravenously (10–20 mg) but has the disadvantage of a relatively slow onset and long duration of action compared with the drugs discussed above. Hydralazine is therefore more suitable for use during the postoperative period.

During the prebypass period systemic pressure may fall for a variety of reasons. Over-enthusiastic vasodilator therapy may be a cause of hypotension, even with meticulous anaesthesia, and rapid withdrawal of autologous blood without adequate colloid replacement is another common reason for a fall in systemic pressure. These events can usually be treated by simple measures such as stopping vasodilator infusions, replacing colloid, lightening the level of inhalational anaesthesia and requesting the surgeons to cease deleterious manipulation within the chest. Occasionally it is necessary to treat these events pharmacologically with a vasoconstrictor agent such as metaraminol (0.5–1 mg i.v.) or phenylephrine (0.25–1 mg i.v.). Used in the above circumstances, for short term treatment, these agents are unlikely significantly to affect the afterload on the heart but will improve coronary and cerebral blood flow. Alternative therapy for hypotension at this stage will include treatment of arrhythmias and correction of acid-base abnormalities. Atropine should be used initially to treat bradycardia in patients with coronary artery disease because the drop in diastolic blood pressure and tachycardia associated with the use of isoprenaline is particularly likely to provoke ischaemia.

It is very uncommon to institute inotropic support *de novo* before cardiopulmonary bypass but some patients will come to surgery as emergencies with infusions running and it may be prudent to start a low-dose dopamine infusion in those with significant renal failure or poor ventricular function. If inotropic therapy is considered necessary at this stage the choice of inotropic can be made on conventional criteria.

Anaesthetic management during cardiopulmonary bypass

In order to manage anaesthesia during bypass it is necessary to have a broad understanding of the haemodynamics involved. Much of this will be found in more detail elsewhere in this book but for completeness a brief résumé is included here.

Conventionally pump flow rates of 2.2–2.4 $l\ min^{-1}\ m^{-1}$ are used during normothermic cardiopulmonary bypass. These flow rates can be considerably reduced as the patient is cooled. Currently, the optimal mean arterial pressure during non-pulsatile cardiopulmonary bypass remains speculative. Many clinicians prefer to maintain mean arterial pressure within the range 50–70 mmHg, accepting lower levels for short periods of time in younger patients not known to have cerebrovascular disease. In children, and in adults during hypothermia (Kolkka and Hilberman, 1980) lower perfusion pressures have been considered acceptable by some workers. Cerebral blood flow during hypothermia is also profoundly influenced by acid–base management as alpha-stat acid–base management appears to preserve autoregulation of cerebral blood flow (Rogers *et al.*, 1988) whereas pH-stat management causes pressure dependent cerebral hyperfusion. Optimal perfusion pressures and flow rates at different temperatures remain controversial. As the brain is the most likely organ to suffer permanent damage if inadequately perfused during bypass the reader is referred to Chapter 13 of this edition (Neurological sequelae of cardiopulmonary bypass) for further discussion on this subject.

Once bypass is established intermittent positive pressure ventilation is discontinued so the patient no longer receives inhalational anaesthetic agents by that route. At the same time haemodilution due to the crystalloid pump-prime lowers the plasma concentration of many drugs including sufentanil and fentanyl. As previously mentioned there is also additional evidence that there can be a far greater decrease in plasma fentanyl levels than expected on purely a haemodilutional basis, probably because of uptake by the membrane oxygenator (Rosen *et al.*, 1988). As a result of these changes there is obviously a possibility of patients becoming 'aware' during bypass and this has been reported.

Relatively little has been written about the management of anaesthesia during bypass but the kinetics of anaesthetic drugs during bypass and their effects on cerebral metabolism and the stress response has been the subject of a recent review (Reves *et al.*, 1989). Hypothermia is important in the control of cerebral blood flow and is the most effective means of attenuating cerebral metabolic activity. It is also likely that hypothermia provides some 'anaesthetic effect' or protection from awareness. This effect cannot be relied on totally, particularly during the rewarming period when many clinicians administer incremental doses of benzodiazepines, and there has been increasing interest in ensuring anaesthesia during bypass by constant infusion techniques and the administration of volatile agents via the oxygenator.

Fentanyl can be given by infusion during bypass to offset the drop in plasma levels detailed above (Hynynen, Lehtinen and Salmenpera, 1986) and this has been shown to block the release of stress hormones. Pharmacologically active concentrations of highly lipid soluble drugs such as the opiod alfentanil remain relatively unchanged at the onset of bypass, but this drug must also be given by infusion because of its short duration of action.

The short-acting induction agent propofol has been used alone or in combination with an opiate to provide anaesthesia during cardiac surgery (Bell and Goodchild, 1989; Russell *et al.*, 1989). The cardiovascular effects of this drug may not be suitable for all patients undergoing cardiac surgery (Stephan *et al.*, 1986) although there seems to be great enthusiasm for its use in clinical situations more than adequately managed by simpler anaesthetic techniques. Propofol, however, with its short duration of action, lack of accumulation and profound venodilator effect may be particularly useful to provide anaesthesia by infusion during cardiopulmonary bypass once an adequate perfusion pressure has been established. A rigid dose regime has not been established when propofol is used in this way but it appears that relatively low infusion rates [3 mg kg^{-1} h^{-1}] can be used to provide hypnosis and amnesia during cardiopulmonary bypass when the drug is used in combination with moderate doses of fentanyl (Ghosh and Bethune, 1989).

There has also been increasing interest in the administration of volatile agents via the oxygenator during cardiopulmonary bypass (Reves *et al.*, 1989). Again, it is difficult to judge dose levels but isoflurane 2% has been shown to significantly reduce the cortisol response during bypass, albeit in combination with a large dose of fentanyl given at the start of surgery (Flezzani *et al.*, 1986). Isoflurane at 1% also attenuates cortisol levels, but to a lesser extent.

In addition to providing anaesthesia during bypass the anaesthetist must control the perfusion pressure and flow rates. At the onset of bypass perfusion pressures are often low due in part to the reduction in viscosity caused by haemodilution, lack of pulsatile flow and to the dilution of circulating catecholamines. This hypotension is often exacerbated when cold cardioplegia is administered. At this stage flow rates are increased and this may elevate the perfusion pressure to some degree. Many clinicians would take no further action if flow rates were adequate at this stage others administer a vasoconstrictor (phenylephrine, methoxamine or metaraminol) if perfusion pressure remains consistently below 35 mmHg. In elderly patients or those with known cerebrovascular disease a higher perfusion pressure (50–60 mmHg, or above) is usually maintained. Once bypass has been established for 20–30 min, mean arterial pressure tends to rise despite a constant flow rate. This is due to peripheral vasoconstriction. Increasing anaesthesia by the methods discussed above may attenuate this rise in pressure but it is often necessary to administer vasodilators at this stage. These can be given as bolus doses (phentolamine, nitroglycerin) or by infusion (sodium nitroprusside, nitroglycerin).

Once the definitive part of the cardiac operation has been completed the aortic cross-clamp is removed following complete de-airing of the heart. Re-warming of the patient is then begun. As warming proceeds it may be necessary to cut down infusion rates of vasodilator drugs because peripheral vasodilation occurs and the perfusion pressure drops.

The early postbypass period

The patient is weaned from bypass once warming is complete, ventilation has been re-established, acid–base status and plasma potassium levels are within normal limits and the cardiac rhythm is stable or satisfactory pacing has been established. Filling of the heart is controlled from the arterial line of the pump with the venous return lines occluded. The flow rate from the arterial line is gradually decreased so that ultimately the heart ejects producing pressure transients on the monitor. Filling of the heart is merely an application of Starling's Law at this stage and is gauged on the central venous pressure, the left atrial pressure and the appearance of the contracting heart. It is unwise to over fill the heart at this stage and it is preferable to accept a relatively low systemic pressure if the heart appears to be contracting comfortably. Systemic pressure recorded in peripheral arteries may be lower than aortic pressure initially but this gradient gradually decreases as peripheral vasodilation occurs and cardiac output improves. Once bypass has been discontinued the venous return lines are removed from the heart and protamine is slowly administered to reverse heparinization. As much blood as possible is returned to the patient from the pump at this stage, providing it is of reasonable quality and the heart is not overdistended. Vasodilators can be used to aid this process in the stable patient with adequate systemic pressure.

The majority of patients do not require any specific support for the circulation after bypass. A minority will require pharmacological support with inotropic agents and vasodilators and even fewer require mechanical support with the intra-aortic balloon pump or even a period of supportive bypass. If the surgery has been carried out satisfactorily with adequate myocardial protection the individuals requiring this type of support can usually be identified from preoperative data including diagnosis, cardiac status, ventricular function and relevant concomitant disease. If there is any doubt about the adequacy of ventricular function it is much safer, in the first instance, to recommence bypass while a biochemical survey is undertaken to exclude hypoxia, hypercapnia, metabolic acidosis or electrolyte abnormalities. Once these abnormalities have been excluded or corrected and surgical causes of poor function have been eliminated then a further attempt at weaning from bypass can be undertaken with moderate inotropic therapy. Choice of inotropic agent at this stage remains a matter of opinion. Many clinicians prefer to use a weaker inotrope such as dopamine or dobutamine initially (Kapur, 1987) whereas others prefer to use a stronger inotrope such as adrenaline from the outset. Other clinicians compromise by giving a bolus dose of adrenaline initially and follow this with an infusion of dopamine. If adrenaline or noradrenaline are used then strong consideration should be given to introducing an infusion of nitroglycerin, providing systemic pressure is maintained, to reduce preload and improve coronary and peripheral flow. When myocardial failure is the major problem and systemic pressure is relatively well maintained the newer phosphodiesterase inhibitors such as enoximone may be useful to increase cardiac output while lowering systemic vascular resistance and pulmonary capillary wedge pressure. This type of drug is, however, often more useful in the intensive care unit where it can be introduced more slowly with serial measurements of cardiac indices.

Large doses of inotropic agents inevitably increase myocardial oxygen consumption and in this situation intra-aortic counter pulsation is indicated, particularly in the presence of left ventricular disease. This should be instituted at an earlier rather than later stage in order to gain maximum benefit.

Transfer to the intensive care unit

After completion of surgery the patient is transferred to the intensive care unit. In most instances the patient remains ventilated initially, although a number of anaesthetists re-establish spontaneous respiration immediately following straightforward bypass surgery.

During transfer the ventilated patient should remain sedated with all infusions maintained via battery-operated pumps. An ECG provides minimal monitoring but if the transfer is of substantial length or includes a lift journey portable arterial monitoring should be available. Resuscitation drugs are kept to hand during the transfer and it is useful to take a capped syringe of propofol or etomidate in case sedation is required on the journey or unacceptable hypertension develops.

Once in the intensive care unit the patient is attached to a ventilator and monitors in the usual way. This should be carefully supervised by the anaesthetist accompanying the patient. No matter how proficient the intensive care staff are it is the responsibility of the clinician involved in the previous 3–4h of surgery to ensure his or her patient is stabilized in the intensive care unit and that the intensivists are aware of any difficulties or problems that arose in the operating theatres.

References

Bashein, G. and Ivey, T.D. (1987) A pulmonary artery catheter is not indicated for all coronary artery surgery. *Journal of Cardiothoracic Anaesthesia*, **1**, 362–365

Becker, L.C. (1987) Is isoflurance dangerous for the patient with coronary artery disease? Editorial. *Anaesthesiology*, **66**, 259–261

Bell, M.D. and Goodchild, C.S. (1989) Hypertrophic obstructive cardiomyopathy in combination with a prolapsing mitral valve. Anaesthesia for surgical correction with propofol. *Anaesthesia*, **44**, 409–411

Buffington, C.W., Davis, K.B., Gillispie, S. and Pettinger, M. (1988) The prevalence of steal-prone coronary anatomy in patients with coronary artery disease. An analysis of the coronary artery surgery study register. *Anesthesiology*, **69**, 721–727

Buffington, C.W., Romson, J.L., Levine, A., *et al.* (1987) Isoflurane induces steal in a canine model of chronic coronary occlusion. *Anesthesiology*, **66**, 280–292

Cason, B.A., Verrier, E.D., London, M.J., *et al.* (1987) Effects of isoflurane and halothane on coronary vascular resistance and collateral myocardial blood flow: their capacity to induce coronary steal. *Anesthesiology*, **67**, 665–675

Conzen, P.F., Hobbhahn, J., Goetz, A.E., *et al.* (1989) Regional blood flow and tissue oxygen pressures of the collateral-dependent myocardium during isoflurane anesthesia in dogs. *Anesthesiology*, **70**, 442–452

English, I.C.W., Frew, R.M., Pigott, J.F. and Zaki, M. (1969) Percutaneous catheterization of the internal jugular vein. *Anaesthesia*, **24**, 521–526

Flezzani, P., Croughwell, N., McIntyre, R.W. and Reves, J.G. (1986) Isoflurane decreases the cortisol response to cardiopulmonary bypass. *Anesthesia and Analgesia*, **65**, 1117–1122

Ghosh, S. and Bethune, D.W. (1989) Propofol infusion for cardiac surgery. Letter. *Anaesthesia*, **44**, 785

Hynyen, M., Lehtinen, A.M. and Salmenpera, M. (1986) Continuous infusion of fentanyl or alfentanil for coronary artery surgery. *British Journal of Anaesthesia*, **58**, 1260–1266

Kapur, P.A. (1987) Potent inotropes are the drugs of choice after cardiopulmonary bypass: An opposing view. *Journal of Cardiothoracic Anesthesia*, **1**, 256–258

Kolkka, R. and Hilberman, M. (1980) Neurological dysfunction following cardiac surgery with low flow, low pressure cardiopulmonary bypass. *Journal of Thoracic and Cardiovascular Surgery*, **79**, 432–437

Larsen, R., Rathgeber, J., Bagdahn, A., *et al.* (1988) Effects of propofol on cardiovascular dynamics and coronary blood flow in geriatric patients. *Anaesthesia*, **43**, 25–31

Liban, B.J. and Davies, D.M. (1986) Elective coronary bypass surgery without pulmonary artery catheter monitoring. Letter. *Anesthesiology*, **64**, 664–665

Mangano, D.T. (1989) Anesthetics, coronary artery disease and outcome: Unresolved controversies. Editorial. *Anethesiology*, **70**, 175–178

Merin, R.G., Lowenstein, E. and Gelman, S. (1986) Is anesthesia beneficial for the ischaemic heart? III. Editorial. *Anesthesiology*, **64**, 137–140

Moffit, E.A. and Sethna, D.H. (1986) The coronary circulation and myocardial oxygenation in coronary artery disease: effects of anesthesia. *Anesthesia and Analgesia*, **65**, 395–410

O'Connor, J.P., Ramsay, J.G., Wynands, J.E., *et al.* (1989) The incidence of myocardial ischaemia during anesthesia for coronary artery bypass surgery in patients receiving pancuronium or vecuronium. *Anesthesiology*, **70**, 230–236

Priebe, H.J. and Foex, P. (1987) Isoflurane causes regional dysfunction in dogs with critical coronary artery stenoses. *Anesthesiology*, **66**, 293–300

Prys-Roberts, C. (1988) Anaesthetic considerations for the patient with coronary artery disease. *British Journal of Anaesthesia*, **61**, 85–96

Reiz, S. (1988) Myocardial ischaemia associated with general anaesthesia. *British Journal of Anaesthesia*, **61**, 68–84

Reiz, S. and Ostman, M. (1985) Regional coronary hemodynamics during isoflurane-nitrous oxide anesthesia in patients with ischemic heart disease. *Anesthesia and Analgesia*, **64**, 570–576

Reves, J.G., Croughwell, N., Jacobs, J.R. and Greeley, W. (1989) Anesthesia during cardiopulmonary bypass: Does it matter? In *Cardiopulmonary Bypass: Current Concepts and Controversies*, (ed. J.H. Tinker), W.B. Saunders, Philadelphia, pp. 69–97

Rogers, A.T., Stump, D.A., Graulee, G.P., *et al.* (1988) Response of cerebral blood flow to phenylephrine infusion during hypothermic cardiopulmonary bypass. *Anesthesiology*, **69**, 547–551

Rosen, D., Rosen, K., Davidson, B. and Broadman, L. (1988) Fentanyl uptake by the Scimed membrane oxygenator. *Journal of Cardiothoracic Anesthesia*, **2**, 619–626

Russell, G.N., Wright, E.L., Fox, M.A., *et al.* (1989) Propofol–fentanyl anaesthesia for coronary artery surgery and cardiopulmonary bypass. *Anaesthesia*, **44**, 205–208

Sill, J.C., Bove, A.A., Nugent, M., *et al.* (1987) Effects of isoflurane on coronary arteries and coronary arterioles in the intact dog. *Anesthesiology*, **66**, 273–279

Slogoff, S. and Keats, A.S. (1989) Randomized trial of primary anaesthetic agents on outcome of coronary bypass operations. *Anesthesiology*, **70**, 179–188

Stephan, H., Sonntag, H.O., Schenck, D., *et al.* (1986) Effects of propofol on cardiovascular dynamics, myocardial blood flow and myocardial metabolism in patients with coronary artery disease. *British Journal of Anaesthesia*, **58**, 969–975

Streisand, J.B. and Wong, K.C. (1988) Anaesthesia for

coronary artery bypass graft. *British Journal of Anaesthesia*, **61**, 97–104

Thomson, I.R. and Putnins, C.L. (1985) Adverse effects of pancuronium during high-dose fentanyl anesthesia for coronary artery bypass grafting. *Anesthesiology*, **62**, 708–713

Tuman, K.J., McCarthy, R.J., Spiess, B.D., *et al.* (1989a) Does choice of anesthetic agent significantly affect outcome after coronary artery surgery? *Anesthesiology*, **70**, 189–198

Tuman, K.J., McCarthy, R.J., Spiess, B.D., *et al.* (1989b) Effect of pulmonary artery catheterisation on outcome in patients undergoing coronary artery surgery. *Anesthesiology*, **70**, 432–437

Wierda, J.M.K.H., Maestrone, E., Bencini, A.F., *et al.* (1989) Haemodynamic effects of vecuronium. *British Journal of Anaesthesia*, **62**, 230–236

8

Intraoperative myocardial protection

Simon J.M. Ledingham

Cardiac physiology

For the understanding of procedures that have been developed to provide intraoperative myocardial protection, it is important to be aware of the metabolism and circulation of the myocardium under both normal and ischaemic conditions and to be aware of the pathophysiological consequences of myocardial ischaemia and reperfusion.

Cardiac metabolism

Under aerobic conditions, oxidation of a variety of substrates, predominantly free fatty acids, but also glucose, pyruvate, acetate, ketone bodies and amino acids, occurs in the mitochondria with the generation of oxidative phosphorylation of the high energy phosphates ATP and creatine phosphate, whose subsequent degradation to ADP, AMP and creatine is associated with energy release in the form of heat and muscle activity, both isometric and isotonic. In this process 1 mole of glucose is consumed in the production of 36 moles of ATP. The rate of metabolism in the contracting heart depends on a number of factors including heart rate, wall tension and the action of catecholamines. There is 75% oxygen extraction from the coronary blood, higher than in any other organ, and an increased demand for oxygen must be met by increasing coronary flow rather than by increasing extraction. When $Pa\text{O}_2$ is reduced to less than 5 mmHg, oxidative phosphorylation ceases and ATP production falls. Glycogenolysis and anaerobic glycolysis take over with the formation of glycolytic intermediaries. Anaerobic glycolysis only yields 2 moles ATP per mole glucose in comparison with aerobic glycolysis.

Coronary circulation

In the beating heart, coronary flow takes place predominantly in diastole, so that if this should shorten through any cause, flow may be compromised. Epicardial arteries function in part as capacitance vessels and phasic flow in the epicardium differs from that within the myocardial wall (Chilian, 1988). Flow is normally adjusted by autoregulatory responses in the coronary arterioles to maintain sufficient flow to meet the metabolic demand for oxygen when perfusion pressure changes within the so-called autoregulatory range or when energy requirements alter (Dole, 1987). The coronary endothelium, like the endothelium throughout the vascular system, has a wide variety of important biological functions (Kaiser and Sparks, 1987), including a crucial role in the modulation of coronary vascular tone (Bassenge and Busse, 1988), and pathological conditions such as arteriosclerosis and ischaemic injury may impair these functions. Endothelial cells respond to an increase in shearing stress as the rate of flow increases by producing endothelial derived relaxing factor (EDRF) (Furchgott and Zawadzki, 1980), and recent evidence indicates that EDRF is probably identical to nitric oxide (Palmer, Ferrige and Moncada, 1987; Ignarro, 1989). However, in the presence of coronary artery disease, aortic pressure falling below the autoregulatory range or a rise in ventricular wall tension, due either to a rise in intraventricular diastolic pressure or reduced wall compliance as in hypertrophy, flow may become impaired. This occurs predominantly in the subendocardial regions which are most vulnerable to ischaemia since flow in these regions occurs exclusively during diastole (Hoffman, 1987). In the surgical setting, low cardiopulmonary bypass perfusion pressures (lower than 50 mmHg), hypothermia (28°C), tachycardia, ventricular fibrillation and ventricular distension, may each result in ischaemia of the subendocardium, even in normal hearts (Hottenrott and Buckberg, 1974; Hottenrott, Maloney and Buckberg, 1974a and b; Baird *et al.*, 1975; McConnell *et al.*, 1977). A small intracardiac collateral circulation exists and is of importance in limiting the extent of ischaemic damage due to regional arterial lesions. In addition, non-coronary collateral flow from mediastinal and bronchial vessels entering the heart via pericardial connections assists in maintaining flow, albeit mainly to the subepicardium. This flow may be disadvantageous in chemical cardioplegia with arrested coronary flow, since it results in washout of the cardioplegic solution (Brazier, 1975). Ischaemia causes coronary vasodilation through the release of a number of agents from endothelial cells (Dole, 1987), including adenosine (Berne, 1963; Zucchi *et al.*, 1989) and prostacyclin (Bassenge and Busse, 1988), but when endothelial cells become severely hypoxic they may release vasoconstrictor substances (Rubanyi and Vanhoutte, 1985).

Myocardial ischaemia

In ischaemia, fatty acid utilization is suppressed and carbohydrate utilization is stimulated through the effects of catecholamines (Mayer, 1974). Aerobic changes to anaerobic metabolism with glycogenolysis and glycolysis, resulting in the production of lactate and hydrogen ions (Rovetto, Whitmer and Neely, 1973). Thus, in the early stages of ischaemia, there is a rapid loss of myocardial energy stores (Hearse and Chain, 1972) accompanied by a rising intracellular acidosis which progressively inhibits the enzymes involved with glycolysis (Rovetto, Lamberton and Neely, 1975) and the maintenance of membrane, contractile and organelle function. ATP dephosphorylation transfers high-energy phosphate via the creatine–creatine phosphate shuttle from the site of production in the mitochondria to the site of usage in the myofibril. Thus, continued contractile activity without ATP production results in a rapid fall in creatine phosphate (Lewardowski, Devous and Nunnally, 1987). There is an immediate reduction in contractile activity, which may be due to ATP and creatine phosphate depletion (Merchant, Feinberg and Levitsky, 1974), interference with cellular calcium homeostasis and other unknown causes. Various dysrhythmias may occur due to alterations of intracellular ionic gradients (Corabeuf, Deroubaix and Hoeter, 1976), accumulation of fatty acid derivatives (Corr, Gross and Sobel, 1984) and adenosine (Belardinelli, Mattas and Berne, 1981). The cells lose potassium and accumulate sodium and chloride. Cell osmolality rises causing cell swelling (Leaf, 1973) and this may contribute to the membrane damage caused by the activation of intracellular hydrolases and lipases (Ricciutti, 1972; Weglicki *et al.*, 1974). Membrane damage causes leakiness and loss of intracellular magnesium (Shen and Jennings, 1972). For example, in rabbit hearts subjected to normothermic ischaemic arrest for 30 min, intracellular pH falls from 7.2 to 5.8 and myocardial creatine phosphate (CP) and ATP fall to 7% and 30% of their normal levels respectively (Ambrosio *et al.*, 1987). As the duration of ischaemia increases, there is progressive mitochondrial malfunction, inhibition of respiration and irreversible damage (Jennings, 1969). Calcium is lost from the mitochondria (Hearse, 1977) and accumulates with cytoplasmic ionized calcium resulting from the dechelation of calcium from ATP. Eventually there is myofibril contracture due to the loss of ATP (Cooley, Reul and Wukasck, 1972), disruption and cytolysis. The full sequence of events in myocardial ischaemia has been reviewed (Hearse, Baimbridge and Jynge, 1981; Hearse, 1987).

If normal coronary flow is restored during the early minutes of ischaemia, the cellular changes that have occurred are fully reversible and will be associated with a rapid and complete recovery of mechanical function, with no cellular death (Jennings and Reimer, 1979). As the duration of ischaemia increases, restoration of coronary flow may not result in immediate full recovery of mechanical function, but after a period of time there will be complete recovery with no cellular death. This temporary failure to regain contractile function, which may last from 1 to 2 weeks, has become known as 'myocardial stunning' (Braunwald and Kloner, 1982). Myocardial stunning may be due solely to specific events occurring during the early seconds or minutes of reperfusion or to a combination of these events and the recovery of depleted nucleotides and nucleosides. During ischaemia ATP is dephosphorylated to ADP and AMP, but these do not accumulate since AMP is further dephosphorylated to adenosine which is then progressively converted to inosine, hypoxanthine and uric acid in the endothelial cells and lost to the system during reperfusion (De Witt, Jochim and Behrendt, 1983). Creatine phosphate is rapidly restored on reperfusion (Lewardowski Devous and Nunnally, 1987), but ATP has to be regenerated either by *de novo* synthesis or by the salvage pathways and, while the latter are at least ten times faster and are the principle route for restoring ATP in normal circumstances, when nucleosides are depleted it may take up to 1 week to return ATP to normal levels (Ward *et al.*, 1984). However, although depressed ATP is used as a criterion of the likelihood of functional recovery (Whitman *et al.*, 1989) and severe depletions are associated with poor recovery (Reibel and Rovetto, 1978; De Witt, Jochim and Behrendt,

1983), moderate depletions have not been shown to correlate with the degree of functional impairment (Taegtmeyer, Roberts and Raine, 1985; Rosenkranz *et al.*, 1986b; Lewardowski, Devous and Nunnally, 1987). Up to this stage, ischaemic cellular injury can be considered to be reversible, but beyond a certain point, possibly related to ATP levels below 10% of normal (Jennings *et al.*, 1978), irreversible cellular injury occurs and cell death results despite reperfusion. Furthermore, reperfusion at this time may actually accelerate the injurious processes (Shen and Jennings, 1972; Hearse, 1977; Jennings and Kloner, 1981). However, irreversible injury is heterogeneous both in relation to time and cellular location (Hearse, 1987) and the ultrastructural changes associated with irreversibility may not be manifested until after reperfusion has commenced (Vinten-Johansen *et al.*, 1988b). In experiments involving regional ischaemia, reperfusion is associated with a degree of endothelial disruption not seen in experiments of comparable duration in which the region is not subjected to reperfusion (Forman, Puett and Virmani, 1989). In these experiments, obstruction of the coronary microvasculature by endothelial cell protrusions and aggregated blood elements have been seen (Kloner, Ganote and Jennings, 1974; Kloner *et al.*, 1980; Engler *et al.*, 1986). It is possible that the severity of the microvascular damage at the start of reperfusion may ultimately determine the extent of cellular injury or death seen in the reperfused myocardium. There are now many reports demonstrating that manipulation of the initial reperfusion conditions will result not only in improved recovery of immediate contractile function, but also in a reduction in the extent of myocardial necrosis in the area at risk.

Reperfusion injury

Myocardial reperfusion injury is a rather vague term. It can be used as a collective description of a number of pathophysiological events that occur during reperfusion of previously ischaemic myocardium, but, more recently, it has been become synonymous with cellular damage or death occurring specifically due to the reperfusion process and implies that the destiny of these cells has changed by the reperfusion process itself. However, it is claimed by some (Jennings, Reimer and Steenbergen, 1986) that reperfusion injury which results in cell death is merely the acceleration of pathological events that would in any case have occurred and does not itself determine irreversibility. This presents a practical dilemma, since cells that are not reperfused are certainly destined to die and cells that are reperfused before irreversibility, whenever that is, are destined to recover at some time, but which cells are destined to die and which are destined to recover can only be truly revealed by allowing reperfusion to take place. Thus, the existence of reperfusion injury *per se* can only be confirmed by demonstrating that an intervention, commenced at the start of reperfusion, alters the severity of a reperfusion associated event (Opie, 1989).

Reperfusion injury is characterized by inability of the heart to utilize oxygen normally (Kane *et al.*, 1975) due to reduced mitochondrial oxygen uptake caused either by functional impairment of oxidative metabolism or by structural damage. Structurally, there is a rapid cellular influx of calcium with the formation of calcium phosphate particles within the mitochondria accompanied by intense myocardial contraction, disruption of myofibrils and sarcolemma, explosive cell swelling and mitochondrial rupture, and extensive haemorrhagic injury (Shen and Jennings, 1972; Ganote et al., 1975; Hearse et al., 1975). The severity and homogeneity of these events are much influenced by the circumstances and length of the preceding ischaemic period and are significantly reduced by hypothermic cardioplegic arrest (Hearse, Braimbridge and Jynge, 1981). The rapid influx of calcium into the mitochondria has been closely linked to the reintroduction of oxygenation (Ganote, Worstell and Kaltenback, 1976), the 'oxygen-paradox', and is very similar to the 'calcium-paradox' seen when calcium is first completely removed from the extracellular space and then reintroduced (Hearse, Humphrey and Bullock, 1978). The uptake of calcium during both these paradoxes both expends and prevents production of ATP. Calcium-free cardioplegic solutions predispose to the calcium-paradox, particularly in the isolated heart in which the supply of small amounts of calcium through non-coronary collateral blood flow, as with the heart *in situ*, is absent. Minute (50 μmol) amounts of calcium (Rich and Langer, 1982) in the cardioplegic solution are sufficient to protect the heart and the risk is further reduced by hypothermia (Baker, Bullock and Hearse, 1983; Ganote and Nayler, 1985). In contrast, the calcium influx associated with the oxygen-paradox is probably initiated by free radical mediated injury.

Hypoxia creates the conditions for the generation of the superoxide radical by the mitochondria (Guarnieri, Flamingni and Caldarera, 1980) and its production is greatly increased by reperfusion. Normally, the superoxide radical is dismutated to hydrogen peroxide which is then metabolized to oxygen and water by catalase or glutathione peroxidase, the latter involving the oxidation of reduced glutathione. Potentially, another source of superoxide radical formation comes from the oxidation of hypoxanthine, which has accumulated during ischaemia, to xanthine (Chambers *et al.*, 1985; McCord, 1985). However, this source requires the enzyme xanthine oxidase, which is formed from xanthine dehydrogenase during ischaemia, and although it is known to be present in the myocardium of the rat and the dog, it appears to be absent or only present in minute quantities in man (Jarasch, Bruder and Heidi, 1986; Eddy *et al.*, 1987). Ischaemia depletes intracellular glutathione (Blaustein *et al.*, 1989), glutathione peroxidase and superoxide dismutase (Guarnieri, Flamigni and Calderera, 1980). and the quantity of free radicals produced during reperfusion overwhelms the free radical scavenging pathways (Gaudel and Duvelleroy, 1984; McCord, 1985). Much of the cytotoxicity of the superoxide and hydrogen peroxide free radicals is thought to be related to their conversion to the highly cytotoxic hydroxyl free radical and its subsequent initiation of lipid peroxidation, both of which involve iron-catalysed reactions (Gutteridge, Richmond and Halliwell, 1979; Halliwell, 1989), Free radical production, during reperfusion, has been measured by electron spin resonance (ESR) spectroscopy directly (Zweier, Flaherty and Weisfeldt, 1987; Garlick *et al.*, 1987) and indirectly either through the use of spin-trap agents (Bolli *et al.*, 1988) or by the quantitation of the products of lipid peroxidation (Romaschin *et al.*, 1987; Weisel *et al.*, 1989).

Experimental studies have linked the temporary depression of myocardial contractile function or 'myocardial stunning', seen after reversible ischaemia, to free radical mediated injury. Indirect evidence has come from the attenuation of stunning by the administration during reperfusion of the free radical scavengers superoxide dismutase and catalase (Gross *et al.*, 1986; Przyklenk and Kloner, 1986; Ambrosio *et al.*, 1987) mercaptopropionylglycine (MPG) (Myers *et al.*, 1985) and dimethylthiourea (Bolli *et al.*, 1987), by the inhibition of xanthine oxidase by allopurinol (Charlat *et al.*, 1987) and by the limitation of iron-catalysed reactions by iron-chelation with desferrioxamine (Ambrosio *et al.*, 1987b; Bolli *et al.*, 1987). Direct evidence has come from the correlation of free radical production, as determined by spin-trapping, with stunning (Bolli *et al.*, 1988) and, recently, from a study which demonstrated that both free radical production and stunning can be reduced by MPG commenced at the start of reperfusion (Bolli *et al.*, 1989). Reperfusion is known to be associated with arrhythmias and these have also been linked to free radical formation and abnormal calcium fluxes (Hearse and Tosaki, 1988). Reperfusion with low calcium concentrations (0.1–0.5 mmol) (Kusuoka *et al.*, 1987) and the administration of the calcium antagonist nifedipine (Przyklenk *et al.*, 1989) have been shown to reduce stunning. However, the role of calcium in the process of stunning is possibly more complex, since it has also been demonstrated that the stunned myocardium will respond to calcium (Ito, Tate and Kobayaski, 1987). It has been proposed that after a period of calcium overload, associated with damage to intracellular membranes and impaired calcium cycling by the sarcoplasmic reticulum, there results a relative insensitivity of the contractile proteins to calcium and that in this state an increase in external calcium may be beneficial. Furthermore, the stunned myocardium has been shown to respond to inotropic agents, such as epinephrine (Becker, Levine and Di Paula, 1986), which are believed to increase intracellular calcium.

Neutrophils are another potential cause of reperfusion injury (Luchessi, Werns and Fantone, 1989). Activated neutrophils release proteolytic enzymes and superoxide, hydrogen peroxide, hydroxyl and hypochlorous free radicals. They also release platelet activating factor and arachidonic acid metabolites, including leukotrienes, which attract and activate other neutrophils. It is well known that neutrophils play a major role in the inflammatory response following myocardial infarction, but they can also become activated during myocardial ischaemia and reperfusion. Furthermore, in the surgical setting, cardiopulmonary bypass predisposes to neutrophil activation and free radical production through complement activation (Kirklin *et al.*, 1983; Cavarocchi, England and Schaff, 1986; Royston, Fleming and Desai, 1986) and may, itself, cause or exacerbate reperfusion injury (Menasche and Piwrica, 1989). Thus, neutrophils have the potential to injure vascular endothelium and myocardium. However, neutrophil-mediated free radical injury is not thought to play a major role in pathogenesis of myocardial stunning associated with reversible cellular injury (Jeremy and Becker, 1989), although it may be important following periods of ischaemia associated with irreversible cellular injury (Kloner, 1989; Reimer, Murray and Richard, 1989). Neutrophils have been linked to endothelial damage and plugging of the microvasculature during reperfusion following prolonged periods of regional ischaemia and contribute to the 'no reflow' phenomenon (Engler *et al.*, 1986; Ambrosio *et al.*, 1989). Neutrophil adherence may be facilitated by the loss, during ischaemia or reperfusion, of various agents in the endothelium, including adenosine, cyclic AMP and prostacyclin, which normally inhibit adherence (Forman, Puett and Virmani, 1989). Various studies have demonstrated that neutrophil depletion by leukocyte filters (Litt *et al.*, 1989) or inhibition of neutrophil function by anti-inflammatory drugs (Bednar *et al.*, 1985), prostacyclin (Simpson *et al.*, 1987), adenosine (Olafsson *et al.*, 1987), perfluorocarbons (Forman *et al.*, 1987) and monoclonal antibodies (Simpson *et al.*, 1988), before or during reperfusion following regional ischaemia, will limit the extent of no reflow and reduce the amount of myocyte necrosis that would have otherwise occurred.

The objectives of intraoperative myocardial protection are to prevent or limit the detrimental effects of myocardial ischaemia and reperfusion described above. The greatest potential for myocardial injury occurs during unmodified normothermic ischaemia under normal cardiac work load. On cardiopulmonary bypass, the factors predisposing to ischaemia and reperfusion damage can be closely controlled and significantly influenced by the method of myocardial protection adopted.

Preischaemic metabolic manipulations

Glycogen loading

Hearts in good nutritional condition, as evidenced by normal or elevated myocardial glycogen stores, have a better tolerance to ischaemia (Scheuer and Stezoski, 1970; Lolley *et al.*, 1979), since glycogen is a principal substrate for the anaerobic production of ATP. In patients undergoing cardiac surgery, reduced preischaemic myocardial glycogen levels have been shown to be associated with increased perioperative mortality (Lolley *et al.*, 1985). In a large clinical study in patients undergoing elective revascularization, preoperative intravenous glucose, insulin and potassium (GIK), intravenous fats, and a combination of oral fat with GIK were all shown significantly to raise intramyocardial glycogen stores (Lolley *et al.*, 1985). All methods of enhancement significantly reduced the need for postoperative inotropic support, but the latter combination had both the greatest effect on glycogen content and appeared to have the best overall clinical result. Also, in three small clinical studies, two randomized (Haider *et al.*, 1984; Oldfield, Commerford and Opie, 1986) and one not (Bormann *et al.*, 1985), in patients undergoing elective valve replacements, preischaemic infusions GIK were shown significantly to raise intramyocardial glycogen (Oldfield, Commerford and Opie, 1986), ATP and CP (Bormann *et al.*, 1985; Haider *et al.*, 1985) contents, but the only positive clinical effect observed was a reduction in serious postoperative arrhythmias (Oldfield, Commerford and Opie, 1986). These clinical observations are supported by a recent experimental study in the isolated rabbit heart undergoing hypothermic cardioplegic arrest (McElroy, Walker and Taegtmeyer, 1989). Preischaemic glycogen loading with glucose and insulin was seen to enhance tolerance to ischaemia and improve functional recovery, while preischaemic glycogen depletion with intravenous epinephrine was seen to reduce tolerance to ischaemia and impair functional recovery, when compared with controls. Glycogen loaded hearts maintained the highest level of ATP and there was a close correlation between intramyocardial glycogen and CP during reperfusion, suggesting that glycogen content is a measure of myocardial metabolic and functional integrity. Presently, the role of glycogen loading in elective cardiac surgical patients has yet to be more widely evaluated in randomized clinical trials (Moulton and Robinson, 1990). However, special consideration should be given to those hearts which are likely to have reduced glycogen stores, for example in patients with low cardiac output, acute coronary insufficiency, inotropic infusions, and intra-aortic balloon counterpulsation support. In these circumstances perioperative infusion of GIK would appear to be advantageous (Coleman, 1989).

β-blockade

Chronic treatment with β-blockers has a number of physiological effects on the myocardium including decreased myocardial oxygen consumption, decreased sympathetic stimulation, increased coronary collateral flow, altered substrate utilization and membrane stabilization. Overall, β-blockers exert a protective effect on the myocardium in ischaemic heart disease, but the exact mechanisms are unclear. In animal studies, pretreatment with propranolol significantly increases the heart's tolerance to ischaemia (Nayler *et al.*, 1978; Pieper *et al.*, 1980; Veronee *et al.*, 1986). Propranolol appears not to preserve ATP, but may enhance its utilisation, slowing anaerobic glycolysis and lactate production, thereby delaying the onset of irreversible injury (Veronee *et al.*, 1986). Propranolol has been shown to preserve myocardial glycogen stores (Ichihara and Abiko, 1977). Clinically, it has been reported that patients who are on β-blockers, before coronary artery bypass surgery, suffer less perioperative myocardial damage (Poirier, Belliveau and Wynands, 1980; Berggren *et al.*, 1983). Of course, most patients undergoing elective coronary revascularization will already be established on β-blockers and should remain on them up to the time of surgery. For patients who are not already on β-blockers, it is recommended that they should be placed on them preoperatively to provide for a stable anaesthetic induction and prebypass period.

Calcium-antagonists

The coronary vasodilator, membrane-stabilizing and calcium homeostatic properties of calcium antagonists also exert a protective effect on the myocardium in ischaemic heart disease. Like β-blockers, pretreatment with calcium antagonists has also been shown to enhance the heart's tolerance to ischaemia (Clark *et al.*, 1977; Lowe *et al.*, 1977; Robb-Nicholson, Currie and Wechsler, 1978; Nayler, Ferrari and Williams, 1980). Similarly, most patients undergoing elective coronary revascularization will also be established on calcium-antagonists and should remain on them up to the time of surgery. Particularly beneficial effects have been reported with preischaemic infusions of lidoflazine in both laboratory (Flameng *et al.*, 1981; Kates *et al.*, 1983; Guvendick *et al.*, 1988) and clinical (Flameng *et al.*, 1983) studies. In the latter, intravenous lidoflazine, before cardiopulmonary bypass, was shown to enhance the preservation of myocardial CP, CP, glycogen and left ventricular function during coronary revascularization with an intermittent aortic cross-clamping technique. Some of the effects of lidoflazine may be attributable to nucleoside transport inhibition (Van Belle, 1985; Van Belle, Goossens and Wynants, 1987).

Nucleoside transport inhibition

During ischaemia, ATP is catabolized to AMP and leaks out of the myocyte into the interstitial space where it is degraded to adenosine by ectonucleotidases (Jennings and Steenbergen, 1985). Adenosine is taken-up from the interstital space into the endothelial cells, by a membrane nucleoside transport mechanism, where it is then metabolized to inosine and hypoxanthine (Van Belle, Goossens and Wynants, 1987). Adenosine, inosine and hypoxanthine constitute a nucleoside pool for the resynthesis of ATP via the salvage pathway (Manfredi and Holmes, 1985). However, leakage into the intravascular lumen and loss through wash-out by cardioplegia, non-coronary collateral flow and reperfusion, reduces the size of the nucleoside pool and could impair the rate of ATP synthesis (De Witt, Jochim and Behrendt, 1983). In addition, the loss of adenosine may have other detrimental effects within the myocardium, in regard to its vasodilator, β-blocker, calcium-antagonistic, anti-platelet and anti-neutrophil actions (Van Belle, 1985; Belardinelli, Linden and Berne, 1989). The metabolism of adenosine to inosine and hypoxanthine and its consequent loss from the nucleoside pool, can be limited by preventing its uptake into endothelial cells by nucleoside transport inhibition (NTI) (Van Belle, 1985; Van Belle, Goossens and Wynants, 1987). Various agents with NTI activity, including dipyridamole, dilazep, lidoflazine, mioflazine and soluflazine, have been shown experimentally to enhance the tolerance of the heart to ischaemia. However, except for lidoflazine (Flameng *et al.*, 1983), the clinical application of NTI in cardiac surgery has been limited due to the various practical problems with these agents, including poor bioavailability, non-parenteral preparations and proportionally greater calcium- antagonistic activities. Recently, a pure NTI for intravenous use (R 75 231, Janssen Research Foundation, Beerse, Belgium) has become available and is presently being evaluated for clinical use. Potentially, it could be administered before subjecting the heart to any form of ischaemic stress and used not only in elective or emergency cardiac surgery but also prophylactically in patients undergoing difficult angioplasty, where it would provide a valuable cardioprotective effect should things go wrong, while surgical intervention is arranged.

Warm cardioplegia

It is the policy of some blood cardioplegic administration protocols to initially infuse the solution at normothermia (Buckberg and Rosenkranz, 1987; Buckberg, 1989). The rationale for this technique is based on experimental studies in ischaemically damaged hearts demonstrating that a period of electromechanical arrest at normothermia would provide conditions whereby oxygen and other metabolic substrates, such as glutamate and aspartate (Rosenkrantz *et al.*, 1986), could be directed to reparative processes (Follette *et al.*, 1977b; Lazar *et al.*, 1979; Rosenkranz and Buckberg, 1983). The metabolic effects of these and other potential additives, such as calcium antagonists and free radical scavengers, are discussed in later sections. When the heart is already depleted of energy reserves before operation, as may occur in cardiogenic shock, recent cardiac arrest or when the heart is hypertrophied, it has been claimed that normothermic blood cardioplegic induction for 5 min, followed by cold blood cardioplegia, results in better postischaemic oxygen uptake and glycolysis, and superior functional recovery, than when cardioplegia is induced by cold blood alone (Rosenkranz *et al.*, 1982 and 1983). This technique can be readily applied to blood cardioplegia and is especially recommended for high risk patients (Buckberg and Rosenkranz, 1987; Buckberg, 1989).

Non-cardioplegic techniques of intraoperative myocardial protection

Hypothermic cardiopulmonary bypass

Electromechanical work accounts for approximately 80–85% of oxygen demand of the myocardium, with the remaining 20–25% representing basal metabolism (Challoner, 1968). Cardiopulmonary bypass reduces myocardial oxygen consumption by approximately 50–70% in the beating, non-tachycardiac, adequately perfused, non-hypertrophied, empty heart at 37°C (Hottenrott *et al.*, 1973; Buckberg *et al.*, 1977; McConnell *et al.*, 1977). As the heart is cooled there is progressive slowing of metabolism and oxygen uptake is further reduced by almost 40% at 28°C and 50% at 22°C (Buckberg *et al.*, 1977). Thus, hypothermic cardiopulmonary bypass can reduce myocardial oxygen consumption to approximately 25% of that of the working heart at 37°C. However, the marked beneficial effects of hypothermia, over and above those of cardiopulmonary bypass, on myocardial oxygen consumption have not been universally confirmed (Archie and Kirklin, 1973), since hypothermia may make the heart more prone to ischaemia due to its adverse effects on contractility, coronary flow reserve and oxygen dissociation (Archie and Kirklin, 1973; McConnell *et al.*, 1977). Hypothermia induces a progressive inotropic response such that oxygen consumption per beat is increased despite a reduction in heart rate. Consumption of high energy phosphate stores are increased and reach a maximum at 20°C. The effect is believed to be due to an increase in cytoplasmic calcium arising from both the inhibition of transport of calcium out of the cell and its sequestration within the cell (Kaufmann and Fleckenstein, 1965; Mattiazzi and Nilsson, 1976). This increase in contractility, coupled with the inability to induce and maintain cardiac arrest without fibrillation, partly explains the relatively poor myocardial protection brought about by hypothermia alone and the benefits to be gained by the combination of hypothermia and cardioplegic arrest (Follette *et al.*, 1978; Rosenfelt *et al.*, 1980), which has been demonstrated to reduce myocardial oxygen consumption at 20°C to only 5% of that of the working heart at 37°C (Bretschneider *et al.*, 1975; Buckberg *et al.*, 1977; Chitwood *et al.*, 1979). The complex relationships of perfusate pressure, temperature, composition and pH, heart rate and rhythm on coronary flow, coronary flow reserve and microvascular perfusion (McConnell *et al.*, 1975 and 1977) may also account for the suboptimal myocardial protection afforded by hypothermic cardiopulmonary bypass alone.

Coronary ostial perfusion

The widespread use of continuous coronary artery perfusion (Kay, Head and Nogueira, 1958) was largely abandoned 10–15 years ago as the benefits of cardioplegic arrest became recognized. Retrospective analysis of clinical results comparing continuous coronary artery perfusion with cold potassium cardioplegia revealed the superiority of the latter (Braimbridge *et al.*, 1977; Follette *et al.*, 1978). However, intermittent coronary ostial perfusion continues as an important technique during operations involving the aortic valve as the means to effectively deliver cardioplegia. The major problem is the avoidance of damage by the cannulae to the coronary ostia and guidelines have been layed down to minimise this risk (Pennington *et al.*, 1982). Early hand-held metal cannulae, with tips that could easily traumatize the coronary intima have been replaced by better designed devices with short, plastic or Silastic tips, and these are held in place only during the infusion of the dose of cardioplegia. Care must be taken to avoid excessive perfusion pressures, particularly when a cardioplegia pumped-delivery system is employed.

Hypothermic intermittent ischaemia and ventricular fibrillation

Intermittent ischaemia, by the simple application of the aortic cross-clamp, combined with systemic and topical hypothermia was the most commonly used procedure for intraoperative myocardial protection until the resurgence of interest in chemical cardioplegia. However, intermittent ischaemia during moderate systemic hypothermia (30–32°C), with or without topical hypothermia, continues to be used for short lasting procedures. Advocates of this technique have stressed its potential superiority in coronary artery bypass grafting, where there is uncertainty concerning the uniform distribution of the cardioplegic solution to all parts of the myocardium due to local obstructive lesions and to an unpredictable degree of non-coronary collateral flow (Olinger, Boncheck and Geiss, 1981; Olinger, Maloney and Mulder, 1985). It is claimed that graft length and orientation can be judged more precisely with a full and beating heart, and that the technique facilitates reconstruction of the heart following ventricular aneursysmectomy. Potential disadvantages include the risk of aortic damage and atheromatous embolization due to repeated cross-clamping. The importance of left ventricle venting (Buckberg, 1975; Olinger and Boncheck, 1978) and spontaneous or brief induction of fibrillation, as opposed to sustained electrical fibrillation (Hottenrott, Maloney and Buckberg, 1974a; Khuri *et al.*, 1985), have been emphasised in a description of an optimum technique (Olinger, 1987). Excellent results have been claimed by those who use this method of myocardial protection during coronary revascularization (Bonchek and Burlingame, 1987).

Hypothermic ventricular fibrillation

In earlier years, before the widespread adoption of cardioplegia, prolonged elective ventricular fibrillation was much favoured because of its relatively still field for surgical manipulation and reduced risk of air embolism, while permitting continuous coronary perfusion. However, the greatly increased oxygen consumption compared with the empty beating heart and the relatively poor perfusion to the subendocardium, particularly in the hypertrophied heart (Hottenrott *et al.*, 1973; Sink *et al.*, 1983) and during sustained electrical fibrillation (Hottenrott and Buckberg, 1974; Hottenrott, Maloney and Buckberg, 1974a and b), swung interest away from this technique, although it is still used by some during coronary revascularization (Akins, 1984 and

1987). The potentially detrimental effects of ventricular fibrillation have been claimed to have been overcome by adequate left ventricle venting, maintenance of cardiopulmonary bypass perfusion pressures between 80 mmHg and 100 mmHg, systemic hypothermia between 25°C and 28°C, topical cooling and the avoidance of electrical fibrillation (Baird *et al.*, 1975: Cox *et al.*, 1977; Vinas *et al.*, 1979; Spadaro *et al.*, 1982). However, these studies were performed in normal animal hearts in which the clinically relevant and potentially harmful effects of coronary artery stenoses and ventricular hypertrophy could not have been assessed. Nevertheless excellent results have been claimed by those who use this method of myocardial protection during coronary revascularization (Akins and Carrolly, 1987).

Conclusions on non-cardioplegic techniques

Despite the bulk of experimental evidence in favour of hypothermic cardioplegic arrest, various techniques based upon hypothermic fibrillation, with or without intermittent global or regional ischaemia, appear to provide satisfactory intraoperative myocardial protection for coronary revascularization. The natural history of coronary artery disease predisposes the myocardium to a degree of ischaemic tolerance and the presence of well developed coronary and non-coronary collaterals may be advantageous to a non-cardioplegic technique. In addition, pretreatment with β-blockers and calcium-antagonists will enhance the tolerance of the heart to limited periods of ischaemia. The potentially beneficial effects arising from the natural history of clinical ischaemic heart disease cannot be evaluated in the experimental animal. Unfortunately, there have been very few reports of clinical comparison, even less randomized, and the various protocols for fibrillation and ischaemia make it difficult to define the optimum technique. Nevertheless, these studies have tended to support the opinion that non-cardioplegic, in comparison with cardioplegic, techniques provide mildly suboptimal myocardial protection as determined by the preservation of myocardial ultrastructure (Flameng *et al.*, 1984; Schaper *et al.*, 1986; Beyersdorf *et al.*, 1990), high energy phosphates (Flameng *et al.*, 1984; Beyersdorf *et al.*, 1990) and glycogen (Flameng *et al.*, 1984), and by the amount of creatine kinase leakage (serum CK-MB) (Beyersdorf *et al.*, 1990), although some studies have reported no significant differences in creatine kinase leakage (Roberts *et al.*, 1981; Pepper *et al.*, 1982; Flameng *et al.*, 1984; Baur *et al.*, 1986). However, what limited haemodynamic studies have been performed have either failed to show any differences between the two techniques (Roberts *et al.*, 1981) or shown only mildly inferior immediate postoperative myocardial function after the non-cardioplegic technique (Flameng *et al.*, 1984; Beyersdorf *et al.*, 1990). Furthermore, what differences have been observed have either been non-significant (Beyersdorf *et al.*, 1990) or have been only temporary, with no differences in the final clinical outcome (Flameng *et al.*, 1984).

In conclusion, for routine revascularization in non-high risk patients, there is little to choose between non-cardioplegic and cardioplegic methods of myocardial protection, provided that they are performed by experienced surgeons. However, which of the two methods preserves the greatest number of myocardial cells and leads to better long-term results cannot be ascertained, since indirect measures of cell death, such as serum creatine kinase (CK-MB) and postoperative Q-waves, are often unreliable (Levitsky, 1987). Certainly, myocardial high energy phosphate and substrate stores are most likely to become depleted with intermittent ischaemia techniques (Levitsky, 1987; Flameng *et al.*, 1984; Beyersdorf *et al.*, 1990). Pretreatment with lidoflazine has been shown to significantly enhance the preservation of these stores, ultrastructure and function during coronary revascularization with intermittent ischaemia (Flameng *et al.*, 1983), and may well have contributed to the excellent results recently reported from the same institution (Kirklin *et al.*, 1989).

Cardioplegic techniques of intraoperative myocardial protection

Cold chemical cardioplegia has now become almost universally adopted by surgeons as the standard intraoperative protective measure (Buckberg, 1979, Rosenfeld, 1987; Miller, Binford and Hessel, 1982) although there are a few situations where other techniques may provide equally acceptable results. However, controversy still exists over the composition of the solutions and over the details of their administration. These include whether the solutions should be blood or crystalloid based, their electrolyte composition and pH, the addition of agents designed to maintain the concentration of high energy phosphates, reduce cell and interstitial oedema, increase coronary flow, avoid accumulation of toxic metabolites and free radicals, and the temperature, frequency, volume and method of administration. The controversy is fuelled when a successful method developed in animal experimentation has not been followed by the predicted equal success in its clinical application and *vice verse*. One explanation for this may lie in the absence of non-coronary collateral flow and consequent washout of the cardioplegic solution in isolated heart experiments. Clinically, this effect could potentially impair the efficacy of a good cardioplegic solution or improve the efficacy of a poor or toxic cardioplegic solution, as predicted by isolated heart studies.

The objectives of cardioplegia are to achieve mechanical and electrical arrest of the heart as quickly as possible, to cool it to the optimal temperature, to provide substrates to meet the reduced metabolic demands, buffer adverse changes in pH and to prevent intracellular and interstitial oedema developing. Cardioplegia may be induced in a number of ways, most commonly by raising the concentration of potassium in the solution, but also by removing calcium, lowering sodium, raising magnesium and adding procaine. In broad terms crystalloid cardioplegic solutions, besides containing potassium in concentrations ranging from 5 to 30 mmol l^{-1}, have developed along two lines. 'Intracellular' solutions containing low concentrations of sodium chloride and absent calcium, as in the Bretschneider (Bretschneider, 1964; Gebhard *et al.*, 1987) and Roe (Roe *et al.*, 1977) solutions, and 'extracellular' solutions containing near-normal concentrations of sodium chloride and mildly reduced calcium, as in the St. Thomas' Hospital (Hearse, Braimbridge and Jynge, 1981; Ledingham, Braimbridge and Hearse, 1987) and Tyers (Tyers *et al.*, 1977) solutions. The roles of potassium, sodium, calcium and magnesium during myocardial ischaemia, their inter-ionic relationships and their inclusion in optimum concentrations in cardioplegic solutions have proven to be of critical importance to successful cardioplegic protection, to which Hearse and colleagues have contributed considerable knowledge (Hearse, Braimbridge and Jynge, 1981).

Electrolyte composition of cardioplegic solutions

Potassium

From the time of its first use in arresting the heart by Melrose (Melrose *et al.*, 1955), potassium has continued as the major cardioplegic agent, albeit at much reduced concentration. Extracellular hyperkalaemia reduces the membrane potential and inactivates the sodium channel, whose opening normally initiates the upstroke of the action potential, thereby rendering the myocardium unexcitable in diastolic arrest. The concentration required to produce arrest is positively correlated with temperature and at 20°C a concentration ranging between 15 and 30 mmol l^{-1} is optimal (Hearse, Braimbridge and Jynge, 1981; Rousou *et al.*, 1981). Higher concentrations of potassium predispose to a cellular influx of calcium that increases wall tension, raises coronary vascular resistance, accelerates ATP consumption and promotes myocardial contracture (Rich and Brady, 1974; Hearse, Stewart and Braimbridge, 1975). It can also cause injury to the coronary endothelium (Saldanha and Hearse, 1989). The adverse effects of high potassium cardioplegia may be less evident in the clinical situation because of washout of the solution by non-coronary collateral blood flow (Buckberg, 1979).

Calcium

The complete removal of calcium from a solution perfusing a heart results in cardioplegic arrest, but is not, on its own, an acceptable method when applied to the isolated heart since calcium is required for cell membrane stabilization (Hearse, Braimbridge and Jynge, 1981). Cardioplegic solutions free from calcium have been shown to result in acute ischaemic contracture after reperfusion, thought to be due to the flooding of calcium back into the cell, the 'calcium-paradox'. However, there are many factors that influence the loss of cell calcium during cardioplegia and *in vivo* this phenomenon is largely avoided, since sufficient calcium derives from the non-coronary collateral blood flow after aortic cross-clamping. In isolated hearts, the occurrence of the calcium paradox depends on the concentration of calcium in the reperfusate and the duration of reperfusion (Baker *et al.*, 1984), the temperature during ischaemia (Baker, Bullock and Hearse, 1983) and on the pH of the cardioplegic solution (Hendren *et al.*, 1987). Thus, in isolated hearts, myocyte damage and functional impairment, attributable to the calcium paradox, has been eliminated by lowering the ischaemic temperature to 4°C and by reducing the pH of a cardioplegic solution from 8.5 to 7.5. The optimal range of calcium concentration for extracellular cardioplegic solutions appears to be very narrow and temperature dependent. In isolated heart experiments, varying the concentration of calcium between 0 and 2.4 mmol l^{-1}, under normothermic conditions, in St. Thomas' Hospital cardioplegic solution No.2, produced the least leakage of creatine kinase and greatest recovery of aortic flow at a calcium concentration of 1.2 mmol l^{-1} (Yamamoto, Braimbridge and Hearse, 1984) and most likely accounts for its better protection when compared under moderate hypothermic (20°C) conditions with the earlier St. Thomas' Hospital solution No.1 (Ledingham, Braimbridge and Hearse, 1987). However, when a similar study was performed under more severe hypothermic (8°C) conditions, but with a different extracellular cardioplegic solution, it was found that the best preservation of ATP and functional recovery occurred in the complete absence of calcium (Boggs *et al.*, 1987).

Calcium-channel blocking drugs have been used for the induction of cardioplegic arrest and reasonable functional recovery has been reported (Barner *et al.*, 1982). However, the recovery is either no better (Magee *et al.*, 1979; Johnson *et al.*, 1982) or inferior to hyperkalaemic cardioplegia (Yamamto *et al.*, 1983), possibly due to residual negative inotropic and chronotropic effects of large dosages, and attention has since focused more on the use of calcium-blocking drugs as additives to other forms of induced cardioplegia.

Magnesium

Magnesium has negative inotropic activity and may be used as a primary cardioplegic agent, but is less effective than potassium. Its negative inotropic action may depend on the reduction of intracellular sodium ion activity which may limit sodium ion-stimulated calcium influx or expedite calcium efflux. Incorporation of magnesium into cardioplegic solutions appears to be beneficial through counteracting the positive inotropic effect of calcium during cardioplegia, thereby permitting the presence of calcium in the solution and avoiding the risk of the calcium paradox. Magnesium in a concentration of 16 mmol l^{-1} has been shown to greatly improve functional recovery from normothermic arrest produced by 16 mmol l^{-1} potassium (Hearse, Stewart and Baimbridge, 1978a) and this has recently been confirmed under hypothermic (8°C) hyperkalaemic arrest in a solution containing only 0.1 mmol l^{-1} calcium and shown to be accompanied by better conservation of CP (Reynolds *et al.*, 1989). Also recently, in the isolated rat heart, low concentrations of calcium (0.1 and 1.2 mmol l^{-1}) during hypothermic (8°C) cardioplegia were shown to cause myocardial contracture, depletion of CP and ATP and depressed functional recovery in comparison with a solution lacking both calcium and magnesium (Geffin *et al.*, 1989). The addition of magnesium to the calcium-containing solutions reversed these effects. The same investigators had previously demonstrated that myocardial contracture, associated with calcium-containing, magnesium-free solutions, causes an increase in coronary vascular resistance during cardioplegia infusion (Torchiana *et al.*, 1987). Thus, when calcium is absent from a cardioplegic solution, there appears to be no great benefit from adding magnesium, but then there is the ever present risk of the calcium paradox, particularly at higher temperatures and longer durations of cardioplegia.

Sodium

As extracellular sodium is reduced, the sodium-calcium exchange promotes either calcium influx (Langer, Nudd and Ricchiuti, 1976) or decreased efflux (Reuter and Seitz, 1968) which results in an increase in cellular calcium. The immediate effect is to produce temporary systolic arrest with contracture, followed by relaxation and diastolic arrest as transmembrane equilibrium is restored. The contracture phase is associated with creatine kinase leakage and can be averted by reducing the availability of calcium. Bretschneider's intracellular solutions, with low sodium and absent calcium, meet this requirement and diastolic arrest is expedited by the incorporation of procaine into the solution. The partial or total exclusion of sodium from a cardioplegic solution leaves a large osmotic capacity available for other protective agents, as for example the histidine buffer included in Bretschneider's solutions (Gebhard *et al.*, 1987). In the extracellular hyperkalaemic cardioplegic solution, it has been shown that creatine kinase leakage is least when the sodium concentration is in the range of 100–110 mmol l^{-1} (Hearse, Braimbridge and Jynge, 1981), the concentration used in St. Thomas' Hospital No.2 solution.

Procaine

Procaine has been widely used in cardioplegic solutions to promote arrest, to reduce oxygen demand in the arrested state and to improve recovery, but the optimum concentration for these effects differs widely (Dudziak and Lochner, 1965). Details on its exact mode of action are uncertain, but, in common with other local anaesthetics, it binds to the lipid components of cellular membranes and blocks the movement of sodium and calcium (Lee, 1976). Thus, it can induce cardiac arrest by inhibiting sodium influx and potentially protects the ischaemic myocardium by inhibiting calcium influx. Procaine, in a concentration of around 10 mmol l^{-1}, in combination with low sodium and absent calcium, forms the basis of a number of cardioplegic solutions and its presence is essential to the cardioplegic action. However, procaine in this concentration has a long lasting action which may delay recovery after reperfusion. Lower concentrations of procaine have been used in combination with hyperkalaemic cardioplegia and a concentration of 1.0 mmol l^{-1}, as used in St. Thomas' Hospital No.1, reduces postischaemic creatine kinase leakage (Hearse, Braimbridge and Jynge, 1981). Functional studies with St. Thomas' Hospital solution No.2 have demonstrated that the optimal concentration of procaine is 0.05 mmol l^{-1}, that this benefit is lost at 1.0 mmol l^{-1} and that it becomes progressively more detrimental at higher concentrations (Hearse, O'Brien and Braimbridge, 1981). It is possible that at higher concentrations the cell membrane is no longer stabilized and becomes leaky, permitting an adverse influx of calcium (Katz, 1980).

Cardioplegia pH and buffering

Ischaemia stimulates anaerobic glycolysis, even in hypothermic conditions, leading to an accumulation of lactic and hydrogen ions. In addition, the hydrolysis of ATP also generates a significant quantity of hydrogen ions. The resulting intracellular acidosis inhibits further anaerobic energy production (Rovett, Lamberton and Neely, 1975) and causes cellular damage by inducing lysosomal enzyme activity. Thus, the provision of a buffering agent in the cardioplegic solution might prevent these detrimental effects. However, the ideal pH for cardioplegia and, in consequence, the ideal buffering agent, are yet undefined. With decreasing temperature, the neutrality point of water (pN) shifts in an alkaline direction and, under physiological conditions, there is a parallel shift in intracellular pH known as the 'Rahn effect' (Rahn, Reeves and Howell, 1975). Accordingly, to maintain cellular metabolism during cooling, the extracellular pH must change in similar proportion to the intracellular pH and thus a slightly alkaline cardioplegic solution might be desirable (McConnell *et al.*, 1975; Hearse, Braimbridge and Jynge, 1981). Thus, if it is important to preserve enzyme activity at 17°C the extracellular pH should theoretically be kept between 8.0 and 8.1. The selection of a buffer depends not only on the buffering capacity, but also on the dissociation constant (pK) value, since this determines the pH range over which a buffering effect will be operative. Cardioplegic solutions may contain no buffer (St. Thomas' No.1), thus permitting the myocardium to adjust its own pH during ischaemia, or buffers whose pK varies from 4.07 (glutamate), 6.04 (histidine, as in Bretschneider's solutions), 6.1 (bicarbonate), 6.7 (imidazole), 7.2 (phosphate) to 8.08 (Tris/THAM). The relative buffering capacities of these agents has been evaluated (Kresh *et al.*, 1987). The concentration of buffer may be relatively low and simply stabilize the various components of the solution (St. Thomas' No.2, with 10 mmol l^{-1} bicarbonate buffer adjusted to pH 7.8) or sufficiently high to counteract acidosis developing in the ischaemic myocardium (Bretschneider's solutions, with 180 mmol l^{-1} histidine-HCL buffer adjusted to pH 7.1). In comparison with non-buffered cardioplegic solutions, the buffering of Bretschneider's solutions have been shown to significantly slow the decay of ATP in ischaemic canine myocardium and this beneficial effect is progressively enhanced by increasing hypothermia (Gebhard *et al.*, 1987). Some evidence in favour of maintaining the intracellular pH either constant or permitting it to fall has been provided by studies in the isolated rat heart subjected to 2h of cardioplegic arrest at 15°C (Bernard *et al.*, 1985). A glutamate-containing solution adjusted to pH 7.0, in comparison with one adjusted to pH 7.7, resulted in higher myocardial creatine phosphate at the end of ischaemia, higher ATP content at the end of reperfusion and a faster recovery, although the final level of aortic flow was no better. With four different buffers, glutamate, bicarbonate, Tris and histidine, all adjusted to pH 7.0 or 7.4, the latter three maintained intracellular pH, measured by ^{31}P NMR spectroscopy, close to the control level throughout ischaemia, whereas that containing glutamate resulted in a fall in intracellular pH, as might be anticipated by its low pK. However, despite this fall, there was marginally better preservation of ATP at the end of both ischaemia and reperfusion with the glutamate buffered cardioplegic solution at pH 7.0 and it was suggested that this might have been due to glutamate acting as a substrate for anaerobic energy production. There was no evidence that a persistently low or even reduced intracellular pH was deleterious. Somewhat contrastingly, in an isolated working rabbit heart preparation, normothermic cardioplegia with an imidazole buffer was shown to be marginally, but significantly, better in preserving functional recovery than a bicarbonate buffer (Vander Woude *et al.*, 1985). The pH of the coronary effluent was higher with imidazole compared with bicarbonate. Whether the improved recovery was attributable to the more effective buffering with imidazole, which has a higher pK than bicarbonate and, being less ionized, traverses cell membranes more readily, or some other property of imidazole, was not established.

In conclusion, it may be said that the question of the optimal buffer and its concentration, or even for the need for a buffer, in a cardioplegic solution remains unresolved. The most effective buffering system appears to be histidine, as used in Bretschneider's solutions, but its use greatly influences the other components of the solution (Del-Nido *et al.*, 1985). What small differences have been described in isolated hearts in the performance of different buffers, may reflect some actions of the buffer other than that of stabilizing pH (Hearse, Braimbridge and Jynge, 1981). Within reasonable limits, finely controlling pH may be irrelevant in the *in vivo* situation because non-coronary collateral blood flow dilutes the cardioplegia and it is thus relatively more important to regularly reinfuse the solution, washout metabolites and rearrest mechanical and metabolic activity.

Conclusions on the electrolyte composition of cardioplegic solutions

No world wide agreement on the optimal composition of a cardioplegic solution has yet been reached, probably because of the very many variables involved, not only in the components, but also in the precise circumstances, including temperature, in which the observations have been conducted. There have been few direct comparisons between widely used cardioplegic solutions. The very complexity of the subject and the controversies surrounding it have led most surgeons to settle on one recommended formula and, finding this gives reasonably good surgical results, restrict themselves to it thenceforth. However, there is no doubt that the search for the optimal composition of cardioplegic solutions should continue, so that high risk cases receive the best possible management leading to good immediate postoperative recovery and a satisfactory long-term outcome.

Comparisons of presently used crystalloid cardioplegic solutions

Although there have been many reported comparisons of blood and crystalloid cardioplegic solutions, there have been relatively few experimental or clinical comparisons of crystalloid solutions, particularly those in current use.

St. Thomas' No.2, Tyers', Roe's and lactated Ringer's solutions were compared in the isolated working rat heart undergoing 3h of arrest at 20°C (Robinson, Braimbridge and Hearse, 1984a). Recovery of aortic flow was 88% with St. Thomas' and only between 9.6% and 20.6% with the other solutions. Furthermore, spontaneous return of sinus rhythm occurred within 1 min in all cases with St. Thomas' solution, whereas the return was delayed or incomplete with the others. Creatine kinase leakage following ischaemia was least with St. Thomas' solution.

St. Thomas' No.1 and No.2 solutions were compared in the isolated working rat heart undergoing 3h of arrest at 20°C (Ledingham, Braimbridge and Hearse, 1987). Solution No.2 was superior in nearly all respects including a faster and spontaneous return to sinus rhythm, greater recovery of aortic flow and lesser leakage of creatine kinase. In contrast, 40% of the hearts receiving solution No.1 could not be defibrillated.

Bretschneider's, St. Thomas' No.2 with procaine and Kirklin's solutions were compared in the isolated dog heart undergoing 3–5h of arrest at 22°C (Schnabel *et al.*, 1987). Bretschneider's solution was two or three times more effective in preserving ATP and ultrastructure than either of the other two. Much endothelial and myocyte oedema occurred during ischaemia with both St. Thomas' and Kirklin's solutions, which did not reverse during perfusion and led to obstructed capillaries and contraction band formation.

Bretschneider's and Roe's solutions were compared in a canine model of cardiopulmonary bypass undergoing 4.5h of arrest at 27°C (Wilson *et al.*, 1990). Bretschneider's solution provided superior preservation of ATP, coronary effluent pH, ultrastructure and function.

Bretschneider's and St. Thomas' No.1 solutions were compared in a randomized series of clinical cases over a range of aortic cross-clamp times by the measurement of several haemodynamic variables in the immediate postoperative period (Gallandat-Huet *et al.*, 1988). Myocardial protection was good with both solutions and no important differences were observed except for a significantly higher incidence of pacemaker insertion after Bretschneider's solution.

Conclusions on comparisons between crystalloid cardioplegic solutions

It is not possible to state which of the crystalloid cardioplegic solutions perform best in the clinical situation, since there have been hardly any direct comparisons. Information concerning the worldwide practice of crystalloid cardioplegia is lacking. The most commonly used solutions tend to be the commercially available ones. In the United Kingdom St. Thomas' No.1 is almost exclusively used, in Europe Bretschneider's and St. Thomas' No.1 solutions are used, and in North America St. Thomas' No.2 (Plegisol) is used. It is acknowledged that various institutions around the world continue to use their own, locally developed, cardioplegia formulations and, presumably, these provide satisfactory results. It is conceivable that the differences in efficacy among currently used crystalloid cardioplegia solutions will never be clearly demonstrated in the clinical environment.

Oxygenated cardioplegic solutions

Oxygenated crystalloid cardioplegia

Although hypothermic cardioplegia greatly reduces the oxygen demand of the heart, it does not inhibit it altogether and this has led to the widespread use of blood cardioplegia in the hope that better recovery of mechanical and metabolic function will result. However, good results are regularly reported from centres employing crystalloid cardioplegia and there is a natural reluctance by these centres to change to blood cardioplegia in view of the additional equipment and procedures required for its use. Furthermore, it has been pointed out that although blood cardioplegia will carry more oxygen per ml than crystalloid cardioplegia, the actual amounts of oxygen available to the myocardium, in clinically applied hypothermia, is similar (Digerness, Vanini and Wideman, 1981). Attempts have therefore been made to explore the possibility of providing more oxygen in crystalloid cardioplegic solutions by equilibrating them with

100% oxygen and increasing their oxygen carrying capacity by the incorporation of perfluorocarbons. Oxygenation can be achieved by bubbling oxygen directly into the vented cardioplegia bag (Merin and Fishman, 1986) or by bubbler or membrane oxygenating systems (Landymore and Myers, 1988). Many laboratory based reports have shown the superiority of oxygenation of multi-dose crystalloid solutions in improving mechanical (Bodenhamer *et al.*, 1983; Coetzee *et al.*, 1986; Oguma, Imai and Eguchi, 1986; De Witt *et al.*, 1988; Ledingham, Braimbridge and Hearse, 1988; Tabayashi *et al.*, 1983) and metabolic functions (Bodenhamer *et al.*, 1983; Coetzee *et al.*, 1986; Oguma, Imai and Eguchi, 1986; De Witt *et al.*, 1988), decreasing creatine kinase release (Ledingham, Braimbridge and Hearse, 1988) and diminishing ultrastructural changes (Bodenhamer *et al.*, 1983; Coetzee *et al.*, 1986). The value of oxygenation has been demonstrated under hypothermic conditions ranging from 4°C to 20°C and shown to be effective during ischaemic periods of 4h or longer (Bodenhamer *et al.*, 1983; Ledingham, Braimbridge and Hearse, 1988). Estimates of the availability of oxygen dissolved in the cardioplegic solution have suggested that oxygenation with 100% oxygen is adequate to meet the demand of the hypothermic cardiopleged heart (Ledingham, Braimbridge and Hearse, 1988) and no further benefit followed from oxygenation of a perfluorocarbon containing solution (Tabayashi *et al.*, 1988). Many cardioplegic solutions contain bicarbonate which may result in a distinctly alkaline pH if oxygenation is performed with 100% oxygen rather than 95% O_2 and 5% CO_2. The effect of this may be to predispose to the calcium paradox on perfusion if the cardioplegic solution is devoid of calcium and may occur even with deep hypothermia, but can be avoided by lowering the pH with a mixture of 95% O_2 and 5% CO_2 (Hendren *et al.*, 1987).

The clinical use of oxygenated crystalloid solutions has not been widely reported and fears have been expressed about the potential risk of oxygen coming out of solution when it is warmed and forming gaseous microemboli in the heart (Engleman *et al.*, 1981). These emboli may affect the uniform distribution of the cardioplegic solution so that some areas are poorly protected, but the practical reality of this danger has never been evaluated. However, it is easily avoided by oxygenating the cardioplegic solution at a higher temperature than that to which it is likely to be warmed when it is infused into the heart, albeit at some loss of its oxygen carrying capacity. This precaution may only be important at the initial cardioplegic infusion, since the temperature of the heart before infusion is likely to be between 25°C and 37°C. A retrospective study of coronary artery bypass surgery showed that 100% oxygenation of the cardioplegic solution was superior to a non-oxygenated solution, as regards postoperative creatine kinase levels, when arrest was longer than 28 min (Guyton *et al.*, 1985).

Blood cardioplegia

Blood cardioplegia has been used extensively in the belief that recovery can be improved by the increased oxygen carriage and the presence of the oncotic activity of plasma proteins limiting the extent of interstitial oedema. Theoretically, further advantages may accrue through the much greater buffering capacity (Bing *et al.*, 1982; Warner *et al.*, 1987 and 1988), the provision of tricarboxylic acid cycle substrates and the presence of catalase systems which are abundant in red blood cells (Illes, 1989). However, although much greater oxygen may be delivered to the heart by blood in comparison with crystalline cardioplegia, the release of oxygen is much reduced since hypothermia shifts the oxyhaemoglobin dissociation curve to the left, although this may be partially offset by the addition of 2,3-DPG to the blood (Valeri *et al.*, 1980; Card *et al.*, 1988). In fact, the release of oxygen from blood at 10°C and 20°C is no greater than that from an oxygenated saline solution (Digerness, Vanini and Wildeman, 1981), and at 4°C the oxygen extracted from a blood cardioplegic solution with an haematocrit up to 24% comes directly from dissolved oxygen (Heitmiller *et al.*, 1985). A recent study comparing functional and metabolic recovery following plasma-based, oxygenated cardioplegia with haematocrits ranging from 0% to 17%, supports the observation that the efficacy of hypothermic (10°C) blood cardioplegia is not solely attributable to oxygen delivery, but to some other physiological role of the red cells (Illes *et al.*, 1989).

There are a number of potential disadvantages to the use of blood cardioplegia. In the first place, the viscosity of blood is much higher than that of a crystalloid solution, particularly in hypothermia. This reduces the rate of flow to the myocardium and it is more difficult to lower the temperature of the heart (Mullen *et al.*, 1987a). Secondly, the capillary perfusion is impaired and it has been shown that even with a blood cardioplegic solution of haematocrit 5% at 10°C, the number of unfilled capillaries on the left ventricular epicardial surface was reduced to 31% of those filled at 37°C due to sludging, despite the fact that coronary vascular resistance, which is determined by precapillary resistance vessels, was reduced (Sakai *et al.*, 1988). Such sludging could result in maldistribution of the blood cardioplegia solution throughout the heart and may have been responsible for frequent postoperative conduction disturbances observed following cold blood cardioplegia (Gundry *et al.*, 1989) and it has been asserted that blood cardioplegia should not be used at a temperature lower than 20°C

(Magovern *et al.*, 1982). Even at 28°C regional myocardial perfusion distal to a stenosis of the left anterior descending coronary artery has been reported to be better with crystalloid than with blood cardioplegia (Eugene *et al.*, 1987). On the other hand, it has been claimed that a very dilute blood cardioplegic solution at 5°C, with a haematocrit of 5%, reduced oedema, doubled oxygen consumption and prevented an increase in coronary vascular resistance (Suaudeau *et al.*, 1982).

In practice, it is usual to take whole blood from the extracorporeal circuit and mix it with a cardioplegic solution containing potassium and other agents to form the blood cardioplegic solution. This can be done by either manually mixing the components in a reservoir or by using a specifically designed delivery system which automatically mixes pump-blood and cardioplegia in pre-defined ratios (Rose, Catinella and Cunningham, 1987; Buckberg, 1989). After mixing, the solution is passed through a cooling circuit prior to its delivery to the patient. No advantage has been observed by using washed red cells rather than whole blood (Bing *et al.*, 1987).

Comparison of blood and crystalloid cardioplegia

There have been very many laboratory and clinical comparisons of the relative merits of blood and crystalloid cardioplegia. The evaluation of these studies is difficult because of a number of variables, including the temperature maintained during cardioplegia, the concentration of red cells in the perfusate, the composition of the crystalloid solution and the many and varied criteria of efficacy applied to haemodynamic, metabolic, structural and clinical consequences of the procedures. In particular, the composition of the crystalloid cardioplegic solutions used are not always stated, and when such information is provided, it is clear that the composition would not be acceptable to many experts regularly using crystalloid cardioplegia, as for example, the not uncommon total absence of calcium from the solution. Furthermore, although the blood solution is almost invariably oxygenated, this is not so in the case of the crystalloid solution. Thus, it is not surprising that in a comparison between a poor crystalloid solution and a blood-based solution the more physiological solution performed better. In the opinion of authors undertaking laboratory studies comparing the two forms of cardioplegia, blood, in comparison with crystalloid solutions, has been considered superior by some (Bing *et al.*, 1982; Catinella *et al.*, 1984; Feindel *et al.*, 1984; Krukenkamp, Silverman and Levitsky, 1987; Prasad, Bharadwaj and Card, 1988) and equal or inferior by others (Magovern *et al.*, 1982; Heitmiller *et al.*, 1985; Goldstein *et al.*, 1986; Card *et al.*, 1988; Rousou *et al.*, 1988). Again, in clinical practice, blood cardioplegia has been considered better by some (Shapira *et al.*, 1980; Fremes *et al.*, 1984; Iverson *et al.*, 1984; Daggett *et al.*, 1987; Mullen *et al.*, 1987b; Khuri *et al.*, 1988) and equal or inferior by others (Engleman *et al.*, 1981; Mullen *et al.*, 1986; Gundry *et al.*, 1989). In conclusion, it is impossible with the evidence currently available to decide which of the two procedures is preferable and more studies are indicated in circumstances where the application of either is considered to be optimal. Thus, there is good evidence that there is little to be gained as regards oxygen availability by the use of a blood solution below 20°C and, at lower temperatures, there is danger of blood sludging and causing poor perfusion of the microvasculature. In the case of a crystalloid solution, this must have been shown to be superior to other crystalloid solutions at the temperature selected for a comparison with blood. In addition, it is reasonable that crystalloid solution should be fully oxygenated and that the equilibration should be undertaken at a temperature no lower than that of the heart, to avoid any risk of gas emboli when the solution is infused. Finally, any additives, for example Krebs cycle intermediates, that supplement the blood cardioplegia and are known to be beneficial in their own right, should, in fairness, also be added to the crystalloid solution under comparison. In the present state of knowledge, there seems generally little to choose between blood or crystalloid solutions for routine intraoperative myocardial protection, but in special circumstances, severe cardiac hypertrophy (Khuri *et al.*, 1988), extensive coronary artery disease, or revascularization and reperfusion following acute ischaemia (Buckberg, 1986), the relative merits would have to be specifically validated. The techniques of warm induction (Rosenkranz *et al.*, 1983; Buckberg and Rosenkranz, 1987; Buckberg, 1989) and warm reperfusion (Teoh *et al.*, 1986; Buckberg and Rosenkranz, 1987; Buckberg, 1989) are unique to some blood cardioplegia administration protocols and may not be comparable with crystalloid cardioplegia techniques due to the oxygen requirements of the heart in normothermic circumstances.

Crystalloid solutions containing perfluorocarbons

Any inferiority of a crystalloid as opposed to a blood cardioplegic solution has been mainly attributed to its low oxygen carrying capacity in simple solution, although this can be much enhanced by oxygenation. The development of perfluorocarbons opened up the possibility that this difficulty could be overcome and an initial report using the rabbit heart (Kanter *et al.*, 1981) claimed higher oxygen uptake during normothermic ischaemia and better recovery of function following an oxygenated perfluorocarbon crystalloid solution than after a non-oxygenated crystalloid solution. However, in a study in pig hearts, although the perfluorocarbon solution maintained better high energy phosphate levels in comparison with a non-oxygenated crystalline solution during hypothermic (10–15°C) ischaemia, the postischaemic recovery of contractility and compliance were similar (Rousou, 1982). In contrast, the importance of oxygen availability to the hypertrophied pig heart, subjected to 3 hours of hypothermic ischaemia, was shown by the superiority of an oxygenated perfluorocarbon solution over a non-oxygenated crystalloid solution in improving haemodynamic recovery and in preventing ultrastructural changes (Novick *et al.*, 1985). Furthermore, the perfluorocarbon solution performed significantly better than a blood solution with a haematocrit of 24%. However, these initially encouraging results have recently been shown to be matched by simply oxygenating a standard crystalloid solution (Tabayashi *et al.*, 1988). In dogs submitted to 2h of arrest at 18°C, the oxygenated crystalloid solution produced as good haemodynamic recovery as an oxygenated perfluorocarbon solution, although the perfluorocarbon solution delivered twice the oxygen content. It remains to be seen whether this difference in oxygen carrying capacity is of importance in higher risk circumstances, such as cardiac hypertrophy. Nevertheless, the importance of oxygen availability during arrest at higher temperatures has been demonstrated in animals receiving an oxygenated crystalloid solution containing a lecithin-based perfluorocarbon. Arrest for 90 minutes (Menasche *et al.*, 1988a) and 180 min (Johnson *et al.*, 1988a) at 30°C was followed by significantly better recovery of dynamic ventricular function than in the absence of the perfluorocarbon. Perfluorocarbons, in addition to binding oxygen, have been shown to reduce neutrophil chemotaxis, adherence and superoxide generation, and thereby may have a role in protecting the endothelium of the microvasculature from reperfusion injury (Forman *et al.*, 1987; Bajaj *et al.*, 1989).

In conclusion, there have been no reports of the clinical use of perfluorocarbons in cardioplegic solutions, probably because the perfluorocarbon emulsions that have been available until recently have possessed adverse complement-activating properties (Vercellotti *et al.*, 1982). However, the newer lecithin-based perfluorocarbon emulsions are free from this disadvantage and clinical trials are awaited.

Effect of cardioplegia on the heart

Hyperkalaemic cardioplegia produces rapid mechanical and electrical arrest of the heart, thereby reducing energy demand to a level depending on the temperature. In combination with hypothermia, energy demand falls further and at 20°C oxygen consumption is only one twentieth of that in the normal working heart (Bretschneider *et al.*, 1975; Buckberg *et al.*, 1977; Chitwood *et al.*, 1979). However, even this small demand cannot be entirely provided by oxygen derived from intermittent oxygenated crystalloid or blood cardioplegia and metabolism shifts progressively from aerobic to anaerobic, which is more than ten times less economical in utilizing glucose for ATP production. Hence myocardial ATP falls, levels of ADP and AMP are largely unaffected, and adenosine, inosine, hypoxanthine and lactate accumulate during ischaemia (Sollevei *et al.*, 1987). Following reperfusion there is several hours delay in the recovery of oxygen and lactate consumption, compliance and ejection fraction (Fremes et al., 1985), and uptake of substrates is, for a while, markedly abnormal with no uptake of fatty acids or carbohydrates (Svensson *et al.*, 1990). Studies have shown that inefficient postischaemic oxygen utilization, when the heart is developing physiological pressures, is a sensitive marker of myocardial injury and of the efficacy of cardioplegic protection (Krukenkamp *et al.*, 1986).

Standard cardioplegic techniques often fail to suppress the electrical activity in the atrioventricular node and bundle of His (Magilligan *et al.*, 1985; Ferguson *et al.*, 1986a and b; Landymore *et al.*, 1986 and 1987). Such activity appears to be responsible for the delayed return of sinus rhythm and the associated metabolic activity appears to be responsible for reduced myocardial ATP, mitochondrial injury and depressed postischaemic functional performance (Landymore *et al.*, 1987). However, this activity can be suppressed by reinfusions of the cardioplegic solution, topical hypothermia or by the addition of a calcium-channel blocker to the solution (Ferguson *et al.*, 1986a and b; 1987).

Potentially detrimental effects of cardioplegia

Cold crystalloid cardioplegia has been observed in man to cause damage to the endothelium of the coronary microvasculature, evidenced by reduced pinocytic vesicles, intracellular oedema and slight nuclear changes (Lindal, Srlie and Jrgenson, 1988). During reperfusion these changes worsen, whereas changes in the myocytes tended to regress. Similar findings were observed in the guinea-pig (Chiavarelli *et al.*, 1989) and sheep (Mattila *et al.*, 1987), but, in the latter, these could be prevented by introducing blood or albumin into the cardioplegic solution. Rewarming after cold cardioplegia has been shown to increase the coronary contractile response to acetylcholine and could predispose to parasympathetically induced intraoperative coronary spasm (Furusho *et al.*, 1989). In the isolated rat heart, coronary vascular responsiveness to 5-hydroxytryptamine (5-HT), an endothelium-dependent vasodilator, was lost following a 30 min hypothermic infusion of a non-oxygenated cardioplegic solution containing either 25 mmol l^{-1} or 40 mmol l^{-1} potassium (Saldanha and Hearse, 1989). Thus, these studies suggest that hyperkalaemic cardioplegic solutions either damage the endothelium or impair its function and this may have unfavourable effects on microvascular perfusion and postischaemic functional recovery. However, recent studies from the author's laboratory (Amrani 1991 – unpublished work), in which the potassium concentration in St. Thomas' No.1 was increased from 20 mmol l^{-1} to 120 mmol l^{-1}, showed that the postischaemic recovery of endothelial function, as assessed by the response to 5-HT, was not affected by the potassium concentration when the solution was administered at 20°C, although the recovery of mechanical function was detrimentally affected at the highest potassium concentration. In contrast, severe hypothermia (4°C), as obtainable during transplantation, may protect both the endothelium and the myocyte from the potentially adverse effects of hyperkalaemic solutions (Ledingham *et al.*, 1990b).

Optimal temperature for cardioplegic protection

Severe hypothermia has a number of effects on cellular homeostasis (Hearse, Braimbridge and Jynge, 1981), including ionic redistribution and cell swelling due to the inactivation of sodium–potassium ATPase (Leaf, 1973), protein denaturalization, enzyme damage and cold-induced injury, which may be detrimental to the myocardium in the absence of cardioplegic protection. However, a reduction in the fluidity of lipid cell membranes during hypothermia (Chapman, 1975) may actually protect against the consequences of inhibition of ion transport and confer protection against reperfusion injury (Hearse, Humphrey and Bullock, 1978). Experimentally it has been shown in the isolated working rat heart that cold cardioplegia produces optimal recovery of function and retention of myocardial ATP at 4°C (Hearse, Stewart and Chain, 1974; Hearse, Stewart and Braimbridge, 1975). However, the outcome was only slightly less good at 15°C and this observation was confirmed in the isolated dog heart (Rosenfeldt, 1982). Other *in vivo* studies also support the observation that temperatures between 10°C and 15°C provide optimal functional recovery following 2h of cardioplegic arrest (Balderman *et al.*, 1983). In a study of postischaemic left ventricular function it was shown that the recovery of myocardial oxygen consumption at peak developed left ventricular pressure was unchanged after cardioplegia at 12°C, but raised after 20°C and further raised after 28°C (Krukenkamp *et al.*, 1986). Clinical observations suggest that a cardiac temperature in the range 11–15°C results in higher myocardial ATP and lower lactate than temperatures in the range of 6–10°C or 16–24°C (Jansson *et al.*, 1987). There is good evidence that cooling the heart to 4°C is well tolerated (Swanson, Dufek and Kahn, 1980) and this temperature has been employed for the preservation of the isolated heart for transplantation with good results (English *et al.*, 1980; Swanson and Meyerowitz, 1987). However, in surgical practice it is most difficult to induce and maintain cardiac cooling much below 15°C and this level is now generally accepted as satisfactory.

Methods of cardiac cooling

Experiments in isolated hearts can ensure uniform cooling, but in the clinical situation the heart is lying in a bed where the surrounding temperature is higher than optimal and, at the same time, it is being warmed by systemic perfusate returning to it via various vascular channels. The problem is to lower the temperature consistently in all parts of the heart and this is particularly difficult in the presence of coronary artery stenoses or ventricular hypertrophy.

Systemic cooling

Systemic cooling limits myocardial rewarming by lowering the temperature gradient between the heart and its surroundings and by reducing the return of systemic perfusate to the heart through collaterals (Rosenfeldt and Watson, 1979). Cooling to a temperature of 22°C can be achieved on cardiopulmonary bypass, but, in practice the time for rewarming from this level is so prolonged that a temperature of 28°C is usually applied.

Cold cardioplegic solution

Cold cardioplegic perfusion at 4°C is the most rapid and effective means of lowering global cardiac temperature. However, in the presence of coronary stenoses, the distribution of the solution to the affected areas may be impaired, although it has been claimed that this can be overcome by increasing the volume of perfusion (Borst and Iverson, 1980). Distribution of the solution in such cases can also be assisted by retrograde coronary sinus perfusion.

Prevention of return of warm systemic blood to the heart

Blood returning from the systemic circulation comes into contact with the right atrium and raises the temperature of the atrioventricular node

(Rosenfeldt and Watson, 1979; Smith *et al.*, 1983a) and appears to be a major cause of postoperative supraventricular arrhythmias and conduction defects (Smith *et al.*, 1983a and b; Magilligan *et al.*, 1985). This problem can be largely overcome by snaring the venae cavae proximal to cannulation, as demonstrated by a reduction in right atrial temperature from 25°C to 17°C following this procedure (Menasche *et al.*, 1987a). This procedure does not overcome the problem of rewarming from non-coronary collateral blood flow entering the right atrium and it has been claimed that an atriocaval cannula to drain the flow results in better temperature control than snaring the vena cavae (Baile *et al.*, 1986). Further measures include draining the aortic root (Schneider, Conti and Kurusz, 1983), pulmonary artery (Little *et al.*, 1984), or left ventricle (Yasuda *et al.*, 1983), but, unless otherwise indicated, their advantages are often outweighed by their disadvantages, particularly the introduction of intracardiac and intracoronary air during coronary artery bypass grafting (Daily, 1984; Grover, 1987).

Topical external cooling

The importance of topical cooling in addition to hypothermic (28°C) systemic perfusion in maintaining a low cardiac temperature has been frequently demonstrated. Surrounding the heart with saline ice slush in the pericardial cavity carries the risk of cooling to below 0°C with consequential damage to the heart and surrounding tissues (Speicher *et al.*, 1962), including phrenic nerve paralysis. If ice slush is to be used, the heart should be first wrapped in cold swabs, which are then kept cold by the periodic application of slush. However, cold saline irrigation of the pericardial well is effective and has been shown in pigs, with experimental occlusion of the left anterior descending artery, to produce a lower temperature in the occluded territory and better preservation of function and wall motion (Lazar and Rivers, 1989). Specially designed cooling jackets have been employed, but these have also been reported to damage the phrenic nerve (Rousou *et al.*, 1985), although this difficulty may be overcome by incorporating insulation into the jacket to protect the surrounding tissues (Daily *et al.*, 1987). Such surface cooling has been claimed to be necessary in coronary artery disease to obtain adequate cooling of the inferior aspect of the left ventricular epicardium, as it lies in contact with the aorta and diaphragm, and that the use of the cooling jacket avoids the necessity for multidose cardioplegia and so shortens bypass time (Daily *et al.*, 1987).

Topical internal cooling

A further means of controlling the temperature of the right atrium by direct topical internal cooling has been evaluated in an experimental study in dogs, comparing the effect of isolated right atrial perfusion with cold blood with three methods of atrial and caval drainage (Chen, Shardey and Rosenfeldt, 1988). The mean atrioventricular node temperature was lowered from 25.1°C to 16.5°C by right atrial perfusion, in comparison with atrial and caval drainage, and similar findings were made in a small series of patients undergoing coronary artery bypass. The procedure was shown experimentally to result in almost complete abolition of electrical activity during arrest and, after reperfusion, less prolongation of atria to bundle of His conduction time, improved preservation of myocardial creatine phosphate and reduced lactate accumulation (Chen, Neuman and Rosenfeldt, 1988). However, no clinical benefit from right heart cooling during coronary artery bypass surgery could be demonstrated in a prospective randomized study, in comparison with single atriocaval cannulation (Cheung *et al.*, 1988).

Conclusions on cardiac cooling

Recommended measures to ensure uniform myocardial cooling include sufficient cold cardioplegic solution, separate venae cavae cannulation with proximal snaring, right atrial irrigation with cold blood or saline, pericardial lavage with cold saline or a cooling jacket, and pulmonary artery or left ventricle venting. It has been emphasised that the success of whatever technique is adopted should be constantly monitored by recording temperature in the subepicardium and subendocardium of both ventricles (Daily *et al.*, 1987). However, it should be recognized that intramyocardial pH may be a more sensitive indicator of the adequacy of myocardial protection than temperature (Khuri and Hearse, 1987) and more closely reflects the metabolic state of the heart, since hydrolysis of ATP causes a progressive rise in intra- and extra-cellular pH. Clinical studies have shown that changes in the on-line measurement of intramyocardial pH reflect the adequacy of cardioplegic protection and the need for reinfusions of the solution (Khuri and Warner, 1987).

Considerations in the administration of cardioplegia

Providing that there is no, or minimal, aortic valve incompetence, cardioplegia can be administered into the aortic root, proximal to the aortic cross-clamp, either through a simple, wide-bore, intravenous needle or cannula, or through a specific, commercially available cannula system (Buckberg, 1989). The latter has the advantage that retrograde, non-coronary collateral blood flow can be readily aspirated from the aortic root during coronary artery surgery. Cardioplegia delivery can be increased by simply applying manual pressure to the cold bag of cardioplegia (Braimbridge, 1979), by pressurising the bag with an encircling sphygmanometer cuff, or by using a purpose designed reservoir, cooling coil and roller pump. Roller pump administration has been reported to achieve faster cooling and higher aortic perfusion pressures than pressure on the bag (Grover *et al.*, 1982).

Distribution of the cardioplegic solution in the heart

In the unobstructed coronary vasculature, a neutral crystalloid solution of 37°C has been shown experimentally to be distributed homogeneously and relative flows to the left ventricle, subendocardium and subepicardium remain unchanged from the prearrested state (Zile *et al.*, 1987). Furthermore, in prolonged ischaemia and despite the development of left ventricular contracture, the relative flows to the left ventricle and subendocardium actually increased. However, in contrast, it has more recently been shown that regional cardioplegia flow in the diastolically arrested, maximally vasodilated, canine heart is heterogeneous even at normal coronary perfusion pressures and the variability increases with lower perfusion pressures (Aldea *et al.*, 1990). Coronary artery stenoses are known to cause heterogeneous distribution of cardioplegic solutions, resulting in sub-optimal myocardial preservation and impaired recovery of regional wall function (Hilton *et al.*, 1979; Dorsey *et al.*, 1983; Heineman *et al.*, 1981). It has been claimed that blood is superior in achieving a better distribution beyond stenoses (Robertson *et al.*, 1983), but this has been questioned (Landymore and Kinley, 1984a and b). Equality of perfusion pressure appears crucial in the comparison and at a perfusion pressure of 100 mmHg there is no difference in distribution, but the flow rate was greater with crystalloid solutions (Landymore and Kinley, 1984b). However, the problem of heterogeneous distribution of cardioplegia to the territories of severely stenosed coronary arteries appears to be largely overcome by retrograde perfusion procedures, either into the right atrium or directly into the coronary sinus.

Pressure and flow of cardioplegic solutions

The potential dangers of high infusion pressures have been recognized for some time (R.E. Johnson *et al.*, 1982). In a recent study in dogs, cold crystalloid cardioplegia was administered every 15 min for 1h. It was found that a pressure greater than 110 mmHg and peak flow rate greater than 1500 ml min^{-1} caused a high incidence of trauma to the vascular endothelium, but cellular protection was good (Molina *et al.*, 1989). Pressures less than 30 mmHg and peak flow less than 125 ml min^{-1} led to higher incidence of myocyte ischaemia, focal necrosis and uneven flow distribution. It was recommended that for a canine heart of mean weight 236 g the optimum infusion pressure should be 61 mmHg and in a peak flow rate of 622 ml min^{-1}, the total flow for the first infusion being 600 ml. The detrimental effect of 'cardioplegia barotrauma' has recently been evaluated, in the author's laboratory, in the normal rat heart (Katayama, 1990 – unpublished work). In contrast to low infusion pressure (44 mmHg), even mildly raised cardioplegia infusion pressures (88–176 mmHg) were associated with impaired functional recovery, after 30 min of hypothermic arrest, and the effects correlated with functional and histological changes in the endothelium. Interestingly, the raised infusion pressures may also have initiated a myogenic, vasoconstrictor response which caused heterogeneous distribution of cardioplegia and consequent reperfusion injury.

Volume and frequency of administration of cardioplegic solutions

When cardioplegia is performed with the heart *in situ*, as in the clinical situation, it is necessary for the maintenance of adequate cooling and of cardioplegia to administer the cardioplegic solution half hourly to overcome the effect of wash-out by noncoronary collateral blood flow. Such multidose administration extends the safe period of ischaemic arrest (Engleman *et al.*, 1978; Hearse, Braimbridge and Jynge, 1981; Braimbridge, 1987), but at the same time leads to wash-out of purine nucleotide degradation products, which are needed for resynthesis of ATP by the salvage pathway and so may retard postischaemic recovery (De Witt, Jochim and Behrendt, 1983). In studies of multidose administration, although increasing the volume increased the loss of nucleotides during ischaemia (De Witt, Jochim and Behrendt, 1983; Saydjari, Asimakis and Conti, 1987), the total loss during ischaemia and the first 5 min of reperfusion appeared independent of the volume, and the loss during the remainder of the reperfusion period was inversely related to the volume (Saydjari, Asimakis and Conti, 1987). At the end of reperfusion, myocardial ATP and CP contents were unrelated to total volume, as was the functional recovery. This finding was recently confirmed in the isolated working rat heart for St. Thomas' cardioplegic solution No.2 and a minimal volume established below which indices of recovery, including cardiac output, creatine kinase leakage and myocardial ATP and CP were reduced (Takahashi *et al.*, 1988). The minimal figure (2 ml g^{-1} wet weight of heart) was the same as that usually employed clinically. There have been a number of studies comparing continuous with intermittent cardioplegia, with either blood or crystalloid solutions (Engleman *et al.*, 1978; Bomfin, 1982; Cunningham, Cantinella and Spencer, 1982), but there appears to be no advantage, and possibly some disadvantages, in attempting continuous perfusion. It must be concluded that multidose administration does not impair the conservation of purine nucleotides and functional recovery, and it is reasonable to administer the cardioplegic solution as often as necessary to achieve complete cardiac arrest throughout the period of ischaemia. Infusing up to 2 litres of St. Thomas' solution No.1 is claimed not to significantly alter either intra- or extra-cellular water content (Braimbridge, 1987). Any concern over excessive quantities of crystalloid solution entering the cardiopulmonary bypass perfusate, causing haemodilution and hyperkalaemia, can be avoided by using bicaval snared cannulae and aspirating the coronary effluent with the waste sucker via a small hole in the right atrium.

Particulate contamination in cardioplegic solutions

For many years the potential risks of particles contaminating intravenous infusions have been recognized. The consequences could be even more serious should particles contaminate solutions for intra-arterial use, as in cardioplegia, and microfiltration of the solutions was suggested (Brown *et al.*, 1973). The presence of particles in cardioplegic solutions was subsequently documented (MacDonald, 1981), but the number and sizes of the particles lay within the then specified limits of the United States and British pharmacoepias. A number of solutions were then examined (Robinson, Braimbridge and Hearse, 1984b) and found to contain amorphous and crystalline debris, the removal of which by a 0.8 μm filter resulted overall in a 50% lesser reduction in coronary flow, compared with the unfiltered solutions, during perfusion of the isolated rat heart at 20°C for 20 min. A similar improvement in flow of the unfiltered solutions was produced by the addition of nifedipine. After 3h of multidose cold cardioplegia, the filtered solutions led to 90% restoration of functional recovery, whereas there was little or no recovery following the unfiltered solutions. It was suggested that the particles triggered vasoconstriction and subsequent studies indicated that the endothelial release of 5-hydroxytryptamine was probably the major factor producing transient vasospasm (Hearse *et al.*, 1985 and 1986). Subsequent to this work, most cardiac surgical units incorporated a microfilter in the cardioplegia delivery line and the manufacturers acted to reduce particulate contamination. Current standards of commercially available cardioplegic solutions probably make intraoperative filtration unnecessary, but it is clearly essential that any hospital-prepared cardioplegic solutions should be microfiltered.

Retrograde administration of cardioplegic solutions

Coronary sinus cardioplegia (CSC)

The technique of retrograde coronary sinus perfusion was introduced before the advent of cardioplegia to permit the repair of the aortic valve in the beating heart (Lillehei *et al.*, 1956), but fell into disuse until revived in association with cold cardioplegia for aortic valve surgery (Menasche *et al.*, 1982), primarily in order to avoid the risk of damage to the coronary ostia produced by intermittent or maintained cannulation. Coronary veins are not liable to atherosclerosis, even if traumatised (Hochberg and Austin, 1980), although rarely the endothelium and walls may be damaged and lead to thrombosis (Guerci *et al.*, 1987) or vein rupture (Menasche *et al.*, 1982). To counter these complications a special balloon-tipped catheter has been developed (Menasche and Piwnica, 1987; Buckberg, 1989). Interest has also focused on the technique because of its promise to overcome non-uniform distribution of the cardioplegic solution in the presence of coronary artery stenoses (Becker *et al.*, 1981; Ekroth *et al.*, 1980). In animal experiments, in the presence of acute coronary artery stenoses, coronary sinus cardioplegia (CSC) has been shown to be superior to antegrade perfusion in achieving more uniform distribution of the solution and in preserving left ventricular function (Solorzano, Taitelbaum and Chiu, 1978; Bolling *et al.*, 1983; Gundry and Kirsh, 1984; Mori *et al.*, 1986) and myocardial ATP, reducing lactic acid accumulation (Masuda *et al.*, 1986), preventing ischaemic fall in intramyocardial pH (Johnson *et al.*, 1988b) and reducing post-ischaemic reactive hyperaemia (Lust *et al.*, 1988). However, it must be recognized that the benefits may be less in clinical coronary artery disease, where the collateral circulation would be expected to be better developed. A further advantage of CSC is that it can be administered continuously and at low pressure and flow, thus avoiding interruption to surgical manipulations at the aortic root, while washing-out harmful metabolic products (La Raia *et al.*, 1981; Walls *et al.*, 1982), maintaining consistent cardioplegia and abolishing the wash-out effects of non-coronary collateral flow. The infusion pressure for CSC should not exceed 40 mmHg (Menasche and Piwnica, 1987) and a pressure of 15–20 mmHg appears to be satisfactory in establishing complete global cardioplegic arrest (Bolling *et al.*, 1983).

The potentially inadequate delivery of cardioplegia to the right atrium, ventricle and septum via the coronary sinus (Solorzano, Taitelbaum and

Chiu, 1978; Shiki *et al.*, 1986; Stirling *et al.*, 1989) remains controversial. This may be caused either by the malpositioning of the balloon-tipped catheter within the coronary sinus, which mechanically blocks veins draining these areas, or due to the fact that veins draining the right atrium and ventricle often empty directly into the right atrium and would, therefore, not be perfused by the CSC technique. However, many studies on CSC distribution have been performed in normal canine hearts and the findings may not be applicable to human hearts, let alone those with coronary artery disease. Human hearts have been shown to have extensive venovenous, arteriovenous and venoluminal anastomoses, connecting the major tributaries of the coronary sinus with other venous networks not draining directly into the coronary sinus (Ratajczyk-Pakalska, and Kolff, 1984), and their frequency is increased in coronary vascular disease (Ratajczyk-Pakalska, 1986).

In a study on specific regional flows in dogs, with and without occlusion of the left anterior descending artery, it was concluded that CSC was superior to antegrade perfusion in delivering nutritive flow to areas supplied by the occluded artery and in maintaining subendocardial flow to these areas after the release of the obstruction (Partington *et al.*, 1989a). Excellent left ventricular septal cooling was achieved by CSC, despite reduced nutritive flow, but flow to the right ventricle was poorly distributed. A further study, in which dogs with the same coronary occlusion were subjected either to antegrade, retrograde or both methods of infusion, showed that a combination was better than either technique alone (Partington *et al.*, 1989b). The combination ensured good cardioplegic distribution to both ventricles, including the areas supplied by the occluded artery, and obviated the problem of inconsistent right ventricle protection seen when CSC was used alone.

Clinical trials of the technique of CSC have been few. In patients undergoing aortic valve replacement, CSC was as effective as antegrade perfusion in preserving left ventricular function as assessed haemodynamically by radionuclides (Menasche *et al.*, 1982). More recently, similar studies have supported the opinion that CSC preserves right ventricular function (Menasche *et al.*, 1989), provided that the balloon-tipped catheter does not obstruct the terminal tributaries of the coronary sinus. The same authors have also recently reported their overall experience of CSC in 500 patients undergoing aortic valve replacement (Menasche, Subayi and Piwnica, 1990). In patients undergoing coronary artery bypass grafting, CSC produced more uniform cooling compared with antegrade perfusion, as assessed by thermovision (Shapira *et al.*, 1987), but no differences between the two techniques have been reported in regard to enzyme indices, haemodynamics, wall motion or clinical outcome (Guirauden *et al.*, 1986; Fiure *et al.*, 1989). Evidence has been presented that CSC reduces the risk of embolization from diseased grafts at redo operations (Snyder *et al.*, 1988). In conclusion, it appears that CSC is as satisfactory in general as antegrade perfusion, but has distinct advantages in the presence of severe or multiple coronary artery stenoses and in ascending aorta and aortic valve operations. Combinations of the two techniques may provide optimal cardioplegic protection (Buckberg, 1988 and 1989) and this is supported by a recent trial in coronary artery bypass surgery, in which improved preservation of left ventricular function when compared with antegrade cardioplegia alone was reported (Bhayana *et al.*, 1989).

Right atrial cardioplegia (RAC)

The technique of right atrial cardioplegia (RAC) was developed to avoid the risk of damage to the coronary sinus, shunting of cardioplegic solution into the right atrium through Thebesian veins and the need for atriotomy (Fabiani *et al.*, 1986 and 1987). The cardioplegic solution is infused into the right atrium at a pressure of 40–60 mmHg while temporarily occluding the pulmonary artery. Blood may be admixed with crystalloid cardioplegic solutions by transiently releasing the vena cavae snares. The method cannot be employed in the presence of an atrial septal defect or a patent foramen ovale. In a large randomized clinical trial comparing RAC with CSC, RAC was followed by significantly fewer conduction defects, reduced creatine kinase leakage and better preservation of function (Fabiani *et al.*, 1987). One potentially harmful effect of RAC arises from the possible overdistension of the right atrium and ventricle. In a detailed experimental study in dogs it was found that right ventricular function was greatly impaired after RAC at a pressure of 40 mmHg, whether the solution was administered continuously or intermittently, in comparison with complete recovery of function following CSC at the same pressure and volume (Salter *et al.*, 1987). Temperature was more effectively lowered with CSC and it was suggested that distension of the right ventricle during RAC might have impaired intramyocardial distribution of the cardioplegic solution. However, a small randomized clinical comparison of cold blood RAC, administered at pressures below 40 mmHg, and antegrade cardioplegia, in patients undergoing myocardial revascularization, revealed no differences in the preservation of right ventricular function and both methods were equally effective in cooling the right ventricle (Diehl *et al.*, 1988). The same investigators have also demonstrated the beneficial effects of RAC in comparison to antegrade cardioplegia in a canine model of acute right ventricular ischaemia

(Diehl *et al.*, 1989). RAC requires a larger volume of solution than antegrade cardioplegia to achieve arrest and arrest may be delayed (Buckberg, 1988). For this reason it has been suggested that RAC be combined with antegrade cardioplegia, but this is considered to be unnecessary by the originators of the technique (Fabiani, Jebara and Carpentier, 1989). Wider experience with the technique of RAC is required before conclusions can be reached.

Pressure-controlled intermittent coronary sinus occlusion (PICSO)

The technique of pressure-controlled intermittent coronary sinus occlusion (PICSO) has been applied mainly with the object of minimizing infarct size and improving regional dysfunction after coronary artery occlusion (Mohl *et al.*, 1984), but it is also been shown to be effective during acute myocardial ischaemia and reperfusion (Mohl, 1987). The objective of the technique is to distribute blood, cardioplegia or reperfusion solutions more effectively to areas beyond coronary artery stenoses or occlusions. A balloon placed in the coronary sinus is cyclically inflated for 10 seconds and deflated for 4 sec. In a pig model of acute left anterior coronary artery occlusion, the performing of PICSO during each of the multidose infusions of cardioplegia was shown to produce significantly faster arrest, lower temperature and higher tissue pH during ischaemia and greater functional recovery after the release of the occlusion, than in the absence of PICSO (Lazar, Khoury and Rivers, 1988). In a similar experiment, the administration of PICSO only during the perfusion period was also shown to have significantly beneficial effects on myocardial pH and functional recovery (Lazar, Rajaii and Roberts, 1988). Interestingly, in a similar sheep model, simple occlusion of the coronary sinus during the periods of infusion of antegrade cardioplegia has been reported to improve postischaemic function and reduce the amount of necrosis in the area at risk (Sun *et al.*, 1988). The technique of PICSO carries similar risks to retrograde coronary sinus perfusion, particularly damage to the coronary sinus, and heart-block and other conduction disturbances have been reported. Its greatest value appears to be during revascularization procedures in patients with acute coronary ischaemia and the results of an early clinical trial of the technique in these circumstances have been promising (Mohl, 1987). The potential role of various coronary sinus interventions during cardiac surgery have been reviewed (Lazar, 1988).

Additives to cardioplegic solutions

The beneficial effects of the addition of oxygen and/or red blood cells to cardioplegic solutions has already been discussed. Theoretically, it would be predicted that the addition of other agents, such as metabolic enhancers to conserve high energy phosphates, calcium antagonists to depress contractile activity and modulate cellular flux, free radical inhibitors and scavengers to reduce the accumulation of toxic oxygen radicals and osmolar and oncotic agents to reduce intracellular and interstitial oedema, might also enhance myocardial preservation and improve postischaemic functional recovery. However, many potentially beneficial agents have been tested and the results have often been controversial, possibly due to the agents being administered in concentrations varying from beneficial to harmful. This emphasizes the importance of deriving dose–response curves and conducting trials under strict control conditions. Such laborious studies involve large numbers of animals and it is here that the isolated working rat heart preparation has been particularly of value (Hearse, Braimbridge and Jynge, 1981). Once an additive and its optimal concentration has been experimentally defined, it has to be tested under carefully controlled randomized trials in clinical surgical practice.

Metabolic enhancers

Creatine phosphate

For many years there have been reports of beneficial effects from adding CP to cardioplegic solutions. The optimal concentration for this purpose was established using the isolated working rat heart undergoing cardioplegic arrest at both 37°C and 20°C with St. Thomas' solution No.2 (Robinson, Braimbridge and Hearse, 1984c). The dose–response curve peaked at 10 mmol l^{-1}, at which concentration there was great improvement in all mechanical functions and uniform return to sinus rhythm. The observation was confirmed in other controlled trials in isolated pig (Thelin *et al.*, 1987c) and rat (Sharov *et al.*, 1987; Thelin *et al.*, 1987a) hearts and in a series of patients undergoing valve replacement (Semenovsky *et al.*, 1987), the dose of CP being 10 mmol l^{-1}, as recommended by the earlier work. In one of the studies P^{31} NMR was employed (Sharov *et al.*, 1987) to show that in addition to almost full functional recovery, myocardial CP recovered completely and ATP to 61% of initial level, in all respects much better than in the control.

Adenosine triphosphate

As in the case of CP, ATP has been administered for several years in an attempt to improve recovery from ischaemia (Hearse, Stewart and Braimbridge, 1976; Thelin *et al.*, 1986), but the results have not been uniformly good (Thelin *et al.*, 1987b) and, on occasion, even detrimental (Brown, Mulder and

Chiu, 1979). The reason for the conflicting experiences is largely explained by the relatively narrow dose–response curve peaking at a concentration of 0.1 mmol l^{-1} (Robinson, Braimbridge and Hearse, 1987). This concentration, in St. Thomas' solution No.2 when administered to rat hearts undergoing arrest at both 37°C and 20°C, produced beneficial functional results similar to those following CP alone, and when both were administered together, the improvement was further enhanced. Since both ATP and CP are impermeable to the cell membrane, the mechanisms underlying their beneficial effects are undetermined and are potentially complex (Hearse, Braimbridge and Jynge, 1981). The effect of ATP may be related to its powerful calcium and magnesium binding characteristics or due to its extracellular degradation to adenosine, which then enters the cell to participate in the salvage pathway for ATP. The authors stressed the need for carefully controlled clinical trials before a general introduction.

Nucleosides

Previous reference has been made of the fact that during ischaemia ATP is catabolized to adenosine, inosine and hypoxanthine, which leak into the intravascular lumen and are lost to the systemic circulation through wash-out by cardioplegia, non-coronary collateral flow and reperfusion. The loss of this nucleoside pool could impair the post-ischaemic recovery of ATP (De Witt, Jochim and Behrendt, 1983) and the loss of adenosine may have other detrimental effects within the myocardium (Van Belle, 1985; Belardinelli, Linden and Berne, 1989). Laboratory experimentation has shown that either the provision of exogenous nucleosides or the limitation of their loss will enhance the heart's tolerance to ischaemia.

Inosine

In experiments with the isolated working rat heart it was shown that myocardial ATP following reperfusion after a period of cold cardioplegic arrest, correlated with functional recovery and that both were enhanced by incorporating inosine (200 μmol l^{-1}) into the cardioplegic solution, and further enhanced by continuing inosine into the reperfusion period (De Witt, Jochim and Behrendt, 1983). Similar beneficial effects of inosine (100 μmol l^{-1}) given before a period of global ischaemia, without cardioplegia, were confirmed in a ^{31}P NMR study in isolated working rabbit hearts (Devous and Lewandowski, 1987).

Adenosine

The administration of adenosine to the normothermic ischaemic heart reduces the rate of ATP degradation and improves postischaemic recovery (Foker, Einzig and Wang, 1980; Ely *et al.*, 1985; Takeo *et al.*, 1988). When added to crystalloid cardioplegic solutions, adenosine (1 mmol l^{-1} maintained myocardial ATP levels during 1h of hypothermic (8°C) arrest and reperfusion in rats (Kao and Magovern, 1986) and in rabbits adenosine (400 μmol l^{-1}) significantly improved the haemodynamic recovery from 2h of mildly hypothermic (32°C) arrest (Bolling *et al.*, 1989). In addition, all hearts defibrillated spontaneously, in contrast to 17% failing to do so in the control group. Bradyarrhythmias did not occur in either group, which is important, since adenosine is known to depress pacemaker automaticity and impair atrioventricular nodal conduction and is considered to be a mediator of post-fibrillation bradyarrhythmia and cardiovascular collapse (Wesley and Belardinelli, 1989). Presumably adenosine was rapidly washed out from the heart at the time of reperfusion. A combination of adenosine (100 μmol l^{-1}) and ribose (2 mmol l^{-1}) has also been reported to enhance myocardial ATP preservation and functional recovery in the dog heart subjected to 1h of normothermic cardioplegic arrest (Wyatt *et al.*, 1989). The author's laboratory has recently defined the dose–response of adenosine as an additive to St. Thomas' cardioplegia, in the isolated working rat heart undergoing 3h of multidose, hypothermic (20°C and 10°C) arrest (Ledingham, Katayama and Yacoub, 1990). Under these clinically relevant conditions adenosine, in its optimal concentration of 10 mmol l^{-1}, improved the efficacy of the cardioplegic solution by almost 75%. ATP, both before and after reperfusion was significantly better preserved in hearts receiving adenosine and was associated with significant changes in other nucleotides that suggested that the effects were mediated through inhibition of ATP catabolism. Thus, it would appear that the addition of adenosine to cardioplegic solutions may be clinically beneficial.

Nucleoside transport inhibition (NTI)

Previous reference has also been made to the limitation of the metabolism of adenosine to inosine and hypoxanthine by preventing its uptake into endothelial cells by nucleoside transport inhibition (NTI) (Van Belle, 1985; Van Belle, Goossens and Wyrants, 1987). Recently, a pure NTI (R 75 231, Janssen Research Foundation, Beerse, Belgium), when added to a crystalloid cardioplegic solution and administered during reperfusion, has been demonstrated dramatically to improve the preservation of the canine heart subjected to 24h of hypothermic ischaemia and transplantation (Flameng *et al.*, 1990). Adenosine and inosine were not washed-out and, after 2h of reperfusion, there was complete restoration of ATP content. Clinically, NTI has the potential to preserve or enhance the recovery of ATP and ameliorate neutrophil-mediated reperfusion injury (Olafsson *et al.*, 1987).

Glucose

Glucose, potassium and insulin have been the basis of many cardioplegic solutions. However, glucose has been claimed to be both beneficial (Roe *et al.*, 1977) and harmful (Hearse, Stewart and Braimbridge, 1978b) when administered to the ischaemic heart. The detrimental findings were made in an isolated rat heart preparation undergoing ischaemic arrest at 28°C with a single infusion of glucose containing cardioplegic solution, and were exacerbated by insulin. It was suggested that accumulation of lactate and protons could be partly responsible by inhibiting glycolysis and it was envisaged that if these metabolites were washed-out by multidose cardioplegia or by non-coronary collateral blood flow in the heart *in situ*, this inhibition would be avoided and some underlying beneficial action revealed. This prediction was confirmed in the isolated working rat heart (Conti and Kao, 1983) when it was shown that although a cardioplegic solution containing 0.5% glucose was of no benefit when it was infused once at 32°C, it was most effective when it was reinfused every 15 min in improving recovery and in preserving ATP and glycogen. Increased lactate in the coronary effluent indicated stimulation of glycolysis. Subsequently, it was reported that double-dose oxygenated cardioplegia containing glucose at 8°C was superior to either single or multiple doses in maintaining ATP and was stated to result in complete functional recovery, though data on the latter were not reported (Kao and Magovern, 1986). Recently, the author's laboratory has re-evaluated the addition of glucose with and without insulin to non-oxygenated St. Thomas' solution No.1, in the isolated rat heart subjected to 3h of multi-dose hypothermic (20°C) arrest (Katayama, 1990, unpublished work). Glucose alone did not improve upon the basic solution, but glucose and insulin together were mildly detrimental. These findings question the advantages of adding glucose to an effective cardioplegic solution when it is used under clinically relevant temperatures. Unfortunately, despite their continued use, there have been no recent reports of experimental evaluations of glucose, potassium and insulin containing cardioplegic solutions. Presumably, in the clinical situation, they are not overtly detrimental (Matsuda *et al.*, 1986). However, it would appear that any reported benefit of glucose only occurs under specific experimental conditions. In support of this contention, a recent study reports the beneficial effects of the addition of glucose and various amino acids to St. Thomas' solution No.2 (Schwalb *et al.*, 1989). Isolated rat hearts were subjected to an initial 10 min infusion of warm oxygenated cardioplegia, followed by 28 min of normothermic ischaemia, followed by 3 min of oxygenated cardioplegia, followed by 27 min of normothermic ischaemia. The marked improvement in functional recovery from the addition of glucose and oxygen, as opposed to oxygen alone, was attributed to enhanced Krebs' cycle and oxidative phosphorylation that met the metabolic demands of the heart under these, specific, ischaemic conditions.

Glutamate and aspartate

The depletion of Krebs cycle intermediates during ischaemia delays the return of normal glycolysis and oxidative phosphorylation upon reperfusion and exogenously applied cycle substrates have the potential to limit this detrimental effect. Under anaerobic conditions, the metabolism of 1 mol of glutamate results in the production of 1 mol ATP. The addition of glutamate (26 mmol l^{-1}) to multidose blood cardioplegia, in the *in situ* dog heart subjected to 4h or arrest at 4–8°C, did not improve on what was an excellent recovery of mechanical function in the absence of glutamate (Robertson *et al.*, 1984). However, it was thought possible that the value of glutamate might only be revealed if the heart was metabolically stressed prior to cardioplegic arrest. The benefits of glutamate were subsequently confirmed in hearts initially subjected to 45 min of unmodified normothermic ischaemia (Rosenkranz *et al.*, 1984). Furthermore, a 5 min period of normothermic induction of glutamate-containing blood cardioplegia resulted in even better metabolic and functional recovery, such that the latter was indistinguishable from control. Under anaerobic conditions, the production of ATP from glutamate is enhanced by the presence of aspartate, such that 1 mol of aspartate results in the additional production of 1 mol of ATP. The advantages of aspartate (13 mmol l^{-1}) and glutamate (13 mmol l^{-1}) in promoting post-reperfusion oxidative metabolism in energy depleted hearts was later demonstrated by the same investigators (Rosenkranz *et al.*, 1986a). The clinical application of normothermic induction of glutamate and aspartate containing blood cardioplegia in patients with cardiogenic shock had previously been reported (Rosenkranz *et al.*, 1983).

Other investigators have examined the metabolic value of the addition of glutamate, succinate, fumarate and malate to unoxygenated crystalloid cardioplegia in a comparison with blood and perfluorocarbon containing cardioplegic solutions, in the pig subjected to 2h of arrest at 15°C (Rousou *et al.*, 1986). Although ATP was better maintained during ischaemia by either oxygenation or Krebs' cycle intermediates, after reperfusion there was no longer any significant difference between these groups and controls.

Calcium antagonists

As mentioned earlier, the removal of calcium from the extracellular milieu is cardioplegic itself, but on reperfusion with a calcium containing solution there is risk of inducing the calcium paradox. The administration of Ca-channel blocker will also produce diastolic arrest and theoretically might be expected to reduce the deleterious influx of calcium during both ischaemia and reperfusion. Furthermore, as an additive to potassium-induced cardioplegia, a Ca-channel blocker would theoretically suppress residual electrochemical activity. Early studies (Clark *et al.*, 1977; Lowe *et al.*, 1977; Robb-Nicholson, Currie and Wechsler, 1987) demonstrated the significant protective properties of Ca-channel blockers in comparison to unmodified ischaemia, when they were used as the sole cardioplegic agent under normothermic or mild hypothermic conditions. Postischaemic functional recovery was reported to be either similar (Magee *et al.*, 1979) or better (Vouhe, Helias and Grondin, 1980) in comparison with simple hyperkalaemic cardioplegia formulations, but it was noted that the initial rate of recovery was often retarded due to persistent negative chronotropic and inotropic effects. Attention turned to the use of Ca-channel blockers as adjuncts to hyperkalaemic cardioplegic solutions and the first clinical report (Clark *et al.*, 1981) indicated their favourable effects in this role. Early reports confirmed that nifedipine could reduce intracellular calcium sequestration and improve postischaemic functional recovery of the dog heart, under both normothermic and hypothermic conditions (Boe *et al.*, 1982; Magovern, Dixon and Burkholder, 1981). Subsequently, the potential role of verapamil as an additive to St. Thomas' cardioplegia was evaluated in a dose–response study in the isolated working rat heart (Yamamoto *et al.*, 1983a). Under normothermic ischaemic conditions, mechanical recovery was enhanced and enzyme leakage reduced, but under hypothermic ischaemia there was no additional benefit. It was surmised that the failure of verapamil to improve on recovery from hypothermic hyperkalaemic cardioplegia might be due to it having a similar action to that of hypothermia itself, such as inhibition of the slow calcium channel. Very similar findings were reported with nifedipine (Yamamoto *et al.*, 1983b) and with a combination of verapamil and nifedipine (Yamamoto *et al.*, 1985). The observation that Ca-channel blockers fail to enhance hypothermic hyperkalaemic cardioplegia is supported by studies with diltiazem in dogs undergoing hyperkalaemic cardioplegic arrest at 20°C (Krukenkamp *et al.*, 1986). However, in contrast to these findings, it has been reported that diltiazem improves cold (5°C) blood cardioplegia (Standeven *et al.*, 1984), possibly through the conservation of energy by more completely abolishing electromechanical activity, and others have demonstrated that verapamil does enhance hypothermic myocardial preservation (Balderman, Chan and Gage, 1984). It has been suggested that the hypothermic response may be species and cardioplegic solution dependent (Clark *et al.*, 1985). A double-blind, placebo-controlled, randomized clinical trial of nifedipine (200 μg l^{-1}) as an adjunct to St. Thomas' cardioplegia, in groups of patients undergoing either coronary artery grafting or aortic valve replacement, demonstrated that nifedipine lessened the degradation of nucleotides when myocardial cooling was inadequate, but did not improve clinical outcome (Flameng *et al.*, 1986). It was noted that weaning from bypass was more difficult in the nifedipine group than the placebo group. A single blind, placebo-controlled, randomized trial of diltiazem (100 μg kg^{-1}) as an adjunct to blood cardioplegia, in patients undergoing coronary artery bypass grafting, demonstrated less CK-MB release and improved cardiac function on the first postoperative day compared with controls (Barner *et al.*, 1987). By the fifth postoperative day, functional indices in the diltiazem group had returned to preoperative values, whereas they remained depressed in the controls. However, it was concluded that the advantages of diltiazem were not only small, but were offset by the prolonged recovery of A–V node function, which necessitated pacing, and these findings were in agreement with others (Christakis *et al.*, 1986). The subject of calcium antagonists in cardioplegia has been reviewed (de Jong, 1986).

In conclusion, experimental work in animals suggests that calcium antagonists moderately improve the protection afforded by some hyperkalaemic cardioplegic solutions, particularly at higher temperatures. Unfortunately, at a dose sufficient to achieve added protection there are invariably persistent postischaemic conduction disturbances and occasionally persistent inotropic effects. Controlled clinical studies are few and largely support the laboratory findings.

Additives that reduce the accumulation of free radicals

The likely involvement of free radical formation in reperfusion injury and during cardiopulmonary bypass (Menasche and Piwnica, 1989), to which previous reference has been made, including some recent clinical evidence (Weisel *et al.*, 1989), raises the possibility that by incorporating an antioxidant in the cardioplegic solution this danger can be averted. Procedures which may overcome the accumulation of free radicals include the use of antioxidant enzyme systems, such as superoxide dismutase, catalase and peroxidase, and organic free radical scavengers, such as ascorbate, reduced glutathione and methionine, all of which occur naturally in the body and rapidly eliminate free radicals providing that their rate of formation is not excessive (Gaudel and Duvelleroy, 1984; McCord, 1985).

Laboratory research has mainly been responsible for demonstrating the potential value of a wide variety of antioxidants including ascorbate, methionine and reduced glutathione (Chambers *et al.*, 1989), allopurinol, an inhibitor of xanthine oxidise (Stewart *et al.*, 1983 and 1985; Myers *et al.*, 1986a; Chambers, Braimbridge and Hearse, 1987; Vinten-Johansen, 1988a), peroxidase, an inhibitor of lipid peroxidation (Menasche *et al.*, 1986b and 1987a), desferrioxamine, an iron-chelator which reduces the iron-catalysed formation of the highly damaging hydroxyl radical (Myers *et al.*, 1986a; Menasche *et al.*, 1987a), and superoxide dismutase and catalase (Shlafer, Kane and Kirsch, 1982; Menasche *et al.*, 1986a; Myers *et al.*, 1986a; Ytrehus *et al.*, 1987; Greenfield, Greenfield and Hess, 1988; Jurmann *et al.*, 1988). From these extensive studies it is clear that antioxidants can significantly improve the postischaemic recovery of myocardial function when added to hypothermic cardioplegic solutions. The agents have been given before, during and after ischaemic stress, but, from the surgical perspective, there is ample evidence that they are most effective when administered throughout the cardioplegic period (Chambers *et al.*, 1989; Menasche and Piwnica, 1989), although it may be prudent to continue them into the first few minutes of reperfusion (Otani *et al.*, 1986; Bergsland *et al.*, 1987; Chambers, Braimbridge and Hearse, 1987a; Zweier, Flaherty and Weisfeldt, 1987; Bando, Tago and Teramoto, 1988; Bolli *et al.*, 1989). These is some evidence that free radical scavengers which permeate cells and act predominantly intracellularly on mitochondria are less effective than those which do not enter cells, suggesting that intracellularly generated free radicals may not be responsible for significant damage (Chambers *et al.*, 1989), and there is a need for further studies to establish dose-response characteristics and define optimal levels.

To date there have been very few reports on the use of antioxidants in clinical cardioplegia. Allopurinol, as an additive to blood cardioplegia, was recently reported to reduce chromosomal damage attributable to free radical injury, although there were no observable differences in the postoperative course between the control and treated groups (Emerit *et al.*, 1988). Also recently, desferrioxamine was administered both intravenously, starting before and ending after bypass, and as an additive to the cardioplegic solution (Menasche *et al.*, 1988b). No functional studies were performed, but evidence was gained that the protective value of desferrioxamine in the clinical situation may to some extent relate to its suppression of neutrophil-mediated free radical production that occurs following complement activation during cardiopulmonary bypass (Kirklin *et al.*, 1983; Cavarocchi, England and Schaff, 1986; Royston, Fleming and Desai, 1986). The pharmacokinetics of human superoxide dismutase during hypothermic cardiopulmonary bypass is presently being evaluated (Lee *et al.*, 1989). In the light of evidence that indicates minimal endothelial xanthine oxidase-mediated free radical production in human hearts (Jarash, Bruder and Heidi, 1986; Eddy *et al.*, 1987; Muxfeldt and Schaper, 1987), the potential role of human superoxide dismutase may arise from the limitation of neutrophil-mediated free radical injury. However, since potentially the greatest amount of cellular damage results from hydroxyl radical formation and lipid peroxidation, which are both iron-catalysed (Gutteridge, Richmond and Halliwell, 1979; Halliwell, 1989), further clinical reports on the use of desferrioxamine are presumed imminent.

Osmolar and oncotic agents

Theoretically, myocardial cell function during and subsequent to cardioplegia could be impaired by cellular oedema or dehydration and also by interstitial oedema interfering with the delivery and removal of metabolites by both compressing capillaries and increasing the distance for diffusion across the interstitial space. Cardioplegic solutions vary from mildly hypotonic (Tyers' solution: 275 mosmol kg^{-1}), iso- or mildly hypertonic (St. Thomas' Hospital solutions: 300–325 mosmol kg^{-1}) to frankly hypertonic (Kirklin's solution with mannitol: 385 mosmol kg^{-1}, Buckberg's blood cardioplegia: 400 mosmol kg^{-1}). Hypotonic cardioplegic solutions have been reported to increase cardiac water content during brief periods of ischaemia (Foglia *et al.*, 1979), presumably mainly through cellular oedema, but, apart from decreasing compliance in the arrested state, had no effect on postischaemic water content or left ventricular function and compliance on reperfusion. Whether or not more prolonged periods of cardioplegia with hypotonic or isotonic solutions are detrimental, permitting mild cellular oedema, has not been established. However, infusing up to 2 litres of St. Thomas' solution No.1 is claimed not to significantly alter either intra- or extracellular water content (Braimbridge, 1987). Mannitol, a common additive in hypertonic solutions, has been reported to impair left ventricular recovery through its osmotic action (Hearse, Stewart and Braimbridge, 1978). In the present state of knowledge, it must be concluded that the tonicity of cardioplegic solutions should be kept near to isotonic. Various oncotic agents, including albumin, dextran, hydroxyethyl starch and gelatine have been added to cardioplegic solutions to counteract the interstitial oedema, but the importance of such measures in improving recovery from intraoperative cardioplegia remains to be established, although there is evidence that they are of value in the hypothermic conditions (4°C) used for cardiac preservation in transplantation (Belzer and Southand, 1988; Ledingham *et al.*, 1990).

Glucocorticoids

Opinions of the value of glucocorticoids given immediately before cardioplegia have been conflicting (Hearse, Braimbridge and Jynge, 1981). In a double-blind controlled trial in patients, the addition of methyl-prednisolone succinate (MPSS) to a cold hyperkalaemic-cardioplegic solution resulted in better preservation of myocardial ultrastructure and reduced need for postoperative inotropic support (Levinsky *et al.*, 1979). However, a recent laboratory study of the dose-response characteristics of MPSS added to a cold (20°C) crystalloid hyperkalaemic cardioplegic solution, revealed no improvement in recovery of mechanical or metabolic function or in the degree of enzyme leakage after 3h of ischaemic arrest (Sellevold and Jynge, 1987a). Furthermore, high concentrations (1000 mg l^{-1}) of MPSS were harmful, possibly because they promoted intracellular calcium accumulation, contracture and excessive nucleotide catabolism. Any benefit that has been observed from its use may possibly be attributable to suppression of particle-induced coronary vasospasm (Sellevold and Jynge, 1987b), complement activation and generation of free radicals, or to better endothelial preservation. In conclusion, there is no clear evidence that glucocorticoids are beneficial additives to cardioplegic solutions.

Conclusions on the use of additives to cardioplegic solutions

Most reports of additives to cardioplegic solutions have been based on laboratory experiments and their value clinically has yet to be tested. Well formulated crystalloid or blood-based cardioplegic solutions, when administered in multi-dose fashion under hypothermic conditions, are considered by many to provide adequate intraoperative protection for most patients. However, there is no doubt that the level of protection can be enhanced by the use of certain additives and this could be of increased importance in high risk patients. To this end, glutamate and aspartate are principally the only additives that have been both shown to be beneficial in the laboratory and are currently used clinically (Buckberg and Rosenkranz, 1987; Buckberg, 1989). ATP, glucose, calcium antagonists, glucocorticoids, osmolar and oncotic agents are of uncertain clinical value. Creatine phosphate, antioxidants, adenosine and nucleoside transport inhibition have been shown in animal studies to have significant benefits and may thus have clinical potential.

Reperfusion procedures and suppression of reperfusion injury following cardioplegia

Concepts of the nature of reperfusion injury have already been mentioned and the potential for damage is at its greatest following a period of unmodified normothermic ischaemia. Although, in the surgical setting, hypothermic cardioplegia markedly attenuates ischaemic damage and reduces the risk of reperfusion injury it may still occur, either because some consequences of the reintroduction of oxygen are inherently unavoidable or because of inadequate myocardial protection due to poor cardioplegic distribution or efficacy. Interest in the suppression of reperfusion injury has focused, for some time, on modulating the re-entry of calcium into myocardial cells and, more recently, on the prevention of formation and the removal of oxygen free-radicals, both of which may be linked. However, there are a number of other factors which are important at this time, including the temperature of the reperfusate, the pressure at which the reperfusate is administered, the rate of recovery from intracellular acidosis, the provision of substrates to restore depleted reserves of CP and ATP, the limitation of oedema formation and restoration of normal or supranormal coronary flow to deliver oxygen and substrates to the heart. In the surgical setting these factors can readily be controlled and, in addition, it may be beneficial to maintain electromechanical arrest during the initial period of reperfusion so that the myocyte can devote all of its resources to the restoration of cellular homeostasis, at a time when it is not necessary to perform external work.

Control of calcium entry

Excessive entry of calcium into the cell at the commencement of reperfusion increases ATP consumption due to activation of ATPase, activates phospholipase and proteases, impairs mitochondrial function and causes maldistribution of ions (Jennings, 1981; Fleckenstein, Frey and Freckenstein-Grun, 1983; Nayler *et al.*, 1983). In the extreme it may cause myocardial contracture and result in the 'stone heart' (Katz and Tada, 1972; Henry *et al.*, 1977). On the other hand a supply of calcium is essential for normal function (Yates and

Dhalla, 1975) and opinions diverge on how best to achieve a balance between the two requirements. The potential injury caused by calcium overload following normothermic ischaemia appears to be at its greatest during the first few minutes of reperfusion (Yano *et al.*, 1987) and the optimal calcium concentration during this period appears to be dependent on its concentration during the ischaemic period (Shine, Douglas and Ricchiuti, 1978). However, hypothermic ischaemia markedly reduces the susceptibility to calcium induced reperfusion injury (Baker, Bullock and Hearse, 1983) and a well formulated hypothermic cardioplegic solution further minimizes the risks (Hearse, Braimbridge and Jynge, 1981). Nearly all the evidence in favour of lowering the concentration of calcium in the reperfusate arises from experiments in reperfusion following unmodified ischaemia and in these circumstances ionic calcium concentrations of 0.5 mmol l^{-1} (Follette *et al.*, 1981) or between 0.15 mmol l^{-1} and 0.25 mmol l^{-1} (Allen *et al.*, 1986b) during initial reperfusion have been shown to be significantly beneficial in the canine heart. The lowering of ionic calcium was achieved by adding citrate to the pump blood directed to coronary perfusion. Considerable care must be exercised to ensure that the ionic calcium level does not become too low, since the same investigators report that lowering the ionic calcium below 0.1 mmol l^{-1} was detrimental. In contrast, it has been shown that an ionic calcium concentration of 1.0 mmol l^{-1} is superior 0.25 mmol l^{-1} following hypothermic cardioplegic arrest in isolated rat hearts (Menasche *et al.*, 1984b). Alternatively, the addition of the calcium-blocker diltiazem to normocalcaemic (1.0–1.2 mmol l^{-1}) pump blood has also been shown to be beneficial (Allen *et al.*, 1986b) and citrate phosphate dextrose (CPD) and diltiazem are used clinically to lower calcium concentration in blood cardioplegia to 0.15–0.25 mmol l^{-1} (Buckberg and Rosenkranz, 1987).

Reperfusate temperature

A recent study in the rat confirmed that calcium-induced reperfusion injury is temperature dependent and recommended an initial reperfusate temperature of under 28°C, since this prevented the impairment of function and lessened the creatine kinase leakage seen at higher temperatures when the calcium concentration lay outside the range of 0.3–0.7 mmol l^{-1} (Hamasaki, Kuroda and Mori, 1988). However, providing the calcium concentration lay within this range, the rate of re-warming was of less importance. Although other studies in this area have not always reported on the concentration of calcium in the perfusate, which is often pump blood, they have invariably demonstrated that initial normothermic reperfusion is superior to initial hypothermic reperfusion and provides for optimal postischaemic recovery conditions (Hedley Brown, Morritt and Hammo, 1982; Rousou *et al.*, 1982; Swanson and Myerowitz, 1983; Metzdorff, Grunkemeier and Star, 1986).

Perfusion pressure

Raised reperfusion pressures following normothermic global ischaemia have, for many years, been known to be associated with excessive post-ischaemic oedema (Engleman, Levitsky and Wyndham, 1977; Todd *et al.*, 1977). In the aforementioned studies of the effect of reperfusion temperature on recovery from hypothermic cardioplegic arrest, the combination of normothermia and normal perfusion pressure, in the region 80–100 mmHg, has been demonstrated by different investigators to be either beneficial (Hedley Brown, Morritt and Hammo, 1982) or detrimental (Swanson and Myerowitz, 1983) to functional recovery. However, more recently, it has been shown in normal canine hearts, subjected to 2h of hypothermic cardioplegic arrest with St. Thomas' solution No.1, that recovery of myocardial contractility, coronary flow, oxygen consumption, lactate flux and ATP is independent of reperfusion pressure when it is maintained in the range of 40–100 mmHg for 30 min (Rosenfeldt *et al.*, 1986), although it may be important gradually to raise the infusion pressure to these levels over the initial 2 min of reperfusion. However, it was emphasized that, in the clinical situation, the presence of coronary artery stenoses or ventricular hypertrophy (Hottenrott *et al.*, 1973) may significantly reduce the perfusion pressure in the distal coronary arteries and it was demonstrated, in a small intraoperative study in patients with coronary artery disease, that distal coronary artery pressures during reperfusion were always below 40 mmHg despite aortic pressures of 52–78 mmHg. Allowances should be made for pressure gradients of up to 60 mmHg and it was recommended that aortic, or radial, pressures should be kept between 70 mmHg and 100 mmHg during reperfusion. This is in contrast to reperfusion after unmodified, normothermic, regional ischaemia, where gradual low pressure reperfusion has been reported to be preferable to sudden high pressure perfusion (Okamoto *et al.*, 1986a; Peng *et al.*, 1989).

Limitation of oedema

Oedema occurring during reperfusion potentially impairs myocardial perfusion and exacerbates ischaemic damage (Engleman, Levitsky and Wyndham, 1977). Although reperfusion oedema is most marked following unmodified ischaemia, it is known to occur after hypothermic cardioplegia (Christlieb and Clark, 1982), particularly when myocardial protection has been poor (Braimbridge, 1987). Furthermore, as referred to above, excessive reperfusion pressure predisposes to oedema. The incorporation of mannitol, to increase the osmolality of the reperfusate, has been reported to improve coronary flow and functional recovery following unmodified ischaemia (Hottenrott *et al.*, 1975), hypothermic ischaemia (Follette *et al.*, 1981) and hypothermic cardioplegic arrest (Magovern *et al.*, 1984). In the latter study, an equally hyperosmotic solution containing glucose was shown to be ineffective and it was suggested that the beneficial effect of mannitol may have been related to its hydroxyl radical scavenging properties (Stewart *et al.*, 1983). Clinically, mannitol has been used to raise the osmolality of the reperfusate to 370 mmol l^{-1} (Menasche *et al.*, 1984a) and glucose to raise the osmolality of the reperfusate to over 400 mmol l^{-1} (Buckberg, 1987 and 1989).

Buffering of reperfusate

By the end of a prolonged period of ischaemia there is potentially severe intracellular acidosis and it has been recommended that a buffered, mildly alkaline reperfusate should be used to accelerate the restoration of normal intracellular pH and optimize conditions for the recovery of postischaemic metabolism and normal calcium ionic flux (Follette *et al.*, 1981; Menasche *et al.*, 1984b). Furthermore, correction of acidosis also reduces coronary vascular resistance (Rovetto, Whitmer and Neely, 1973). A reperfusate pH of 7.8 has been shown to provide for optimal functional recovery (Follette *et al.*, 1977a) and the addition of THAM (Folletto *et al.*, 1981) or glutamic acid–sodium hydroxide buffers (Menasche *et al.*, 1984b) to the reperfusate, following hypothermic ischaemia, have been demonstrated to be beneficial in animal studies and have also been used clinically (Menasche *et al.*, 1984a; Buckberg and Rosenkranz, 1987).

Substrate provision

At the start of reperfusion there is temporary inhibition of the oxidative pathways for ATP production (Mochizuki and Neely, 1980) and the heart has to rely on anaerobic metabolism provided by endogenous energy stores. Immediate postischaemic infusions of glutamate (Menasche *et al.*, 1984b; Rosenkranz *et al.*, 1984) and aspartate (Rosenkrantz *et al.*, 1986) are claimed to be beneficial during this period since they accumulate in the cytosol and enter the Krebs cycle to produce ATP through anaerobic pathways (Rau *et al.*, 1979). Furthermore, positron emission tomography has revealed that the postischaemic myocardium uses glucose rather than fatty acids as the principle substrate for energy production (Schwaiger *et al.*, 1985). A recent study, in patients undergoing coronary artery bypass surgery, has shown that the uptake of most myocardial substrates, including fatty acids, glucose, lactate and pyruvate, is markedly reduced for several hours after reperfusion, with no uptake of fatty acids or glucose (Svensson *et al.*, 1990). The investigators proposed that there was a profound resistance to insulin following cardiopulmonary bypass and, in a randomized trial, demonstrated that exogenous insulin significantly increased the uptake of these substrates. Other investigators have reported that glucose-insulin-potassium (GIK) infusion is significantly beneficial for the treatment of left ventricular failure following coronary artery bypass surgery (Coleman *et al.*, 1989; Gradinac *et al.*, 1989). In other studies, exogenous lactate has been shown to promote fatty acid oxidation following hypothermic cardioplegic arrest (Mickle *et al.*, 1986) and it has been suggested that lactate may be the preferred substrate for postischaemic oxidative metabolism. Ringer's lactate, added to the pump perfusate during coronary artery bypass surgery, has been demonstrated to reduce creatine kinase leakage and improve metabolic and functional recovery (Teoh *et al.*, 1988).

Replacement of depleted T_3 (tri-iodothyronine)

Cardiopulmonary bypass is associated with a reduction in circulating T_3 (Brummer, Taylor and Baird, 1978; Robuschi, Medici and Fesani, 1986) and this may adversely affect postischaemic myocardial recovery by impairing mitochondrial function (Sterling, 1986). Metabolic events may be similar to those observed following brain death, where a fall in circulating T_3 is associated with a shift from aerobic to anaerobic metabolism and results in decreased myocardial energy stores and haemodynamic instability which can be reversed by exogenous T_3 (Novitzky *et al.*, 1988a). The administration of T_3 to pigs at the time of reperfusion, after 2–3h of cardiopulmonary bypass and hypothermic cardioplegic arrest, resulted in a significant difference in survival in comparison with untreated pigs, there being uniform survival in all eleven treated and only five survivors in eleven untreated (Novitzky, Human and Cooper, 1988b). Recently, the same investigators reported similar beneficial effects of T_3 infusion when applied clinically in two small, randomized, blind studies (Novitzky *et al.*, 1989).

Reduction of free radical mediated damage

There is now much evidence that the formation of oxygen free radicals during cardiopulmonary bypass and during myocardial ischaemia and reperfusion is potentially an important cause of intraoperative myocardial damage (Menasche and Piwnica, 1989). Reference has already been made to the value of agents either suppressing the formation of or scavenging free radicals, when used as additives to cardioplegic solutions. However, the addition of such agents to the reperfusate alone has now been shown to result in improved functional recovery, which strongly supports the concept that myocardial injury does not exclusively occur during ischaemia and that damage at the time of reperfusion is paramount (Bolli *et al*., 1988; Opie, 1989). Although the majority of evidence for pharmacological modulatation of free radical damage during reperfusion has resulted from unmodified normothermic ischaemic models (Przyklenk and Kloner, 1986; Gross *et al*., 1986; Ambrosio *et al*., 1987a and b; Bolli *et al*., 1987a and b; Bolli *et al*., 1989), demonstrating their amelioration of 'stunning', there is experimental evidence demonstrating that superoxide dismutase and catalase (Otani *et al*., 1986; Bergsland *et al*., 1987; Chambers, Braimbridge and Hearse, 1987b; Bando, Tago and Teramoto, 1988) will enhance functional recovery from hypothermic cardioplegic arrest when they are administered at the time of reperfusion. The potentially beneficial effect of the infusion of desferrioxamine, throughout cardiopulmonary bypass, upon the suppression of hydroxyl radical formation, lipid peroxidation and neutrophil-mediated free radical production has been referred to previously (Menasche *et al*., 1988b) and, more recently, has been shown to improve functional recovery when added to blood cardioplegia following a period of regional, unmodified, normothermic ischaemia (Illes *et al*., 1989a).

Vasodilators to improve coronary flow

It has been shown that a variety of vasodilators, whose mode of action differed, produced supranormal coronary flows and an equal improvement in myocardial functional recovery following normothermic ischaemia (Stahl, Aversano and Becker, 1986). The addition of adenosine, a potent coronary vasodilator and substrate for ATP, to the reperfusate carries the risk of inducing bradyarrhythmias, but in low concentration this complication does not occur. Recently, the effect of reperfusion with 1 mg l^{-1} adenosine following 3h of hypothermic (20°C) arrest with multidose infusion of St. Thomas' solution No.1 was examined in the isolated working rat heart (Ledingham *et al*., 1990a). In comparison with hearts receiving ordinary reperfusate, those receiving adenosine had 50% greater coronary flow and 100% better recovery of cardiac output in the postischaemic period. It was suggested that the beneficial effect was mediated through enhanced coronary flow to the microvasculature rather than an increase in intramyocardial ATP and, if applied clinically, there may be additional benefits from the protective action of adenosine on neutrophil-mediated endothelial damage (Olafsson *et al*., 1987).

Maintaining cardioplegic arrest

Although rapid and spontaneous return of sinus rhythm during reperfusion is an indication of the efficacy of hypothermic cardioplegic protection, since is it associated with good recovery of function (Robinson, Braimbridge and Hearse, 1984a; Ledingham, Braimbridge and Hearse, 1987), it may actually be beneficial to pharmacologically maintain diastolic arrest during the initial period of reperfusion (Levitsky, 1988). Early studies evaluating the benefits of cardioplegic reperfusion arose from the observation that ischaemically damaged hearts have a limited capacity to utilise oxygen during reperfusion (Kane *et al*., 1975) and that maintaining arrest would provide conditions whereby oxygen and other metabolic substrates could be directed to reparative processes rather than towards unnecessary electromechanical work (Folletto *et al*., 1977b; Lazar *et al*., 1979; Rosenkranz and Buckberg, 1983). Potassium-containing, blood-based, oxygenated cardioplegic solutions would appear to be particularly applicable to this procedure, since they will deliver optimal concentrations of oxygen under normothermic conditions. However, a hyperkalaemic, asanguineous, hypoxic cardioplegic solution, administered at 28°C, has been used clinically and claimed not only to be beneficial, but to have advantages over modified blood reperfusion in these circumstances (Menasche *et al*., 1984a). With the equipment employed to administer blood cardioplegia it is a simple matter to switch the heat-exchanger to warm the cardioplegic infusion and terminal warm blood cardioplegia, prior to the removal of the cardiac cross-clamp, has become part of the blood cardioplegia administration protocol (Buckberg and Rosenkranz, 1987; Buckberg, 1989). In a small prospective randomised trial, in patients undergoing coronary artery bypass grafting, cold blood cardioplegia with terminal warm blood cardioplegia (500 ml delivered over 1 min) accelerated myocardial metabolic recovery, preserved high energy phosphates and improved the metabolic response to postoperative haemodynamic stresses, when compared with cold blood cardioplegia alone (Teoh *et al*., 1986). With terminal warm blood cardioplegia, postoperative left atrial pressures and diastolic compliance tended to be better in response to volume loading, but there were no significant differences in myocardial performance as determined by nuclear ventriculography. In contrast, another small clinical series reported no significant differences in perioperative myocardial function in a comparison of blood cardioplegia alone and with either additional warm blood cardioplegia induction or reperfusion, although hearts subjected to the latter were more likely to exhibit spontaneous defibrillation (Roberts *et al.*, 1985). However, both these studies were with low risk patients and it is possible that the real benefit from this reperfusion procedure is only seen in high risk patients in combination with normothermic induction (Rosenkranz *et al.*, 1982) and with the use of additional substrates (Rosenkranz *et al.*, 1986a).

Conclusion on reperfusion procedures

With few exceptions, most of the work referred to in this section has been undertaken in experimental animals and controlled clinical trials of reperfusion procedures or reperfusate additives have not been widely reported. Furthermore, most of the evidence for the beneficial effects of modified reperfusion has come from experimental work involving reperfusion following periods of unmodified ischaemia, rather than following periods of cardioplegia arrest. The technique of blood cardioplegia is readily adaptable to controlling the reperfusion conditions and many of the potentially beneficial procedures or additives, referred to above, have been used clinically with terminal warm blood cardioplegia (Buckberg and Rosenkranz, 1987; Buckberg, 1989). However, the technique of crystalloid cardioplegia is simpler and to provide equipment specifically to control the reperfusion conditions would significantly complicate the procedure. There is no clinical evidence that modifying the reperfusion conditions following an efficacious crystalloid cardioplegic solution, which has been used meticulously, is advantageous. Thus, it may be argued that controlling the reperfusion conditions after routine cardioplegic arrest is unnecessary and that the currently reported degree of cardiac recovery is satisfactory without such refinements. However, in circumstances where the myocardium may be metabolically compromised, either because of its preischaemic condition or due to inadequate intraoperative protection, for example in severe coronary artery disease, cardiac hypertrophy, neonatal cyanotic states or long periods of cardioplegia, these measures may be particularly beneficial by enhancing the rate of metabolic and functional recovery.

Reperfusion of acutely compromised myocardium: cardiogenic shock

The surgical management of the acutely metabolically and functionally compromised myocardium, in a manner that will both accelerate recovery and result in the greatest salvage of functioning myocardium, utilizes the principles of the preceding section. In fact, most of the evidence in favour of controlling the postischaemic reperfusion conditions has evolved from experimentation in this clinically challenging area, to which Buckberg and colleagues have contributed considerable knowledge. Broadly speaking, there are two areas where the application of these principles may significantly enhance myocardial recovery and survival. Firstly, in those patients with severe left ventricular failure due, for example, to acute valvular incompetence, acute ischaemic ventricular septal defect or acute coronary insufficiency caused either by pre-existing coronary artery disease or by iatrogenic coronary artery occlusion in the cardiac catheter room, all of which require urgent life-saving surgical intervention. Secondly, in those patients with severe left ventricular failure due to evolving myocardial infarction in whom surgical intervention may provide a more favourable outcome as opposed to presently used methods of medical management, including thrombolytic therapy. Blood cardioplegia techniques are, again, particularly suitable for this role and their use in these circumstances is termed 'secondary cardioplegia'.

In the surgical management of the first group of patients, a 5 min period of normothermic induction of blood cardioplegia has been demonstrated to enhance the recovery from the subsequent hypothermic, multidose, cold blood cardioplegia protocol, both experimentally (Rosenkranz *et al.*, 1982) and clinically (Rosenkranz *et al.*, 1983). Laboratory experimentation has shown that the composition of the blood cardioplegia is very important and, in addition to potassium, that it should contain THAM, glucose, aspartate, glutamate, coenzyme Q_{10}, citrate phosphate dextrose (CPD) and diltiazem (Buckberg and Rosenkranz, 1987; Buckberg, 1989). Aspartate and glutamate are only used during warm induction and reperfusion (Rosenkranz *et al.*, 1986a) and the calcium content is further reduced during these periods by altering the concentration of CPD (Buckberg and Rosenkranz, 1987; Buckberg, 1989). Longer periods of normothermic asystole, during warm induction or warm reperfusion, may allow greater metabolic recovery (Allen *et al.*, 1987e; Addetia *et al.*, 1988), provided the ventricle does not become distended (Allen *et al.*, 1986c).

The surgical management of the second group of patients is debatable since the mortality rate from surgical intervention in evolving myocardial infarction with left ventricular failure is known to be high, although it is not as high as with solely medical treatment (Allen *et al.*, 1989). Furthermore, the impact of thrombolytic therapy on improving the medical management, in comparison with surgical management, has yet to be determined. However, the studies of Buckberg and colleagues indicate that controlling the reperfusion conditions, as may occur during surgical revascularization, will result in better immediate functional recovery and improved myocardial salvage than can be obtained with thrombolytic therapy (Buckberg, 1986). They have shown in a series of experiments in dogs, subjected to regional ischaemia, that reperfusion with ordinary blood is detrimental to recovery, whether or not it is achieved medically or on cardiopulmonary bypass without the use of cardioplegia (Vinten-Johansen *et al.*, 1986a). In contrast, the administration of warm blood cardioplegia, both in the ischaemic region and to the rest of the heart, for 5 min before multidose cold blood cardioplegia, followed by warm blood cardioplegia for 5 min prior to the removal of the aortic cross-clamp, resulted in substantial immediate functional recovery and greater muscle salvage. Considerable emphasis has been placed on the composition of the cardioplegia (Allen *et al.*, 1986b; Okamoto *et al.*, 1986c), its supplementation with coenzyme Q_{10}, a free radical scavenger and phospholipase inhibitor (Okamoto *et al.*, 1986b), the duration (Allen *et al.*, 1986e) and pressure of administration (Okamoto *et al.*, 1986a), and the importance of total ventricular decompression during reperfusion (Allen *et al.*, 1986c). Using these reperfusion techniques, they report significantly beneficial effects on myocardial recovery and salvage following periods of regional ischaemia in dogs up to 6h (Allen *et al.*, 1986d) and in patients up to 45h (Allen *et al.*, 1986a and 1989). In the latter, warm, substrate-enriched, blood cardioplegia is perfused down the graft to the infarcting area for 20 min (at 50 ml min^{-1} or 50 mmHg), while the proximal anastomoses of the other grafts are constructed. Others have confirmed the advantages of surgical reperfusion, with modified blood cardioplegia, over medical reperfusion in providing sustained myocardial salvage one week after two hours of acute regional ischaemia (Cheung *et al.*, 1989), and the clinical implications have been discussed (Bergmann and Sobel, 1989). Although blood cardioplegia has been claimed to be superior to non-oxygenated asanguineous cardioplegia as a reperfusate in these circumstances (Vinten-Johansen *et al.*, 1986b), it has been shown that a brief period of reperfusion with 500 ml of St. Thomas' cardioplegia is preferable to initial reperfusion with unmodified pump-blood (Rebeyka *et al.*, 1989) and further benefits may be gained by the addition of free radical scavengers (Gharagozloo *et al.*, 1988).

Finally, it has recently been recognized that the function of the remote, non-ischaemic, myocardium is the primary determinant of early survival after an otherwise non-lethal coronary occlusion (Beyersdorf *et al.*, 1989b). Cardiogenic shock develops when the remote muscle fails to develop or sustain compensatory hypercontractility, due either to autoregulatory failure or substrate depletion, and this is more likely to occur in the presence of multivessel coronary artery disease. In a dog model of complete left anterior descending coronary artery occlusion and 50% stenosis of the circumflex artery, an intravenous infusion of glutamate, aspartate, glucose-insulin-potassium (GIK), coenzyme Q_{10}, and 2-mercapto-propionyl-glycine (MPG), commenced 2h after the onset of ischaemia and continued for 4h, was shown to restore compensatory hypercontractility, improve stroke-work index to within normal limits, maintain high energy phosphates and improve survival (Beyersdorf *et al.*, 1989a). These interesting observations may have clinical application not only in the management of acute regional ischaemia, but also in the treatment of postoperative cardiac failure.

In conclusion, the successful surgical management of cardiogenic shock may depend on an operative strategy that encompasses many principles of myocardial protection and reperfusion, all of which have been shown to be beneficial in laboratory experimentation at some time.

Paediatric myocardial protection

The optimum method for protection of the neonatal and infant myocardium is still uncertain and there has recently been much investigative work in this area (Ledingham, 1988). It is important to recognize that there are major physiological differences between the neonatal and adult myocardium (Anderson *et al.*, 1990). Whereas the adult myocardium can utilize a wide variety of substrates with fatty acid providing the dominant energy source, the neonatal heart, due to the delayed maturation of specific enzymes and a physiological tolerance to hypoxaemia, directs metabolism away from fatty acids and towards substrates such as glucose and lactate. Immature hearts have larger glycogen stores compared with the adult heart and thus have a greater capacity for anaerobic glycolysis. The potential to produce more high energy phosphates under anaerobic conditions is believed to be the reason why the immature myocardium has a better tolerance to ischaemia than the mature myocardium (Bove and Stammers, 1986; Grice, Konishi and Apstein, 1987; Yano, Braimbridge and Hearse, 1987). In addition, the neonatal myocardium possesses different isoforms of the myofilament regulatory proteins which are more resistant to the effects of acidosis (Solaro *et al.*, 1988). Furthermore, the immaturity of enzymes concerned with the metabolism of nucleotides and nucleosides helps to preserve myocardial ATP and purine base pool during ischaemia and reperfusion (Achterberg *et al.*, 1988; Mask *et al.*, 1989). However, on the other hand, the relative immaturity of transmembrane sodium-calcium exchange mechanisms (Pridjian *et al.*, 1988), antioxidant defence systems and synthesis of membrane phospholipids (Otani *et al.*, 1987) may make the neonatal heart more vulnerable to reperfusion injury.

The interpretation of experimental studies in paediatric myocardial protection is complicated by the inherent resistance of the immature myocardium to ischaemia, the variety of animal species and ages investigated, the differing experimental temperature and protocols employed, and the various indices of preservation examined. Nevertheless, assuming that there are similarities between neonatal animal and neonatal human hearts, some conclusions can be drawn from these studies at this time. They support the opinion that the neonatal heart is more resistant to normothermic ischaemia than the adult heart (Avkiran and Hearse, 1989) and demonstrate that topical hypothermia (10°C) alone provides a remarkable degree of protection (Corno *et al.*, 1987; Kempsford and Hearse, 1990). They also demonstrate that cardioplegia significantly enhances the preservation of the neonatal heart (Bove, Stammers and Gallagher, 1987; Ganzel, Katzmart and Mavroudis, 1988; Avkiran and Hearse, 1989; Konishi and Apstein, 1989) and in comparisons between currently used crystalloid cardioplegic solutions, that St. Thomas' Hospital, Tyers, and Hospital Lariboisiere solutions provide good protection (Kempsford and Hearse, 1989; Konishi and Apstein, 1989), although better protection may be afforded by blood cardioplegia (Corno *et al.*, 1987). However, there is uncertainty concerning the optimum temperature and frequency of cardioplegia infusion, and multidose cardioplegia has been claimed to be detrimental (Baker, Boerboom and Olinger, 1988; Magovern, Pae and Waldhausen, 1988; Sawa *et al.*, 1989; Watanabe *et al.*, 1989). These variables were evaluated in a series of experiments in neonatal rabbits undergoing cardioplegic arrest with St. Thomas' Hospital solution No. 2 (Kempsford and Hearse, 1990). It was demonstrated that under moderate hypothermia (20°C) multidose cardioplegia was superior to single dose cardioplegia, but under severe hypothermia (10°C) multidose cardioplegia was detrimental. The investigators concluded that it was not the frequency of infusion that was critical, but a combination of extended ischaemia (greater than 6 h), severe hypothermia, and repeated cardioplegic infusions. The mechanism involved remains to be resolved, as does its possible clinical relevance.

Clinical evaluation of different methods of paediatric myocardial protection is lacking, reflecting not only the difficulties of undertaking comparative trials in the face of established techniques, but of the difficulties in choosing what variables to assess when dealing with a variety of congenital conditions. Unlike the healthy animal model, the protection of the human paediatric myocardium will not only be affected by the immaturity of its metabolic pathways, but may be influenced by coexisting hypoxia, cardiac failure and their treatment. Animal models attempting to mimic these conditions (Silverman *et al.*, 1984; Del Nido *et al.*, 1987; Fujiwara *et al.*, 1988), indicate that 'pathological' changes in metabolism and morphology accompanying the defect may make the immature heart more susceptible to ischaemic injury and prone to inadequate intraoperative myocardial protection.

References

Acterberg, P.W., Nieukoop, A.S., Schoutsen, B. and De Jong, J.W. (1988) Different ATP–catabolism in reperfused adult and newborn rat hearts. *American Journal of Physiology*, **254**, H1091–H1098

Addetia, A.M., O'Reilly, B.F., Walsh, G.W. and Reid, P. (1988) Prolonged asystole during intraoperative myocardial reperfusion: an experimental study. *Annals of Thoracic Surgery*, **45**, 482–488

Akins, C.W. (1984) Noncardioplegic myocardial preservation for coronary revascularization. *Journal of Thoracic and Cardiovascular Surgery*, **88**, 174–181

Akins, C.W. (1987) Fibrillatory arrest. In *Myocardial Protection in Cardiac Surgery*, (ed. A.J. Roberts), Marcel Dekker Inc., New York, pp. 221–228

Akins, C.W. and Carroll, D.L. (1987) Event-free survival following nonemergency myocardial revascularization during hypothermic fibrillatory arrest. *Annals of Thoracic Surgery*, **43**, 628–633

Aldea, G.S., Austin, R.E., Flynn, A.E., *et al.* (1990) Heterogeneous distribution of cardioplegic solution in the absence of coronary artery disease. *Journal of Thoracic and Cardiovascular Surgery*, **99**, 354–353

Allen, B.S., Buckberg, G.D., Schwaiger, M., *et al.* (1986a) Early recovery of regional wall motion in patients following revascularization after eight hours of acute coronary occlusion. *Journal of Thoracic and Cardiovascular Surgery*, **92**, 636–648

Allen, B.S., Okamoto, F., Buckberg, G.D., *et al.* (1986b) Reperfusate composition: benefits of marked hypocalcaemia and diltiazem on regional recovery. *Journal of Thoracic and Cardiovascular Surgery*, **92**, 564–572

Allen, B.S., Okamoto, F., Buckberg, G.D., *et al.* (1986c) Reperfusion conditions: critical importance of total ventricular decompression during regional reperfusion. *Journal of Thoracic and Cardiovascular Surgery*, **92**, 605–612

Allen, B.S., Okamoto, F., Buckberg, G.D., *et al.* (1986d) Immediate functional recovery after six hours of regional ischemia by careful control of conditions of reperfusion and composition of reperfusate. *Journal of Thoracic and Cardiovascular Surgery*, **92**, 621–635

Allen, B.S., Okamoto, F., Buckberg, G.D., *et al.* (1986e) Effects of 'duration' of reperfusate administration versus reperfusate 'dose' on regional functional, biochemical, and histochemical recovery. *Journal of*

Thoracic and Cardiovascular Surgery, **92**, 594–604

Allen, B.S., Rosenkranz, E., Buckberg, G.D., *et al.* (1989) Studies on prolonged acute regional ischemia. VI. Myocardial infarction with left ventricular power failure: a medical/surgical emergency requiring urgent revascularization with maximal protection of remote muscle. *Journal of Thoracic and Cardiovascular Surgery*, **98**, 691–703

Ambrosio, G., Weisfeldt, M.L., Jacobus, W.E. and Flaherty, J.T. (1987a) Evidence for a reversible oxygen radical-mediated component of reperfusion injury: reduction by recombinant human superoxide dismutase administered at the time of reflow. *Circulation*, **75**, 282–291

Ambrosio, G., Weisman, H.F., Mannisi, J.A. and Becker, L.C. (1989) Progressive impairment of regional myocardial perfusion after initial restoration of postischemic blood flow. *Circulation*, **80**, 1846–1861

Ambrosio, G., Zweier, H.F., Jacobus, W.E., *et al.* (1987b) Improvement of postischemic myocardial function and metabolism induced by administration of deferoxamine at the time of reflow: the role of iron in the pathogenesis of reperfusion injury. *Circulation*, **76**, 906–915

Anderson, P.A.W. (1990) Fetal and neonatal physiology and pharmacology. *Current Opinion in Cardiology*, **5**, 3–16

Archie, J.P. and Kirklin, J.W. (1973) Effect of hypothermic perfusion on myocardial oxygen consumption and coronary resistance. *Surgical Forum*, **24**, 186–188

Avkiran, M. and Hearse, D.J. (1989) Protection of the myocardium during global ischemia. Is crystalloid cardioplegia effective in the immature myocardium? *Journal of Thoracic and Cardiovascular Surgery*, **97**, 220–228

Baile, E.M., Ling, H., Miyagishima, R.T., *et al.* (1986) Cardiac temperature and cardioplegic volume during cardiopulmonary bypass. *Journal of Surgical Research*, **41**, 388–393

Baird, R.D., Dutka, F., Okumori, M., *et al.* (1975) Surgical aspects of regional myocardial blood flow and myocardial pressure. *Journal of Thoracic and Cardiovascular Surgery*, **69**, 17–29

Bajaj, A.K., Cobb, M.A., Virmani, R., *et al.* (1989) Limitation of myocardial reperfusion injury by intravenous perfluorochemicals: role of neutrophil activation. *Circulation*, **79**, 645–656

Baker, J.E., Boerboom, L.E. and Olinger, G.N. (1988) Age-related changes in the ability of hypothermia and cardioplegia to protect ischemic rabbit myocardium. *Journal of Thoracic and Cardiovascular Surgery*, **96**, 717–724

Baker, J.E., Bullock, G.R. and Hearse, D.J. (1983) The temperature dependence of the calcium paradox: enzymatic, functional and morphological correlates of cellular injury. *Journal of Molecular and Cellular Cardiology*, **15**, 393–411

Baker, J.E., Kemmenoe, B.H., Hearse, D.J. and Bullock, G.R. (1984) Calcium delivery and time: factors affecting the progression of cellular damage during the calcium paradox in the rat heart. *Cardiovascular Research*, **18**, 361–370

Balderman, S.C., Binette, J.P., Chan, A.W. and Gage, A.A. (1983) The optimal temperature for preservation of the myocardium during global ischemia. *Annals of Thoracic Surgery*, **35**, 605–614

Balderman, S.C., Chan, A.K. and Gage, A.A. (1984) Verapamil cardioplegia: improved myocardial preservation during global ischemia. *Journal of Thoracic and Cardiovascular Surgery*, **88**, 57–66

Bando, K., Tago, M. and Teramoto, S. (1988) Prevention of free radical-induced myocardial injury by allopurinol. Experimental study in cardiac preservation and transplantation. *Journal of Thoracic and Cardiovascular Surgery*, **95**, 465–473

Barner, H.B., Jellinek, M., Standeven, J.W., *et al.* (1982) Cold blood-diltiazem cardioplegia. *Annals of Thoracic Surgery*, **33**, 55–63

Barner, H.B., Swartz, M.T., Devine, J.E., *et al.* (1987) Diltiazem as an adjunct to cold blood potassium cardioplegia: a clinical assessment of dose and prospective randomization. *Annals of Thoracic Surgery*, **43**, 191–197

Bassenge, E. and Busse, R. (1988) Endothelial modulation of coronary tone. *Progress in Cardiovascular Diseases*, **30**, 349–380

Baur, H.R., Peterson, T.A., Yasmineh, W.G. and Gobel, F.L. (1986) Cold potassium cardioplegia versus topical hypothermia and intermittent aortic occlusion for myocardial protection during coronary artery surgery: a randomized clinical study. *Annals of Thoracic Surgery*, **41**, 511–514

Becker, H., Vinten-Johansen, J., Buckberg, G.D., *et al.* (1981) Critical importance of ensuring cardioplegic delivery with coronary stenoses. *Journal of Thoracic and Cardiovascular Surgery*, **81**, 507–515

Becker, L.C., Levine, J.H. and DiPaula, A.F. (1986) Reversal of dysfunction in postischemic stunned myocardium by epinephrine and postextrasystolic potentiation. *Journal of the American College of Cardiology*, **7**, 580–589

Bednar, M., Smith, B., Pinto, A. and Mullane, K.M. (1985) Nafazatrom-induced salvage of ischemic myocardium is mediated through inhibition of neutrophil function. *Circulation Research*, **57**, 131–141

Belardinelli, L., Linden, J. and Berne, R.M. (1989) The cardiac effects of adenosine. *Progress in Cardiovascular Diseases*, **32**, 73–97

Belardinelli, L., Mattos, E.C. and Berne, R.M. (1981) Evidence for adenosine mediation of atrioventricular block in the ischemic canine myocardium. *Journal of Clinical Investigation*, **68**, 195–205

Belzer, F.O. and Southard, J.H. (1988) Principles of solid-organ preservation by cold storage. *Transplantation*, **45**, 673–697

Berggren, H., Ekroth, R., Herlitz, J., *et al.* (1983) Myocardial protective effect of maintained beta-blockade in aorto-coronary bypass surgery. *Scandinavian Journal of Thoracic and Cardiovascular Surgery*, **17**, 29

Bergmann, S.R. and Sobel, B.E. (1989) Surgical recanalization for treatment of evolving myocardial infarction. *Annals of Thoracic Surgery*, **48**, 319–321

Bergsland, J., LoBalsamo, L., Lajos, P., *et al.* (1987) Allopurinol in prevention of reperfusion injury of hypoxically stored rat hearts. *Journal of Heart Transplantation*, **6**, 137–140

Bernard, M., Menasche, P., Canioni, P., *et al.* (1985) Influence of the pH of cardioplegic solutions on intracellular pH, high-energy phosphates, and postarrest performance. Protective effects of acidotic, glutamate-containing cardioplegic perfusates. *Journal of Thoracic and Cardiovascular Surgery*, **90**, 235–242

Berne, R.M. (1963) Cardiac nucleotides in hypoxia: possible role in regulation in coronary blood flow. *American Journal of Physiology*, **204**, 317–322

Beyersdorf, F., Acar, C., Buckberg, G.D., *et al.* (1989a) Studies on prolonged acute regional ischemia. V. Metabolic support of remote myocardium during left ventricular power failure. *Journal of Thoracic and Cardiovascular Surgery*, **98**, 567–579

Beyersdorf, F., Acar, C., Buckberg, G.D. *et al.* (1989b) Studies on prolonged acute regional ischemia. III. Early natural history of stimulated single and multivessel disease with emphasis on remote myocardium. *Journal of Thoracic and Cardiovascular Surgery*, **98**, 368–380

Beyersdorf, F., Krause, E., Sarai, K., *et al.* (1990) Clinical evaluation of hypothermic ventricular fibrillation, multidose blood cardioplegia, and single-dose Bretschneider cardioplegia in coronary surgery. *Thoracic Cardiovascular Surgeon*, **38**, 20–29

Bhayana, J.N., Kalmbach, T., Booth, F.V., *et al.* (1989) Combined antegrade/retrograde cardioplegia for myocardial protection: a clinical trial. *Journal of Thoracic and Cardiovascular Surgery*, **98**, 956–960

Bing, O.H., Hayman, J.A., LaRaia, P.J., *et al.* (1987) Comparison of washed blood and oxygenator whole blood as vehicles for sanguinous multidose cardioplegia. *Journal of Surgical Research*, **43**, 179–186

Bing, O.H., LaRaia, P.J., Gaasch, W.H., *et al.* (1982) Independent protection provided by red blood cells during cardioplegia. *Circulation*, **66** (suppl I), I-81–I-84

Blaustein, A., Deneke, S.M., Stolz, R.I., *et al.* (1989) Myocardial glutathione depletion impairs recovery after short periods of ischemia. *Circulation*, **80**, 1449–1457

Bodenhamer, R.M., DeBoer, L.W., Geffin, G.A., *et al.* (1983) Enhanced myocardial protection during ischemic arrest. Oxygenation of a crystalloid cardioplegic solution. *Journal of Thoracic and Cardiovascular Surgery*, **85**, 769–780

Boe, S.L., Dixon, C.M., Sakert, T.A. and Magovern, G.J. (1982) The control of myocardial Ca^{++} sequestration with nifedipine cardioplegia. *Journal of Thoracic and Cardiovascular Surgery*, **84**, 678–684

Boggs, B.R., Torchiana, D.F., Geffin, G.A., *et al.* (1987) Optimal myocardial preservation with an acalcemic crystalloid cardioplegic solution. *Journal of Thoracic and Cardiovascular Surgery*, **93**, 838–846

Bolli, R. (1988) Oxygen-derived free radicals and postischemic myocardial dysfunction ('stunned myocardium'). *Journal of the American College of Cardiology*, **12**, 239–249

Bolli, R., Jeroudi, M.O., Patel, B.S., *et al.* (1989) Marked reduction of free radical generation and contractile dysfunction by antioxidant therapy begun at the time of reperfusion. *Circulation Research*, **65**, 607–622

Bolli, R., Patel, B.S., Jeroudi, M.O., *et al.* (1988) demonstration of free radical generation in 'stunned' myocardium of intact dogs with the use of the spin trap alpha-phenyl N-tert-butyl nitrone. *Journal of Clinical Investigation*, **82**, 476–485

Bolli, R., Patel, B.S., Zhu, W.X., *et al.* (1987) The iron chelator desferrioxamine attenuates postischemic ventricular dysfunction. *American Journal of Physiology*, **253**, H1372–H1380

Bolli, R., Zhu, W.X., Hartley, C.J., *et al.* (1987) Attenuation of dysfunction in the postischemic 'stunned' myocardium by dimethylthiourea. *Circulation*, **76**, 458–468

Bolling, S.F., Bies, L.E., Gallagher, K.P. and Bove, E.L. (1989) Enhanced myocardial protection with adenosine. *Annals of Thoracic Surgery*, **47**, 809–815

Bolling, S.F., Flaherty, J.T., Bulkley, B.H., *et al.* (1983) Improved myocardial preservation during global ischemia by continuous retrograde coronary sinus perfusion. *Journal of Thoracic and Cardiovascular Surgery*, **86**, 659–666

Bomfin, V. (1982) Continuous blood cardioplegia–a unique approach. In *A Textbook of Clinical Cardioplegia*, (eds R.M. Engleman and S. Levitsky), Futura Publishing, Mt. Kisco, New York, pp. 265–276

Bonchek, L.I. and Burlingame, M.W. (1987) Coronary artery bypass without cardioplegia. *Journal of Thoracic and Cardiovascular Surgery*, **93**, 261–267

Bormann, B., Scheld, H.H., Podzuweit, T., *et al.* (1985) Enhancement of myocardial energy potentials in man by glucose-insulin treatment before and after ischaemia heart arrest. *Journal of Cardiovascular Surgery*, **26**, 182–186

Borst, H.G. and Iversen, S. (1980) Myocardial temperatures in clinical cardioplegia. *Thoracic Cardiovascular Surgeon*, **28**, 29–33

Bove, E.L. and Stammers, A.H. (1986) Recovery of left ventricular function after hypothermic global ischemia: age-related differences in the isolated working rabbit heart. *Journal of Thoracic and Cardiovascular Surgery*, **91**, 115–122

Bove, E.L., Stammers, A.H. and Gallagher, K.P. (1987) Protection of the neonatal myocardium during hypothermic ischemia. Effect of cardioplegia on left ventricular function in the rabbit. *Journal of Thoracic and Cardiovascular Surgery*, **94**, 115–123

Braimbridge, M.V. (1979) Equipment for inducing cold cardioplegic arrest. *Journal of Thoracic and Cardiovascular Surgery*, **77**, 323–324

Braimbridge, M.V. (1987) The St. Thomas' Solution: magnesium containing, high-potassium, crystalloid cardioplegia. In *Myocardial Protection in Cardiac Surgery* (ed. A.J. Roberts), Marcel Dekker Inc., New York, pp. 121–128

Braimbridge, M.V., Chayen, J., Bitensky, L., *et al.* (1977) Cold cardioplegia or continuous coronary perfusion? Report on preliminary clinical experience as assessed cytochemically. *Journal of Thoracic and Cardiovascular Surgery*, **74**, 900–906

Braunwald, E. and Kloner, R.A. (1982) The stunned myocardium: prolonged, postischemic ventricular dysfunction. *Circulation*, **66**, 1146–1149

Brazier, J., Hottenrott, E., Buckberg, G.D. (1975) Non-coronary collateral myocardial blood flow. *Annals of Thoracic Surgery*, **19**, 426–442

Bremmer, W.F., Taylor, K.M. and Baird, S. (1978) Hypothalamo-pituitary-thyroid axis function during cardiopulmonary bypass. *Journal of Thoracic and Cardiovascular Surgery*, **75**, 392–399

Bretschneider, H.J. (1964) Uberlebenszeit und Wiederbelebungszeit des Herzens bei Normo-und Hypothermie. *Verhandlungen der Deutschen Gesellschaft fur Kreislaufforsch*, **30**, 11–34

Bretschneider, H.J., Hubner, G., Knoll, D., *et al.* (1975) Myocardial resistance and tolerance to ischemia: physiological and biochemical basis. *Journal of Cardiovascular Surgery*, **16**, 241–260

Brown, H.A., Niles, N.R., Braimbridge, M.V. and Austen, W.G. (1973) Preservation of the myocardium by means of cold physiological solutions, as assessed by ventricular function, histochemistry and birefringence. *Journal of Surgical Research*, **14**, 46–57

Brown, P.R., Mulder, D.S. and Chiu, R.C. (1979) Effects of hypothermic K-cardioplegia and ATP-Mg solution on myocardial ATP content and function. *Surgical Forum*, **30**, 248–250

Buckberg, G.D. (1975) The importance of venting the left ventricle. *Annals of Thoracic Surgery*, **20**, 488–490

Buckberg, G.D. (1979) A proposed 'solution' to the cardioplegic controversy. *Journal of Thoracic and Cardiovascular Surgery*, **77**, 803–815

Buckberg, G.D. (1986) Studies of controlled reperfusion after ischemia. I. When is cardiac muscle damaged irreversibly? *Journal of Thoracic and Cardiovascular Surgery*, **92**, 483–487

Buckberg, G.D. (1988) Antegrade cardioplegia, retrograde cardioplegia, or both? *Annals of Thoracic Surgery*, **45**, 589–590

Buckberg, G.D. (1989) Antegrade/retrograde blood cardioplegia to ensure caardioplegic distribution: operative techniques and objectives. *Journal of Cardiac Surgery*, **4**, 216–238

Buckberg, G.D. and Rosenkranz, E.R. (1987) Principles of cardioplegic myocardial protection. In *Myocardial Protection in Cardiac Surgery*, (ed. A.J. Roberts), Marcel Dekker Inc., New York, pp. 71–94

Buckberg, G.D., Brazier, J.R., Nelson, R.L., *et al.* (1977) Studies of the effects of hypothermia on regional myocardial blood flow and metabolism during cardiopulmonary bypass. I. The adequately perfused beating, fibrillating, and arrested heart. *Journal of Thoracic and Cardiovascular Surgery*, **73**, 87–94

Card, R.T., Prasad, K., Bharadwaj, B., *et al.* (1988) High 2,3-DPG blood cardioplegia and myocardial preservation during cardiopulmonary bypass. *Angiology*, **39**, 123–131

Catinella, F.P., Cunningham, J.N. and Spencer, F.C. (1984) Myocardial protection during prolonged aortic cross-clamping. Comparison of blood and crystalloid cardioplegia. *Journal of Thoracic and Cardiovascular Surgery*, **88**, 411–423

Cavarocchi, N.C., England, M.D. and Schaff, H.V. (1986) Oxygen free radical generation during cardiopulmonary bypass: correlation with complement activation. *Circulation*, **74** (suppl 3), 130–133

Challoner, D.R. (1968) Respiration in myocardium. *Nature*, **217**, 78–79

Chambers, D.E., Parks, D.A., Patterson, G., *et al.* (1985) Xanthine oxidase as a source of free radical damage in myocardial ischemia. *Journal of Molecular and Cellular Cardiology*, **17**, 145–152

Chambers, D.J., Astras, G., Takahashi, A., *et al.* (1989) Free radicals and cardioplegia: organic anti-oxidants as additives to the St. Thomas' Hospital cardioplegic solution. *Cardiovascular Research*, **23**, 351–358

Chambers, D.J., Braimbridge, M.V. and Hearse, D.J. (1987a) Free radicals and cardioplegia: allopurinol and oxypurinol reduce myocardial injury following ischemic arrest. *Annals of Thoracic Surgery*, **44**, 291–297

Chambers, D.J., Braimbridge, M.V. and Hearse, D.J. (1987b) Free radicals and cardioplegia: free radical scavengers improve post-ischaemic function of the rat myocardium. *European Journal of Cardiothoracic Surgery*, **1**, 37–45

Chapman, D. (1975) Phase transition and fluidity characteristics of lipids and cell membranes. *Quarterly Review of Biophysics*, **8**, 185–235

Charlat, M.L., O'Neill, P.G., Egan, J.M., *et al.* (1987) Evidence for pathogenic role of xanthine oxidase in the 'stunned' myocardium. *American Journal of Physiology*, **252**, H566–H577

Chen, X.Z., Newman, M. and Rosenfeldt, F.L. (1988) Internal cardiac cooling improves atrial preservation: electrophysiological and biochemical assessment. *Annals of Thoracic Surgery*, **46**, 406–411

Chen, X.Z., Shardy, G.C. and Rosenfeldt, F.L. (1988) A new technique of internal cardiac cooling improves atrial protection. *Annals of Thoracic Surgery*, **46**, 401–405

Cheung, E.H., Arcidi, J.M., Dorsey, L.M.A., *et al.* (1989) Reperfusion of infarcting myocardium: benefit of surgical reperfusion in a chronic model. *Annals of Thoracic Surgery*, **48**, 331–338

Cheung, E.H., Arcidi, J.M., Jackson, E.R., *et al.* (1988) Intracavitary right heart cooling during coronary bypass surgery. A prospective randomized trial. *Circulation*, **78**, III173–III179

Chiavarelli, R., Macchiarelli, G., Familiari, G., *et al.* (1989) Ultrastructural changes of coronary artery endothelium induced by cardioplegic solutions. *Thoracic and Cardiovascular Surgeon*, **37**, 151–157

Chilian, W.M., Eastman, C.L., Layne, S.M. and Marcus, M.L. (1988) Small vessel phenomena in the coronary microcirculation: phasic intramyocardial perfusion and coronary microvascular dynamics. *Progress in Cardiovascular Diseases*, **31**, 17–38

Chitwood, W.R., Sink, J.D., Hill, R.C., *et al.* (1979) The effects of hypothermia on myocardial oxygen consumption and transmural coronary blood flow in the potassium-arrested heart. *Annals of Surgery*, **190**, 106–116

Christakis, G.T., Fremes, S.E., Weisel, R.D., *et al.* (1986) Diltiazem cardioplegia. A balance of risk and benefit. *Journal of Thoracic and Cardiovascular Surgery*, **91**, 647–661

Christlieb, I.Y. and Clark, R.E. (1982) Adequacy of the perfusate: its influence on successful myocardial protection. *Journal of Thoracic and Cardiovascular Surgery*, **84**, 689–695

Clark, R.E., Christlieb, I.Y., Ferguson, T.B., *et al.* (1981) The first American clinical trial of nifedipine in cardioplegia. A report of the first 12 month experience. *Journal of Thoracic and Cardiovascular Surgery*, **82**, 848–859

Clark, R.E., Christlieb, I.Y., Vander Woude, J.C. and Henry, P.D. (1985) Use of nifedipine to decrease ischemic-reperfusion injury in the surgical setting. *American Journal of Cardiology*, **55**, 125B–138B

Clark, R.E., Ferguson, T.B. West, P.N., *et al.* (1977) Pharmacological preservation of the ischemic heart. *Annals of Thoracic Surgery*, **24**, 307–314

Coetzee, A., Kotze, J., Louw, J. and Lochner, A. (1986) Effect of oxygenated crystalloid cardioplegia on the functional and metabolic recovery of the isolated perfused rat heart. *Journal of Thoracic and Cardiovascular Surgery*, **91**, 259–269

Coleman, G.M., Gradinac, S., Taegtmeyer, H., *et al.* (1989) Efficacy of metabolic support with glucose-insulin-potassium for left ventricular pump failure after aortocoronary bypass surgery. *Circulation*, **80** (suppl I), I-91–I-96

Conti, V.R. and Kao, R.L. (1983) Metabolic and functional effects of carbohydrate substrate with single-dose and multiple-dose potassium cardioplegia. *Annals of Thoracic Surgery*, **36**, 320–327

Cooley, D.A., Reul, G.J. and Wukasch, D.C. (1972) Ischemic contracture of the heart: 'stone heart'. *American Journal of Cardiology*, **29**, 575–577

Coraboeuf, E., Deroubaix, E. and Hoerter, J. (1976) Control of ionic permeabilities in normal and ischemic hearts. *Circulation Research*, **38** (suppl I), I-92–I-98

Corno, A.F., Bethencourt, D.M., Laks, H., *et al.* (1987) Myocardial protection in the neonatal heart. A comparison of topical hypothermia and crystalloid and blood cardioplegic solutions. *Journal of Thoracic and Cardiovascular Surgery*, **93**, 163–172

Corr, P.B., Gross, R.W. and Sobel, B.E. (1984) Amphipathic metabolites and membrane dysfunction in ischemic myocardium. *Circulation Research*, **55**, 135–154

Cox, J.L., Anderson, R.W., Pass, H.I., *et al.* (1977) The safety of induced ventricular fibrillation during cardiopulmonary bypass in nonhypertrophied hearts. *Journal of Thoracic and Cardiovascular Surgery*, **74**, 423–432

Cunningham, J.N., Cantinella, F.P. and Spencer, F.C. (1982) Blood cardioplegia–experience with prolonged cross-clamping. In *A Textbook of Clinical Cardioplegia* (eds R.M. Engleman, S. Levitsky), Futura Publishing, Mt. Kisco, New York, pp. 241–264

Daggett, W.M. jr., Randolph, J.D., Jacobs, M., *et al.* (1987) The superiority of cold oxygenated dilute blood cardioplegia. *Annals of Thoracic Surgery*, **43**, 397–402

Daily, P.O. (1984) Discussion on the use of the pulmonary artery for left ventricular venting during cardiac operations. *Journal of Thoracic and Cardiovascular Surgery*, **87**, 537

Daily, P.O., Pfeffer, T.A., Wisniewski, J.B., *et al.* (1987) Clinical comparisons of methods of myocardial protection. *Journal of Thoracic and Cardiovascular Surgery*, **93**, 324–336

De Jong, J.W. (1986) Cardioplegia and calcium antagonists: a review. *Annals of Thoracic Surgery*, **42**, 593–598

De Witt, L., Coetzee, A., Kotze, J. and Lochner, A. (1988) Oxygen requirements of the isolated rat heart during hypothermic cardioplegia. Effect of oxygenation on metabolic and functional recovery after five hours of arrest. *Journal of Thoracic and Cardiovascular Surgery*, **95**, 310–320

Del Nido, P.J., Benson, L.N., Mickle, D.A., *et al.* (1987) Impaired left ventricular postischemic function and metabolism in chronic right ventricular hypertrophy. *Circulation*, **76** (suppl V), V-168–V-173

Del Nido, P.J., Wilson, G.J., Mickle, D.A., *et al.* (1985) The role of cardioplegic solution buffering in myocardial protection. A biochemical and histopathological assessment. *Journal of Thoracic and Cardiovascular Surgery*, **89**, 689–699

Devous, M.D. and Lewandowski, E.D. (1987) Inosine preserves ATP during ischemia and enhances recovery during reperfusion. *American Journal of Physiology*, **253**, H1224–H1233

De Witt, D.F., Jochim, K.E. and Behrendt, D.M. (1983) Nucleotide degradation and functional impairment during cardioplegia: amelioration by inosine. *Circulation*, **67**, 171–178

Diehl, J.T., Eichhorn, E.J., Konstam, M.A., *et al.* (1988) Efficacy of retrograde coronary sinus cardioplegia in patients undergoing myocardial revascularization: a propsective randomized trial. *Annals of Thoracic Surgery*, **45**, 595–602

Diehl, J.T., Kaplan, E., Dresdale, A.R., *et al.* (1989) Effects of atrial cardioplegia on the ischemic right ventricle after acute coronary artery occlusion and reperfusion. *Annals of Thoracic Surgery*, **48**, 829–834

Digerness, S.B., Vanini, V. and Wideman, F.E. (1981) In vitro comparison of oxygen availability from asanguinous and sanguinous cardioplegic media. *Circulation*, **64** (suppl II), II-80–II-83

Dole, W.P. (1987) Autoregulation of the coronary circulation. *Progress in Cardiovascular Diseases*, **29**, 293–323

Dorsey, L.M., Colgan, T.K., Silverstein, J.I., *et al.* (1983) Alterations in regional myocardial function after heterogeneous cardioplegia. *Journal of Thoracic and Cardiovascular Surgery*, **86**, 70–79

Dudziak, R. and Lochner, W. (1965) Under die Wirkung des Procain und des Ca^{++}-Entzuges auf den Sauerstoffverbrauch und die electromechanische Koppelung des Warmbluterherzens. *Pflugers Archiv. European Journal of Physiology*, **285**, 160–168

Eddy, L.J., Stewart, J.R., Jones, H.P., *et al.* (1987) Free radical-producing enzyme, xanthine oxidase, is undetectable in human hearts. *American Journal of Physiology*, **253**, H709–H711

Ekroth, R., Berggren, H., Sudow, G., *et al.* (1980) Thermographic demonstration of uneven myocardial cooling in patients with coronary lesions. *Annals of Thoracic Surgery*, **29**, 341–345

Ely, S.W., Mentzer, R.M., Lasley, R.D., *et al.* (1985) Functional and metabolic evidence of enhanced myocardial tolerance to ischemia and reperfusion with adenosine. *Journal of Thoracic and Cardiovascular Surgery*, **90**, 549–556

Emerit, I., Fabiani, J.N., Panzio, O., *et al.* (1988) Clastogenic factor in ischemia-reperfusion injury during open-heart surgery: protective effect of allopurinol. *Annals of Thoracic Surgery*, **46**, 619–624

Engelman, R.M., Levitsky, S. and Wyndham, C.R. (1977) Optimal conditions for reperfusion during cardiopulmonary bypass. *Circulation*, **56** (suppl II), II-148–II-156

Engelman, R.M., Auvil, J., O'Donoghue, M.J. and Levitsky, S. (1978) The significance of multidose cardioplegia and hypothermia in myocardial preservation during ischemic arrest. *Journal of Thoracic and Cardiovascular Surgery*, **75**, 555–563

Engelman, R.M., Rousou, J.H., Lemeshow, S. and Dobbs, W.A. (1981) The metabolic consequences of blood and crystalloid cardioplegia. *Circulation*, **64** (suppl II), II-67–II-74

Engler, R.L., Dahlgren, M.D., Morris, D., *et al.* (1986) Role of leukocytes in the response to acute myocardial ischemia and reflow in dogs. *American Journal of Physiology*, **251**, H314–H323

English, T., Cooper, D.K.C., Medd, R. and Wheeldon, D. (1980) Orthotopic heart transplantation after 16 hours of ischaemia. *British Heart Journal*, **43**, 721–722

Eugene, J., Lyons, K.P., Ott, R.A. *et al.* (1987) Regional myocardial perfusion of cardioplegic solutions. *Annals of Thoracic Surgery*, **43**, 522–526

Fabiani, J.N., Deloche, A., Swanson, J. and Carpentier, A. (1986) Retrograde cardioplegia through the right atrium. *Annals of Thoracic Surgery*, **41**, 101–102

Fabiani, J.N., Jebara, V. and Carpentier, A. (1989) Right atrial cardioplegia: a safe procedure for myocardial protection (letter). *Annals of Thoracic Surgery*, **47**, 331–332

Fabiani, J.N., Swanson, J., Deloche, A. and Carpentier, A.F. (1987) Right atrial cardioplegia. In *Myocardial Protection in Cardiac Surgery* (ed. A.J. Roberts), Marcel Dekker Inc., New York, pp. 505–514

Feindel, C.M., Tait, G.A., Wilson, G.J., *et al.* (1984) Multidose blood versus crystalloid cardioplegia. Comparison by quantitative assessment of irreversible myocardial injury. *Journal of Thoracic and Cardiovascular Surgery*, **87**, 585–595

Ferguson, T.B., Damiano, R.J., Smith, P.K., *et al.* (1986a) The electrophysiological effects of calcium channel blockade during standard hyperkalemic hypothermic cardioplegic arrest. *Annals of Thoracic Surgery*, **41**, 622–629

Ferguson, T.B., Smith, P.K., Lofland, G.K., *et al.* (1986b) The effects of cardioplegic potassium concentration and myocardial temperature on electrical activity in the heart during elective cardioplegic arrest. *Journal of Thoracic and Cardiovascular Surgery*, **92**, 755–765

Ferguson, T.B., Smith, L.S., Smith, P.K., *et al.* (1987) Electrical activity in the heart during hyperkalemic hypothermic cardioplegic arrest: site of origin and relationship to specialized conduction tissue. *Annals of Thoracic Surgery*, **43**, 373–379

Fiore, A.C., Naunheim, K.S., Kaiser, G.C., *et al.* (1989) Coronary sinus versus aortic root perfusion with blood cardioplegia in elective myocardial revascularization. *Annals of Thoracic Surgery*, **47**, 684–688

Flameng, W., Borgers, M., Van der Vusse, G.J., *et al.* (1983) Cardioprotective effects of lidoflazine in extensive aorta-coronary bypass grafting. *Journal of Thoracic and Cardiovascular Surgery*, **85**, 758–768

Flameng, W., Daenen, W., Borgers, M., *et al.* (1981) Cardioprotective effects of lidoflazine during 1-hour normothermic global ischemia. *Circulation*, **64**, 796–807

Flameng, E., De Meyere, R., Daenen, W., *et al.* (1986) Nifedipine as an adjunct to St. Thomas' Hospital cardioplegia. A double-blind, placebo-controlled, randomized clinical trial. *Journal of Thoracic and Cardiovascular Surgery*, **91**, 723–731

Flameng, W., Mollhoff, T., Sukehiro, S., *et al.* (1990) A new concept for donor heart preservation: nucleoside transport inhibition. *Journal of Molecular and Cellular Cardiology*, **22** (suppl III), S.99 (abstract)

Flameng, W., Van der Vusse, G.J., De Meyere, R., *et al.* (1984) Intermittent aortic cross-clamping versus St. Thomas' Hospital cardioplegia in extensive aorta-coronary bypass grafting. *Journal of Thoracic and Cardiovascular Surgery*, **88**, 164–173

Fleckenstein, A., Frey, M. and Fleckenstein-Grun, G. (1983) Consequences of uncontrolled calcium entry and its prevention with calcium antagonists. *European Heart Journal*, **4** (suppl 2), 241–255

Foglia, R.P., Steed, D.L., Follette, D.M., *et al.* (1979) Iatrogenic myocardial edema with potassium cardioplegia. *Journal of Thoracic and Cardiovascular Surgery*, **78**, 217–222

Foker, J.E., Einzig, S. and Wang, T. (1980) Adenosine metabolism and myocardial preservation. *Journal of Thoracic and Cardiovascular Surgery*, **80**, 506–516

Follette, D., Fey, K., Livesay, J., *et al.* (1977a) Studies on myocardial reperfusion injury. I. Favorable modification by adjusting reperfusate pH. *Surgery*, **82**, 149–155

Follette, D., Steed, D., Foglia, R., *et al.* (1977b) Reduction of postischemic myocardial damage by maintaining arrest during initial reperfusion. *Surgical Forum*, **28**, 281–283

Follette, D.M., Fey, K., Buckberg, G.D., *et al.* (1981) Reducing postischemic damage by temporary modification of reperfusate calcium, potassium, pH, and osmolarity. *Journal of Thoracic and Cardiovascular Surgery*, **82**, 221–238

Follette, D.M., Mulder, D.G., Maloney, J.V. and Buckberg, G.D. (1978) Advantages of blood cardioplegia over continuous coronary perfusion or intermittent ischemia. Experimental and clinical study. *Journal of Thoracic and Cardiovascular Surgery*, **76**, 604–619

Forman, M.B., Puett, D.W., Bingham, S.E., *et al.* (1987) Preservation of endothelial cell structure and function by intracoronary perfluorochemical in canine preparation of reperfusion. *Circulation*, **76**, 469–479

Forman, M.B., Puett, D.W. and Virmani, R. (1989) Endothelial and myocardial injury during ischemia and reperfusion: pathogenesis and therapeutic implications. *Journal of the American College of Cardiology*, **13**, 450–459

Fremes, S.E., Christakis, G.T., Weisel, R.D., *et al.* (1984) A clinical trial of blood and crystalloid cardioplegia. *Journal of Thoracic and Cardiovascular Surgery*, **88**, 726–741

Fremes, S.E., Weisel, R.D., Mickle, D.A., *et al.* (1985) Myocardial metabolism and ventricular function following cold potassium cardioplegia. *Journal of Thoracic and Cardiovascular Surgery*, **89**, 531–546

Fujiwara, T., Kurtts, T., Anderson, W., *et al.* (1988) Myocardial protection in cyanotic neonatal lambs. *Journal of Thoracic and Cardiovascular Surgery*, **96**, 700–710

Furchgott, R.F. and Zawadzki, J.V. (1980) The obligatory role of endothelial cells in the relaxation of arterial smooth muscle by acetylcholine. *Nature*, **288**, 373–376

Furusho, N., Araki, H., Nishi, K. and Miyauchi, Y. (1989) Effect of cold cardioplegic solution and hypothermia on response to acetylcholine in perfused epicardial coronary artery of pig. *Annals of Thoracic Surgery*, **47**, 287–292

Gallandat-Huet, R.C., Karliczek, G.F., van der Heidi, J.N., *et al.* (1988) Clinical effect of Bretschneider-HTK and St. Thomas' cardioplegia on hemodynamic performance after bypass measured using an automatic datalogging database system. *Thoracic and Cardiovascular Surgeon*, **36**, 151–156

Ganote, C.E. and Nayler, W.G. (1985) Contracture and the calcium paradox. *Journal of Molecular and Cellular Cardiology*, **17**, 733–745

Ganote, C.E., Seabra-Gomes, R., Nayler, W.G. and Jennings, R.B. (1975) Irreversible myocardial injury in anoxic perfused rat hearts. *American Journal of Pathology*, **80**, 419–450

Ganote, C.E., Worstell, J. and Kaltenbach, J.P. (1976) Oxygen-induced enzyme release after irreversible myocardial injury: effects of cyanide in reperfused rat hearts. *American Journal of Pathology*, **84**, 327–350

Ganzel, B.L., Katzmark, S.L. and Mavroudis, C. (1988) Myocardial preservation in the neonate. Beneficial effects of cardioplegia and systemic hypothermia on piglets undergoing cardiopulmonary bypass and myocardial ischemia. *Journal of Thoracic and Cardiovascular Surgery*, **96**, 414–422

Garlick, P.B., Davies, M.J., Hearse, D.J. and Slater, T.F. (1987) Direct detection of free radicals in the reperfused rat heart using electron spin resonance spectroscopy. *Circulation Research*, **61**, 757–760

Gaudel, Y. and Duvelleroy, M.A. (1984) Role of oxygen radicals in cardiac injury due to reoxygenation. *Journal of Molecular and Cellular Cardiology*, **16**, 459–470

Gebhard, M.M., Bretschneider, H.J., Gersing, E. and Schnabel, P.A. (1987) Bretschneider's histidine-buffered cardioplegic solution: concept, application, and efficiency. In *Myocardial Protection in Cardiac Surgery* (ed A.J. Roberts), Marcel Dekker, Inc., New York, pp. 95–119

Geffin, G.A., Love, T.R., Hendren, W.G., *et al.* (1989) The effects of calcium and magnesium in hyperkalemic cardioplegic solutions on myocardial preservation. *Journal of Thoracic and Cardiovascular Surgery*, **98**, 239–250

Gharagozloo, F., Melendez, F.J., Hein, R.A., *et al.* (1988) The effect of oxygen free radical scavengers on the recovery of regional myocardial function after acute coronary occlusion and surgical reperfusion. *Journal of Thoracic and Cardiovascular Surgery*, **95**, 631–636

Goldstein, J.P., Salter, D.R., Murphy, C.E., *et al.* (1986) The efficacy of blood versus crystalloid coronary sinus cardioplegia during global myocardial ischemia. *Circulation*, **74** (suppl III), III-9–III-104

Gradinac, S., Coleman, G.M., Taegtmeyer, H., *et al.* (1989) Improved cardiac function with glucose-insulin-potassium after aortocoronary bypass grafting. *Annals of Thoracic Surgery*, **48**, 484–489

Greenfield, D.T., Greenfield, L.J. and Hess, M.L. (1988) Enhancement of crystalloid cardioplegic protection against global normothermic ischemia by superoxide dismutase plus catalase but not diltiazem in the isolated, working rat heart. *Journal of Thoracic and Cardiovascular Surgery*, **95**, 799–813

Grice, W.N., Konishi, T. and Apstein, C.S. (1987) Resistance of neonatal myocardium to injury during normothermic and hypothermic ischemic arrest and reperfusion. *Circulation*, **76** (suppl V), V-150–V155

Gross, G.L., Farber, N.E., Hardman, H.F. and Warltier, D.C. (1986) Beneficial actions of superoxide dismutase and catalase in stunned myocardium of dogs. *American Journal of Physiology*, **259**, H372–H377

Grover, F.L. (1987) The relative efficacy of venous drainage and venting techniques in myocardial protection. In *Myocardial Protection in Cardiac Surgery* (ed A.J. Roberts), Marcel Dekker Inc., New York, pp. 269–281

Grover, F.L., Fewel, J.G., Ghidoni, J.J., *et al.* (1982) Comparison of roller pump versus pressurized bag administration of potassium cardioplegic solution. *Annals of Thoracic Surgery*, **34**, 278–286

Guarnieri, C., Flamigni, F. and Caldarera, C.M. (1980) Role of oxygen in the cellular damage induced by reoxygenation of hypoxic heart. *Journal of Molecular and Cellular Cardiology*, **12**, 797–808

Guerci, A.D., Ciuffo, A.A., DiPaula, A.F. and Weisfeldt, M.L. (1987) Intermittent coronary sinus occlusion in dogs: reduction in infarct size 10 days after reperfusion. *Journal of the American College of Cardiology*, **9**, 1075

Guiraudon, G.M., Campbell, C.S., McLellan, D.G., *et al.* (1986) Retrograde coronary sinus versus aortic root perfusion with cold cardioplegia: randomized study of levels of cardiac enzymes in 40 patients. *Circulation*, **74** (suppl III), III-105–III-115

Gundry, S.R. and Kirsh, M.M. (1984) A comparison of retrograde cardioplegia versus antegrade cardioplegia in the presence of coronary artery obstruction. *Annals of Thoracic Surgery*, **38**, 124–127

Gundry, S.R., Sequeira, A., Coughlin, T.R. and McLaughlin, J.S. (1989) Postoperative conduction disturbances: a comparison of blood and crystalloid cardioplegia. *Annals of Thoracic Surgery*, **47**, 384–390

Gutteridge, J.M.C., Richmond, R. and Halliwell, B. (1979) Inhibition of the iron-catalysed formation of hydroxyl radicals from superoxide and of lipid peroxidation by desferrioxamine. *Biochemical Journal*, **184**, 469–472

Guvendik, L., Hynd, J., Drake-Holland, A. and Parker, D.J. (1990) Myocardial protective effects of lidoflazine during ischemia and reperfusion. *Thoracic and Cardiovascular Surgeon*, **38**, 15–19

Guyton, R.A., Dorsey, L.M., Craver, J.M., *et al.* (1985) Improved myocardial recovery after cardioplegic arrest with an oxygenated crystalloid solution. *Journal of Thoracic and Cardiovascular Surgery*, **89**, 877–887

Haider, W., Benzer, H., Schutz, W. and Wolner, E. (1984) Improvement of cardiac preservation by preoperative high insulin supply. *Journal of Thoracic and Cardiovascular Surgery*, **88**, 294–300

Halliwell, B. (1989) Superoxide, iron, vascular endothelium and reperfusion injury. *Free Radical Research Communications*, **5**, 315–318

Hamasaki, T., Kuroda, H. and Mori, T. (1988) Temperature dependency of calcium-induced reperfusion injury in the isolated rat heart. *Annals of Thoracic Surgery*, **45**, 306–310

Hearse, D.J. (1977) Reperfusion of the ischemic myocardium. *Journal of Molecular and Cellular Cardiology*, **9**, 605–616

Hearse, D.J. (1987) The pathophysiology of myocardial ischemia. In *Myocardial Protection in Cardiac Surgery* (ed A.J. Roberts), Marcel Dekker Inc., New York, pp. 7–28

Hearse, D.J. and Chain, E.B. (1972) The role of glucose in the survival and 'recovery' of the anoxic isolated perfused rat heart. *Journal of Biochemistry*, **128**, 1125–1133

Hearse, D.J. and Tosaki, A. (1988) Free radicals and calcium: simultaneous interacting triggers as determinants of vulnerability to reperfusion-induced arrhythmias in the rat heart. *Journal of Molecular and Cellular Cardiology*, **20**, 213–223

Hearse, D.J., Braimbridge, M.V. and Jynge, P. (1981) *Protection of the Ischaemic Myocardium: Cardioplegia.* Raven Press, New York

Hearse, D.J., Erol, C., Robinson, L.A., *et al.* (1985) Particle-induced coronary vasoconstriction cardioplegic infusion. Characterization and possible mechanisms. *Journal of Thoracic and Cardiovascular Surgery*, **89**, 428–438

Hearse, D.J., Humphrey, S.M. and Bullock, G.R. (1978) The oxygen paradox and the calcium paradox: two facets of the same problem? *Journal of Molecular and Cellular Cardiology*, **10**, 641–668

Hearse, D.J., Humphrey, S.M., Nayler, W.G., *et al.* (1975) Ultrastructural damage associated with reoxygenation of the anoxic myocardium. *Journal of Molecular and Cellular Cardiology*, **7**, 315–324

Hearse, D.J., O'Brien, K. and Braimbridge, M.V. (1981) Protection of the myocardium during ischemic arrest. Dose-response curves for procaine and lignocaine solutions. *Journal of Thoracic and Cardiovascular Surgery*, **81**, 873–879

Hearse, D.J., Sonmez, B., Saldanha, C., *et al.* (1986) Particle-induced coronary vasconstriction in the rat heart: pharmacological investigation of underlying mechanisms. *Thoracic and Cardiovascular Surgeon*, **34**, 316–325

Hearse, D.J., Stewart, D.A. and Braimbridge, M.V. (1975) Hypothermic arrest and potassium arrest, metabolic and myocardial protection during elective cardiac arrest. *Circulation Research*, **36**, 481–489

Hearse, D.J., Stewart, D.A. and Braimbridge, M.V. (1976) Cellular protection during myocardial ischemia. The development and characterization of a procedure for the induction of reversible ischemic arrest. *Circulation*, **54**, 193–202

Hearse, D.J., Stewart, D.A. and Braimbridge, M.V. (1978a) Myocardial protection during ischemic cardiac arrest. The importance of magnesium in cardioplegic infusates. *Journal of Thoracic and Cardiovascular Surgery*, **75**, 877–885

Hearse, D.J., Stewart, D.A. and Braimbridge, M.V. (1978b) Myocardial protection during ischemic cardiac arrest. Possible deleterious effects of glucose and mannitol in coronary infusates. *Journal of Thoracic and Cardiovascular Surgery*, **76**, 16–23

Hearse, D.J., Stewart, D.A. and Chain, E.B. (1974) Recovery from cardiac bypass and elective cardiac arrest. The metabolic consequences of various cardioplegic procedures in the isolated rat heart. *Circulation Research*, **35**, 448–457

Hedley Brown, A., Morritt, G.N. and Hammo, M. (1982) Avoidance of reperfusion injury after cardioplegia. *Thorax*, **37**, 275–279

Heineman, F.W., MacGregor, D.C., Wilson, G.J. and Ninomiya, J. (1981) Regional and transmural myocardial temperature distribution in cold chemical cardioplegia: significance of critical coronary arterial stenosis. *Journal of Thoracic and Cardiovascular Surgery*, **81**, 851–859

Heitmiller, R.F., DeBoer, L.W., Geffin, G.A., *et al.* (1985) Myocardial recovery after hypothermic arrest: a comparison of oxygenated crystalloid to blood cardioplegia. The role of calcium. *Circulation*, **72** (suppl II), II-241–II-253

Hendren, W.G., O'Keefe, D.D., Geffin, G.A., *et al.* (1987) Maximal oxygenation of dilute blood cardioplegia solution. *Annals of Thoracic Surgery*, **44**, 48–52

Henry, P.D., Shuchleib, R., Davis, J., *et al.* (1977) Myocardial contracture and accumulation of mitochondrial calcium in ischemic rabbit heart. *American Journal of Physiology*, **223**, 677–684

Hilton, C.J., Teubl, W., Acker, M., *et al.* (1979) Inadequate cardioplegic protection with obstructed coronary arteries. *Annals of Thoracic Surgery*, **28**, 323–334

Hochberg, M.S. and Austen, W.G. (1980) Selective retrograde coronary venous perfusion. *Annals of Thoracic Surgery*, **29**, 578–588

Hoffman, J.I.E. (1987) Transmural myocardial perfusion. *Progress in Cardiovascular Diseases*, **29**, 429–464

Hottenrott, C.E. and Buckberg, G.D. (1974) Studies of the effects of ventricular fibrillation on the adequacy of regional myocardial flow: II. Effects of ventricular distention. *Journal of Thoracic and Cardiovascular Surgery*, **68**, 626–633

Hottenrott, C.E., Maloney, J.V. and Buckberg, G.D. (1974a) Studies of the effects of ventricular fibrillation on the adequacy of regional myocardial flow: I. Electrical vs. spontaneous fibrillation. *Journal of Thoracic and Cardiovascular Surgery*, **68**, 615–625

Hottenrott, C.E., Maloney, J.V. and Buckberg, G.D. (1974b) Studies of the effects of ventricular fibrillation on the adequacy of regional myocardial flow: III. Mechanisms of ischemia. *Journal of Thoracic and Cardiovascular Surgery*, **68**, 634–645

Hottenrott, C., Nelson, R.L., McConnell, D.H., *et al.* (1975) The effect of mannitol on the distribution and adequacy of coronary flow in ventricles made ischemic by fibrillation or arrest during bypass. *Surgical Forum*, **26**, 266

Hottenrott, C.E., Towers, B., Kurkji, H.J., *et al.* (1973) The hazard of ventricular fibrillation in hypertrophied ventricles during cardiopulmonary bypass. *Journal of Thoracic and Cardiovascular Surgery*, **66**, 742–753

Ichihara, K. and Abiko, Y. (1977) Inhibition of endo- and epicardial glycogenolysis by propranolol in ischemic hearts. *American Journal of Physiology*, **232**, H353

Ignarro, L.J. (1989) Biological actions and properties of endothelium-derived nitric oxide formed and released from artery and vein. *Circulation Research*, **65**, 1–21

Illes, R.W., Silverman, N.A., Krukenkamp, I.B., *et al.* (1989a) Amelioration of postischemic stunning by deferoxamine blood cardioplegia. *Circulation*, **80** (suppl III), III-30–III-35

Illes, R.W., Silverman, N.A., Krukenkamp, I.B., *et al.* (1989b) The efficacy of blood cardioplegia is not due to oxygen delivery. *Journal of Thoracic and Cardiovascular Surgery*, **98**, 1051–1056

Ito, B.R., Tate, H. and Kobayashi, M. (1987) Reversibly injured, postischemic canine myocardium retains normal contractile reserve. *Circulation Research*, **61**, 834–846

Iverson, L.I., Young, J.N., Ennix, C.L., *et al.* (1984) Myocardial protection: a comparison of cold blood and cold crystalloid cardioplegia. *Journal of Thoracic and Cardiovascular Surgery*, **87**, 509–516

Jansson, E., Bomfim, V., Schmidt, W. and Kaijser, L. (1987) Myocardial energy metabolism in the induction phase of cardioplegia in relation to myocardial temperature during open heart surgery. *Clinical Physiology*, **7**, 43–49

Jarasch, E.D., Bruder, G. and Heid, H.W. (1986) Significance of xanthine oxidase in capillary endothelial cells. *Acta Physiologica Scandinavica. Supplement*, **548**, 39–46

Jennings, R.B. (1969) Early phase of myocardial ischemic injury and infarction. *American Journal of Cardiology*, **24**, 753–765

Jennings, R.B. and Kloner, K.A. (1981) Lethal myocardial ischemic injury. *American Journal of Pathology*, **102**, 241–255

Jennings, R.B. and Reimer, K.A. (1979) Biology of experimental, acute myocardial ischemia and infarction. In *Enzymes in Cardiology: Diagnosis and Research* (eds D.J. Hearse and J. de Leris), John Wiley, Chichester, pp. 21–57

Jennings, R.B. and Steenbergen, C. (1985) Nucleotide metabolism and cellular damage in myocardial ischemia. *Annual Review of Physiology*, **47**, 727–749

Jennings, R.B., Hawkins, H.K., Lowe, J.E. *et al.* (1978) Relation between high-energy phosphate and lethal injury in myocardial ischemia in the dog. *American Journal of Pathology*, **92**, 187–214

Jennings, R.B., Reimer, K.A. and Steenbergen, C. (1986) Myocardial ischemia revisited: the osmolar load, membrane damage, and reperfusion. *Journal of Molecular and Cellular Cardiology*, **18**, 769–780

Jeremy, R.W. and Becker, L.C. (1989) Neutrophil depletion does not prevent myocardial dysfunction after brief coronary occlusion. *Journal of the American College of Cardiology*, **13**, 1155–1163

Johnson, D.L., Greene, P.S., Gott, V.L. and Gardner, T.J. (1988a) New pluronic-free perfluorocarbon cardioplegia improves myocardial oxygenation. *Circulation*, **78** (suppl III), III-153–III-157

Johnson, D.L., Lahorra, J.A., Gott, V.L and Gardner, T.J. (1988b) Reducing intraoperative myocardial acidosis by continuous cardioplegic perfusion via the coronary sinus. *Journal of Surgical Research*, **44**, 625–630

Johnson, R.E., Dorsey, L.M., Moye, S.J., *et al.* (1982) Cardioplegic infusion: the safe limits of pressure and temperature. *Journal of Thoracic and Cardiovascular Surgery*, **83**, 813–824

Johnson, R.G., Jacocks, M.A., Aretz, T.H., *et al.* (1982) Comparison of myocardial preservation with hypothermic potassium and nifedipine arrest. *Circulation*, **66** (suppl I), 73–80

Jurmann, M.J., Schaefers, H.J., Dammenhayn, L. and Haverich, A. (1988) Oxygen-derived free radical scavengers for amelioration of reperfusion damage in heart transplantation. *Journal of Thoracic and Cardiovascular Surgery*, **95**, 368–377

Kaiser, L. and Sparks, H.V. (1987) Endothelial cells. Not just a cellophane wrapper. *Archives of Internal Medicine*, **147**, 569–573

Kane, J.J., Murphy, M.L., Bissett, K.J., *et al.* (1975) Mitochondrial function, oxygen extraction, epicardial S-T segment changes and tritiated digoxin distribution after reperfusion of ischemic myocardium. *American Journal of Cardiology*, **36**, 218–224

Kanter, K.R., Jaffin, J.H., Ehrlichman, R.J., *et al.* (1981) Superiority of perfluorocarbon cardioplegia over blood or crystalloid cardioplegia. *Circulation*, **64** (suppl II), II-75–II-80

Kao, R.L. and Magovern, G.J. (1986) Prevention of reperfusional damage from ischemic myocardium. *Journal of Thoracic and Cardiovascular Surgery*, **91**, 106–114

Kates, R.A., Dorsey, L.M., Kaplan, J.A., *et al.* (1983) Pretreatment with lidoflazine, a calcium-channel blocker. *Journal of Thoracic and Cardiovascular Surgery*, **85**, 278–286

Katz, A.M. and Tada, M. (1972) The 'stone heart': a challenge to the biochemist. *American Journal of Cardiology,* **29**, 578–580

Katz, A.M. (1980) A basic scientist reacts to the discussions of surgery. In *Proceedings of Cardioplegia Workshop–an International Exchange of Ideas.* Travenol Laboratories, Deerfield, pp. 31–34

Kaufmann, R. and Fleckenstein, A. (1965) Die bedeutung der Aktionspotential-Dauer und der Ca^{++} lonen beim Zustandekommen der positiv-inotropen Kaltewirkungen am Warmbluter-Myokard. *Pfluegers Archiv. European Journal of Physiology*, **285**, 1–18

Kay, E.B., Head, L.R. and Nogueira, C. (1958) Direct coronary artery perfusion for aortic valve surgery. *JAMA*, **168**, 1967

Kempsford, R.D. and Hearse, D.J. (1989) Protection of the immature myocardium during global ischemia. A comparison of four clinical cardioplegic solutions in the rabbit heart. *Journal of Thoracic and Cardiovascular Surgery*, **97**, 856–863

Kempsford, R.D. and Hearse, D.J. (1990) Protection of the immature heart. Temperature-dependent beneficial or detrimental effects of multidose crystalloid cardioplegia in the neonatal rabbit heart. *Journal of Thoracic and Cardiovascular Surgery*, **99**, 269–279

Khuri, S.F. and Warner, K.G. (1987) Intraoperative pH monitoring for the detection of progresssive myocardial ischemia. In *Myocardial Protection in Cardiac Surgery*, (ed. A.J. Roberts), Marcel Dekker Inc., New York, pp. 399–412

Khuri, S.F., Marston, W.A., Josa, M., *et al.* (1985) Observations on 100 patients with continuous intraoperative monitoring of intramyocardial pH. The adverse effects of ventricular fibrillation and reperfusion. *Journal of Thoracic and Cardiovascular Surgery*, **89**, 170–182

Khuri, S.F., Warner, K.G., Josa, M., *et al.* (1988) The superiority of continuous cold blood cardioplegia in the metabolic protection of the hypertrophied human heart. *Journal of Thoracic and Cardiovascular Surgery*, **95**, 442–454

Kirklin, J.K., Westaby, S., Blackstone, E.H., *et al.* (1983) Complement and the damaging effects of cardiopulmonary bypass. *Journal of Thoracic and Cardiovascular Surgery*, **86**, 845–857

Kirklin, J.W., Naftel, D.C., Blackstone, E.H. and Pohost, G.M. (1989) Summary of consensus concerning death and ischemic events after coronary artery bypass grafting. *Circulation*, **79** (suppl I), I-81–I-91

Kloner, R.A. (1989) Do neutrophils mediate the phenomenon of stunned myocardium? *Journal of the American College of Cardiology*, **13**, 1164–1166

Kloner, R.A., Ganote, C.E. and Jennings, R.B. (1974) The 'no-reflow' phenomenon after temporary occlusion in the dog. *Journal of Clinical Investigation*, **54**, 1496–1508

Kloner, R.A., Rude, R.E., Carlson, N., *et al.* (1980) Ultrastructural evidence of microvascular damage and myocardial cell injury after coronary occlusion: which come first? *Circulation*, **62**, 945–952

Konishi, T. and Apstein, C.S. (1989) Comparison of three cardioplegic solutions during hypothermic ischemic arrest in neonatal blood-perfused rabbit hearts. *Journal of Thoracic and Cardiovascular Surgery*, **98**, 1132–1137

Kresh, J.Y., Nastala, C., Bianchi, P.C., *et al.* (1987) The relative buffering power of cardioplegic solutions. *Journal of Thoracic and Cardiovascular Surgery*, **93**, 309–311

Krukenkamp, I.B., Silverman, N.A. and Levitsky, S. (1987) The effect of cardioplegic oxygenation on the correlation between the linearized Frank-Starling relationship and myocardial energetics in the ejecting postischemic heart. *Circulation*, **76** (suppl V), V-122–V-128

Krukenkamp, I., Silverman, N., Sorlie, D., *et al.* (1986) Myocardial energetics after thermally graded hyperkalemic crystalloid cardioplegic arrest. *Journal of Thoracic and Cardiovascular Surgery*, **92**, 56–62

Krukenkamp, I.B., Silverman, N.A., Sorlie, D., *et al.* (1986) Temperature-specific effect of adjuvant diltiazem therapy on myocardial energetics following potassium cardioplegic arrest. *Annals of Thoracic Surgery*, **42**, 675–680

Kusuoka, H., Porterfield, J.K., Weiseman, H.F., *et al.* (1987) Pathophysiology and pathogenesis of stunned myocardium: depressed Ca^{++} activation of contraction as a consequence of reperfusion-induced cellular calcium overload in ferret hearts. *Journal of Clinical Investigation*, **79**, 950–961

Landymore, R.W. and Kinley, C.E. (1984a) The effect of viscosity on poststenotic distribution of cardioplegic solutions (letter). *Journal of Thoracic and Cardiovascular Surgery*, **87**, 944–946

Landymore, R.W. and Kinley, C.E. (1984b) Effects of crystalloid and blood cardioplegic solutions on myocardial cooling during myocardial revascularization. *Canadian Journal of Surgery*, **27**, 257–259

Landymore, R.W. and Myers, G. (1988) Evaluation of delivery systems for oxygenated cardioplegia. *Canadian Journal of Surgery*, **31**, 346–348

Landymore, R.W., Marble, A.E., Trillo, A., *et al.* (1987) Prevention of myocardial electrical activity during ischemic arrest with verapamil cardioplegia. *Annals of Thoracic Surgery*, **43**, 534–538

Landymore, R.W., Marble, A.E., Trillo, A., *et al.* (1986) Effect of small-amplitude electrical activity on myocardial preservation in the cold potassium-arrested heart. *Journal of Thoracic and Cardiovascular Surgery*, **91**, 684–689

Langer, G.A., Nudd, L.M. and Ricchiuti, N.V. (1976) The effect of sodium deficient perfusion on calcium exchange in cardiac tissue culture. *Journal of Molecular and Cellular Cardiology*, **8**, 321–328

LaRaia, P.J., Bing, O.H.L., Gasch, W.H., *et al.* (1981) Myocardial protection by coronary washout during global ischemic cardiac arrest. *Journal of Surgical Research*, **31**, 179–187

Lazar, H.L. (1988) Coronary sinus interventions during cardiac surgery. *Annals of Thoracic Surgery*, **46**, 475–482

Lazar, H.L. and Rivers, S. (1989) Importance of topical hypothermia during heterogeneous distribution of cardioplegic solution. *Journal of Thoracic and Cardiovascular Surgery*, **98**, 251–257

Lazar, H.L., Buckberg, G.D., Manganaro, A.J. *et al.* (1979) Reversal of ischemic damage with secondary blood cardioplegia. *Journal of Thoracic and Cardiovascular Surgery*, **78**, 688–697

Lazar, H.L., Khoury, T. and Rivers, S. (1988) Improved distribution of cardioplegia with pressure-controlled intermittent coronary sinus occlusion. *Annals of Thoracic Surgery*, **46**, 202–207

Lazar, H.L., Rajaii, A. and Roberts, A.J. (1988) Reversal of reperfusion injury after ischemic arrest with pressure-controlled intermittent coronary sinus occlusion. *Journal of Thoracic and Cardiovascular Surgery*, **95**, 637–642

Leaf, A. (1973) Cell swelling, a factor in ischemic tissue injury. *Circulation*, **48**, 455–458

Ledingham, S.J.M. (1988) Intraoperative protection of the paediatric myocardium. *Current Opinion in Cardiology*, **3**, 741–747

Ledingham, S.J., Braimbridge, M.V. and Hearse, D.J. (1987) The St. Thomas' Hospital cardioplegic solution. A comparison of the efficacy of two formulations. *Journal of Thoracic and Cardiovascular Surgery*, **93**, 240–246

Ledingham, S.J., Braimbridge, M.V. and Hearse, D.J. (1988) Improved myocardial protection by oxygenation of St. Thomas' Hospital cardioplegic solutions. Studies in the rat. *Journal of Thoracic and Cardiovascular Surgery*, **95**, 103–111

Ledingham, S.J.M., Katayama, O. and Yacoub, M. (1990) Adenosine enhances the efficacy of hypothermic cardioplegic arrest. *British Heart Journal*, **64**, 89 (abstract)

Ledingham, S., Katayama, O., Lachno, D., *et al.* (1990a) Beneficial effect of adenosine during reperfusion following prolonged cardioplegic arrest. *Cardiovascular Research*, **24**, 247–253

Ledingham, S.J.M., Katayama, O., Lachno, D.R. and Yacoub, M. (1990b) Prolonged cardiac preservation: evaluation of the University of Wisconsin preservation solution by comparison with the St. Thomas' Hospital cardioplegic solutions in the rat. *Circulation*, **82** (suppl IV), IV-351–IV-358

Lee, A.G. (1976) Model for action of local anaesthetics. *Nature*, **262**, 545–548

Lee, R.B., Stewart, J.R., Merrill, W.H., *et al.* (1989) Pharmacokinetics of superoxide dismutase during hypothermic cardiopulmonary bypass. *Circulation*, **80**, (suppl III), III-25–III-29

Levinsky, L., Schimert, G., Lajos, T.Z., *et al.* (1979) The use of steroids as a potentiator of hypothermic myocardial preservation in man. *Journal of Surgical Research*, **26**, 629–651

Levitsky, S. (1987) Is hypothermic fibrillatory arrest a rational alternative to cardioplegic arrest? *Annals of Thoracic Surgery*, **43**, 127–128

Levitsky, S. (1988) Another look at reperfusion asystole. *Annals of Thoracic Surgery*, **45**, 471–472

Lewandowski, E.D., Devous, M.D. and Nunnally, R.L. (1987) High-energy phosphates and function in isolated, working rabbit heart. *American Journal of Physiology*, **253**, H1215–H1223

Lillehei, C.W., Dewall, R.A., Gott, V.A.L. and Varco, R.L. (1956) The direct-vision correction of calcific aortic stenosis by means of pump-oxygenator and retrograde coronary sinus perfusion. *Diseases of the Chest*, **30**, 123–127

Lindal, S., Srlie, D. and Jrgensen, L. (1988) Endothelial cells of the cardiac microvasculature during and after cold cardioplegic ischaemia. Comparison of endothelial and myocyte damage. *Scandinavian Journal of Thoracic and Cardiovascular Surgery*, **22**, 257–265

Litt, M.R., Jeremy, R.W., Weisman, H.F., *et al.* (1989) Neutrophil depletion limited to reperfusion reduces myocardial infarct size after 90 minutes of ischemia. Evidence for neutrophil-mediated reperfusion injury. *Circulation*, **80**, 1816–1827

Little, A.G., Lin, C., Wernly, J.A., *et al.* (1984) Use of the pulmonary artery for left ventricular venting during cardiac operations. *Journal of Thoracic and Cardiovascular Surgery*, **87**, 532–538

Lolley, D.M., Myers, W.O., Ray, J.F., *et al.* (1985) Clinical experience with preoperative myocardial nutrition management. *Journal of Cardiovascular Surgery*, **26**, 236–243

Lolley, D.M., Ray, J.F., Myers, W.O., *et al.* (1979) Importance of preoperative myocardial glycogen levels in human cardiac preservation. *Journal of Thoracic and Cardiovascular Surgery*, **78**, 678–687

Lowe, J.E., Kleinman, L.H., Reimer, K.A., *et al.* (1977) Effects of cardioplegia produced by calcium flux inhibition. *Surgical Forum*, **28**, 279–280

Lucchesi, B.R., Werns, S.W. and Fantone, J.C. (1989) The role of the neutrophil and free radicals in ischemic myocardial injury. *Journal of Molecular and Cellular Cardiology*, **21**, 1241–1251

Lust, R.M., Beggerly, C.E., Morrison, R.F., *et al.* (1988)

Improved protection of chronically inflow-limited myocardium with retrograde coronary sinus cardioplegia. *Circulation*, **78** (suppl III), III-217–III-223

McConnell, D.H., Brazier, J.R., Cooper, N. and Buckberg, G.D. (1977) Studies of the effects of hypothermia on regional myocardial blood flow and metabolism during cardiopulmonary bypass. II. Ischemia during moderate hypothermia in continually perfused beating hearts. *Journal of Thoracic and Cardiovascular Surgery*, **73**, 95–101

McConnell, D.H., White, F., Nelson, R.L., *et al.* (1975) The importance of alkalosis in maintenance of 'ideal' blood pH during hypothermia. *Surgical Forum*, **26**, 263

McCord, J.M. (1985) Oxygen-derived free radicals in post ischemic tissue injury. *New England Journal of Medicine*, **312**, 159–163

MacDonald, J.L. (1981) Is crystalloid cardioplegia a source of particulate debris? *American Academy of Cardiovascular Perfusion Proceedings*, **2**, 20–24

McElroy, D.D., Walker, W.E. and Taegtmeyer, H. (1989) Glycogen loading improves left ventricular function of the rabbit heart after hypothermic ischemic arrest. *Journal of Applied Cardiology*, **4**, 455–465

Magee, P.G., Flaherty, J.T., Bixler, T.J., *et al.* (1979) Comparison of myocardial protection with nifedipine and potassium. *Circulation*, **60**, 151–157

Magilligan, D.J., Vij, D., Peper, W., *et al.* (1985) Failure of standard cardioplegic techniques to protect the conducting system. *Annals of Thoracic Surgery*, **39**, 403–408

Magovern, G.J., Bolling, S.F., Casale, A.S., *et al.* (1984) The mechanism of mannitol in reducing ischemic injury: hyperosmolarity or hydroxyl scavenger? *Circulation*, **70** (suppl I), I-91–I-95

Magovern, G.J., Dixon, C.M. and Burkholder, J.A. (1981) Improved myocardial protection with nifedipine and potassium-based cardioplegia. *Journal of Thoracic and Cardiovascular Surgery*, **82**, 239–244

Magovern, G.J., Flaherty, J.T., Gott, V.L., *et al.* (1982) Failure of blood cardioplegia to protect myocardium at lower temperatures. *Circulation*, **66**, I60–I67

Magovern, J.A., Pae, W.E. and Waldhausen, J.A. (1988) Protection of the immature myocardium. An experimental evaluation of topical cooling, single-dose, and multiple-dose administration of St. Thomas' Hospital cardioplegic solution. *Journal of Thoracic and Cardiovascular Surgery*, **96**, 408–413

Manfredi, J.P. and Holmes, E.W. (1985) Purine salvage pathways in myocardium. *Annual Review of Physiology*, **47**, 691–705

Mask, W.K., Abd-Elfattah, A.S., Jessen, M., *et al.* (1989) Embryonic versus adult myocardium: adenine nucleotide degradation during ischemia. *Annals of Thoracic Surgery*, **48**, 109–112

Masuda, M., Yonenaga, K., Shiki, K., *et al.* (1986) Myocardial protection in coronary occlusion by retrograde cardioplegic perfusion via the coronary sinus in dogs. Preservation of high-energy phosphates and regional function. *Journal of Thoracic and Cardiovascular Surgery*, **92**, 255–263

Matsuda, H., Maeda, S., Hirose, H., *et al.* (1986) Optimum dose of cold potassium cardioplegia for patients with chronic aortic valve disease: determination by left ventricular mass. *Annals of Thoracic Surgery*, **41**, 22–26

Mattiazzi, A.R. and Nilssson, E. (1976) The influence of temperature on the time course of the mechanical activity in rabbit papillary muscle. *Acta Physiologica Scandinavica*, **97**, 310–318

Mattila, S., Harjula, A., Mattila, I., Myllarniemi, H., *et al.* (1987) Coronary endothelium and cardioplegic solutions. *Annales Chirugiae et Gynaecologiae*, **76**, 46–50

Mayer, S.E. (1974) Effect of catecholamines on cardiac metabolism. *Circulation Research*, **34/35** (suppl III), III-129–III-137

Melrose, D.G., Dreyer, B., Bentall, H.H. and Baker, J.B.E. (1955) Elective cardiac arrest. *Lancet*, **ii**, 21–22

Menasche, P. and Piwnica, A. (1987) Retrograde cardioplegia through the coronary sinus. *Annals of Thoracic Surgery*, **44**, 214–216

Menasche, P. and Piwnica, A. (1989) Free radicals and myocardial protection: a surgical viewpoint. *Annals of Thoracic Surgery*, **47**, 939–945

Menasche, P., Dunica, S., Kural, S., *et al.* (1984a) An asanguineous reperfusion solution. An effective adjunct to cardioplegic protection in high-risk valve operations. *Journal of Thoracic and Cardiovascular Surgery*, **88**, 278–286

Menasche, P., Grousset, C., De Boccard, G. and Piwnica, A. (1984b) Protective effect of an asanguineous reperfusion solution on myocardial performance following cardioplegic arrest. *Annals of Thoracic Surgery*, **37**, 222–228

Menasche, P., Grousset, C., Gauduel, Y., *et al.* (1986a) Enhancement of cardioplegic protection with the free-radical scavenger peroxidase. *Circulation*, **74** (suppl III), III-138–III-144

Menasche, P., Grousset, C., Gauduel, Y., *et al.* (1987a) Prevention of hydroxyl radical formation: a critical concept for improving cardioplegia. Protective effects of deferoxamine. *Circulation*, **76** (suppl V), V-180–V-185

Menasche, P., Grousset, C., Gauduel, Y. and Piwnica, A. (1986b) A comparative study of free radical scavengers in cardioplegic solutions. Improved protection with peroxidase. *Journal of Thoracic and Cardiovascular Surgery*, **92**, 264–271

Menasche, P., Grousset, C., Mouas, C., *et al.* (1988a) Enhancement of cardioplegic protection with a lecithin-based perfluoroadamantane emulsion. *Biomaterials, Artificial Cells, and Artificial Organs*, **16**, 607–616

Menasche, P., Kucharski, K., Mundler, O., *et al.* (1989) Adequate preservation of right ventricular function after coronary sinus cardioplegia. A clinical study. *Circulation*, **80** (suppl III), III-19–III-24

Menasche, P., Kural, S., Fauchet, M., *et al.* (1982) Retrograde coronary sinus perfusion: a safe alternative for ensuring cardioplegic delivery in aortic valve surgery. *Annals of Thoracic Surgery*, **34**, 647–658

Menasche, P., Maisonblanche, P., Bousseau, D., *et al.*

(1987b) Decreased incidence of supraventricular arrhythmias achieved by selective atrial cooling during aortic valve replacement. *European Journal of Cardiothoracic Surgery*, **1**, 33–36

Menasche, P., Pasquier, C., Bellucci, S., *et al.* (1988a) Deferoxamine reduces neutrophil-mediated free radical production during cardiopulmonary bypass in man. *Journal of Thoracic and Cardiovascular Surgery*, **96**, 582–589

Menasche, P., Subayi, J.B. and Piwnica, A. (1990) Retrograde coronary sinus cardioplegia for aortic valve operations: a clinical report on 500 patients. *Annals of Thoracic Surgery*, **49**, 556–564

Merchant, F.J., Feinberg, H. and Levitsky, S. (1974) Sequential analysis of altered myocardial metabolism and contractility induced by normothermic arrest and reperfusion. *Journal of Surgical Research*, **16**, 153–158

Merin, G. and Fishman, N.H. (1986) Preparation of oxygenated cold crystalloid cardioplegic solution. *Annals of Thoracic Surgery*, **41**, 679–679

Metzdorff, M.T., Grunkemeier, G.L. and Starr, A. (1986) Effect of initial reperfusion temperature on myocardial preservation. *Journal of Thoracic and Cardiovascular Surgery*, **91**, 545–550

Mickle, D.A., Del Nido, P.J., Wilson, G.J., *et al.* (1986) Exogenous substrate preference of the post-ischaemic myocardium. *Cardiovascular Research*, **20**, 256–263

Miller, D.W., Binford, J.M. and Hessel, E.A. (1982) Results of a survery of the professional activities of 811 cardiopulmonary perfusionists. *Journal of Thoracic and Cardiovascular Surgery*, **83**, 385–389

Mochizuki, S. and Neely, J.R. (1980) Energy metabolism during reperfusion following ischemia. *Journal de Physiologie (Paris)*, **76**, 805–812

Mohl, W. (1987) Pressure-controlled intermittent coronary sinus occlusion in cardiac surgery. In *Myocardial Protection in Cardiac Surgery* (ed. A.J. Roberts), Marcel Dekker Inc., New York, pp. 495–503

Mohl, W., Glogar, D., Mayr, H., *et al.* (1984) Reduction of infarct size by pressure controlled intermittent coronary sinus occlusion. *American Journal of Cardiology*, **53**, 923

Molina, J.E., Galliani, C.A., Einzig, S., *et al.* (1989) Physical and mechanical effects of cardioplegic injection on flow distribution and myocardial damage in hearts with normal coronary arterties. *Journal of Thoracic and Cardiovascular Surgery*, **97**, 870–877

Mori, F., Ivey, T.D., Tabayashi, K., *et al.* (1986) Regional myocardial protection by retrograde coronary sinus infusion of cardioplegic solution. *Circulation*, **74** (suppl III), III-116–III-124

Moulton, A.L. and Robinson, L.A. (1990) Cardiac function with glucose-insulin-potassium solution. *Annals of Thoracic Surgery*, **49**, 1025–1026 (letter)

Mullen, J.C., Christakis, G.T., Weisel, R.D., *et al.* (1986) Late postoperative ventricular function after blood and crystalloid cardioplegia. *Circulation*, **74** (suppl III), III-89–III-98

Mullen, J.C., Fremes, S.E., Weisel, R.D., *et al.* (1987a) Right ventricular function: a comparison between blood and crystalloid cardioplegia. *Annals of Thoracic Surgery*, **43**, 17–24

Mullen, J.C., Khan, N., Weisel, R.D., *et al.* (1987b) Atrial activity during cardioplegia and postoperative arrhythmias. *Journal of Thoracic and Cardiovascular Surgery*, **94**, 558–565

Muxfeldt, M. and Schaper, W. (1987) The activity of xanthine oxidase in heart and liver of rats, guinea pigs, pigs, rabbits and human beings. *Circulation*, **76** (suppl IV), IV-98 (abstract)

Myers, C.L., Weiss, S.J., Kirsh, M.M., *et al.* (1986a) Effects of supplementing hypothermic crystalloid cardioplegic solution with catalase, superoxide dismutase, allopurinol, or deferozamine on functional recovery of globally ischemic and reperfused isolated hearts. *Journal of Thoracic and Cardiovascular Surgery*, **91**, 281–289

Myers, M.L., Bolli, R., Lekich, R.F., *et al.* (1986b) N-2-mercaptopropionyglycine improves recovery of myocardial function following reversible regional ischemia. *Journal of the American College of Cardiology*, **8**, 1161–1168

Nayler, W.G., Ferrari, R. and Williams, A. (1980) Protective effect of pretreatment with verapamil, nifedipine and propranolol on mitochondrial function in the ischemic and reperfused myocardium. *American Journal of Cardiology*, **46**, 242

Nayler, W.G., Yepez, C.E., Fassold, E. and Ferrari, R. (1978) Prolonged protective effect of propranolol on hypoxic heart muscle. *American Journal of Cardiology*, **42**, 217–225

Novick, R.J., Stefaniszyn, H.J., Michel, R.P., *et al.* (1985) Protection of the hypertrophied pig myocardium. A comparison of crystalloid, blood, and Fluosol-DA cardioplegia during prolonged aortic clamping. *Journal of Thoracic and Cardiovascular Surgery*, **89**, 547–566

Novitsky, D., Cooper, D.K.C., Barton, C.I., *et al.* (1989) Triiodothyronine as an inotropic agent after open heart surgery. *Journal of Thoracic and Cardiovascular Surgery*, **98**, 972–978

Novitsky, D., Cooper, D.K.C., Morrell, D. and Isaacs, S. (1988a) Change from aerobic to anaerobic metabolism after brain death, and reversal following triiodothyronine therapy. *Transplantation*, **45**, 32–36

Novitsky, D., Human, P.A. and Cooper, D.K. (1988b) Inotropic effect of triiodothyronine following myocardial ischemia and cardiopulmonary bypass: an experimental study in pigs. *Annals of Thoracic Surgery*, **45**, 50–55

Oguma, F., Imai, S. and Eguchi, S. (1986) Role played by oxygen in myocardial protection with crystalloid cardioplegic solution. *Annals of Thoracic Surgery*, **42**, 172–179

Okamoto, F., Allen, B.S., Buckberg, G.D., *et al.* (1986a) Reperfusion conditions: importance of ensuring gentle versus sudden reperfusion during relief of coronary occlusion. *Journal of Thoracic and Cardiovascular Surgery*, **92**, 613–620

Okamoto, F., Allen, B.S., Buckberg, G.D., *et al.* (1986b) Reperfusate composition: supplemental role of intravenous and intracoronary coenzyme Q_{10} in avoiding reperfusion damage. *Journal of Thoracic and Cardiovascular Surgery*, **92**, 573–582

Okamoto, F., Allen, B.S., Buckberg, G.D., *et al.* (1986c) Reperfusate composition: interaction of marked hyperglycemia and marked hyperosmolarity in allowing immediate contractile recovery after four hours of regional ischemia. *Journal of Thoracic and Cardiovascular Surgery*, **92**, 583–593

Olafsson, B., Forman, M.B., Puett, D.W., Pou, A., *et al.* (1987) Reduction of reperfusion injury in the canine preparation by intracoronary adenosine: importance of the endothelium and the no-reflow phenomenon. *Circulation*, **76**, 1135–1145

Oldfield, G., Commerford, P.J. and Opie, L.H. (1986) Effects of preoperative glucose-insulin-potassium on myocardial glycogen levels and on complications of mitral valve replacement. *Journal of Thoracic and Cardiovascular Surgery*, **91**, 874–878

Olinger, G.N. (1987) Intermittent ischemic arrest. In *Myocardial Protection in Cardiac Surgery*, (ed A.J. Roberts), Marcel Dekker Inc., New York, pp. 207–219

Olinger, G.N. and Boncheck, L.I. (1978) Ventricular venting during coronary revascularization: assessment of benefit by intraoperative ventricular function curves. *Annals of Thoracic Surgery*, **26**, 525–534

Olinger, G.N., Boncheck, L.I. and Geiss, D.M. (1981) Noncoronary collateral distribution in coronary artery disease. *Annals of Thoracic Surgery*, **32**, 554–557

Olinger, G.N., Maloney, J.V. and Mulder, D.G. (1985) Coronary revascularization in 'high' versus 'low-risk' patients. *Annals of Surgery*, **182**, 293–301

Opie, L.H. (1989) Reperfusion injury and its pharmacological modification. *Circulation*, **80**, 1049–1062

Otani, H., Engleman, R.M., Rousou, J.A., *et al.* (1987) Mechanism of myocardial reperfusion injury in neonates. *Circulation*, **76** (suppl V), V-161–V-167

Otani, H., Umemoto, M., Kagawa, K., *et al.* (1986) Protection against oxygen-induced reperfusion injury of the isolated canine heart by superoxide dismutase and catalase. *Journal of Surgical Research*, **41**, 126–133

Palmer, R.M.J., Ferrige, A.G. and Moncada, S. (1987) Nitric oxide release accounts for the biological activity of endothelium-derived relaxing factor. *Nature*, **327**, 524–526

Partington, M.T., Acar, C., Buckberg, G.D., *et al.* (1989a) Studies of retrograde cardioplegia. I. Capillary blood flow distribution to myocardium supplied by open and occluded arteries. *Journal of Thoracic and Cardiovascular Surgery*, **97**, 605–612

Partington, M.T., Acar, C., Buckberg, G.D. and Julia, P.L. (1989b) Studies of retrograde cardioplegia. II. Advantages of antegrade/retrograde cardioplegia to optimize distribution in jeopardized myocardium. *Journal of Thoracic and Cardiovascular Surgery*, **97**, 613–622

Peng, C.F., Murphy, M.L., Colwell, K. and Straub, K.D. (1989) Controlled versus hyperemic flow during reperfusion of jeopardized ischemic myocardium. *American Heart Journal*, **117**, 515–522

Pennington, D.G., Dincer, B., Bashiti, H., *et al.* (1982) Coronary artery stenosis following aortic valve replacement and intermittent intracoronary cardioplegia. *Annals of Thoracic Surgery*, **33**, 576–584

Pepper, J.R., Lockey, E., Cankovic-Darracott, S. (1982) Cardioplegia versus intermittent ischaemic arrest in coronary bypass surgery. *Thorax*, **37**, 887–892

Pieper, G.M., Todd, G.L., Wu, S.T., *et al.* (1980) Attenuation of myocardial acidosis by propranolol during ischaemic arrest and reperfusion. Evidence with 31-P nuclear magnetic resonance. *Cardiovascular Research*, **14**, 646

Poirier, N.L., Belliveau, P.J. and Wynands, J.E. (1980) Effect of cardioplegic solution and of propranolol on perioperative infarction after cardiac surgery for unstable angina. *Canadian Journal of Surgery*, **23**, 387

Prasad, K., Bharadwaj, B. and Card, R.T. (1988) Effects of blood and crystalloid cardioplegia on cardiac function at organ and cellular levels during hypothermic cardiac arrest. *Angiology*, **39**, 23–33

Pridjian, A.K., Levitsky, S., Krukenkamp, I., *et al.* (1988) developmental changes in reperfusion injury. Comparison of intracellular ion accumulation in ischemic and cardioplegic arrest. *Journal of Thoracic and Cardiovascular Surgery*, **96**, 577–581

Przyklenk, K. and Kloner, R.A. (1986) Superoxide dismutase plus catalase improve contractile function in the canine model of the 'stunned' myocardium. *Circulation Research*, **58**, 148–156

Przyklenk, K., Ghafari, G.B., Eitzman, D.T. and Kloner, R.A. (1989) Nifedipine administered after reperfusion ablates systolic contractile dysfunction of postischemic 'stunned' myocardium. *Journal of the American College of Cardiology*, **13**, 1176–1183

Rahn, H., Reeves, R.B. and Howell, B.J. (1975) Hydrogen ion regulation, temperature and evolution. *American Review of Respiratory Disease*, **112**, 165–172

Ratajczyk-Pakalska, E. (1986) Thebesian veins in the human hearts with atherosclerotic lesions in the coronary arteries. In *Clinics of CSI* (eds W. Mohl, D. Faxon and E. Wolner), Springer-Verlag, New York, pp. 141–145

Ratajczyk-Pakalska, E. and Kolff, W.J. (1984) Anatomical basis for the coronary venous outflow. In *The Coronary Sinus* (eds W. Mohl, E. Wolner and D. Glogar), Springer-Verlag, New York, pp. 40–46

Rau, E.E., Shine, K.I., Gervais, A., *et al.* (1979) Enhanced mechanical recovery of anoxic and ischemic myocardium by amino acid perfusion. *American Journal of Physiology*, **236**, H873–H879

Rebeyka, I.M., Wilson, G.J., Axford-Gatley, R.A., *et al.* (1989) Asanguineous reperfusion in a canine model of cardiopulmonary bypass and controlled postischemic work. *Annals of Thoracic Surgery*, **48**, 397–403

Reibel, D.K. and Rovetto, M.J. (1978) Myocardial ATP synthesis and mechanical function following oxygen deficiency. *American Journal of Physiology*, **234**, H620–H624

Reimer, K.A., Murry, C.E. and Richard, V.J. (1989) The role of neutrophils and free radicals in the ischemic-reperfused heart: why the confusion and controversy. *Journal of Molecular and Cellular Cardiology*, **21**, 1225–1239

Reuter, H. and Seitz, N. (1968) The dependence of calcium efflux from cardiac muscle on temperature and external ion composition. *Journal of Physiology*, **195**, 451–470

Reynolds, T.R., Geffin, G.A., Titus, J.S., *et al.* (1989) Myocardial preservation related to magnesium content of hyperkalemic cardioplegic solutions at 8°C. *Annals of Thoracic Surgery*, **47**, 907–913

Ricciutti, M.A. (1972) Lysosomes and myocardial cellular injury. *American Journal of Cardiology*, **30**, 498–502

Rich, T. and Brady, A.J. (1974) Potassium contraction and utilization of high-energy phosphates in rabbit heart. *American Journal of Physiology*, **226**, 105–113

Rich, T. and Langer, G.A. (1982) Calcium depletion in rabbit myocardium. Calcium paradox protection by hypothermia and cation substitutions. *Circulation Research*, **51**, 131–141

Robb-Nicholson, C., Currie, W.D. and Wechsler, A.S. (1978) Effects of verapamil on myocardial tolerance to ischemic cardiac arrest. *Circulation*, **58** (suppl I), 119-124

Roberts, A.J., Sanders, J.H., Moran, J.M., *et al.* (1981) Nonrandomized matched pair analysis of intermittent ischemic arrest versus potassium crystalloid cardioplegia during myocardial revascularization. *Annals of Thoracic Surgery*, **31**, 502–511

Roberts, A.J., Woodhall, D.D., Knauf, D.G. and Alexander, J.A. (1985) Coronary artery bypass graft surgery: clinical comparison of cold blood potassium cardioplegia, warm cardioplegic induction, and secondary cardioplegia. *Annals of Thoracic Surgery*, **40**, 483–487

Robertson, J.M., Buckberg, G.D., Vinten-Johansen, J. and Leaf, J.D. (1983) Comparison of distribution beyond coronary stenoses of blood and asanguineous cardioplegic solutions. *Journal of Thoracic and Cardiovascular Surgery*, **86**, 80–86

Robertson, J.M., Vinten-Johansen, J., Buckberg, G.D., *et al.* (1984) Safety of prolonged aortic clamping with blood cardioplegia. I. Glutamate enrichment in normal hearts. *Journal of Thoracic and Cardiovascular Surgery*, **88**, 395–401

Robinson, L.A., Braimbridge, M.V. and Hearse, D.J. (1984a) Comparison of the protective properties of four clinical crystalloid cardioplegic solutions in the rat heart. *Annals of Thoracic Surgery*, **38**, 268–274

Robinson, L.A., Braimbridge, M.V. and Hearse, D.J. (1984b) The potential hazard of particulate contamination of cardioplegic solutions. *Journal of Thoracic and Cardiovascular Surgery*, **87**, 48–58

Robinson, L.A., Braimbridge, M.V. and Hearse, D.J. (1984c) Creatine phosphate: an additive myocardial protective and antiarrhythmic agent in cardioplegia. *Journal of Thoracic and Cardiovascular Surgery*, **87**, 190–200

Robinson, L.A., Braimbridge, M.V. and Hearse, D.J. (1987) Enhanced myocardial protection with high-energy phosphates in St. Thomas' Hospital cardioplegic solution. Synergism of adenosine triphosphate and creatine phosphate. *Journal of Thoracic and Cardiovascular Surgery*, **93**, 415–427

Robuschi, G., Medici, D. and Fesani, F. (1986) Cardiopulmonary bypass: a low T4 and T3 syndrome with blunted thyrotropin (TSH) response to thyrotropin-releasing hormone (TRH). *Hormone Research*, **23**, 151–158

Roe, B.B., Hutchinson, J.C., Fishman, N.H., *et al.* (1977) Myocardial protection with cold, ischemic, potassium-induced cardioplegia. *Journal of Thoracic and Cardiovascular Surgery*, **73**, 366–374

Romaschin, A.D., Rebeyka, I., Wilson, G.J. and Mickle, D.A.G. (1987) Conjugated dienes in ischemic and reperfused myocardium: an in vivo chemical signature of oxygen free radical mediated injury. *Journal of Molecular and Cellular Cardiology*, **19**, 239–302

Rose, D.M., Catinella, F.P. and Cunningham, J.N. (1987) Experimental, clinical, and technical considerations for the use of blood cardioplegia. In *Myocardial Protection in Cardiac Surgery* (ed. A.J. Roberts), Marcel Dekker Inc., New York, pp. 155–179

Rosenfeldt, F.L. (1982) The relationship between myocardial temperature and recovery after experimental cardioplegic arrest. *Journal of Thoracic and Cardiovascular Surgery*, **84**, 656–666

Rosenfeldt, F.L. (1987) Myocardial preservation 1987: what is the state of the art. *Australian and New Zealand Journal of Surgery*, **57**, 349–353

Rosenfeldt, F.L. and Watson, D.A. (1979) Interference with local myocardial cooling by heat gain during aortic cross-clamping. *Annals of Thoracic Surgery*, **27**, 13–16

Rosenfeldt, F.L., Hearse, D.J., Cankovic-Darracott, S. and Braimbridge, M.V. (1980) The additive protective effects of hypothermia and chemical cardioplegia during ischemic cardiac arrest in the dog. *Journal of Thoracic and Cardiovascular Surgery*, **79**, 29–38

Rosenfeldt, F.L., Rabinov, M., Little, P. and Campbell, G. (1986) The relationship between coronary pressure during reperfusion and myocardial recovery after hypothermic cardioplegia. *Journal of Thoracic and Cardiovascular Surgery*, **92**, 414–424

Rosenkranz, E.R. and Buckberg, G.D. (1983) Myocardial protection during surgical coronary reperfusion. *Journal of the American College of Cardiology*, **1**, 1235–1246

Rosenkranz, E.R., Buckberg, G.D., Laks, H. and Mulder, D.G. (1983) Warm induction of cardioplegia with glutamate-enriched blood in coronary patients with cardiogenic shock who are dependent on inotropic drugs and intra-aortic balloon support. *Journal of Thoracic and Cardiovascular Surgery*, **86**, 507–518

Rosenkranz, E.R., Okamoto, F., Buckberg, G.D., *et al.* (1986a) Safety of prolonged aortic clamping with blood cardioplegia. III. Aspartate enrichment of glutamate-blood cardioplegia in energy-depleted hearts after ischemic and reperfusion injury. *Journal of Thoracic and Cardiovascular Surgery*, **91**, 428–435

Rosenkranz, E.R., Okamoto, F., Buckberg, G.D., *et al.* (1986b) Biochemical studies: failure of tissue adenosine triphosphate levels to predict recovery of contractile function after controlled reperfusion. *Journal of Thoracic and Cardiovascular Surgery*, **92**, 488-501

Rosenkranz, E.R., Okamoto, F., Buckberg, G.D., *et al.* (1984) Safety of prolonged aortic clamping with blood cardioplegia. II. Glutamate enrichment in energy-depleted hearts. *Journal of Thoracic and Cardiovascular Surgery*, **88**, 402–410

Rosenkranz, E.R., Vinten-Johansen, J., Buckberg, G.D., *et al.* (1982) Benefits of normothermic induction of blood cardioplegia in energy-depleted hearts, with maintenance of arrest by multidose cold blood cardioplegic infusions. *Journal of Thoracic and Cardiovascular Surgery*, **84**, 667–677

Rousou, J.H., Dobbs, W.A., Meeran, M.K. and Engleman, R.M. (1982) The temperature dependence of recovery of metabolic function following hypothermic potassium cardioplegic arrest. *Journal of Thoracic and Cardiovascular Surgery*, **83**, 117–121

Rousou, J.H., Dobbs, W.A. and Engleman, R.M. (1982a) Fluosol cardioplegia – a method of optimizing aerobic metabolism. *Circulation,* **66** (Suppl. I), I55–I59

Rousou, J.A., Engleman, R.M., Anisimowicz, L., *et al.* (1986) Metabolic enhancement of myocardial preservation during cardioplegic arrest. *Journal of Thoracic and Cardiovascular Surgery*, **91**, 270–276

Rousou, J.A., Engleman, R.M., Breyer, R.H., *et al.* (1988) The effect of temperature and hematocrit level of oxygenated cardioplegic solutions on myocardial preservation. *Journal of Thoracic and Cardiovascular Surgery*, **95**, 625–630

Rousou, J.H., Engleman, R.M., Dobbs, W.A. and Lemeshow, S. (1981) The optimal potassium concentration in cardioplegic solutions. *Annals of Thoracic Surgery*, **32**, 75–79

Rousou, J.A., Parker, T., Engleman, R.M. and Breyer, R.H. (1985) Phrenic nerve paresis associated with the use of iced slush and the cooling jacket for topical hypothermia. *Journal of Thoracic and Cardiovascular Surgery*, **89**, 921–925

Rovetto, M.J., Lamberton, W.F. and Neely, J.R. (1975) Mechanisms of glycolytic inhibition in ischemic rat hearts. *Circulation Research*, **37**, 742–751

Rovetto, M.J., Whitmer, J.T. and Neely, J.R. (1973) Comparison of the effects of anoxia and whole heart ischemia on carbohydrate utilization in isolated working rat hearts. *Circulation Research*, **32**, 699–711

Royston, D., Fleming, J.S. and Desai, J.B. (1986) Increased production of lipid peroxidation products associated with cardiac operations. Evidence for free radical generation. *Journal of Thoracic and Cardiovascular Surgery*, **91**, 759–756

Rubanyi, G.M. and Vanhoutte, P.M. (1985) Hypoxia releases a vasoconstrictor substance from the canine vascular endothelium. *Journal of Physiology*, **364**, 45–56

Sakai, A., Miya, J., Sohara, Y., *et al.* (1988) Role of red blood cells in the coronary microcirculation during cold blood cardioplegia. *Cardiovascular Research*, **22**, 62–66

Saldanha, C. and Hearse, D.J. (1989) Coronary vascular responsiveness to 5-hydroxytryptamine before and after infusion of hyperkalemic crystalloid cardioplegic solution in the rat heart. *Journal of Thoracic and Cardiovascular Surgery*, **98**, 783–787

Salter, D.R., Goldstein, J.P., Abd-Elfattah, A., *et al.* (1987) Ventricular function after atrial cardioplegia. *Circulation*, **76** (suppl V), V-129–V-140

Sawa, Y., Matsuda, H., Shimazaki, Y., *et al.* (1989) Comparison of single dose versus multiple dose crystalloid cardioplegia in neonate. Experimental study with neonatal rabbits from birth to 2 days of age. *Journal of Thoracic and Cardiovascular Surgery*, **97**, 229–234

Saydjari, R., Asimakis, G. and Conti, V.R. (1987) Effect of increasing volume of cardioplegic solution on postischemic myocardial recovery. *Journal of Thoracic and Cardiovascular Surgery*, **94**, 234–240

Schaper, J., Scheld, H.H., Schmidt, U. and Hehrlein, F. (1986) Ultrastructural study comparing the efficacy of five different methods of intraoperative myocardial protection in the human heart. *Journal of Thoracic and Cardiovascular Surgery*, **92**, 47–55

Scheuer, J. and Stezoski, S.W. (1970) Protective role of increased myocardial glycogen stores in cardiac anoxia in the rat. *Circulation Research*, **27**, 835–849

Schnabel, P.A., Gebhard, M.M., Pomykaj, T., *et al.* (1987) Myocardial protection: left ventricular ultrastructure after different forms of cardiac arrest. *Thoracic and Cardiovascular Surgeon*, **35**, 148–156

Schneider, B., Conti, V.R. and Kurusz, M. (1983) A technique for cardioplegic infusion and left heart venting during coronary artery bypass grafting. *Annals of Thoracic Surgery*, **36**, 105–107

Schwaiger, M., Schelbert, H.R., Ellison, D., *et al.* (1985) Sustained regional abnormalities in cardiac metabolism after transient ischemia in the chronic dog model. *Journal of the American College of Cardiology*, **6**, 336–347

Schwalb, H., Izhar, U., Yaroslavsky, E., *et al.* (1989) The effect of amino acids on the ischemic heart. Improvement of oxygenated crystalloid cardioplegic solution by an enriched branched chain amino acid formulation. *Journal of Thoracic and Cardiovascular Surgery*, **98**, 551–556

Sellevold, O.F. and Jynge, P. (1987a) Protection of the ischemic myocardium: dose-response relationships with glucocorticoids in filtered cardioplegic solutions. *Thoracic and Cardiovascular Surgeon*, **35**, 108–114

Sellevold, O.F. and Jynge, P. (1987b). Steroids and cardioplegia: effects of glucocorticoids upon vascular resistance during cardioplegic perfusion. *Thoracic and Cardiovascular Surgeon*, **35**, 307–311

Semenovsky, M.L., Shumakov, V.I., Sharov, V.G., *et al.* (1987) Protection of ischemic myocardium by exogenous phosphocreatine. II. Clinical, ultrastructural, and biochemical evaluations. *Journal of Thoracic and Cardiovascular Surgery,* **94**, 762–769

Shapira, N., Kirsh, M., Jochim, K. and Behrendt, D.M. (1980) Comparison of the effect of blood cardioplegia to crystalloid on myocardial contractility in man. *Journal of Thoracic and Cardiovascular Surgery*, **80**, 647–655

Shapira, N., Lemole, G.M., Spagna, P.M., *et al.* (1987) Antegrade and retrograde infusion of cardioplegia: assessment by thermovision. *Annals of Thoracic Surgery*, **43**, 92–97

Sharov, V.G., Saks, V.A., Kupriyanov, V.V., *et al.* (1987) Protection of ischemic myocardium by exogenous phosphocreatine. I. Morphologic and phosphorus 31-nuclear magnetic resonance studies. *Journal of Thoracic and Cardiovascular Surgery*, **94**, 749–761

Shen, A. and Jennings, R.B. (1972) Myocardial calcium and magnesium in acute ischemic injury. *American Journal of Pathology*, **67**, 417–440

Shiki, K., Masuda, M., Yonenaga, K., *et al.* (1986) Myocardial distribution of retrograde flow through the coronary sinus of the excised normal canine heart. *Annals of Thoracic Surgery*, **41**, 265–271

Shine, K.I., Douglas, A.M. and Ricchiuti, N.V. (1978) Calcium, barium and strontium movements during ischemia and reperfusion in rabbit ventricle. Implications for myocardial preservation. *Circulation Research*, **43**, 712–720

Shlafer, M., Kane, P.F. and Kirsh, M.M. (1982) Superoxide dismutase plus catalase enhances the efficacy of hypothermic cardioplegia to protect the globally ischemic, reperfused heart. *Journal of Thoracic and Cardiovascular Surgery*, **83**, 830–839

Silverman, N.A., Kohler, J., Levitsky, S., *et al.* (1984) Chronic hypoxemia depresses global ventricular function and predisposes to the depletion of high-energy phosphates during cardioplegic arrest: implications for surgical repair of cyanotic congenital heart defects. *Annals of Thoracic Surgery*, **37**, 304–308

Simpson, P.J., Mitsos, S.E., Ventura, A., *et al.* (1987) Prostacyclin protects ischemic reperfused myocardium in the dog by inhibition of neutrophil activation. *American Heart Journal*, **113**, 129–137

Simpson, P.J., Todd, R.F., Fantone, J.C., *et al.* (1988) Reduction of experimental canine myocardial reperfusion injury by a monoclonal antibody (anti-Mol, anti-CD11b) that inhibits leukocyte adhesion. *Journal of Clinical Investigation*, **81**, 624–629

Sink, J.D., Hill, R.C., Attarian, D.E. and Wechsler, A.S. (1983) Myocardial blood flow and oxygen consumption in the empty-beating, fibrillating, and potassium-arrested hypertrophied canine heart. *Annals of Thoracic Surgery*, **35**, 372–379

Smith, P.K., Buhrman, W.C., Ferguson, T.B., *et al.* (1983a) Conduction block after cardioplegic arrest: prevention by augmented atrial hypothermia. *Circulation*, **68**, II41–II48

Smith, P.K., Buhrman, W.C., Levett, J.M., *et al.* (1983b) Supraventricular conduction abnormalities following cardiac operations. A complication of inadequate atrial preservation. *Journal of Thoracic and Cardiovascular Surgery*, **85**, 105–115

Snyder, H.E., Smithwick, W., Wingard, J.T. and Agnew, R.C. (1988) Retrograde coronary sinus perfusion. *Annals of Thoracic Surgery*, **46**, 389–390

Solaro, R.J., Lee, J.A., Kentish, J.C. and Allen, D.G. (1988) Effects of acidosis on ventricular muscle from adult and neonatal rats. *Circulation Research*, **63**, 779–787

Sollevi, A., Schmidt, W., Jansson, E., *et al.* (1987) Adenine nucleotide degradation in the human myocardium during cardioplegia. *Cardiovascular Research*, **21**, 358–361

Solorzano, J., Taitelbaum, G. and Chiu, R.C. (1978) Retrograde coronary sinus perfusion for myocardial protection during cardiopulmonary bypass. *Annals of Thoracic Surgery*, **25**, 201–208

Spadaro, J., Bing, O.H.L., Gaarsch, W.H., *et al.* (1982) Effects of perfusion pressure on myocardial performance, metabolism, wall thickness, and compliance. *Journal of Thoracic and Cardiovascular Surgery*, **84**, 398–405

Speicher, C.E., Ferrigan, L., Wolfson, S.K., *et al.* (1962) Cold injury of the myocardium and pericardium in cardiac hypothermia. *Surgery, Gynecology and Obstetrics*, **114**, 659–665

Stahl, L.D., Aversano, T.R. and Becker, L.C. (1986) Selective enhancement of function of stunned myocardium by increased flow. *Circulation*, **74**, 843–851

Standeven, J.W., Jellinek, M., Menz, L.J., *et al.* (1984) Cold blood potassium diltiazem cardioplegia. *Journal of Thoracic and Cardiovascular Surgery*, **87**, 201–212

Sterling, K. (1986) The molecular mechanism of thyroid hormone action at the cellular level. In *The Thyroid Gland: Practical Clinical Treatise* (ed. L.C. van Middlesworth), Year Book Medical Publishers, Chicago, pp. 203–229

Stewart, J.R., Blackwell, W.H., Crute, S.L., *et al.* (1983) Inhibition of surgically induced ischemia/reperfusion injury by oxygen free radical scavengers. *Journal of Thoracic and Cardiovascular Surgery*, **86**, 262–272

Stewart, J.R., Crute, S.L., Loughlin, V., *et al.* (1985) Prevention of free radical-induced myocardial reperfusion injury with allopurinol. *Journal of Thoracic and Cardiovascular Surgery*, **90**, 68–72

Stirling, M.C., McClanahan, T.B., Schott, R.J., *et al.* (1989) Distribution of cardioplegic solution infused antegradely and retrogradely in normal canine hearts. *Journal of Thoracic and Cardiovascular Surgery*, **98**, 1066–1076

Suaudeau, J., Shaffer, B., Daggett, W.M., *et al.* (1982) Role of procaine and washed red cells in the isolated dog heart perfused at 5°C. *Journal of Thoracic and Cardiovascular Surgery*, **84**, 886

Sun, S.C., Raza, S.T., Tam, S.K., *et al.* (1988) Effects of antegrade cardioplegic infusion with simultaneously controlled coronary sinus occlusion on preservation of regionally ischemic myocardium after acute coronary artery occlusion and reperfusion. *Journal of Thoracic and Cardiovascular Surgery*, **96**, 626–633

Svensson, S., Svedjeholm, R., Ekroth, R., *et al.* (1990) Trauma metabolism and the heart. Uptake of substrates and effects of insulin early after cardiac operations. *Journal of Thoracic and Cardiovascular Surgery*, **99**, 1063–1073

Swanson, D.K. and Myerowitz, P.D. (1983) Effect of

reperfusion temperature and pressure on the functional and metabolic recovery of preserved hearts. *Journal of Thoracic and Cardiovascular Surgery*, **86**, 242–251

Swanson, D.K. and Myerowitz, P.D. (1987) Heart preservation for transplanation. In *Heart Transplanation* (ed. P.D. Myerowitz), Futura Publishing, New York, pp. 339–355

Swanson, D.K., Dufek, J.H. and Kahn, D.R. (1980) Improved myocardial preservation at 4°C. *Annals of Thoracic Surgery*, **30**, 518–526

Tabayashi, K., McKeown, P.P., Miyamoto, M., *et al.* (1988) Ischemic myocardial protection. Comparison of nonoxygenated crystalloid, oxygenated crystalloid, and oxygenated fluorocarbon cardioplegic solutions. *Journal of Thoracic and Cardiovascular Surgery*, **95**, 239–246

Taegtmeyer, H., Roberts, A.F.C. and Raine, A.E.G. (1985) Energy metabolism in reperfused heart muscle: metabolic correlates to return of function. *Journal of the American College of Cardiology*, **6**, 864–870

Takahashi, A., Chambers, D.J., Braimbridge, M.V. and Hearse, D.J. (1988) Optimal myocardial protection during crystalloid cardioplegia. Interrelationship between volume and duration of infusion. *Journal of Thoracic and Cardiovascular Surgery*, **96**, 730–740

Takeo, S., Tanonaka, K., Miyake, K. and Imago, M. (1988) Adenine nucleotide metabolites are beneficial for recovery of cardiac contractile force after hypoxia. *Journal of Molecular and Cellular Cardiology*, **20**, 187–199

Teoh, K.H., Christakis, G.T., Weisel, R.D., *et al.* (1986) Accelerated myocardial metabolic recovery with terminal warm blood cardioplegia. *Journal of Thoracic and Cardiovascular Surgery*, **91**, 888–895

Teoh, K.H., Mickle, D.A., Weisel, R.D., *et al.* (1988) Improving myocardial metabolic and functional recovery after cardioplegic arrest. *Journal of Thoracic and Cardiovascular Surgery*, **95**, 788–798

Thelin, S., Hultman, J., Ronquist, G. and Hansson, H.E. (1986) Enhanced protection of rat hearts during ischemia by phosphoenolpyruvate and ATP in cardioplegia. *Thoracic and Cardiovascular Surgeon*, **34**, 104–109

Thelin, S., Hultman, J., Ronquist, G. and Hansson, H.E. (1987a) Metabolic and functional effects of creatine phosphate in cardioplegic solution. Studies on rat hearts during and after normothermic ischemia. *Scandinavian Journal of Thoracic and Cardiovascular Surgery*, **21**, 39–45

Thelin, S., Hultman, J., Ronquist, G. and Hansson, H.E. (1987b) Interrelated effects of nucleoside mono-and triphosphates and phosphoenolpyruvate on rat hearts subjected to cardioplegic arrest at normothermia. *Scandinavian Journal of Thoracic and Cardiovascular Surgery*, **21**, 33–38

Thelin, S., Hultman, J., Ronquist, G., *et al.* (1987c) Improved myocardial protection by creatine phosphate in cardioplegic solution. An in vivo study in the pig during normothermic ischemia. *Thoracic and Cardiovascular Surgeon*, **35**, 137–142

Todd, E.P., Koster, J.H., Utley, J.R., *et al.* (1977) The effect of coronary perfusion pressure on recovery of myocardial function following normothermic ischemia. *Journal of Surgical Research*, **22**, 667–670

Torchiana, D.F., Love, T.R., Hendren, W.G., *et al.* (1987) Calcium-induced ventricular contraction during cardioplegic arrest. *Journal of Thoracic and Cardiovascular Surgery*, **94**, 606–613

Tyers, G.F.O., Manley, N.J., Williams, E.H., *et al.* (1977) Preliminary clinical experience with isotonic hypothermic potassium-induced arrest. *Journal of Thoracic and Cardiovascular Surgery*, **74**, 674–681

Valeri, C.R., Yarnoz, M., Vecchione, J.J., *et al.* (1980) Improved oxygen delivery to the myocardium during hypothermia by perfusion with 2,3 DPG-enriched red blood cells. *Annals of Thoracic Surgery*, **30**, 527–535

Van Belle, H. (1985) Myocardial purines during ischemia, reperfusion and pharmacological protection. *Molecular Physiology*, **8**, 615–630

Van Belle, H., Goossens, F. and Wynants, J. (1987) Formation and release of purine catabolites during hypoperfusion, anoxia, and ischemia. *American Journal of Physiology*, **252**, H886–H893

Vander Woude, J.C., Christlieb, I.Y., Sicard, G.A. and Clark, R.E. (1985) Imidazole-buffered cardioplegic solution. Improved myocardial preservation during global ischemia. *Journal of Thoracic and Cardiovascular Surgery*, **90**, 225–234

Vercellotti, G.M., Hammerschmidt, D.E., Craddock, P.R. and Jacob, H.S. (1982) Activation of plasma complement by perfluorocarbon artificial blood: probable mechanism of adverse pulmonary reactions in treated patients and rationale for corticosteriod prophylaxis. *Blood*, **59**, 1299–1304

Veronee, C.D., Lewis, W.R., Takla, M.W., *et al.* (1986) Protective metabolic effects of propranolol during total myocardial ischemia. *Journal of Thoracic and Cardiovascular Surgery*, **92**, 425–433

Vinas, J.F., Fewel, J.G., Arom, K.V., *et al.* (1979) Effects of systemic hypothermia on myocardial metabolism and coronary blood flow in the fibrillating heart. *Journal of Thoracic and Cardiovascular Surgery*, **77**, 900–907

Vinten-Johansen, J., Buckberg, G.D., Okamoto, F., *et al.* (1986a) Superiority of surgical versus medical reperfusion after regional ischemia. *Journal of Thoracic and Cardiovascular Surgery*, **92**, 525–534

Vinten-Johnasen, J., Chiantella, V., Faust, K.B., *et al.* (1988a) Myocardial protection with blood cardioplegia in ischemically injured hearts: reduction of reoxygenation injury with allopurinol. *Annals of Thoracic Surgery*, **45**, 319–326

Vinten-Johansen, J., Edgerton, T.A., Hansen, K.J., *et al.* (1986b) Surgical revascularization of acute (1 hour) coronary occlusion: blood versus crystalloid cardioplegia. *Annals of Thoracic Surgery*, **42**, 247–254

Vinten-Johansen, J., Johnson, W.E., Mills, S.A., *et al.* (1988b) Reperfusion injury after temporary coronary occlusion. *Journal of Thoracic and Cardiovascular Surgery*, **95**, 960–968

Vouhe, P.R., Helias, J. and Grondin, C.M. (1980) Myocardial protection through cold cardioplegia using diltiazem, a calcium channel blocker. *Annals of Thoracic Surgery*, **30**, 342–348

Walls, J.T., Nasser, F.N., Baron, D.W., *et al.* (1982) Beneficial effects of multidose coronary artery washout during elective cardiac arrest and cardiopulmonary bypass. Biochemical and hemodynamic evaluation. *Journal of Thoracic and Cardiovascular Surgery*, **83**, 772–778

Ward, H.B., St. Cyr, J.A., Cogordan, J.A., *et al.* (1984) Recovery of adenine nucleotide levels after global myocardial ischemia in dogs. *Surgery*, **96**, 248–255

Warner, K.G., Josa, M., Butler, M.D., *et al.* (1988) Regional changes in myocardial acid production during ischemic arrest: a comparison of sanguineous and asanguineous cardioplegia. *Annals of Thoracic Surgery*, **45**, 75–81

Warner, K.G., Josa, M., Marston, W., *et al.* (1987) Reduction in myocardial acidosis using blood cardioplegia. *Journal of Surgical Research*, **42**, 247–256

Watanabe, H., Yokosawa, T., Eguchi, S. and Imai, S. (1989) Functional and metabolic protection of the neonatal myocardium from ischemia. Insufficient protection by cardioplegia. *Journal of Thoracic and Cardiovascular Surgery*, **97**, 50–58

Weglicki, W.B., Owens, K., Ruth, R.C. and Sonnenblick, E.H. (1974) Activity of endogenous myocardial lipases during incubation at acid pH. *Cardiovascular Research*, **8**, 237–242

Weisel, R.D., Mickle, D.A., Finkle, C.D., *et al.* (1989) Myocardial free-radical injury after cardioplegia. *Circulation*, **80** (suppl III), III-14–III-18

Wesley, R.C. and Belardinelli, L. (1989) Role of endogenous adenosine in postdefibrillation bradyarrhythmia and hemodynamic depression. *Circulation*, **80**, 128–137

Whitman, G.J., Kieval, R.S., Brown, J., *et al.* (1989) Optimal hypothermic preservation of arrested myocardium in isolated perfused rabbit hearts: a ^{31}P NMR study. *Surgery*, **105**, 100–108

Wilson, G.J., Axford-Gatley, R.A., Bush, B.G., *et al.* (1990) European versus North American cardioplegia: comparison of Bretschneider's and Roe's cardioplegic solutions in a canine model of cardiopulmonary bypass. *Thoracic and Cardiovascular Surgeon*, **38**, 10–14

Wyatt, D.A., Ely, S.W., Lasley, R.D., *et al.* (1989) Purine-enriched asanguineous cardioplegia retards adenosine triphosphate degradation during ischemia and improves postischemic ventricular function. *Journal of Thoracic and Cardiovascular Surgery*, **97**, 771–778

Yamamoto, F., Braimbridge, M.V. and Hearse, D.J. (1984) Calcium and cardioplegia. The optimal calcium content of St. Thomas' Hospital cardioplegic solution. *Journal of Thoracic and Cardiovascular Surgery*, **87**, 908–912

Yamamoto, F., Manning, A.S., Braimbridge, M.V. and Hearse, D.J. (1983a) Cardioplegia and slow calcium-channel blocker. Studies with verapamil. *Journal of Thoracic and Cardiovascular Surgery*, **86**, 252–261

Yamamoto, F., Manning, A.S., Braimbridge, M.V. and Hearse, D.J. (1983b) Nifedipine and cardioplegia: rat heart studies with the St. Thomas' cardioplegic solution. *Cardiovascular Research*, **17**, 719–727

Yamamoto, F., Manning, A.S., Crome, R., *et al.* (1985) Calcium antagonists and myocardial protection: a comparative study of the functional, metabolic and electrical consequences of verapamil and nifedipine as additives to the St. Thomas' cardioplegic solution. *Thoracic and Cardiovascular Surgeon*, **33**, 354–359

Yano, Y., Braimbridge, M.V. and Hearse, D.J. (1987) Protection of the pediatric myocardium. Differential susceptibility to ischemic injury of the neonatal rat heart. *Journal of Thoracic and Cardiovascular Surgery*, **94**, 887–896

Yano, Y., Riggs, T.R., Milam, D.F. and Alexander, J.C. (1987) Calcium-accentuated ischemic damage during reperfusion: the time course of the reperfusion injury in the isolated working rat heart model. *Journal of Surgical Research*, **42**, 51–55

Yasuda, R.K., Fewel, J.G., Ghidoni, J.J., *et al.* (1983) Effect of venting on myocardial protection by hypothermic cardioplegic arrest. *Journal of Surgical Research*, **34**, 347–357

Yates, J.C. and Dhalla, N.S. (1975) Structural and functional changes associated with failure and recovery of hearts after perfusion with Ca^{++} free medium. *Journal of Molecular and Cellular Cardiology*, **7**, 91–103

Ytrehus, K., Gunnes, S., Myklebust, R. and Mjs, O.D. (1987) Protection by superoxide dismutase and catalase in the isolated rat heart reperfused after prolonged cardioplegia: a combined study of metabolic, functional, and morphometric ultrastrucutral variables. *Cardiovascular Research*, **21**, 492–499

Zile, M.R., Neill, W.A., Gaasch, W.H., *et al.* (1987) Distribution of a neutral cardioplegic vehicle during the development of ischemic myocardial contracture. *Journal of Molecular and Cellular Cardiology*, **19**, 977–989

Zucchi, R., Limbruno, U., Poddighe, R., *et al.* (1989) The adenosine hypothesis revisited: relation between purine release and coronary flow in the isolated rat heart. *Cardiovascular Research*, **23**, 125–131

Zweier, J.L., Flaherty, J.T. and Weisfeldt, M.L. (1987) Direct measurement of free radical generation following reperfusion of ischemic myocardium. *Proceedings of the National Academy of Sciences of the USA*, **84**, 1404–1407

9

Postoperative management following cardiopulmonary bypass

Martin K.G. Boylan

The survival of patients who have undergone cardiac surgery or general surgery in the presence of cardiac disease is mainly determined by preoperative risk factors (Goldman *et al.*, 1977; Kennedy *et al.*, 1980; Kouchokos *et al.*, 1980; Urzua *et al.*, 1981; Paiement *et al.*, 1983), the skill of the surgeon, and the quality of the anaesthetic and postoperative care. Postoperative management following cardiopulmonary bypass has four main components: good nursing, accurate monitoring, support of the cardiopulmonary system and other vital organs, and the prevention or treatment of complications. The postoperative period is a continuation of the preoperative and operative phases and begins with the last skin suture.

Transfer of the patient to the intensive care unit

The transfer of any patient to and from an intensive care unit can be hazardous (Braman *et al.*, 1987). Monitoring of vital signs must be continued and portable monitors now permit continuous display of the ECG, arterial and venous pressure and pulse oximetry. Equipment for resuscitation, including a battery-powered defibrillator should accompany the patient. Any circulatory support should be continued using battery powered infusors for inotropic drugs and a battery powered circulatory assist device may also be necessary. Safe transfer to the intensive care unit is best achieved with the patient in a stable condition, with minimal disturbance and accompanied by the surgeon and anaesthetist responsible for the patient in the operating room (Table 9.1).

Most patients are transferred sedated and ventilated and a manual method of ventilating with

Table 9.1 Transfer checklist

Notify ITU
Cardiovascular
- Haemodynamically stable?
- Pacemaker in use?
  - functional?
  - demand mode?
- Volume status optimal?
- Cardiac output adequate?
- Blood pressure within correct limits?
- Electrolytes (K^+, Ca^{2+}) normal?
- Drug infusions?
- i.v. Fluids or blood available for administration?
- Monitoring?
  - ECG
  - arterial pressure
  - central venous pressure

Ventilation
- Blood gases acceptable?
- Endotracheal tube patent and secure?
- Portable ventilator working?
- Oxygen supply?
- Monitoring?
  - Pulse oximeter
  - Stethoscope
  - Airway pressure
- Self inflating manual rebreathing circuit?

Sedation
- Adequately anaesthetized?

Coagulation
- ACT normal?
- Blood drainage from chest drains acceptable?
- Coagulation screen required?
- Administration of clotting factors, platelets?

Other
- All lines, drains, catheters etc. clear?
- Chest drains functional?
- Circulatory assist device – battery check?
- Case records and X-rays?
- Ventilator and haemodynamic parameters known?
- Appropriate personnel available?

oxygen must be available even if a portable ventilator is being used.

The intensive care unit

The postoperative cardiac surgery intensive care unit should be sited close to the operating rooms to reduce the hazards of transfer and the treatment of complications such as tamponade and haemorrhage. Standards for intensive care units have been defined (Hoyt, 1988; Standards for Intensive Care Units, 1990) specifying the area required for each patient bed and the necessary support systems. All patient areas should be visible from a central nursing station. Some individual rooms should be included for the nursing of patients with infections or, if appropriate, for transplant patients needing reverse barrier nursing (Grebenik and Robinson, 1985). The most common fault with any intensive care unit design is lack of space – around the patient area, for storage of equipment, drugs, intravenous fluids and disposable items. There must be adequate space for a surgical scrub sink, a laboratory, relatives' waiting room, resident medical staff accommodation, offices, equipment maintenance, waste disposal, food preparation, staff rest room and changing facilities. Proper ventilation systems, temperature control and lighting are essential. Sterile surgical instruments and sutures for emergency re-sternotomy and a portable operating lamp must be immediately available.

Arrival on ITU

On arrival from the operating room the first priorities are to establish mechanical ventilation according to the anaesthetist's instruction (Table 9.2). Typical values are an FIO_2 of 50%, tidal volume of 10 ml kg^{-1}, rate of 10 breaths per minute, PEEP of 2 cmH_2O and SIMV mode. The chest should be examined to ensure that both sides are moving and the trachea is central. Auscultation of the lungs and heart should confirm breath sounds as the first indication of adequate function of the endotracheal tube and ventilator system.

Monitoring should be established rapidly but do not disconnect the ECG and the arterial pressure at the same time. This maintains some continuity of monitoring during this transition phase. Integrated monitoring systems with transportable multiparameter modules offer significant advantages.

Basic monitoring of ECG, pulse oximetry, direct arterial blood pressure, central venous pressure, peripheral and core temperatures, urine output and blood loss from chest drains is routine. Pulmonary artery pressure, left atrial pressure and cardiac output monitoring may be required.

Table 9.2 ITU arrival checklist

Immediate
- Ventilator
  - assess ventilator function
  - check connection
  - check settings (FIO_2, MV, PEEP, Paw)
  - auscultate chest – bilaterally
  - pulse oximeter
- Haemodynamics
  - ECG (rate, rhythm, ST segment)
  - arterial BP
  - CVP
  - pulmonary artery pressure
- Drug infusion – drug and response
- Coagulation status
- Blood availability
- Communication of all relevant information to ITU staff

Soon after arrival
- Chest drains – amount
- Urine output
- Temperature – core, peripheral
- Other haemodynamic monitoring – cardiac output
- Patient CNS status
- Fine tune ventilator according to blood gases

Investigations on arrival
- Arterial blood gases
- Serum K^+
- PCV
- ECG – 12-lead
- Coagulation screen (if indicated)
- Chest X-ray (if indicated)

As monitoring is established, the ideal parameters for the patient should be communicated to the staff on the ITU who will be in attendance.

Blood specimens should be sent for analysis. Blood gases, serum potassium, serum ionized calcium, serum glucose and haematocrit should be measured at the on site ITU laboratory. If indicated by excessive bleeding or by a history of perioperative risk factors, e.g. reoperation, a clotting profile should be sent to the haematology laboratory.

Sedation and analgesia

Patients require ventilatory support for a variable time after cardiac surgery and usually require sedative drugs to facilitate mechanical ventilation. As surgical and anaesthetic techniques have improved there has been a trend towards earlier discontinuation of ventilatory support (Foster *et al.*, 1984). Until recently, sedation of patients in intensive care has been regarded as an extension of anaesthetic practice but potential hazards of this approach have been recognized (Watt and Ledingham, 1984). The aims of sedating the patients in intensive care who require ventilating after cardiopulmonary bypass should be clearly defined.

An objective form of assessment should be made of the depth and quality of sedation related to the severity of illness.

An ideal level of sedation can be defined as that which causes the patient to be free from pain and anxiety while tolerating medical procedures including mechanical ventilation and from which the patient can easily be roused from light sleep. Depth of sedation can be assessed by response to certain stimuli as a simple measure on the nursing chart. Measures of quality of sedation are more difficult to derive. Linear analogue scales require practice in their use but provide useful data especially if assessments are made of depth of sedation, degree of distress and level of comprehension.

Physiological disturbance affects cerebral function and may result in apparent changes attributed to sedative drugs. A measurement of severity of illness is important and the APACHE II score based on 12 physiological variables (Wagner, Knaus and Draper, 1986) shows that increasing severity of illness has a significant effect on the level of consciousness (Bion *et al.*, 1986). The cerebral function analysing monitor (Sebel *et al.*, 1983) is an alternative although expensive way of assessing the brain and provides further evidence that physiological disturbance affects cerebral function (Jackson *et al.*, 1983).

The commonest drug therapy to achieve sedation on intensive care is a combination of opiates and benzodiazepines. Light sedation is generally the preferred level for patients undergoing mechanical ventilation and there has been a marked reduction in the use of muscle relaxants (Bion and Ledingham, 1987).

Morphine is metabolized by the liver to 3- and 6-glucuronides. Morphine-6-glucuronide has potent opioid activity and accumulates in renal failure (Osborne, Joel and Slevin, 1986). Continuous infusions provide stable conditions but require regular review to prevent excessive dosing. Patient controlled analgesia systems offer a logical route of administration of opiates in the awake patient. High doses of morphine suppress the response to infection in experimental animals (Tubaro *et al.*, 1983). Opiate withdrawal is not usually a problem unless high doses have been used for more than 5 days in patients without physical pain.

The use of short acting opiates over several days may confer no advantages. Alfentanil infusion has been used for sedation of critically ill patients (Cohen and Kelly, 1987) but demonstrated similar quality of analgesia and sedation when compared with pethidine in ventilated cardiac surgery patients (Yate *et al.*, 1986).

Midazolam has replaced diazepam in many intensive care units because of its superior pharmacokinetic properties (Lowry *et al.*, 1985). It has a shorter half life of approximately 2h in healthy people and is metabolized by the liver to 1-(OH)-midazolam with an even shorter half life. Midazolam clearance may be prolonged in critically ill patients (Mathews *et al.*, 1987) and in some patients after cardiopulmonary bypass (Shelly, Mendel and Park, 1987). Benzodiazepines are potent amnesics and can make reassurance and patient co-operation difficult. They are probably best used in conjunction with opiates. Flumazenil (Rodrigo and Rosenquist, 1987) a specific benzodiazepine antagonist enables reversal of benzodiazepines.

Propofol (2, 6-di-isopropylphenol) is now used extensively for the induction of anaesthesia (Sebel and Lowdon, 1989). Studies have shown a virtual lack of accumulation (Glen, 1980) with rapid recovery when administered as a continuous infusion for over 2h (Coppel and Johnston, 1988). Propofol provided effective sedation with haemodynamic stability in patients after cardiac surgery (Grounds *et al.*, 1987; McMurray *et al.*, 1990). The sedation was easily controlled and associated with very rapid recovery. The redistribution and elimination half-lives, and clearance of propofol were prolonged compared with subjects who did not undergo cardiopulmonary bypass and hypothermia.

The attractions of the drug are leading to its widespread use for sedation in intensive care. The reports on the haemodynamic effects of propofol are conflicting. Most authors agree that propofol has a vasodilating effect and that systemic vascular resistance is decreased (Patrick *et al.*, 1985; Stephan *et al.*, 1986; Kaplan *et al.*, 1988) but others have reported significant decreases in cardiac index (Van Aken *et al.*, 1988; Lepage *et al.*, 1988; Coetzee *et al.*, 1989). The cardiovascular effects of propofol are more marked than those following the usual intravenous anaesthetic agents (Sebel and Lowdon, 1990).

Management of ventilation

Improvement in materials and techniques of cardiopulmonary bypass have virtually eliminated the postperfusion lung syndrome. There are still many factors which may give rise to pulmonary dysfunction in the postoperative period. Pre-existing lung disease is increased in cigarette smokers and pulmonary hypertension is a finding in many patients with valvular heart disease.

Vital capacity, total lung capacity, inspiratory capacity and functional residual capacity are significantly decreased post cardiopulmonary bypass and these changes may persist for more than 2 weeks. The reduction in functional residual capacity is associated with closure of small airways and pulmonary dysfunction. Atelectasis and functional residual capacity reduction is multifactorial. Inadequate lung re-expansion after cardiopulmonary bypass, reduced surfactant production, decreased clearance of secretions, ventilation with small tidal volumes, pleural effusion and increased extravascular lung water are among some of the factors.

Intrapulmonary shunting of blood is increased after heart surgery and is indicated by an increase in the alveolar-arterial oxygen gradient. This may persist for several days. Pulmonary dysfunction is maximal 24h postoperatively.

Pulmonary compliance decreases postoperatively. Increased extravascular lung water is a common cause of atelectasis. Extravascular lung water increases on the first postoperative day and may be related to oncotic and hydrostatic pressure changes throughout the postoperative period (Byrick, Kay and Noble, 1977). The work of breathing increases after heart surgery (Elia *et al.*, 1985). The oxygen cost of breathing spontaneously is inversely related to the preoperative vital capacity. All these factors must be considered when planning postoperative respiratory care.

Drugs that depress respiration may have residual effects and high doses of centrally acting drugs may lead to apnoea. Narcotic antagonists can cause severe hypertension and acute left ventricular failure and should be used only rarely. Anticholinergic drugs may result in an increase in the physiological deadspace and impair minute ventilation.

Pulmonary vascular resistance is maximally increased after cardiopulmonary bypass becoming normal on the first postoperative day. The mechanism of the increase in pulmonary vascular resistance is not well defined. Postulated mechanisms include the absence of pulmonary circulation during bypass, air embolus, pulmonary vasoconstriction, microaggregates and the release of vasoactive substances. The incidence is decreased if membrane oxygenators are used during bypass (Byrick and Noble, 1978). Many drugs used during the postoperative period can affect the pulmonary vasculature. Any drug with α-agonist activity may cause pulmonary vasoconstriction independently of hypoxic pulmonary vasoconstriction (Mentzer, Alegre and Nolan, 1976). Drugs with β-agonist activity may increase the shunt fraction by abolishing hypoxic pulmonary vasoconstriction. Reversal of hypoxic pulmonary vasoconstriction must be considered when other vasodilators are used. Both nitroprusside and nitrates worsen intrapulmonary shunting under hypoxic conditions (D'Oliveira *et al.*, 1981; Castheley *et al.*, 1982).

Weaning from mechanical ventilation

Whether extubating patients early or late following cardiac surgery certain guidelines should be followed (Table 9.3). The ideal choice of ventilator should be one that is volume cycled and able to be set as in a (synchronized) intermittent mandatory mode. Intermittent mandatory ventilation allows the patient to breathe spontaneously between machine delivered breaths. This is more efficient, safer and pleasant for the patient. Synchronized intermittent mandatory ventilation may reduce the risk of pulmonary barotrauma (Heenan *et al.*, 1980).

Table 9.3 Criteria for weaning

Clinical status
Awake and alert
No residual effects of repiratory depressants
No residual effects of muscle relaxants
No gross neurological deficit
Haemodynamically stable
No significant arrhythmia
Not oedema
Low dose or no inotropic support.
Normothermia
Not shivering
Peripheral–core temperature difference < 3°C
Bleeding from drains<30 ml h^{-1}
Lung mechanics
Normal arterial blood gases
pH > 7.35
$Pa\text{CO}_2$ < 6.0 kPa
$Pa\text{O}_2$ > 10.0 kPa at $F\text{IO}_2$ < 0.4
Pulmonary function
Respiratory rate < 30 breaths min^{-1}
Forced vital capacity >15 ml kg^{-1}
Inspiratory force > −28 cmH_20
Minute volume < 100 ml $kg^{-1}min^{-1}$

Intermittent mandatory ventilation allows the level of mechanical support to be gradually reduced in patients who are difficult to wean. If the inspired gas for intermittent mandatory ventilation is supplied through a demand valve the workload of breathing may be increased as inspiratory force must be generated to open the valve and the resulting flow rate delivered may be inadequate for the patient. This can be overcome by using a ventilator with inspiratory pressure support. Inspiratory work is minimized by augmenting each breath with additional gas flow up to a pressure limit (Sassoon *et al.*, 1989; Cox, Tinbi and Farrimond, 1988). Improvements in ventilator design have been done much to reduce the workload imposed by the machine and this is important in the patient with impaired respiratory function.

Patients ventilated with positive end-expiratory pressure have quicker reversal of the changes in functional residual capacity after cardiopulmonary bypass compared with those ventilated without (Downs and Mitchell, 1976). Except where specifically contraindicated, e.g. severe bronchospasm, positive end-expiratory pressure up to +5 cmH_2O should be routinely supplied. Clinically it is useful to be able to calculate oxygen delivery when applying positive end-expiratory pressure, as high levels may cause a decrease in cardiac output or fall in mixed venous oxygen saturation (Qvist *et al.*, 1975).

Although clinical assessment of patients is fundamental, modern intensive care unit ventilators have a comprehensive set of alarms to indicate if patients are not breathing adequately, even in the spontaneous mode and these alarms are extremely valuable in protecting patients.

References

Anon (1990) *Standards for Intensive Care Units*. The Intensive Care Society, 9 Bedford Square, London.

Bion, J.F. and Ledingham, I. McA. (1987) Sedation in intensive care – a postal survery. *Intensive Care Medicine*, **13**, 215–216

Bion, J.F., Logan, B.K., Newman, P.M., *et al.* (1986) Sedation in intensive care: Morphine and renal function. *Intensive Care Medicine*, **12**, 359–365

Braman, S.S., Dunn, S.M., Amico, C.A., *et al.* (1987) Complications of intrahospital transport in critically ill patients. *Annals of Internal Medicine,* **107**, 469–473

Byrick, R.J., Kay, J.C. and Noble, W.H. (1977) Extravascular lung water accumulation in patients following coronary artery surgery. *Canadian Anaesthetists Society Journal*, **24**, 332–345

Byrick, R.J. and Noble, W.H. (1978) Postperfusion lung syndrome: comparison of Travenol bubble and membrane oxygenators. *Journal of Thoracic and Cardiovascular Surgery*, **76**, 685–693

Castheley, P.A., Lear, S., Cottrell, J.E., *et al.* (1982) Intrapulmonary shunting during induced hypotension. *Anaesthesia and Analgesia*, **61**, 231–235

Coetzee, A., Fourie, P., Coetzee, J., *et al.* (1989) Effect of various propofol plasma concentrations on regional myocardial contractility and left ventricular afterload. *Anaesthesia and Analgesia*, **69**, 573–583

Cohen, A.T. and Kelly, D.R. (1987) Assessment of alfentanil by intravenous infusion as long-term sedation in intensive care. *Anaesthesia*, **42**, 545–548

Coppel, D.L. and Johnston, J.R. (1988) The use of propofol as a total intravenous anaesthetic agent for thoracic surgery. *Anaesthesia*, **43** (suppl), 118

Cox, D., Tinbi, F.S. and Farrimond, J.G. (1988) Investigation of the spontaneous modes of breathing of different ventilators. *Intensive care Medicine,* **14**, 532–537

D'Oliveira, M., Sykes, M.K., Chakrabarti, M.K., *et al.* (1981) Depression of hypoxic pulmonary vasoconstriction by sodium nitroprusside and nitroglycerin. *British Journal of Anaesthesia*, **53**, 11–18

Downs, J.B. and Mitchell, L.A. (1976) Pulmonary effects of ventilatory pattern following cardiopulmonary bypass. *Critical Care Medicine*, **4**, 295–300

Elia, S., Liu, P. and Mastrocostopoulos, G., *et al.* (1985) Oxygen cost of breathing in postoperative cardiac surgical patients. *Anesthesiology*, **63**, A141

Foster, G.H., Conway, W., Pamulkov, N., *et al.* (1984) Early extubation after coronary artery bypass: brief report. *Critical Care Medicine*, **12**, 994–996

Glen, J.B. (1980) Animal studies of the anaesthetic activity of ICI 35 868. *British Journal of Anaesthesia*, **52**, 731–741

Goldman, L., Caldera, D.L., Nussbaum, S.R., *et al.* (1977) Multifactorial index of risk in non-cardiac surgical procedures. *New England Journal of Medicine*, **297**, 845–850

Grebenik, C.R. and Robinson, P.N. (1985) Cardiac transplantation at Harefield. *Anaesthesia*, **40**, 131–140

Grounds, R.M., Lalor, J.M., Lumley, J., *et al.* (1987) Propofol infusion for sedation in the intensive care unit: a preliminary report. *British Medical Journal*, **294**, 397–400

Heenan, T.J., Downs, J.B., Douglas, M.E., *et al.* (1980) Intermittent mandatory ventilation: is synchronization important? *Chest*, **77**, 598–602

Hoyt, J.W. (1988) Complications of design and construction of the intensive care unit. In *Complications in Critical Care Medicine*, (eds P.D. Lumb and C.W. Bryan-Brown), Year Book Medical Publ Inc, Chicago, pp. 317–318

Jackson, A.C., Boulton, C.F., Young, G.B. *et al.* (1983) The encephalopathy of sepsis. *Annals of Neurology*, **14**, 141

Kaplan, J.A., Guffin, A.V., Mikula, S., *et al.* (1988) Comparative hemodynamic effects of propofol and thiamylal sodium during anaesthetic induction for myocardial revascularization. *Journal of Cardiothoracic Anesthesia*, **3**, 297–302

Kennedy, J.W., Kaiser, G.C., Fisher, L.D. *et al.* (1980) Multivariate discriminant analysis of the clinical and angiographic predictors of operative mortality from the Collaborative Study in Coronary Artery Surgery (CASS). *Journal of Thoracic and Cardiovascular Surgery*, **80**, 876–887

Kouchoukos, N.T., Oberman, A., Kirklin, J.W., *et al.* (1980) Coronary bypass surgery: analysis of factors affecting hospital mortality. *Circulation*, **62**, 184–189

Lepage, J.-Y. M., Pinaud, L.M., Helias, J.H., *et al.* (1988) Left ventricular function during propofol and fentanyl anesthesia in patients with coronary artery disease. Assessment with a radionuclide approach. *Anesthesia and Analgesia*, **67**, 949–955

Lowry, K.G., Dundee, J.W., McClean, E., *et al.* (1985) Pharmacokinetics of diazepam and midazolam when used for sedation following cardiopulmonary bypass. *British Journal of Anaesthesia*, **57**, 883–885

Mathews, H.M.L., Carson, I.W., Collier, P.S., *et al.* (1987) Midazolam sedation following open heart surgery. *British Journal of Anaesthesia*, **59**, 557–560

McMurray, T.J., Collier, P.S., Carson, I.W., *et al.* (1990) Propofol sedation after open heart surgery. A clinical and pharmacokinetic study. *Anaesthesia*, **45**, 322–326

Mentzer, R.M., Alegre, C.A. and Nolan, S.P. (1976) The effects of dopamine and isoproterenol on the pulmonary circulation. *Journal of Thoracic and Cardiovascular Surgery*, **71**, 807–814

Osborne, R.J., Joel, S.P., Slevin, M.L. (1986) Morphine intoxication in renal failure: the role of morphine-6-glucuronide. *British Medical Journal*, **292**, 1548–1549

Paiement, B., Pelletier, C., Dyrda, I., *et al.* (1983) A simple classification of the risk in cardiac surgery. *Canadian Anaesthetists Society Journal*, **30**, 61–68

Patrick, M.R., Blair, I.J., Feneck, R.O., *et al.* (1985) A comparison of the haemodynamic effects of propofol ('Diprivan') and thiopentone in patients with coronary artery disease. *Postgraduate Medical Journal*, **61**, 23–27

Qvist, J., Pontopiddan, H., Wilson, R.S., *et al.* (1975) Hemodynamic responses to mechanical ventilation with PEEP: the effect of hypovolaemia. *Anesthesiology*, **42**, 45–55

Rodrigo, M.R.C. and Rosenquist, J.B. (1987) The effect of Ro15-1788 (Annexate) on conscious sedation produced with midazolam. *Anaesthesia and Intensive Care*, **15**, 185–192

Sassoon, C.H.S., Giron, A.E., Ely, E.A., *et al.* (1989) Inspiratory work on flow-by and demand flow from continuous positive airway pressure. *Critical Care Medicine*, **17**, 1108–1114

Sebel, P.S. and Lowdon, J.D. (1989) Propofol: a new intravenous anesthetic. *Anesthesiology*, **71**, 260–277

Sebel, P.S. and Lowdon, J.D. (1990) In reply. (Letter) *Anesthesiology*, **72**, 396

Sebel, P.S., Maynard, D.E., Major, E., *et al.* (1983) The cerebral function analysing monitor. *British Journal of Anaesthesia*, **55**, 1265–1270

Shelly, M.P., Mendel, L. and Park, G.R. (1987) Failure of critically ill patients to metabolise midazolam. *Anaesthesia*, **42**, 619–626

Stephan, H., Sonntag, H., Schenk, H.D., *et al.* (1986) Effects of propofol on cardiovascular dynamics, myocardial blood flow, and myocardial metabolism in patients with coronary artery disease. *British Journal of Anaesthesia*, **58**, 969–975

Tubaro, E., Borelli, G., Croce, C., *et al.* (1983) Effect of morphine on resistance to infection. *Journal of Infectious Diseases*, **148**, 656–666

Urzua, J., Dominguez, P., Quiroga, M., *et al.* (1981) Preoperative estimation of risk in cardiac surgery. *Anesthesia and Analgesia*, **60**, 625–628

Van Aken, H., Meinshausen, E., Prien, T., *et al.* (1988) The influence of fentanyl and tracheal intubation on the hemodynamic effects of anesthesia induction with propofol/N_2O in humans. *Anesthesiology*, **68**, 157–163

Wagner, D.P., Knaus, W.A. and Draper, E.A. (1986) Physiologic abnormalities and outcome from acute disease. *Archives of Internal Medicine*, **146**, 1389–1396

Watt, I., Ledingham, I. McA. (1984) Mortality amongst multiple trauma patients admitted to an intensive care unit. *Anaesthesia*, **39**, 973–981

Yate, P.M., Thomas, D., Short, S.M., *et al.* (1986) Comparison of infusions of alfentanil or pethidine for sedation of ventilated patients on the ITU. *British Journal of Anaesthesia*, **58**, 1091–1099

10

Haematological aspects of extracorporeal circulation

Mano S. Rajah and Alan F. Penny

Introduction

Denaturation of blood is a significant factor in extracorporeal circulation (ECC). This occurs by mechanical pumping and continuous exposure to large foreign surfaces such as metal, silicone and gas interface. In addition, the use of large amounts of blood, pump prime fluids, heparinization and reversal with protamine, introduces complex changes in haemostasis. Excessive postoperative bleeding due to haemostatic failure is an important complication of ECC. The contributory factors to the aetiology of postoperative bleeding and the prevention of microemboli by filtration will be considered in this chapter. In the current climate, the prefered use of autologous blood will also be discussed.

Haematological effects of extracorporeal circulation for open heart surgery

Despite a normal clotting mechanism before operation (Trimble *et al.*, 1966) many patients suffer postoperative haemorrhage while laboratory measurements of haemostasis show only mild abnormalities and no specific deficiency (Salzman and Britten, 1965; Bachmann *et al.*, 1975). It is not surprising that exposing blood to a hostile environment produces certain changes, best classified as pump related. If the changes proceed beyond acceptable levels, it is not uncommon to develop additional bleeding. It is important to ascertain that there is no surgical cause before proceeding to investigate further and treat a haemostatic problem. Prompt diagnosis of a surgical bleed and immediate correction prevents the use of additional amounts of blood and blood products as the latter can produce an iatrogenic bleeding diathesis.

Pump prime

Buffered electrolyte solutions are now extensively used for priming with consequent haemodilution. It has been demonstrated in dog experiments that this does not cause serious haematological derangements (Hora *et al.*, 1967). This has been confirmed during many surgical procedures (Verska, Ludington and Brewer, 1974). Haemodilution also has beneficial effects; it reduces viscosity, improves microcirculation and reduces haemolysis (Pierce, 1956) and decreases postoperative bleeding (Verska, Ludington and Brewer, 1974). Venesection (for subsequent autologous transfusion) combined with haemodilution, produces improved postoperative haemostasis in cardiopulmonary bypass (CPB) patients when compared with haemodilution alone (Dale, Lilleasen and Erikssen, 1987). These procedures have been used extensively without donor blood replacement on religious grounds (Gollub and Bailey, 1969) and many of the early problems (Neville, Faber and Peacock, 1964; Roe, Hutchinson and Swenson, 1965) have been overcome. It is no longer considered necessary to use fresh blood in the prime even for children unless the patient's haematocrit is low, in which case bank blood is suitable.

Massive blood transfusion

Massive transfusion can be defined as the replacement of the patient's blood volume by homologous bank blood in less than 24h. Many patients who undergo open heart surgery may require several units of blood due to unexpected blood loss and bleeding problems, even when the whole pump volume is returned.

The rapid loss of a large amount of blood impairs tissue perfusion and requires immediate correction (Hewitt and Machin, 1990). Management comprises maintenance of blood volume, the oxygen carrying capacity of blood, haemostasis, colloid osmotic pressure (COP) and biochemical equilibrium. The complications of massive blood transfusion can be exacerbated by pre-existing liver and kidney disease, which superimpose already present abnormalities of haemostasis, plasma protein concentration and renal function.

With postoperative bleeding, as soon as blood loss and fluid replacement reach 40% of blood volume, replacement of red cells is required. Although red cell concentrate or red cells in additive solution such as saline–adenine–glucose–manitol (SAGM) can be used, it is advisable to use whole blood after infusion of the first 4 units of a massive transfusion because the plasma will ensure provision of coagulation factors essential for haemostasis and proteins to maintain COP. As the blood group and antibody screen is routinely done before operation, ABO and RhD compatible blood can be transfused as a rapid compatibility test is being done in the laboratory. The present citrate, phosphate, dextrose with adenine (CPD.A) anticoagulant used to preserve blood ensures adequate concentrations of 2,3-diphosphoglycerate and hence oxygen carrying capacity for up to 2 weeks after collection of blood. Hence it is advisable to use blood under 14 days old.

The metabolic disturbances associated with infusion of large volumes of blood include hyperkalaemia, usually transient and not significant. However, the hyperkalaemia exacerbated by hypothermia caused by the rapid transfusion of blood stored at 4°C can cause cardiac irregularities. Although stored blood has a reduced pH, acidosis is rare unless there is hypoperfusion and shock. The need for alkalizing agents must be based on laboratory tests and not the amount of bank blood transfused. The concept of citrate toxicity and hypocalcaemia will be discussed later. In the management of excess postoperative bleeding, large amounts of crystalloids, colloid solutions and red cell concentrates are administered. This can invariably result in the fall of plasma COP leading to respiratory distress syndrome. If the concentration of plasma albumin falls significantly, infusion of albumin may be necessary to raise the COP hence ensuring adequate renal function and alleviating pulmonary oedema.

Alterations of blood during cardiopulmonary bypass

In the extracorporeal circuit, blood is subjected to an abnormal physical and chemical environment. The resulting trauma includes denaturation of both cellular and plasma components.

Damage to erythrocytes

Significant haemolysis can occur as a result of pump action in the oxygenator, due to surface tension effects or sudden changes in pressure. Membrane oxygenators induce much less haemolysis than bubble oxygenators due to reduced surface tension forces. The level of free haemoglobin actually reached is moderated by the ability of the patient to remove it. Normally the reticuloendothelial system is able to remove approximately 0.1 mgHb kg^{-1} min^{-1} (equivalent to 5 mg dl^{-1} h^{-1} for an adult patient) (Bernstein, Blackshear and Keller, 1967). Haemoglobinuria due to filtration of haemoglobin by the kidneys occurs at plasma concentrations above 100 mg dl^{-1}, but actual renal damage is probably produced only when very high levels (300 mg dl^{-1}) are reached (Clowes, 1960). Several bioengineering studies have been carried out in relation to the factors influencing erythrocyte destruction in artificial organs. Bernstein and colleagues (Bernstein, Blackshear and Keller, 1967; Bernstein *et al.*, 1967) demonstrated the haemolytic effect of the shear forces resulting from sudden dimensional changes in tubing and cannulae and from the jet forces at velocities of 2000 cm s^{-1}. According to Blackshear, Dorman and Steinback (1965), shear stresses must reach the level of 10^4 dynes cm^{-2} to induce significant haemolysis. More recently, it was pointed out that haemolytic mechanisms are mostly surface related (Sutera, Croce and Mekrjardi, 1972). Negative pressures also produce haemolysis when they fall below one-third of an atmosphere (Bernstein, Blackshear and Keller, 1967; Bernstein *et al.*, 1967).

Besides immediate lysis of erythrocytes, perfusion leads to increased mechanical cell fragility (Galletti, 1965). Postperfusion anaemia (Kusserow and Clapp, 1966) and shortened erythrocyte life (Indeglia *et al.*, 1966) are both related to delayed haemolysis. The sublethal trauma is believed to be more important than the immediate haemolysis (Bernstein *et al.*, 1967); for each erythrocyte lysed, 500 cells could be altered. The magnitude of delayed haemolysis in the first 24h after perfusion, may be five times that of the immediate haemolysis. This haemolysis is paralleled by a rise of plasma lactate dehydrogenase released from erythrocytes (Bernstein, Blackshear and Keller, 1967).

Damage to leucocytes

In general the leucocytes decrease with the onset of perfusion and rise as the perfusion is prolonged more than 1–2h. Subsequently, leucocytosis occurs and persists in the absence of infection for over a week (Laufman and Ericson, 1970). During CPB, there is activation of leucocytes with release of granular contents. The released leucoattractants can lead to margination of leucocytes especially in the microvasculature (Bull *et al.*, 1988), perhaps because of complement activation (Hammerschmidt *et al.*, 1981; Kirklin *et al.*, 1983). Activated leucocytes release liposomal enzymes and generate thromboxanes, leucotrienes and oxygen free radicals which may induce tissue damage (Sacks *et al.*, 1978). Pulmonary dysfunction has been associated with pulmonary sequestration of activated leucocytes (Bolanowski *et al.*, 1977). Leucocyte deposition has also been noted in the myocardium after coronary bypass operation and this has been reduced by the antiplatelet drug dipyridamole (Teoh *et al.*, 1986). Dipyridamole may preserve leucocyte count by reducing platelet activation and preventing the release of chemotactic factors (Bolanowski *et al.*, 1977; Fountain *et al.*, 1980).

Damage to platelets

Thrombocytopenia and platelet dysfunction are well described as complications of CPB (Addonizio *et al.*, 1980; Harker *et al.*, 1980). The aetiology is multifactorial, damage to platelets at the blood gas interface (Dutton *et al.*, 1974; Edmunds *et al.*, 1982), dilutional factor due to the priming fluids and use of bank blood. The damaged platelets are invariably deposited in the systemic circulation and ECC (Hope *et al.*, 1981; Peterson, Dewanjee and Kaye, 1982). However, a proportion of platelets undergo temporary sequestration in the liver and spleen and return to the circulation in the postoperative phase (de Leval, Hill and Mielke, 1976). This spontaneous recovery of functioning platelets must be taken into account when evaluating antiplatelet agents during CPB. Platelet-inhibiting agents may preserve platelet count during CPB by preventing platelet aggregation on foreign surfaces and at sites of endothelial damage. One such drug, aspirin, which inhibits platelet adhesion and other haemostatic functions, may unfortunately increase postoperative bleeding. However, agents such as dipyridamole, which preserve platelet adhesion, may reduce postoperative bleeding and decrease the incidence of early coronary bypass graft occlusion (Teoh *et al.*, 1988). Dipyridamole inhibits platelet phosphodiesterase activity, thereby increasing the concentration of cyclic AMP and decreasing calcium mobilization in the platelets (Mills and Smith, 1971; Best *et al.*, 1979). This results in limiting of platelet activation, aggregation and granular release but preserves platelet adhesion. Haemostatic functions of the platelets are, therefore, preserved (Emmons *et al.*, 1965). Perioperative dipyridamole cover with postoperative dipyridamole and aspirin has successfully improved early bypass graft patency (Chesebro *et al.*, 1982). Dipyridamole has been administered both orally and intravenously, the latter maintaining more consistent plasma concentrations (Teoh *et al.*, 1988), preserving platelet counts and reducing postoperative blood loss. Intravenous dipyridamole also reduces myocardial platelet deposition and release of thromboxanes (Teoh *et al.*, 1986), potent coronary vasoconstrictors that may contribute to myocardial ischaemic injury (Teoh *et al.*, 1987).

Alterations in the coagulation and fibrinolytic systems

Several acquired coagulation disorders are commonly found after cardiovascular surgery (Bachmann *et al.*, 1975). However, interpretation of coagulation tests during and after bypass surgery is complicated by the use of heparin and protamine and by the great variation in the nature and volume of priming fluid and the amount of blood used. Normal haemostasis requires that the blood concentration of any clotting factor is at least 20% of normal (Laufman and Ericson, 1970). The replacement of one blood volume by donor blood or priming fluid leaves 34–40% of the patient's own blood and the replacement of two blood volumes leaves only 13%. Hence addition of further fluids during bypass, other than plasma, may produce a hypocoagulable state.

Pre-existing coagulation disorders are not uncommon in children with cyanotic congenital heart disease (Ekert *et al.*, 1970). Defective clot retraction due to high haematocrit, prolonged bleeding time (BT), prolonged prothrombin time (PT) and partial thrombin time (PTT), low fibrinogen with accelerated fibrinolysis, have all been reported. We have observed accelerated fibrinolysis due to fasting, stress, anaesthesia, in addition to perfusion in these children (Pike *et al.*, 1975). Similarly, pre-existing liver disease can account for mild coagulation disorders such as prolonged PT. Although the condition of the liver may impair the ability to restore the clotting factors after bypass, these patients usually do not bleed excessively (Salzman and Britten, 1965) and transfusion during ECC will correct the abnormality (Salzman and Britten, 1965). During operation, excessive oozing may occur; this may be due to the use of preoperative medication such as aspirin. Exceptionally, haemoglobinuria occurs due to excessive haemolysis during perfusion which can cause increased bleeding. The bleeding is due to a limited form of diffuse intravascular coagulation (DIC), effectively controlled by the heparin used during perfusion.

In the postoperative phase, it is not uncommon to find low fibrinogen levels with increased fibrin degradation products and depleted clotting factors II, V, VII, VIII and X due to consumption during ECC (Woods *et al.*, 1967; Bachmann *et al.*, 1975). In addition, prolonged BT with abnormal platelet functions is commonly observed in some patients. There is a direct association between the BT and the number of units of blood transfused during surgery (McKenna *et al.*, 1975; Crow, Kaul and Rajah, 1979).

Following heparin neutralization, any excessive postoperative bleeding is best managed as follows: any patient who bleeds more than 600 ml during the first 3h after open heart surgery, should be evaluated with a coagulation screen, platelet count and BT. If the coagulation screen is normal but BT prolonged and/or platelet count is low, an infusion of 6 units of platelet concentrate is suggested and if the haematocrit is also low, fresh whole blood should be transfused. If the coagulation screen and BT are normal, an exploration of the operative site should be performed without delay as the commonest cause of postoperative bleeding after bypass is inadequate surgical haemostasis. Exceptionally, if depletion of specific coagulation factors is present, this should be corrected. A small number of patients, especially following reoperation, may tend to ooze and bleed excessively; they benefit from fresh whole blood, fresh frozen plasma, cryoprecipitate and platelet concentrate.

If the bleeding is excessive in spite of the above measures, there is then the option for the judicious use of an antifibrinolytic agent such as Cyklokapron (tranexamic acid) with close monitoring and laboratory control. Recent work has shown that the naturally occurring enzyme inhibitor aprotonin, given in high doses, reduced intra and postoperative bleeding (Dietrich, Jochim and Schram, 1989). There is evidence that this is achieved by a reduction of fibrinolysis and contact activation during bypass. Aprotonin is now sometimes included with heparin in the priming fluid for CPB. A further therapeutic approach to minimize postoperative bleeding in patients undergoing complex cardiac operations, is the use of desmopressin (DDAVP). This is a synthetic analogue of vasopressin without vasoconstrictor activity. It is administered after the neutralization of heparin by protamine sulphate (Salzman *et al.*, 1986).

Heparin administered during ECC and its reversal with protamine sulphate

Heparinization of patients under going CPB operations should be according to an individualized protocol rather than a 'fixed' dose protocol (Table 10.1) (Bull *et al.*, 1975; Kaul, 1979). In most instances, an initial heparin dose of 3 mg kg^{-1} body weight with confirmation that this has achieved an activated cephalin time (ACT) of at least 400 s, should be optimum (Figure 10.1). A high heparin dose may be needed in paediatric patients, patients with infective endocarditis and patients who have been on long term heparin treatment (Claes, 1989). Regular ACT measurements during CPB should guide the heparin supplementation needed to maintain ACT in the optimum range of 400–900 s.

The protamine dose needed for reversal of the heparin effect is still debatable. A working approach would be to give 0.75 g per 100 units of initial heparin needed to reach an ACT of over 400 s, supplemented with repeat small doses of protamine. The supplementary doses should be based on measurement of plasma heparin levels; due to the short half life, there is no advantage in giving excess protamine. Protamine is well tolerated by most patients; however, arterial hypotension is reported to have occurred in patients with poor left ventricular function. The rate of administration seems to be of no significance (Claes, 1989).

The term heparin rebound implies reappearance of heparin in blood following its neutralization at the end of bypass as demonstrated in Figure 10.2. There is a correlation between the rebound of

Table 10.1 Comparison of protocols for heparinization of patients during cardiopulmonary bypass.

	Protocol 1 *Arbitrary*	*Protocol 2* *Individual 3 mg kg^{-1}*
No of patients	44	27
Age (years)	21/12–67 (29.6 mean)	5/12–65 (31.4 mean)
Weight (kg)	7.5–81.5 (43.6 mean)	3.8–84 (47.4 mean)
No. of adults >14 years	24	15
No. of children <14 years	20	12
Total heparin dose (mg)	25–500 (231 mean)	18–380 (182 mean)
Total protamine dose (mg)	70–600 (327 mean)	40–600 (311 mean)
Heparin in prime (mg)	57–180 (127 mean)	21–76 (66 mean)
Time on perfusion (min)	19–165 (112 mean)	42–152 (104 mean)
Times between heparin given (min) and commencing perfusion	2–30 (13.7 mean)	2–21 (11.9 mean)
No. patients given extra heparin	26 (59%)	13 (48%)

From Kaul *et al.*, 1979, by courtesy of *Journal of Thoracic and Cardiovascular Surgery*

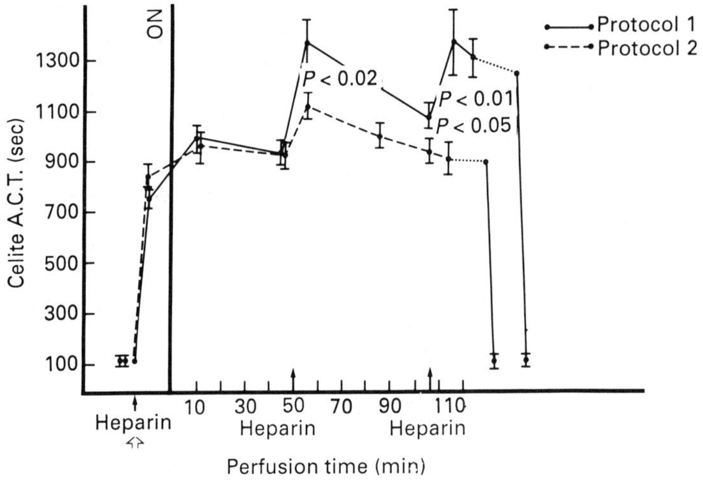

Figure 10.1 Anticoagulation monitored by celite activated cephalin time (ACT) during extracorporeal circulation (ECC). (From Kaul *et al.*, 1979, by courtesy of *Journal of Thoracic and Cardiovascular Surgery*)

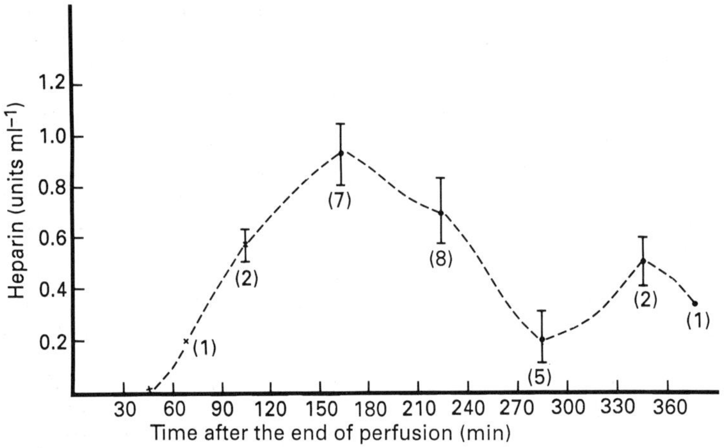

Figure 10.2 Mean heparin levels in ten patients with heparin rebound for 6h postperfusion; (*n*) number at any one time. (From Kaul *et al.*, 1979, by courtesy of *Journal of Thoracic and Cardiovascular Surgery*)

heparin and increased postoperative bleeding (Kaul *et al.*, 1979); an example is shown in Table 10.2. The incidence of heparin rebound after ECC has varied from 0 to 50% (Claes *et al.*, 1989). The mechanism of rebound of heparin is not quite clear, however it is thought to be due to the release of heparin into the extravascular compartment and later returning into circulating blood via the lymphatics.

Blood and blood component therapy

Most of the hazards of CPB are eclipsed by the danger of transfusing incompatible blood. The outcome of a mismatched transfusion can range from mild haemolytic reaction, through pyrexia, to severe haemolytic reaction which can often lead to DIC and renal failure. It is imperative that all members of the surgical and intensive care team are fully aware of the serious consequences that may follow. There is also the growing fear of transmission of human immunodeficiency virus (HIV) and to a lesser degree, hepatitis. For these reasons, an increasing number of cardiac surgeons now operate with little or no donor blood. However, sufficient blood and blood products should always be available and cross-matched when necessary in case of

Table 10.2 Incidence of heparin rebound and postoperative blood loss according to protocol. (From Kaul *et al.*, 1979 by courtesy of *Journal of Thoracic and Cardiovascular Surgery*)

Protocol 1 *Arbitrary*		*Protocol 2* *Individual 3 mg* kg^{-1}	
Rebound (10 patients)	No rebound (14 patients)	Rebound (0 patients)	No rebound (20 patients)
Blood loss 575 ml m^2	Blood loss 183 ml m^2		Blood loss 120 ml m^2

Rebound (Protocol 1) vs no rebound (Protocol 1): *P*<0.001

Rebound (Protocol 1) vs no rebound (Protocol 2): *P*<0.001

emergency. All donations are now tested for antibodies to the viral agents of HIV, hepatitis A, B and C (non-A, non-B). This greatly reduces the risk of transmitted infection, but does not eliminate it. Very little whole blood is now transfused, because of their different storage potentials and optimal conditions, components are separated soon after collection and stored until required. Fresh frozen plasma (FFP) is stored below –40°C for many months with minimal deterioration of coagulation factor function. Platelet concentrates (PC) are stored at 22°C (Slichter, 1981) in sufficient plasma to sustain their metabolism (Archer *et al.*, 1982; Murphy *et al.*, 1982; Rock and Blanchette, 1982), an average unit of platelet concentrate contains about 0.55×10^{11} platelets in 50 ml plasma. Current techniques allow PCs to be stored for up to 7 days and retain viability, as determined by *in vitro* tests and survival studies (Hogge and Schiffer, 1983; Penny *et al.*, 1984; Robinson *et al.*, 1985). Because of the short life of platelets relative to erythrocytes, many transfusion centres now collect PC and FFP by machine apheresis returning the surplus erythrocytes and leucocytes to the donor immediately (Hogge and Schiffer, 1983; Robinson *et al.*, 1985). Much of the FFP is fractionated in bulk to yield purified clotting factors VIII and IX and human albumin solution (HAS) with a very low antigenicity. However, a small proportion of FFP is processed to cryoprecipitate which contains factor VIII, fibrinogen and fibronectin. Packed red cells, in a solution of SAGM, are stored at 4°C for 35 days – this synthetic medium preserves erythrocyte function and maintains isotonicity.

Although there is some loss of function of formed elements and deterioration in clotting factors in stored blood which can contribute to postoperative bleeding, the primary event most probably occurs in the patient or extracorporeal circuit. It has, however, been demonstrated that prophylactic administration of FFP does not reduce blood loss (Kaplan *et al.*, 1977; Roy *et al.*, 1988). Even when diluted by the priming fluid, the circulating clotting factors remain more than adequate (Milam *et al.*, 1981). Platelet dysfunction, not coagulation protein deficiency, appears to be the most likely non-surgical cause of bleeding problems after bypass (Harker *et al.*, 1980; Harker, 1986). There is substantial evidence that despite the damage to platelets during bypass, there is no benefit to be gained from prophylactic administration of PC or fresh blood. These should be reserved for patients who develop thrombocytopenia as well as haemorrhagic complications (Harding, Shakoor and Grindon, 1975).

Microemboli and blood filtration

Microemboli have been implicated in the pathogenesis of pulmonary and cerebral dysfunction after ECC. Hill *et al.* (1969) demonstrated a high incidence of cerebral emboli in patients who died after open heart surgery. Lee *et al.* (1971) have documented the occurrence of neurological deficits and acute mental aberration in the postoperative phase. A third of their patients demonstrated some form of cerebral dysfunction on careful clinical assessment and objective analysis.

The emboli are usually composed of platelet aggregates, leucocytes, fat, denaturated protein or air. The extracorporeal circuit and banked blood are the main source of microemboli which are usually removed when blood passes through the capillary beds of the body. Platelet and leucocyte aggregates form in stored blood with heparin or citrate anticoagulant, within a few hours in heparin but delayed for 2–10 days in acid citrate dextrose (ACD) (Swank, 1961). However, because of the higher pH, aggregates form more rapidly in CPD.A (Solis and Gibbs, 1972). The standard red cell product now available is packed cells resuspended in optimal additive solution (SAGM). However, SAGM blood contains microaggregates (Robertson *et al.*, 1985) as well as macroaggregates; the latter would be removed by a clot screen (170–230 μm) present in blood giving sets (Robertson *et al.*, 1985; Bolton and Peeters, 1988). However, microaggregates pass through these screens and are present in significant numbers in all SAGM and CPD.A blood which, therefore, continue to present a problem. Microaggregates can be detected using either a coulter counter or a laser microphotometer, for instance, aggregates in size range 20–200μm have been estimated at $25–35 \times 10^6$ microaggregates per unit in 1 week old blood and $5–25 \times 10^7$ at 10–15 days storage (Solis and Gibbs, 1972; Eisart, Ostertag and Nieman, 1976). An alternative to counting aggregates is the measurement of screen filtration pressure (SFP) as described by Swank and Porter, 1963). This is the pressure required to force blood of standardized haematocrit through a micropore filter of known pore size. Simple measurement of the peak SFP does not correlate with microaggregate counting (Risberg, 1980), but analysis of the SFP curve and slope is a reproducible measure of microaggregates both in stored and fresh blood (McCollum and Campbell, 1979).

In the ECC during oxygenation, the process of microaggregate formation from leucocytes and platelets is speeded up. The direct oxygen–blood interface is incriminated in this effect, as the SFP is normal if no oxygen is passed through the bubble oxygenator or a membrane oxygenator is used (Ashmore, Svitek and Ambrose, 1968). An increase in SFP has also been demonstrated when the patient's blood mixes with priming blood in the ECC. Blood from the mediastinum and pericardium returned via the cardiotomy suckers is another source of emboli. Hence to eliminate the risk of embolization, several experts studied the use of filters during ECC. Swank and Porter (1963) showed that aggregates pass through the stainless steel mesh filters (pore size 100–150 μm) used in early pump oxygenators. They were successfully removed by filtration through packed fibreglass wool or Dacron wool (pore size 20 μm) (Swank and Porter, 1963) or stainless steel mesh filters (pore size 25 μm) (Patterson, Kessler and Bergland, 1971). However, stainless steel filters do not have sufficient surface area for the flow rates required in adult cardiac surgery and Dacron wool cylindrical depth filters proved most effective (McNamara, Burran and Suchiro, 1972; Solis and Gibbs, 1972).

Following the introduction of microporous filtration, significant improvements were reported in perioperative deaths, postoperative mental state and incidence of fat emboli to the brain (Egeblad *et al.*, 1972). In current practice, screen filters, usually made of biocompatible polyesters of about 28 μm pore size, are used. These allow rapid flow for a longer period without clogging than depth filters and without inducing haemolysis (Buley and Lumley, 1975). As an additional precaution, ultrasonic detectors are used on the arterial line to identify air bubbles.

Biocompatibility of materials in contact with blood

In recent years much interest has centred on the propensity of materials, notably nylon, used in ECC to activate the complement system and release anaphylotoxins C3a and C5a (Chenoweth *et al.*, 1981; Kirklin *et al.*, 1983; Hill *et al.*, 1984). The complex circuit of the pump oxygenator and associated peripherals offers an ideal model for activation of complement (Cavarocchi *et al.*, 1986; Tamiya *et al.*, 1988), involving both the classical and alternative pathways (Jones *et al.*, 1982). New materials with improved biocompatibility are being sought (Chenoweth, 1987) to reduce the contact effects.

Autologous blood transfusion and blood salvage autotransfusion

A combination of these procedures has reduced the demand for homologous transfusion (compatible donor blood). They also reduce the risk of transmission of hepatitis and HIV but do not eliminate it since a large proportion of CPB patients still require homologous blood. They reduce the risk of alloimmunization in patients who may need a repeat blood transfusion at a later date. Most of the blood in an extracorporeal circuit can be returned to the patient at the end of surgery. If a relatively small amount of the patient's own blood can also be obtained before operation (predeposit), the complete transfusion requirement can sometimes be met without adverse effects (Cove *et al.*, 1976). Patients who, for example, refuse homologous transfusion on religious grounds, may make predeposit donations to be returned after the operation, in addition to blood salvage during the operation, this can meet their transfusion requirements.

There are, however, limitations to the autologous predeposit donations in practice. The collection, labelling and storage of the donations is time consuming and can be expensive. In addition, meticulous care is mandatory in identifying the appropriate predeposit and routine check of blood group and cross-matching is essential as the patient who was the donor has now become the recipient of a blood transfusion. If the surgical procedure is delayed for any reason, the blood will soon become outdated. Only a limited amount of blood can be withdrawn from the patient within the short period of time before operation. The recommended maximum is 500 ml every 3 days, provided the haematocrit is above 34% and the haemoglobin is over 11.4 g dl^{-1}. There is also a small but serious risk that the patient on medication may develop an allergy between donation and transfusion, hence all but essential medication should be stopped a few days before donation.

The practice of intra- and perioperative blood salvage has increased more rapidly and more widely than predeposit donation. Shed blood is collected from a wound or body cavity during or after surgery and reinfused after a varying degree of processing to reduce complications. In the mid 1960s, a centrifugal cell washing system was introduced to prepare shed erythrocytes for reinfusion (Wilson and Taswell, 1968). Since then a number of systems have been developed, tested and made commercially available (Gilcher and Orr, 1979). The early systems did not concentrate the cells before infusion

Table 10.3 Reduction in platelet count and function during vascular surgery and cell salvage using Solcotrans

	Preoperative	*Postheparinization*	*In operative pool*	*In Solcotrans reservoir*
Count (×10^9)	210 ± 91	165 ± 34	141 ± 26	108 ± 29
Collagen (%)	72 ± 8	58 ± 17	22 ± 22	4 ± 3
ADP (%)	69 ± 9	50 ± 13	22 ± 21	5 ± 9
ATP (nmols)	3.84 ± 1.9	1.47 ± 0.9	1.15 ± 1.2	0.47 ± 0.52
Hb (mg%)				359 ± 198
APTT (s)	47.6 ± 6	528 ± 112	399 ± 109	261 ± 134
Heparin (units ml^{-1})		1.46 ± 0.35	1.04 ± 0.33	0.51 ± 0.16

Values are mean ± s.d.

and often plasma containing activated clotting factors was infused. This was probably responsible for induction of disseminated intravascular coagulation. Possibly microemboli of fat, platelet, leucocytes, tissue products, activated complement and kinins were also infused. In the simple salvage system, there is a significant decrease in platelet numbers, aggregation and ATP content in the acidic, hypocalcaemic and highly haemolysed environment of the blood reservoir (Table 10.3). When large volumes of salvaged blood are transfused, additional fresh platelet concentrates may be required. Several systems now wash and concentrate the erythrocytes before reinfusion and microporous filters should always be incorporated. Their safety has been well established when used under careful management (McKenzie *et al.*, 1978; Orr, 1978) and is most effective when used regularly (Giordano *et al.*, 1988).

There are contraindications to blood salvage, two of these are absolute: recovery of blood exposed to a source of bacteria (Younes and Samuelson, 1978) or possibly contaminated with tumour cells (Yaw *et al.*, 1975). There is the possibility of introducing procoagulant and leucoattractant products from platelets activated by recent exposure to thrombin in partially clotted blood just before washing (Bull *et al.*, 1988). However, substantially clotted blood collected during and after cardiac operation from the mediastinum has been used safely and effectively (Schaff *et al.*, 1978; Cosgrove, Amiot and Meserko, 1985; Hartz, Smith and Green, 1988). The delay in these procedures allowed activated clotting factors and platelets to be inactivated, the transfusion being effectively erythrocytes suspended in serum.

Citrate toxicity

Citrate is an excellent anticoagulant for storing blood: preventing clotting by binding ionized calcium, not being consumed during storage, yet rapidly metabolized by the recipient after transfusion. At moderate infusion rates, its anticoagulant effect is neutralized almost immediately by the recipient's own ionized calcium. However, because the avidity is fairly low, a tenfold excess of citrate is necessary to keep ionized calcium levels low enough to prevent coagulation during storage. A transfusion, therefore, introduces free citrate into the circulation and rapid infusion of citrated blood can be harmful by significantly lowering the recipient's ionized calcium (Collins, 1976). Reaction to citrate can easily be reversed by stopping or slowing the transfusion.

There is uncertainty as to whether these changes interfere with cardiac function and represent an abnormality that should be treated by infusion of calcium. Little evidence of impaired cardiac function, despite ionized calcium concentrations as low as one-third normal, has been found in at least one study (Howland *et al.*, 1977). Administration of calcium chloride pre- or posttransfusion did not always correct the anomalies but simultaneous administration was always effective (Cooper *et al.*, 1973). The 'routine' supplementation with calcium can be harmful (Wolf, McCarthy and Hafleigh, 1970), even with documentation of decreased ionized calcium levels (Carlon *et al.*, 1978).

Monitoring of ionized calcium is advocated in situations where it is likely to be severely depressed or calcium administration considered since both hyper- and hypocalcaemia (ionized) can cause cardiovascular problems. Critical limits have been recommended for ionized calcium as not more than 0.4 mmol l^{-1} above or below the mean normal of 1.18 mmol l^{-1} (Kost *et al.*, 1986). Calcium should be infused with caution in patients with alkalosis, hypoalbuminaemia and hypokalaemia, as rapid infusion of calcium may result in a sudden rise of ionized calcium, exaggerating the effects of hypokalaemia and triggering arrhythmias.

Conclusion

The refinements in materials, technique and technology have made ECC a safe and efficient procedure. Complex cardiac abnormalities are corrected using hypothermia and prolonged circulation.

The blood–gas interface, the cardiotomy sucker and salvage of blood from the operation site, the use of priming fluids, homologous blood and heparin, all induce complex interactions to produce haematological changes.

These changes can be anticipated and countered; however, in the event of unexpected change, postoperative bleed may occur. Postoperative bleeding is investigated and managed from re-exploration of operation site to neutralization of heparin and by the use of blood and blood products.

A case has been made to minimize the use of homologous blood and an alternative strategy using predeposit autologous blood and salvage has been discussed.

Finally, the significance of emboli from air bubbles and aggregates is highlighted and the use of filters discussed.

References

Addonizio, V.P. Jr, Smith, J.B., Strauss, J.F. III, *et al.* (1980) Thromboxane synthesis and platelet secretion during cardiopulmonary bypass with a bubble oxygenator. *Journal of Thoracic and Cardiovascular Surgery*, **79**, 91–96

Archer, G.T., Grimsley, P.G., Jindra, J., *et al.* (1982) Survival of transfused platelets collected into new formulation packs. *Vox Sanguinis*, **43**, 223–230

Ashmore, P.G., Svitek, V. and Ambrose, P. (1968) The incidence and effects of particulate aggregation and microembolism in pump oxygenator systems. *Journal of Thoracic and Cardiovascular Surgery*, **55**, 691–697

Bachmann, F., McKenna, R., Cole, E.R. and Najafi, H. (1975) The hemostatic mechanism after open heart surgery. *Journal of Thoracic and Cardiovascular Surgery*, **70**, 76–85

Bernstein, E.F., Blackshear, P.L. and Keller, K.H. (1967) Factors influencing erythrocyte destruction in artificial organs. *American Journal of Surgery*, **114**, 126–138

Bernstein, E.F., Indeglia, R., Shea, M. and Varco, R. (1967) Sublethal damage to the red blood cell from pumping. *Circulation*, **45** (suppl 1), 226–233

Best, L.C., McGuire, M.B., Jones, P.B.B., *et al.* (1979) Mode of action of dipyridamole on human platelets. *Thrombosis Research*, **16**, 367–377

Blackshear, P.L., Dorman, R. and Steinback, J.H. (1965) Some mechanical effects that influence haemolysis. *Transactions of the American Society for Artificial Internal Organs*, **11**, 112–117

Bolanowski, P.J.P., Bauer, J., Machiedo, G. and Neville, W.E. (1977) Prostaglandin influence on pulmonary intravascular leukocytic aggregation during cardiopulmonary bypass. *Journal of Thoracic and Cardiovascular Surgery*, **73**, 221–224

Bolton, D.T. and Peeters, A. (1988) Microaggregates and filtration. *Anaesthesia*, **43**, 330–331

Buley, R. and Lumley, J. (1975) Some observation on blood microfilters. *Annals of the Royal College of Surgeons of England*, **57**, 262–267

Bull, B.S., Korpman, R.A., Huse, W.M. and Briggs, B.D. (1975) Heparin therapy during extracorporeal circulation: 1 Problems inherent in existing heparin protocols. *Journal of Thoracic and Cardiovascular Surgery*, **69**, 674–684

Bull, M.H., Bull, B.S., Van Arsdell, G.S. and Smith, L.L. (1988) Clinical implications of procoagulant and leucoattractant formation during intraoperative blood salvage. *Archives of Surgery*, **123**, 1073–1078

Carlon, G.C., Howland, W.S., Goldiner, P.L., *et al.* (1978) Adverse effects of calcium administration. *Archives of Surgery*, **113**, 882–885

Cavarocchi, N.C., Pluth, J.R., Schaff, H.V. *et al.* (1986) Complement activation during cardiopulmonary bypass: comparison of bubble and membrane oxygenators. *Journal of Thoracic and Cardiovascular Surgery*, **91**, 252–258

Chenoweth, D.E. (1987) Complement activation in extracorporeal circuits. *Annals of the New York Academy*, **33**, 306–313

Chenoweth, D.E., Cooper, S.W., Hugli, T.E. *et al.* (1981) Complement activation during cardiopulmonary bypass: evidence for generation of C3a and C5a anaphylotoxins. *New England Journal of Medicine*, **304**, 497–533

Chesebro, J.H., Clements, J.P., Fuster, V., *et al.* (1982) A platelet-inhibitor drug trial in coronary artery bypass operations: benefit of perioperative dipyridamole and aspirin therapy on early postoperative vein graft patency. *New England Journal of Medicine*, **307**, 73–78

Claes, A. (1989) Heparin and protamine during cardiac surgery. *Perfusion*, **4**, 171–181

Clowes, G.H.R. (1960) Extracorporeal maintenance of circulation and respiration. *Physiology Reviews*, **40**, 826–919

Collins, J.A. (1976) Massive blood transfusion. *Clinical Haematology*, **5**, 201

Cooper, N., Brazier, J.R., Hottenrott, C., *et al.* (1973) Myocardial depression following citrated blood transfusion. *Archives of Surgery*, **107**, 756–763

Cosgrove, D.M., Amiot, D.M. and Meserko, J.J. (1985) An improved technique for autotransfusion of shed mediastinal blood. *Annals of Thoracic Surgery*, **40**, 519–520

Cove, H., Matloff, J., Sacks, H.J., *et al.* (1976) Autologous blood transfusion in coronary artery bypass surgery. *Transfusion*, **16**, 245

Crow, M.J., Kaul, T.K. and Rajah, S.M. (1979) Blood products in the treatment of acute bleeding complications following open heart surgery. *Thrombosis and Haemostasis*, **42**, 149

Dale, J., Lilleason, P. and Erikssen, J. (1987) Hemostasis after open-heart surgery with extreme or moderate hemodilution. *European Surgical Research*, **19**, 339–347 deLeval, M.R., Hill, J.D. and Mielke, C.H. (1976) Haematological aspects of extracorporeal circulation. In *Current Techniques in Extracorporeal Circulation* (ed M.I. Ionescu and G.H. Wooler), Butterworths, London, pp. 297–319

Dietrich, W., Jochim, M., Schram, W., *et al.* (1989) Reduction of homologous blood requirement in cardiac surgery using high dose Aprotinin. *Anesthesiology*, **71**, Abstract 7

Dutton, R.C., Edmunds, L.H. Jr, Hutchinson, J.C. and Roe, B.B. (1974) Platelet aggregate emboli produced in patients during cardiopulmonary bypass with membrane and bubble oxygenators and blood filters. *Journal of Thoracic and Cardiovascular Surgery*, **67**, 258–265

Edmunds, L.H., Jr, Ellison, N., Colman, R.W. *et al.* (1982) Platelet function during cardiac operations: comparison of membrane and bubble oxygenators. *Journal of Thoracic and Cardiovascular Surgery*, **83**, 805–812

Egeblad, K., Osborn, J.J. and Burns, W. (1972) Blood filtration during cardiopulmonary bypass. *Journal of Thoracic and Cardiovascular Surgery*, **63**, 384–390

Eisart, W.G., Ostertag, R. and Nieman, E.G. (1976) High speed flow through laser microphotometry: a new tool for particle and cell analysis. *Electron Optics Laser International*, **765**, 173

Ekert, H., Gilchrist, G., Stratan, R. and Hammond, D. (1970) Haemostasis in cyanotic congenital heart disease. *Journal of Pediatrics*, **76**, 221–230

Emmons, P.R., Harrison, M.J.G., Honour, A.J. and Mitchell, J.R.A. (1965) Effect of dipyridamole on human platelet behaviour. *Lancet*, **ii**, 603–606

Fountain, S.W., Martin, B.A., Musclow, C.E. and Cooper, J.D. (1980) Pulmonary leukostasis and its relationship to pulmonary dysfunction in sheep and rabbits. *Circulation Research*, **46**, 175–180

Galletti, P.M. (1965) Laboratory experience with 24 hour partial heart-lung bypass. *Journal of Surgical Research*, **5**, 97–104

Gilcher, R.O. and Orr, M. (1979) Intraoperative blood salvage. In *Hemotherapy in Trauma Surgery* (ed. A. Barnes), Washington D.C., American Association of Blood Banks

Giordano, G.F., Goldman, D.S., Mammana, R.B., *et al.* (1988) Intraoperative autotransfusion in cardiac operations: Effect on intraoperative and postoperative transfusion requirements. *Journal of Thoracic and Cardiovascular Surgery*, **96**, 382–386

Gollub, S. and Bailey, C.P. (1969) Management of major surgical blood loss without transfusion. *JAMA*, **198**, 1171–1174

Hammerschmidt, D.E., Stroncek, D.F., Bowers, T.K., *et al.* (1981) Complement activation and neutropenia occurring during cardiopulmonary bypass. *Journal of Thoracic and Cardiovascular Surgery*, **81**, 370–377

Hara, M., Maris, M., Crumpler, J., *et al.* (1967) Effect of various priming solutions upon red cell mass, plasma volume and extracellular fluid volume of dogs following haemodilution techniques of extracorporeal circulation. *Journal of Thoracic and Cardiovascular Surgery*, **53**, 353–359

Harding, S.A., Shakoor, M.A. and Grindon, A.J. (1975) Platelet support for cardiopulmonary bypass surgery. *Journal of Thoracic and Cardiovascular Surgery*, **70**, 350–353

Harker, L.A. (1986) Bleeding after cardiopulmonary bypass (editorial). *New England Journal of Medicine*, **314**, 1446–1448

Harker, L.A., Malpass, T.W., Bronson, H.E., *et al.* (1980) Mechanism of abnormal bleeding in patients undergoing cardiopulmonary bypass: acquired transient platelet dysfunction associated with selective a-granule release. *Blood*, **56**, 824–834

Hartz, R.S., Smith, J.A. and Green, D. (1988) Autotransfusion after cardiac operation: Assessment of hemostatic factors. *Journal of Thoracic and Cardiovascular Surgery*, **96**, 178–182

Hewitt, P.E. and Machin, S.J. (1990) ABC of transfusion: massive blood transfusion. *British Medical Journal*, **300**, 107–109

Hill, J.D., Aquilar, M.J., Baranco, A., *et al.* (1969) Neuropathological manifestations of cardiac surgery. *Annals of Thoracic Surgery*, **7**, 409–419

Hill, A.G., Groom, R.C., Smith, D., *et al.* (1984) Complement activation during cardiopulmonary bypass: polyester vs nylon tricot in the oxygenator. *Proceedings of the American Academy of Cardiovascular Perfusion*, **4**, 17–19

Hogge, D.E. and Schiffer, C.A. (1983) Collection of platelets depleted of red and white cells with the 'surge pump' adaptation of a blood cell separator. *Transfusion*, **23**, 177–181

Hope, A.F., Heyns, A.duP., Lotter, M.G. *et al.* (1981) Kinetics and site of sequestration of indium 111–labeled human platelets during cardiopulmonary bypass. *Journal of Thoracic and Cardiovascular Surgery*, **81**, 880–886

Howland, W.S., Schweizer, O., Carlon, G.C. and Goldiner, P.L. (1977) The cardiovascular effects of low ionized calcium during massive transfusion. *Surgery Gynecology and Obstetrics*, **145**, 581–586

Indeglia, R.A., Dorman, F.D., Castaneda, A.R., *et al.* (1966) Use of GBH-coated Tygon tubing for experimental prolonged perfusions without systemic heparinization. *Transactions of the American Society for Artifical Internal Organs*, **12**, 166–173

Jones, H.M., Matthews, N., Vaughan, R.S. and Stark, J.M. (1982) Cardiopulmonary bypass and complement activation: involvement of classical and alternative pathways. *Anesthesia*, **37**, 629–633

Kaplan, J.A., Cannarella, C., Jones, E.L. *et al.* (1977) Autologous blood transfusion during cardiac surgery. *Journal of Thoracic and Cardiovascular Surgery*, **74**, 4–10

Kaul, T.K., Crow, M.J., Rajah, S.M., *et al.* (1979) Heparin administration during extracorporeal circulation: heparin rebound and post-operative bleeding. *Journal of Thoracic and Cardiovascular Surgery*, **78**, 95–102

Kirklin, J.K., Westaby, S., Blackstone, E.H. *et al.* (1983)

Complement and the damaging effects of cardiopulmonary bypass. *Journal of Thoracic and Cardiovascular Surgery*, **86**, 845–857
Kost, G.J., Jammal, M.A., Ward, R.E. and Safwat, A.M. (1986) Monitoring of ionized calcium during human hepatic transplantation. *American Journal of Clinical Pathology*, **86**, 61–70
Kusserow, B.K. and Clapp, J.F. (1966) Red blood cell survival after prolonged perfusion with a blood pump. *Transactions of the American Society for Artificial Internal Organs*, **12**, 121–123
Laufman, H. and Ericson, R.B. (1970) *Haematological Problems in Surgery*, WB Saunders, Philadelphia
Lee, W.H., Brady, M.P., Rowe, J.M. and Miller, W.C. (1971) Effects of extracorporeal circulation upon behaviour, personality and brain function. Part II. Haemodynamic, metabolic and psycometric correlations. *Annals of Surgery*, **173**, 1013–1023
McCollum, C.N. and Campbell, I.T. (1979) Value of measuring intravascular aggregates in the prediction of postoperative pulmonary dysfunction. *British Journal of Surgery*, **66**, 703–707
McKenna, R., Bachmann, F., Whittaker, B., *et al.* (1975) The hemostatic mechanism after open-heart surgery: II Frequency of abnormal platelet functions during and after extracorporeal circulation. *Journal of Thoracic and Cardiovascular Surgery*, **70**, 298–308
McKenzie, F.N., Heimbecker, R.D., Wall, W., *et al.* (1978) Intraoperative autotransfusion in elective and emergency vascular surgery. *Surgery*, **83**, 470–475
McNamara, J.J., Burran, E.L. and Suchiro, G. (1972) Effective filtration of banked blood. *Surgery (St. Louis)*, **71**, 594–597
Milam, J.D., Austin, S.F., Martin, R.F., *et al.* (1981) Alteration of coagulation and selected clinical chemistry parameters in patients undergoing open heart surgery without transfusion. *American Journal of Clinical Pathology*, **76**, 155–161
Mills, D.C.B., and Smith, J.B. (1971) The influence on platelet aggregation of drugs that affect the accumulation of adenosine 3:5-cyclic monophosphate in platelets. *Biochemical Journal*, **121**, 185–196
Murphy, S., Kahn, R.A., Holme, S., *et al.* (1982) Improved storage of platelets for transfusion in a new container. *Blood*, **60**, 194–200
Neville, W.E., Faber, L.P. and Peacock, H. (1964) Total prime of the disc oxygenator with Ringer's and Ringer's lactate solution for cardiopulmonary bypass: clinical and experimental observations. *Diseases of the Chest*, **45**, 320–327
Orr, M. (1978) Autotransfusion: the use of washed red cells as an adjunct to component therapy. *Surgery*, **84**, 728–730
Patterson, R.H., Kessler, J. and Bergland, R.M. (1971) A filter to prevent cerebral damage during experimental cardiopulmonary bypass. *Surgery, Gynecology and Obstetrics*, **132**, 71–74
Peirce, E.C., II. (1956) *Extracorporeal Circulation for Open-heart Surgery*, Thomas, Springfield
Penny, A.F., Townley, A., Robinson, E.A.E., *et al.* (1984) Pilot study of an automated dual component plasmapheresis collection system. *Apheresis Bulletin*, **2**, 3–12
Peterson, K.A., Dewanjee, M.K. and Kaye, M.P. (1982) Fate of indium 111-labeled platelets during cardiopulmonary bypass performed with membrane and bubble oxygenators. *Journal of Thoracic and Cardiovascular Surgery*, **84**, 39–43
Pike, G.J., Turner, R.L., Manohitharajah, S.M. and Deverall, P.B. (1975) Fibrinolysis in cyanotic and acyanotic children before and after open intracardiac operations with the Bentley Temptrol oxygenator. *Journal of Thoracic and Cardiovascular Surgery*, **69**, 922–926
Risberg, B. (1980) The intriguing relationship between screen filtration pressure, quantity of microaggregates and amount of debris in stored human blood. *Folia Haematologia*, **107**, 273–379
Robertson, M., Boulton, F.E., Doughty, R., *et al.* (1985) Macroaggregates formation in optimum additive red cells. *Vox Sanguinis*, **49**, 259–266
Robinson, E.A.E., Penny, A.F., Norfolk, D.R., *et al.* (1985) Combined high quality platelet and plasma procurement by automated apheresis. *Plasma Therapy and Transfusion Technology*, **6**, 749–760
Rock, G. and Blanchette, V. (1982) Storage of platelets obtained by apheresis techniques. *Plasma Therapy and Transfusion Technology*, **3**, 305–308
Roe, B.B., Hutchinson, J.C. and Swenson, C.E. (1965) High flow body perfusion with calculated hemodilution. *Annals of Thoracic Surgery*, **1**, 581
Roy, C., Stafford, M.A., Hudspeth, M.D. and Meredith, J.W. (1988) Failure of prophylaxis with fresh frozen plasma after cardiopulmonary bypass. *Anesthesiology*, **69**, 254–257
Sacks, T., Moldow, C.F., Craddock, P.R., *et al.* (1978) Oxygen radicals mediate endothelial cell damage by complement-stimulated granulocytes: an *in vitro* model of immune vascular damage. *Journal of Clinical Investigation*, **61**, 1161–1167
Salzman, E. and Britten, A.F.H. (1965) *Hemorrhage and Thrombosis*, Little, Brown and Co., Boston
Salzman, E.W., Weinstein, M.J., Weintrub, R.M., *et al.* (1986) Treatment with desmopressin acetate to reduce blood loss after cardiac surgery. *New England Journal of Medicine*, **314**, 1402–1406
Schaff, H.V., Hauer, J.H., Bell, W.R., *et al.* (1978) Autotransfusion of shed mediastinal blood after cardiac surgery: a prospective study. *Journal of Thoracic and Cardiovascular Surgery*, **75**, 632–641
Slichter, S.J. (1981) *In vitro* measurement of platelet concentrates stored at 4 and 22°C: Correlation with post transfusion platelet viability and function. *Vox Sanguinis*, **40**, (suppl 1), 72–86
Solis, R.T. and Gibbs, M.B. (1972) Filtration of the microaggregates in stored blood. *Transfusion*, **12**, 245–250
Sutera, S.P., Croce, P.A. and Mehrjardi, M. (1972) Hemolysis and subhemolytic alterations of human red blood cells induced by turbulent shear flow. *Transactions of*

the American Society for Artificial Internal Organs, **18**, 335–341

Swank, R.L. (1961) Alterations of blood on storage: measurement of adhesiveness of aging platelets and leukocytes and their removal by filtration. *New England Journal of Medicine*, **265**, 728–733

Swank, R.L. and Porter, G.A. (1963) Disappearance of the microemboli transfused into patients during cardiopulmonary bypass. *Transfusion*, **3**, 192–197

Tamiya, T., Yamasaki, M., Maeo, Y., *et al.* (1988) Complement activation in cardiopulmonary bypass, with special reference to anaphylotoxin production in membrane and bubble oxygenators. *Annals of Thoracic Surgery*, **46**, 47–57

Teoh, K.H., Christakis, G.T., Weisel, R.D. *et al.* (1986) Prevention of myocardial platelet deposition and thromboxane release with dipyridamole. *Circulation*, **74** (5 part 2): III, 145–152

Teoh, K.H., Christakis, G.T., Weisel, R.D. *et al.* (1988) Dipyridamole preserved platelets and reduced blood loss after cardiopulmonary bypass. *Journal of Thoracic and Cardiovascular Surgery*, **96**, 332–341

Teoh, K.H., Fremes, S.E., Weisel, R.D., *et al.* (1987) Cardiac release of prostacyclin and thromboxane A2 during coronary bypass surgery. *Journal of Thoracic and Cardiovascular Surgery*, **93**, 120–126

Trimble, A., Herst, R., Grady, M. and Crookston, J. (1966) Blood loss in open-heart surgery: correlation with laboratory tests for haemostatic function. *Archives of Surgery*, **93**, 323–326

Verska, J.J., Ludington, L.G. and Brewer, L.A. (1974) A comparative study of cardiopulmonary bypass with non-blood and blood prime. *Annals of Thoracic Surgery*, **18**, 72–80

Wilson, J.D. and Taswell, H.F. (1968) Autotransfusion: historical review and preliminary report on a new method. *Mayo Clinic Proceedings*, **43**, 26–35

Wolf, P.L., McCarthy, L.J. and Hafleigh, B. (1970) Extreme hypercalcemia following blood transfusions combined with intravenous calcium. *Vos Sanguinis*, **19**, 544–545

Woods, J.E., Kirklin, J.W., Owens, C.A., *et al.* (1967) Effects of bypass surgery on coagulation-sensitive clotting factors. *Mayo Clinic Proceedings*, **42**, 724–735

Yaw, P.B., Sentani, M., Link, W.J., *et al.* (1975) Tumour cells carried through autotransfusion. Contraindications to intraoperative blood recovery? *JAMA*, **231**, 490

Younes, H.J. and Samuelson, P.N. (1978) Bacteriologic examination of autologous blood. *Southern Medical Journal*, **71**, 1232–1233

11

The role of the complement system during cardiopulmonary bypass

R.S. Bonser and D. Vergani

The development of an extracorporeal method of gas exchange connected to the human circulation and capable of functioning as an artificial heart and lung in order to facilitate cardiac surgery is undoubtedly one of the major milestones of modern medical practice (Dennis *et al.*, 1951; Gibbon, 1953). This extracorporeal circulation consisting of the 'pump' and an oxygenator was the forerunner of commercially available systems of fully disposable oxygenators, reservoirs and tubing systems for heart–lung machines (Bartlett and Gazzaniga, 1981). One consequence of these developments is the obligatory exposure of blood and its constituents to foreign materials and surfaces. Additionally, rotating pumps to maintain flow, suction apparatus to conserve and return blood to the circuit and the phenomena of direct blood–gas interfaces have contributed to a number of postoperative sequelae including anaemia, platelet damage and consumption and complex effects on plasma proteins (Wildevuur, 1980; de Leval *et al.*, 1981). Clinically major pathophysiological changes have been observed including coagulopathies (Gans and Krivit, 1962; Gomes and McGoon, 1970) and profound disturbances of cardiac, pulmonary, renal and cerebral function (Kouchokos and Karp, 1981). These disturbances can to some extent be explained by the interaction of the heart–lung machine with circulating blood (Wildevuur, 1981; Weegmuller, Kazatchkine and Nydegger, 1983; Kirklin, 1986). In addition a systemic inflammatory response, consisting of fever, increased capillary permeability, accumulation of interstital fluid and leucocytosis has been observed (Kirklin *et al.*, 1983; Westaby, 1983). The similarities between this pathophysiology and the known biological activity of the complement-derived anaphylotoxins has prompted extensive investigation of the changes detectable in the complement cascade before, during and after cardiopulmonary bypass. The extent, pathways of activation and consequences of complement activation during cardiopulmonary bypass have been partially determined and this report reviews these findings. As studies of complement activation during cardiopulmonary bypass have evolved, different workers have used different methods of estimation of complement activation and this has led to debate and confusion regarding the nature and extent of activation during cardiopulmonary bypass (Boralessa *et al.*, 1982; Collett *et al.*, 1984). This review is divided into several parts. Firstly, the structure, function and pathways of complement activation are described. Secondly a brief section discusses the methods of assaying complement activation and their interpretation. Following this, the results of studies of complement activation during cardiopulmonary bypass are reviewed including the role of heparin and protamine. The evidence connecting complement activation during cardiopulmonary bypass and postoperative morbidity are presented and possible methods of attenuating the complement activation responses are discussed.

The pathways of complement activation

Long before its contribution to the human immune system was elucidated the existence of complement was known. A bactericidal action of non-sensitized serum was discovered in the late nineteenth century (Loos, 1982). This action is destroyed by heating and is no longer present in serum left to stand at room temperature for many hours. Initially this heat-labile activity of serum which complemented the heat-stable action of antibody was named 'alexine' though this was gradually replaced by the name *complement*. Pillemer (1943) defined complement as that 'portion of the fresh blood, serum or plasma which is not increased on immunisation and which, when added to certain sensitised cells combines with these sensitised cells and under appropriate conditions results in their destruction or death'.

It is now known that the complement system consists of at least 20 distinct proteins capable of interacting with one another, with antibody and with cell membranes. The component proteins circulate in an inactive state and activation proceeds along a cascading pathway analogous to the cascades of blood coagulation, fibrinolysis and kinin formation (Sundsmo and Fair, 1983). In the complement activation sequence, cleavage and complex reassembly of parent protein components occurs, the product of one reaction becoming a catalyst for the next (Lachmann and Peters, 1982; Müller-Eberhard and Miescher, 1985; Roitt *et al.*, 1986). Inherent in the properties of such biological cascades is the ability for signal amplification to occur, the production and release of biologically active fragments and control of activation within the body afforded by positive and negative feedback loops and naturally occurring circulating chemical inhibitors (Sundsmo and Fair, 1983).

The primary role of the complement system is to mediate and amplify antigen–antibody reactions (Lachmann and Peters, 1982; Müller-Eberhard and Miescher, 1985; Ross, 1986; Cooper, 1987; Whaley, 1987; Law and Reid, 1988). Its beneficial and harmful effects are dependent upon antibody specificity. Thus if the complement-fixing antibody is directed to a pathogenic micro-organism, the result will be beneficial to the host organism. Alternatively if the complement cascade is either unrestrained or directed against autologous tissue, the result will be ultimately harmful to the host (Ruddy and Austen, 1970; Fauci, Haynes and Katz, 1978; Williams and Peters, 1982).

Terminology

There exists a standard nomenclature for the designation of complement proteins (Law and Reid, 1988). The native precursors of the classical and common pathways are designated by the capital letter C followed by a numeral e.g. C1, C2, C9. Proteins of the alternative pathway are given capital letters e.g. factor B, D, P, etc. Fragments derived from enzymatic cleavage of the parent molecule are identified by a small letter following the designation of the original parent molecule e.g. $C4_a$, $C4_b$, B_a, B, where 'a' denotes the smaller fragment. The prefix 'i' indicates enzymatic inactivation of a moiety e.g. $iC3_b$, whereas activation is denoted by an overbar above the symbols of the moiety e.g. $\overline{C4_b2_a}$.

Complement activation

The complement cascade contributes to the innate immunity in man and is one of the principal effectors of the humoral arm of the immune system (Lachmann and Peters, 1982; Müller-Eberhard and Miescher, 1985; Ross, 1986; Cooper, 1987; Whaley, 1987; Law and Reid, 1988). The role of the complement system in human disease is exemplified in two ways. Firstly individuals deficient in one or more components of the cascade have an increased susceptibility to a range of diseases (Agnello, 1978; Frank, 1987). Secondly in various disorders in which tissue damage has an immune basis, involvement of the complement system as a pathogenic effector is demonstrated by evidence of activation of the cascade (Ruddy and Austen, 1970; Fauci, Haynes and Katz, 1978; Williams and Peters, 1982).

The proteins which comprise the complement cascade represent 3–4 $g\,l^{-1}$ of the total protein content of human serum, making them one of the largest constituents (Lachmann and Peters, 1982). Circulating complement components are synthesized in the liver (Alper *et al.*, 1980) a fact well demonstrated by a change in allotype between recipient and donor complement molecules following liver transplantation. Others cells, including macrophages are capable of secreting complement proteins and may contribute to the supply of complement proteins at the sites of acute inflammation (Colten, 1985). The cascade unfolds in a similar manner to the other well characterized pathways such as blood coagulation, fibrinolysis and kinin formation, all of which share certain features in common (Sundsmo and Fair, 1983).

There are three recognized pathways of complement activation (Figure 11.1); the classical (Porter and Reid, 1979; Loos, 1982), alternative (Kazatchkine and Nydegger, 1982; Pangburn and Müller-Eberhard, 1984) and common pathways (Müller-Eberhard, 1984). Detailed descriptions of the sequential activation of the complement cascade can be found elsewhere (Lachmann and Hugh-Jones, 1985; Pangburn, 1986; Reid, 1986) but the following will briefly cover this report. Most of the complement components exist as inactive precursors and when activated they function as proteolytic enzymes cleaving the next parent molecular component and thereby activating the next step of the cascade. In this way, triggering of a single molecule at the beginning of the cascade can lead to activation of thousands of later components as the activated enzyme is capable of processing multiple substrate molecules.

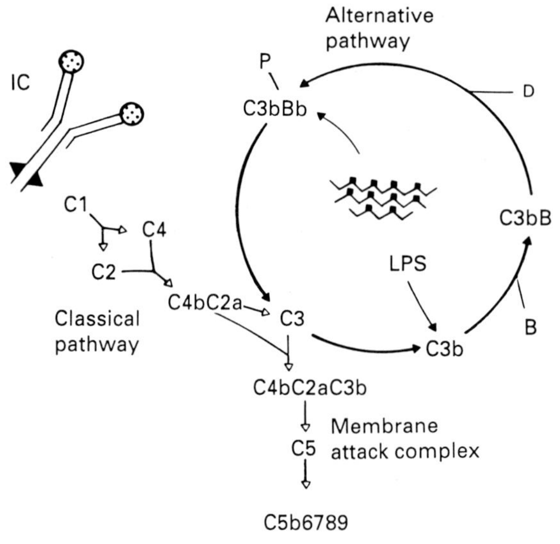

Figure 11.1 Diagram of pathways of complement activation. Classical pathway activation initiated by immune complex (IC) formation is shown. Alternative pathway activation by bacterial lipopolysaccharides or extracorporeal circuit polymers is depicted within the alternative pathway positive feedback loop. (Reproduced with permission from Vergani, D. (1986) Complement, *Diabetic Medicine*, John Wiley)

Classical pathway

The first component of complement C1 consists of three subcomponents named $C1_q$, $C1_r$ and $C1_s$ which are capable of reassociating into the functionally active C1 when exposed to Ca^{++} ions but not Mg^{++} ions. The predominant *in vivo* activating mechanism of C1 is by its exposure to the immunoglobulins IgG or IgM in complex with antigen. Other immunoglobulin classes including IgA, IgD, IgE and certain subclasses of IgG are incapable of activating the classical pathway. The Fc fragment of the immunoglobulin is capable of binding the $C1_q$ moiety of complement. IgM, which exists as a pentamer, has several Fc regions available for binding $C1_q$. These are only accessible for reaction when a configurational change in the IgM molecule has occurred upon combination with antigen. Thus a single antigen-bound IgM molecule is capable of activating the first complement component and the classical complement activation sequence. Similarly, the $C1_q$ binding site of IgG is also located on the Fc portion of the antibody but at least two IgG molecules, bound to antigen in close proximity, are necessary to activate a single C1 molecule (Loos, 1982). The separate human IgG subclasses have different binding affinities for $C1_q$ and C1.

Once the heavy chains of antigen-bound immunoglobulin are exposed to $C1_q$ a change occurs such that $C1_r$ is activated to $\overline{C1_r}$, which in turn activates $C1_s$ to form the serine esterase $\overline{C1_s}$. This esterase subsequently activates and cleaves two further complement parent molecules C4 and C2. C4 is primarily divided into $C4_a$ and $C4_b$. The major component $C4_b$ remains attached to the antigen-containing cell membrane surface. C2 is cleaved into two fragments $C2_a$ and $C2_b$. $C2_a$ combines with $C4_b$ and is added to the developing complex on the membrane surface. This complex depicted $C4_b2_a$ is relatively unstable and may spontaneously release its C2 component rendering it inactive. Under favourable conditions, however, the $\overline{C4_b2_a}$ complex acts as a C3 convertase i.e. an enzyme capable of cleaving and thus activating the C3 parent molecule into $C3_b$, the larger component which becomes principally membrane bound and $C3_a$, an anaphylatoxin, which is released into the fluid phase. Additional molecules of $C3_b$ bind to the membrane surface and form an opsonic coat for immune adherence and phagocytosis. The complex $\overline{C4_b2_a3_b}$ acts as a C5 amplification convertase, cleaving C5 into $C5_a$ and $C5_b$ and proceeding thence as part of the common pathway of activation, common to both classical and alternative pathways. The classical pathway is controlled in its initial stages by the circulating inhibitor C1 esterase inhibitor which blocks the function of activated C1 and which when deficient leads to a chronic situation of unbridled classical pathway activity and the clinical syndrome of angioneurotic oedema (Metzger *et al.*, 1984). C1 esterase inhibitor is capable of inhibiting not only activated $\overline{C1}$ but also its sub-components $\overline{C1_r}$ and $\overline{C1_s}$. It is also capable of inhibiting plasmin, kallikrein, activated plasma thromboplastin antecedent (factor XIa) and activated Hageman factor (factor XIIa). It is thus a multi-specific inhibitor of the complement, coagulation, kinin and fibrinolytic cascades. The effective inhibitory contribution of C1 esterase inhibitor on each of the cascades will vary according to its potency in each specific inhibitory reaction. Although other, more specific inhibitors, exist for the coagulation and fibrinolytic systems, C1 inhibitor is of great importance in the control of complement activation and kinin formation (Cooper, 1985).

The alternative pathway

The alternative pathway also converges on the C3 activation stage. Unlike the classical pathway it is in a state of continuous low grade activation caused by the tendency of C3 to undergo hydrolysis to $C3_b$ (Kazatchkine and Nydegger, 1982). The alternative pathway represents a natural system of infection resistance and recognition of foreign substances even in the absence of antibody. A variety of microbial polysaccharides, such as zymosan from yeast (Pillemer *et al.*, 1954), lipopolysaccharide from

Gram-negative bacteria (Marcus *et al.*, 1981) and teichoic acid from pneumococci (Winklestein and Thomasz, 1978) are recognized and lead to alternative pathway activation. A number of viral, helminthic and protozoal organisms may also be killed by the alternative pathway mechanisms without immune complex reactions. Alternative pathway activation may also occur during contact between plasma and artificial materials (Jacob, 1980; Weegmuller *et al.*, 1983; McLeod, Viernes and Sassett, 1983; Craddock *et al.*, 1977a).

The most important step in the activation of the alternative pathway is the formation of the amplification C3 convertase $\overline{C3_b,B_b}$. This convertase ($\overline{C3_b,B_b}$) is able to cleave the parent molecule C3 thereby producing $C3_b$ and $C3_a$. The major fragment $C3_b$ is capable of binding to cell membranes and surfaces and once bound may recruit the alternative pathway components. Protein B is acted upon enzymatically by factor D, leading to the assembly of more $\overline{C3_b,B_b}$ complexes and releasing the small fragment B_a, in a positive feedback mechanism. This amplification is restrained by circulating inhibitory proteins H and I. Factors H and B appear to compete for a common site on the $C3_b$ molecule. Inhibition or activation of $C3_b$ depends upon the nature of the surface to which $C3_b$ is bound. In the fluid phase, or when bound to non-activating surfaces, factor H binding occurs. When bound to activating surfaces such as zymosan, factor B binding leads to the formation of cell-bound C3 convertase. The binding of factor H to $C3_b$ exposes $HC3_b$ to enzymatic degradation by the $C3_b$ inactivator, factor I, leading to loss of haemolytic and immunoadherence activity. Proteins H and I, prevent the amplification of C3 cleavage in plasma and by regulating the function of the surface-bound convertase allow discrimination between activating and non-activating cells and particles for the alternative pathway. These finely tuned interactions prevent massive alternative pathway activation occurring as may happen in experimental situations e.g. following zymosan or insulin injection. Although the alternative pathway phylogenetically precedes the classical pathway and is capable of proceeding independently there are several interdependent features. Activation of the classical pathway and deposition of $C3_b$ on the cell surface membrane or immune complex is capable of recruiting the alternative pathway proteins to form $\overline{C3_b,B_b}$. In addition, although the alternative pathway represents a humoral defence mechanism in a non-immune host it can in certain circumstances be recruited by antigen-antibody complexes.

The role of C3

The complement parent molecule C3 acts as the hub of the complement cascade. Once either the classical or alternative pathway has resulted in the formation of a C3 convertase, cleavage of C3 occurs, the biologically active products of the complement cascade are produced and further activation proceeds via the common pathway. C3 is the most abundant complement component in serum and is the specific substrate for classical and alternative pathway C3 convertase. Cleavage of C3 generates a small fragment $C3_a$, known as an anaphylatoxin because of its ability to trigger the degranulation of mast cells and to release mediators of inflammation (Hughli and Müller-Eberhard, 1978). The other product of cleavage is $C3_b$. $C3_b$ as previously mentioned binds to cell surfaces and has a number of functions. Firstly it can bind factor B and serve as a subunit of cell-bound alternative pathway C3 amplification convertase $\overline{C3_b,B_b}$. It also facilitates the cleavage of C5 by $\overline{C3_b(n),B_b}$ convertase, binds the regulatory proteins P and H and acts as an opsonin by mediating immune adherence of cells expressing $C3_b$ receptor. Inactivation of plasma $C3_b$ occurs upon its proteolytic fragmentation by factor I and results in its ability to form further cell bound C3 amplification convertase. Inactive $C3_b$, $iC3_b$, is further broken down by a variety of naturally available proteases including, trypsin, plasmin and leucocyte elastase, generating the less biologically active split products $C3_c$ and $C3_d$. Further degradation and production of mildly active further fragments such as $C3_e$ may occur.

The common pathway

The C3 convertase of the classical and alternative pathways are both capable of binding additional molecules of $C3_b$ and forming the C5 amplification convertase. The classical pathway enzyme is denoted $\overline{C4_b2_b3_b}$ and the alternative pathway enzyme $\overline{C3_bB_b3_b}$ or $\overline{C3_b(n),B_b}$. C5 is split by either of these enzymes into $C5_a$ and $C5_b$ fragments. $C5_a$ is another anaphylatoxin capable of increasing vascular permeability both directly and via mast cell degranulation. It is also the most potent chemotactic agent for polymorphs of the complement cascade and activates neutrophils leading to a burst of cytotoxic oxygen-derived free radical production, extracellular release of lysosomal enzymes and other vascular permeability factors. The larger $C5_b$ fragment binds to the surface membrane and complexes with protein C6 and C7 leading to the assembly of a cytolytic membrane insertion complex. Recruitment of the component C8 leads to polymerization of C9 and formation of the membrane attack complex capable of creating 'holes' or transmembrane channels in the cell membrane. This leads to full permeability of the affected cell membrane and subsequent osmotic lysis.

The role of complement in host defence

Cytolysis

Completion of the complement cascade with formation of the membrane attack complex leads to the lysis of certain Gram-negative organisms and other organisms, whether induced by classical pathway activation with antigen–antibody reactions or via the alternative pathway activation due to cell wall endotoxin lipopolysaccharide (Müller-Eberhard, 1984).

Immune adherence

This would appear to be the major biological role of the complement system. The deposition of $C3_b$ and to a lesser extent $C4_b$ on the micro-organism cell surface facilitates the adherence of cells with $C3_b$ receptors. $C3_b$ receptors are present on neutrophils, eosinophils and macrophages including monocytes, Kupffer cells and alveolar macrophages. Immunoadherence promotes subsequent phagocytosis. $C3_b$ bound to cell membrane undergoes a change in antigenic configuration which can provoke the formation of immunoconglutinin, a circulating antibody. This may play a role in the agglutination of small complexes making them more susceptible to phagocytosis (Lachmann, 1966) and may be an important marker of chronic complement activation.

Immune complex solubilization

The alternative pathway C3 convertase once stabilized on surface membranes is capable of covalently binding to immunoglobulin molecules, preventing and reversing the formation of large antibody–antigen aggregates which may be difficult for phagocytes to digest and may provoke hypersensitivity reactions. In addition a role for $C3_b$ in the regulation of the antibody production responses of B cells is speculated.

Production of biologically active inflammatory fragments

The fragments $C3_a$, $C5_a$ and to a lesser extent $C4_a$ act as anaphylatoxins and stimulate two helpful inflammatory reactions in controlled conditions (Hughli and Müller-Eberhard, 1978; Hughli, 1984). Chemotactic activity leads to an influx of neutrophil polymorphonuclear leucocytes to the site of the complement activation. Anaphylatoxins precipitate mast cell degranulation releasing histamine and other vasoactive substances leading to increased blood flow and vascular permeability at the site of microbial invasion (Hughli, 1979).

Methods of measuring complement activation

Assessment of complement activation involves estimation of both the extent of activation and the pathways involved. Interpretation of reports depends upon the factors measured to assess activation and the analytical technique used for its determination. Only fresh blood is suitable for complement estimations and requires immediate arrest of clotting by the addition of ethylenediaminine-tetracetic acid (EDTA) which chelates Ca^{++} and Mg^{++}, to prevent *in vitro* activation. Prompt separation and storage at –70°C if not lower temperatures is necessary. Serum levels of complement components reflect a balance between synthesis, utilization and catabolism. Parent molecule concentrations may be elevated in the acute phase response obscuring the presence of consumption through activation. The absence of parent molecule depletion is not confirmation of the absence of complement activation. Commonly used laboratory assays fall into four groups:

1. functional complement assays,
2. measurement of intact components of complement,
3. measurement of biologically active fragments and
4. measurement of split products.

Functional complement assays

The complement cascade is capable of mediating the lysis of red blood cells coated with a specific antierythrocyte antibody. This ability has been exploited as the Complement Haemolytic 50 (CH50) assay (Mayer, 1961). Reduced activity in serum suggests complement activation but could also be the result of reduced synthesis or non-activated consumption or denaturation of any molecule in the C1–C9 sequence. These assays assess the whole of the classical and common pathways but require a 50% reduction in a component to compromise the haemolytic activity (Cooper, 1987). Similar assays can be used to measure haemolytic activity for single factors or pathways but require extreme care in specimen handling.

Measurement of intact components of complement

Information can also be derived by the measurement of intact complement parent molecule concentrations (Cooper, 1986). A reduced level of serum complement factors such as C3 and C4 may indicate complement consumption due to activation of the cascades. Accurate interpretation of parent molecule concentrations may be limited as there is a wide variation in concentrations even within individuals and extensive activation is required to deplete concentrations below the normal range (Whicher, 1978; Frank, 1987). Significant complement activation may occur with a 50% reduction in parent molecule concentration but which may still lie in the normal range. In addition, increased synthesis of parent molecules, as seen in acute phase reactions may mask complement consumption due to activation (Downton and Colten, 1988). Commercially available specific antisera allow the detection of the majority of parent molecules using such immunochemical methods as radial immunodiffusion, counter-current electrophoresis, rocket immunoelectrophoresis and nephelometry in a semi-quantitative way (Cooper, Nemerow and Meyers, 1983).

Measurement of biologically active fragments

Measurement of haemolytic activity or parent molecule concentrations alone is insufficient to allow informed interpretation of the extent, pathways and occasionally even the presence of complement activation. Measurement of the biologically active fragments of complement activation allows a very direct assessment of complement activation. Sensitive radioimmunoassays have been developed for the demonstration of $C3_a$, $C4_a$ and $C5_a$ which can be detected in blood and body fluids (Chenoweth *et al.*, 1981; Gorski, 1981; Hughli and Chenoweth, 1981). With these techniques there are certain disadvantages including cost and the use of radioactive substances. In addition these fragments exert their full biological effect at the site of their release and have a very short half-life. Their circulating levels may, therefore be low or undetectable despite strong circumstantial evidence suggesting their formation (Chenoweth *et al.*, 1981).

Measurement of split products

The problems of measurement of short-life, biologically active anaphylatoxins is to some extent overcome by the measurement of other biologically inert split products with longer half-lives and which are produced at the same time as anaphylatoxins and remain in the circulation in higher concentration (Charlesworth *et al.*, 1974). They are generated at a rate directly proportional to the rate of cleavage of the parent molecule on a unit for unit basis. The demonstration of increased levels of these split products, with or without parent molecule depletion is unequivocal evidence of activation-derived consumption of the parent molecule. As many complement fragments have antigenic determinants also present on their precursors, *in vitro* separation is necessary before immunoassay can be performed and differences in molecular size, electrical charge and differential solubility in polyethylene glycol are all methods that have been exploited to separate the fragments before the use of commercially available antisera in assay techniques (Morse, Müller-Eberhard and Kunkel, 1962; Müller-Eberhard and Lepow, 1965; West *et al.*, 1966; Perrin, Lambert and Miescher, 1975; Perrin *et al.*, 1975). Although initially only qualitative information regarding the presence of split products could be obtained more recent techniques of laser nephelometry and enzyme-linked immunosorbent assays allow sensitive quantitative assays (Vergani *et al.*, 1983; Peakman *et al.*, 1987; Senaldi *et al.*, 1987; Davies *et al.*, 1988). Evaluation of the serum levels of split products allows assessment of activation through the classical, alternative and common pathways. In addition, determination of the parent molecule concentration in a matched sample allows the fragment level–parent molecule concentration ratio to be calculated. This ratio e.g. $C4_d/C4$, $C3_d/C3$, B_a/B, is extremely valuable and represents a sensitive index of fragment production and parent molecule consumption. It has been shown to correlate most closely with the fractional catabolic rate of the intact component as measured in *in vivo* studies in health and disease (Milgrom *et al.*, 1980; Swaak *et al.*, 1985).

The role of complement activation as an effector in disease processes

It is clear that controlled complement activation in the presence of microbial infection is beneficial to the host organism. Equally evident is the potential for wholesale inflammation and tissue damage, if unrestrained complement activation occurred. The release of anaphylatoxins $C3_a$ and $C5_a$ triggers the degranulation of mast cells releasing highly active preformed mediators including histamine, heparin, 5-hydroxytryptamine, platelet activating factor, lysosomal enzymes and factors leading to chemotaxis of eosinophils and neutrophils. The vasodilator and capillary permeability response to histamine is well known but other substances including the arachidonic acid derivatives, thromboxanes, other prostaglandins and leukotrienes, are also produced following mast cell stimulation by anaphylatoxins. $C3_a$ and $C5_a$ are cleaved from C3 and C5 respectively by the classical and alternative pathways C3 and C5 amplification convertases. Both anaphylatoxins have spasminogen properties dependent upon the possession of an arginine residue at the carboxyterminal of the peptide chain. Removal of the arginine group by peptidases destroys all the biological functions of $C3_a$. Although produced in much smaller quantities $C5_a$ is more potent on a molar basis. In addition to vasospastic properties it is the most potent chemotactic factor for neutrophils known. $C5_a$ causes neutrophil margination and chemotaxis leading to a circulating neutropenia. It is also capable of activating neutrophils and triggering a bactericidal oxidative burst. Loss of the $C5_a$ arginine residue leads to the production of $C5_a$desArg. This retains some cell activation properties, but like $C3_a$ loses its spasminogenic effects. In the Arthus reaction, for example, immune complexes are formed in the presence of antibody excess and are deposited in tissues and lead to complement activation, chemotaxis and release of mast cell mediators. Frustrated phagocytosis occurs when complexes attached to basement membrane cannot be engulfed and this leads to increasing tissue damage and immune vasculitis. Complement depletion abrogates this disease process. Complement depletion is also capable of reducing the vasculitis and tissue damage response in a number of animal models of human disease including serum sickness and experimental forms of glomerulonephritis. The demonstration of complement components and evidence of the membrane attack complex in the glomeruli of patients with lupus nephritis implicates complement activation in the kidney produced by immune complexes containing anti-DNA antibodies. Serological evidence of complement activation and demonstration of complement components in the bronchoalveolar lavage fluid of cases of the adult respiratory distress syndrome suggest a possible aetiological role, although the extent of complement activation cannot necessarily be correlated to the severity of the disease process.

Surprisingly congenital deficiency of complement components is not automatically related to a profound predisposition to septic illness. Individuals with isolated deficiencies of factors C6–C9 have an increased susceptibility to *Neisseria* infection whereas deficiencies of other factors are associated with pyogenic infections. Protection against other infections is presumably afforded by other opsonins, antibodies and immune adherence mechanisms. Deficiency of the C1 esterase inhibitor may lead to unrestrained activation of the classical pathway and recurring episodes of angioneurotic oedema (Lachmann and Peters, 1982).

Any process that leads to unbridled complement activation and production of anaphylatoxins is likely to be detrimental to the host organism. The venom of the Malayan pit viper contains a factor (CVF) closely resembling $C3_b$ which is capable of combining with factor B and forming an amplification convertase and decomplementing a victim via the alternative pathway (Lachmann and Peters, 1982). In experimental animal studies such massive complement activation is capable of causing severe haemodynamic and whole body inflammatory reactions similar to the changes seen in septic shock and adult respiratory distress syndrome (Brigham, 1982; Schirmer *et al.*, 1988).

Before the investigation of complement activation during cardiopulmonary bypass, Kaplow *et al.* (1968) noted the appearance of severe leucopenia during the early stages of haemodialysis using cellophane dialyser membranes. Although it was initially thought that this was due to the sequestration of leucocytes within the cellophane coils of the dialyser it was noted that injection of autologous serum, incubated with dialyser cellophane, into experimental animals also produced a prompt leukopenia (Craddock *et al.*, 1977a; Craddock *et al.*, 1977b). Further investigations demonstrated the development of pulmonary vascular leucocyte sequestration with elevation of pulmonary vascular resistance and this was attributed to the activation of the alternative pathway of complement by exposure to the polysaccharide cellophane of the dialyser membrane. The production of $C5_a$, capable of producing polymorphonuclear leucocyte aggregation *in vitro* and *in vivo*, was demonstrated and associated with adherence of activated neutrophils to pulmonary endothelial cells leading to endothelial damage and haemodynamic changes due to a number of mechanisms including leukocyte aggregates plugging small vessels, release of cytototoxic oxygen-derived free radicals and release of lysosomal enzymes following neutrophil degranulation (Craddock *et al.*, 1977c). The potential for such injury is well reviewed by several authors (Jacob, 1983; Hakim *et al.*, 1984). The discovery of complement activation and neutrophil effects in haemodialysis prompted investigation of other forms of extracorporeal circulation including cardiopulmonary bypass (Hammerschmidt *et al.*, 1981) and leukapheresis (McLeod, Viernes and Sassetti, 1983a; McLeod, Viernes and Sassetti, 1983b).

In animal models of *in vivo* complement activation (Till *et al.*, 1982) infusions of anaphylatoxin or complement-derived chemotactic activity are able to reproduce manifestations of an acute lung injury bearing close resemblance to the adult respiratory distress syndrome (ARDS). A full review of the role of complement activation in the production of this syndrome is beyond the scope of this chapter. It is sufficient to point out that it is not known, in the clinical situation, if complement activation alone, from whatever cause, is capable of inducing acute lung injury or if other mediators such as prostaglandins, platelet-derived factors, kinins or changes in endothelial elements (Ryan and Ryan, 1983) are necessary and more important in the development of adult respiratory distress syndrome (Rinaldo and Rogers, 1982). It is known that elevated levels of $C5_a$ are associated with increasing risk of ARDS but that $C5_a$ levels alone cannot discriminate between patients at risk and those who proceed to the full syndrome (Hammerschmidt *et al.*, 1980; Duchateau *et al.*, 1984).

Complement changes during cardiopulmonary bypass

Abnormalities of complement during cardiopulmonary bypass were first reported by Hairston *et al.* (1969). A fall in complement haemolytic activity was detected associated with a decrease in immunoglobulin levels, suggesting a reduction in the capacity for immunological competence following extracorporeal circulation. Other workers (Pruitt, Stroud and Scott, 1971) demonstrated the capacity for disc oxygenators and other air–liquid interfaces to alter and denature immunoglobulin, leading to aggregate formation and classical pathway activation. The reduction of immunological competence was confirmed experimentally by Subramanian *et al.* (1969), who demonstrated a reduction in the opsonic activity of blood following cardiopulmonary bypass. Subsequently other workers have confirmed this effect and have demonstrated changes in immunity in humoral and cell-mediated immune systems following bypass (Roth *et al.*, 1980). Parker *et al.* (1971) detected maximal complement consumption as demonstrated by a fall in the haemolytic activity (CH50) 4h following bypass surgery before returning to normal levels by the second postoperative day. Presumably, this occurred with replenishment of complement parent molecules as part of an acute phase reaction. Adjusting measured values for simultaneous haemoglobin concentrations excluded haemodilution as the cause for the reduction of complement activity. Reduced levels of circulating IgG and IgM were also detected suggesting the possibility that denatured immunoglobulin might lead to *in vivo* complement activation (Parker *et al.*, 1971). In a further study, (Parker, Cook and Turner-Warwick, 1975) more direct evidence for complement activation was found using crossed immunoelectrophoresis techniques to detect conversion of C3 and $C3_b$. Maximal C3 conversion was present 1h postoperatively and appeared independent of haemodilution and transfusion. Using a more refined immunoassay technique Haslam, Townsend and Branthwaite (1980) demonstrated C3 conversion within 30 min of commencing cardiopulmonary bypass in a series of patients undergoing cardiopulmonary bypass using a membrane oxygenator. Some change may have been due to transfusion of stored blood in which spontaneous complement activation was detected. C3 conversion was also demonstrable, perioperatively, in 25% of patients undergoing thoracotomy without bypass and appeared to be associated with extensive dissection and substantial use of cautery haemostasis. Hammerschmidt *et al.* (1981) studied 34 patients undergoing coronary artery surgery and detected significant leucopenia within 30 min of commencing cardiopulmonary bypass followed by a rebound neutrophilia by the end of the operation. Complement haemolytic activity also fell significantly during bypass but C3 conversion and $C5_a$ production could not be demonstrated. These findings were reminiscent of the early transient and profound neutropenia seen during haemodialysis with cellophane membrane dialysers (Craddock *et al.*, 1977a). In haemodialysis patients, neutropenia was found to coincide with temporary hypoxia and the changes in both white cells and gas exchange could be reproduced in experimental animals in which complement activation had been induced by zymosan or by the infusion of autologous plasma previously incubated with cellophane. Complement and leucocyte depletion abrogated the response (Craddock *et al.*, 1977b). In the context of cardiopulmonary bypass *in vitro* studies demonstrated polymorphonuclear aggregation following exposure of neutrophils to plasma incubated with a variety of different oxygenator membranes *in vitro*, including silicone, Teflon and polypropylene (Hammerschmidt *et al.*, 1981). It was also found that that ability to cause *in vitro* white cell aggregation could be blocked by decomplementing plasma but not by classical pathway inhibition, suggesting a major role of the alternative complement pathway in this process.

The first study to measure biologically active complement fragments by sensitive radioimmunoassay techniques was performed by Chenoweth *et al.* (1981). Measuring $C3_a$ and $C5_a$ they demonstrated significant elevation of $C3_a$ within 10 min of commencing cardiopulmonary bypass. Maximal elevation of this fragment was seen at the end of bypass, levels then fell towards preoperative levels but remained significantly elevated for 3h after surgery. The maximal level of generated $C3_a$ appeared to correlate with the duration of cardiopulmonary bypass. In contrast plasma levels of $C5_a$ did not change significantly during or after perfusion. Leucocyte sequestration within the lungs was also noted and the transpulmonary white cell count gradient appeared to be most closely associated with factors other than the extent of anaphylatoxin production, including the duration of aortic cross-clamping, the duration of the re-warming period and the degree of rebound neutrophilia. No correlation between the degree of leucocyte sequestration or $C3_a$ levels and postoperative pulmonary performance could be demonstrated. In an attempt to identify the cause of complement activation during bypass the authors performed several *in vitro* experiments assessing anaphylatoxin generation during exposure of serum and blood to the nylon mesh of bubble oxygenators and to direct oxygen–blood interfaces during vigorous bubble oxygenation. Incubation of either serum or heparinized blood with nylon mesh resulted in immediate and time-dependent generation of $C3_a$. $C5_a$ generation was also detectable following serum but not blood incubation with nylon. This effect and the failure to demonstrate elevated $C5_a$ during bypass was attributed to interactions between $C5_a$ and neutrophils. Earlier studies had demonstrated that $C5_a$ binds avidly to neutrophils following which it is degraded to products which are no longer detectable by immunoassay (Craddock *et al.*, 1977c; Jacob *et al.*, 1980). Even if $C5_a$ was produced during cardiopulmonary bypass it may not be detectable until all receptor sites on neutrophils have been occupied, allowing excess $C5_a$ to be detected in the fluid phase. Vigorous *in vitro* bubble oxygenation of heparinized whole blood also led to time-dependent $C3_a$ but not $C5_a$ generation.

The mechanisms and pathways of complement activation during cardiopulmonary bypass were further investigated by Jones *et al.* (1982). Activation products of C3 were demonstrable in plasma within 30 min of commencing cardiopulmonary bypass, but were not detectable perioperatively in non-bypass patients. In addition reduced serum concentrations of C4 and factor B were detected with a more profound depletion of C4 than B, implicating both classical and alternative pathways. Depressed levels of IgM and detection of IgM aggregates in certain cases provided an explanation for $C1_q$ binding. Boralessa *et al.* (1982) studied total haemolytic complement activity (CH50), alternative pathway haemolytic activity, C3, C4 and $C3_d$ concentrations in ten patients subjected to cardiopulmonary bypass. Serum transferrin concentrations, measured as a non-specific protein marker, fell significantly during bypass in parallel with changes in C3 and C4. Following bypass transferrin levels returned rapidly to normal while C3 and C4 levels continued to fall. The authors questioned whether complement activation occurred at all during bypass, suggesting that the changes in parent molecule and split product concentrations might be attributable to dilution, denaturation and other non-specific but generalized effects on proteins occurring during extracorporeal perfusion. In the period following bypass, the sustained and continuing fall in parent molecule concentrations appeared incompatible with declining levels of anaphylatoxins demonstrated previously by Chenoweth *et al.* (1981). The sustained fall in C3 concentrations, accompanied by depression of IgG and fibronectin levels, was confirmed by Gandhi, Salm and Szymanski (1983). It is possible that the reduction in parent molecule concentrations following bypass could be attributable to decreased synthesis or release, although this is unlikely as they might be expected to rise in an acute phase response. Increased, low grade, spontaneous turnover and catabolism at a rate of 1–2% per hour might also contribute (Ruddy *et al.*, 1976). Significant rises in $C3_d$ levels were not demonstrable at any time during or after cardiopulmonary bypass in the study of Boralessa *et al.* (1982) but the sensitivity of the radial immunodiffusion technique used for $C3_d$ assay has subsequently been questioned (Vergani *et al.*, 1983; Collett *et al.*, 1984).

The fall in C4 levels during bypass in several studies (Boralessa *et al.*, 1982; Chiu and Samson, 1984; Collett *et al.*, 1984; Bonser *et al.*, 1990a) strongly suggests a role of the classical pathway in addition to alternative pathway activation in the production of complement activation during cardiopulmonary bypass. Immunoglobulin depletion during bypass has been reported (Hairston *et al.*, 1969; Parker *et al.*, 1971) and immune aggregates may accumulate (Jones *et al.*, 1982). Antigammaglobulin antibodies have been detected following bypass (Pretty *et al.*, 1968) and some denaturation of gammaglobulin may occur on exposure to oxygenator materials *in vitro* (Pruitt, Stroud and Scott, 1971). Whether classical pathway activation occurs because of immune aggregates formation, other immunoglobulin changes or interaction of C-reactive protein with $C1_q$, a reaction capable of causing classical pathway activation *in vitro*, or other factors (Dodds *et al.*, 1981) is not clear. Although elevated levels of the acute phase reactant C-reactive protein have been detected following open heart surgery (Ghoneim, McGoldrick and Ionescu, 1982), concentrations do not change during cardiopulmonary bypass (Collett *et al.*, 1984) arguing against a significant role for C-reactive protein in classical pathway activity during bypass. More recently the presence of significant activation of the classical pathway has been confirmed by the demonstration of $C4_a$ (Tamiya *et al.*, 1988) and $C4_d$ (Bonser *et al.*, 1990a) generation during perfusion with a progressive rise in the $C4_d$/C4 ratio. Direct gas–blood interfaces may be an important cause of classical pathway activation (Tamiya *et al.*, 1988).

Further information regarding the alternative pathway activation of complement during cardiopulmonary bypass was provided by Collett *et al.* (1984). Demonstration of elevated levels of alternative pathway produced fragment, B_a, within 90 s of commencing cardiopulmonary bypass provided strong evidence for the predominant role of this pathway in bypass-associated complement activation. Maximal elevation of B_a levels occurs 10 min after exposure of blood to the polymers of the extracorporeal circuit (Bonser *et al.*, 1990a). Further complement activation may occur after protamine administration (Loubser, 1987).

Recent assays have been developed allowing differentiation of the cytolytic, membrane bound, terminal complement complex ($C5_b$–9) and inactive, non-lytic fluid phase $C5_b$–9 complexes (Mollnes, Lee and Harboe, 1984; Mollnes, 1985). Terminal complement complex components have been demonstrated during cardiopulmonary bypass, bound to circulating blood elements (Salama *et al.*, 1988). Fluid phase terminal complement complexes have also been found. Using an enzyme linked immunosorbent assay Fosse, Mollnes and Ingvaldsen (1987) demonstrated an abrupt rise in the fluid phase complex soon after commencing cardiopulmonary bypass. Levels appeared maximal after 1h of bypass before falling to preoperative values 4h after surgery. These changes occur in parallel with elevation of C3-derived split products.

The occurrence of neutropenia during bypass has been demonstrated by several studies (Chenoweth *et al.*, 1981; Hammerschmidt *et al.*, 1981; Collett *et al.*, 1984). In contrast to haemodialysis, where the generation of $C3_a$ and the occurrence of leucopenia are temporally associated, in cardiopulmonary bypass maximal neutropenia precedes maximal production of $C3_a$ (Chenoweth *et al.*, 1981). This discrepancy may be partially explained by the appearance in blood of stimulus-specific deactivated neutrophils and enhanced marrow release of neutrophils activated by agents such as $C3_e$ and leukotrienes despite the tendency of hypothermia to reduce the numbers of circulating mature and immature neutrophils (Biggar, Bohn and Kent, 1983; Quiroga *et al.*, 1985).

There have been few accounts of complement activation in patients with congenital or acquired abnormalities of the complement cascade. Umebayashi *et al.* (1987) were able to successfully perform cardiopulmonary bypass in a patient with biochemical evidence of hereditary C1 esterase inhibitor deficiency but no clinical history of angioneurotic oedema using pretreatment with anabolic steroids. An exaggerated complement activation response to cardiopulmonary bypass was noted in a case of acquired C1 esterase inhibitor deficiency, with a strong history of angioneurotic oedema, despite the administration of steroids, danazol, fresh frozen plasma and epsilon-amino caproic acid (Bonser *et al.*, 1991).

The demonstration of circulating split products, anaphylatoxins and terminal complement complexes during cardiopulmonary bypass confirm the occurrence of complement activation. The exact contribution of the individual pathways and the pathophysiological consequences of this remains unclear.

The effects of heparin, protamine and the heparin–protamine reaction on complement activation during cardiopulmonary bypass

Heparin: serological studies

In addition to immunoglobulins, certain polyanions including heparin are capable of interacting with the $C1_q$ component of complement, presumably because of their negative charge reacting with the highly cationic $C1_q$ (Loos, 1982). Certain of these polyanions including dextran sulphate, polyvinyl sulphate and polyanethol sulphate result in dose-dependent activation of the classical pathway (Loos *et al.*, 1974; Raepple, Hill and Loos, 1976). There is evidence that heparin binds to $C1_q$ but only causes a small and dose-related activation of the macromolecular C1 (Rent *et al.*, 1975).

Heparin has been demonstrated to inhibit the generation of the alternative pathway C3 amplification convertase at a final concentration in serum comparable to those required for heparin anticoagulant activity (Kazatchkine and Nydegger, 1982). Heparin inhibits the formation of the amplification convertase in both fluid and membrane surface phases by inhibiting the binding of factor B to $C3_b$ (Kazatchkine *et al.*, 1979). The inhibitory effect of heparin on convertase formation is independent of its antithrombin III cofactor activity and it requires maintenance of the integrity of its sulphate groups (Kazatchkine *et al.*, 1982). Neutralization of the negative charges of the sulphate groups by fluid phase polycations abolishes the inhibition of the convertase (Kazatchkine and Maillet, 1981).

The exact effects of heparin on the complement system are multiple and complex. Heparin has long been known as an 'anti-complementary' or complement consuming agent (Gross and Ecker, 1928; Ecker and Gross, 1929; Ecker and Pillemer, 1941). Various investigators have reported that the preincubation of serum with heparin results in the depletion of C1, and C2 (Rent *et al.*, 1975). Heparin may also potentiate C1 inhibitor activity reducing classical pathway activation (Myhrman, Monckton and Gewürz, 1973). The heparin-induced consumption of common pathway components C3 to C9 is independent of and not potentiated by protamine (Rent *et al.*, 1975). Since certain polysaccharides are potent activators of the alternative complement pathway and the heparin-like mucopolysaccharide, polyanethol sulphate has been reported to induce conversion of C3 via the alternative pathway, it is possible that one of the complex effects of heparin includes independent alternative pathway activation or component consumption (Loos *et al.*, 1974).

Heparin: clinical studies

The majority of studies of complement activation during cardiopulmonary bypass have paid little attention to complement changes associated with heparinization. Collett *et al.* (1984) detected significant elevation of B_a fragment levels within 90 s of commencing cardiopulmonary bypass and suspected that some increase may have occurred even before the institution of bypass. More recently significant elevation of B_a fragment levels and the B_a/B ratio have been detected within 5 min of systemic heparinization before the institution of cardiopulmonary bypass. These changes are followed by a significant rise in $C3_d$ levels and $C3_d/C3$ ratio, 10 min after heparinization. These changes suggest early alternative pathway complement activation before bypass temporally associated with the administration of heparin (Bonser *et al.*, 1990a). In certain other forms of non-bypass major vascular surgery, using limited heparinization, a low degree of complement activation has also been detected (Lew *et al.*, 1985; Fosse, Mollnes and Ingvaldsen, 1987). It is not known if heparin is responsible for complement activation in these cases but other surgical procedures in which heparin is not used have also been associated with a mild degree of complement activation in certain cases (Hahn-Pedersen, Sorensen and Kehlet, 1978; Halsam, Townsend and Branthwaite, 1980; Hällgren, Samuellson and Modig, 1987).

Heparin–protamine: serological studies

It has already been mentioned that although classical pathway activation is a consequence of immune complex formation, a number of substances including polyanionic proteins such as C-reactive protein and polynucleotides are capable of binding $C1_q$ and causing classical pathway activation (Loos, 1982). Classical pathway activation is also seen in a reaction independent of antibody, following the interaction of certain polyanions and polycations, the most important of which are heparin and protamine (Rent *et al.*, 1975; Fiedel *et al.*, 1976; Claus *et al.*, 1977; Best *et al.*, 1984). Protamine alone, in normal serum, does not activate complement (Rent *et al.*, 1975), but may react with C-reactive protein to activate the classical pathway strongly (Siegel, Rent and Gewürz, 1974). This reaction is unlikely to be relevant in clinical bypass as C-reactive protein concentrations do not change during bypass (Collett *et al.*, 1984) and only increase as part of the acute phase response following surgery (Ghoneim, McGoldrick and Ionescu, 1984) whereas heparin–protamine interaction is an essential component of almost every open heart procedure. *In vitro* investigations have demonstrated that heparin and protamine in fresh serum enhance the depletion of haemolytic C1 far in excess of any additive effect of each agent individually (Rent *et al.*, 1975). In the situation of slight protamine excess marked complement activation via the classical pathway with consumption of C2 and C4 is observed. In the presence of heparin excess C4 and C2 consumption is not seen possibly because of the potentiation of C1 esterase inhibition by extra heparin. It is necessary for the heparin–protamine reaction to take place in the presence of serum for maximal complement activation to occur suggesting the necessity for a serum-contained cofactor to effect the process. Further investigations in animal models have demonstrated classical pathway activation, intravascular generation of $C5_a$ and transient neutropenia in animals exposed to polyanion–polycation complexes (Fehr and Rohr, 1983).

Heparin–protamine: *in vivo* studies

The cardiovascular effects of protamine neutralization of heparin anticoagulation have been well described (Jastrzebiski, Sykes and Woods. 1974; Conahan, Andrews and McVaugh, 1981; Shapira *et al.*, 1982; Michaels and Barash, 1983; Frater *et al.*, 1984). Mild systemic vasodilation is partially compensated by an increase in cardiac output but may be associated with a depression of myocardial contractility and elevation of pulmonary arteriolar resistance (Jastrzebinski, Sykes and Woods, 1974; Olinger, Becker and Bonchek, 1980; Kirklin *et al.*, 1986; Maggart, 1987). Occasionally profound cardiovascular disturbance occurs with permeability pulmonary oedema (Olinger, Becker and Bonchek, 1980). The exact biochemical mediation of these events remains to a large extent unknown (Nordstrom, Fletcher and Pavek, 1978; Lowenstein *et al.*, 1983). Although a direct non-cytotoxic, non-immune effect on mast cells has been suggested it is possible to invoke a role for the complement cascade in certain cases (Olinger, Becker and Bonchek, 1980). Protamine is a highly positively charged polypeptide isolated commercially from salmon sperm. Its efficacy in reversing the effects of heparin anticoagulation has lead to its clinical use since 1939. In common with intravenous agents severe anaphylactic reactions with circulatory shock have been reported after its administration, which in most circumstances follows the prior administration of heparin during a procedure requiring anticoagulation (Nordstrom, Fletcher and Pavek, 1978; Olinger, Becker and Bonchek, 1980; Westaby, Turner and Stark, 1985). It is possible that many instances of haemodynamic instability are caused by Type I hypersensitivity reactions and high circulating levels of IgE have been found in certain patients previously exposed to protamine e.g. previous cardiac surgery, vascular surgery, haemodialysis, cardiac catheterization, leukapheresis, or in insulin-dependent diabetic patients using protamine–insulin–zinc suspensions (Lakin *et al.*, 1978; Stewart *et al.*, 1984; Sharath *et al.*, 1985).

The temporal relationship of protamine administration and haemodynamic deterioration following weaning from cardiopulmonary bypass has prompted investigation of a role of complement and activated leucocytes in these effects. Olinger, Becker and Bonchek (1980) described four cases of circulatory collapse following the administration of protamine and questioned the role of complement activation in this response. Although a heparin–protamine interaction has been suspected following cardiopulmonary bypass (White, 1981; Kirklin, 1982; Chenoweth, 1981) early work failed to show additional C3 or C4 consumption after the administration of protamine (Boralessa *et al.*, 1982; Chiu and Samson, 1984). Chiu and Samson (1984) suspected that further activation of complement did not occur after protamine injection but in this study no measurements of split products were made also the potentially insensitive assay methods for parent molecule concentrations may have been unable to detect the small reduction in parent molecule concentration occurring as a result of activation. Best *et al.* (1984) studied five patients after cardiopulmonary bypass, measured the split products $C3_c$ and $C3_d$. $C3_d$ levels increased significantly, compared with end of bypass levels, after the administration of protamine. Circulating $C3_c$ was only demonstrable in those samples taken immediately following protamine. *In vitro* experiments suggested that the complement activation was attributable to dose-related heparin–protamine interaction. In a study of 100 patients undergoing cardiopulmonary bypass (Cavarocchi *et al.*, 1985) measured $C3_a$ and the biologically active classical pathway fragment $C4_a$ levels by radioimmunoassay, before and after the administration of protamine. During cardiopulmonary bypass $C3_a$ rose significantly and a further significant rise in $C3_a$ levels was demonstrated postprotamine sulphate injection. In contrast $C4_a$ levels did not rise significantly during cardiopulmonary bypass but were significantly elevated 10 min following protamine reversal of heparin. In a separate subset of patients, the administration of protamine was delayed for 45 min following the discontinuation of bypass. In this set the elevation of $C4_a$ and the secondary peak in $C3_a$ levels did not occur until skin closure soon after the administration of protamine. Kirklin *et al.* (1986) studied the effects of protamine administration on complement activation, white cell kinetics and haemodynamic changes and detected significant elevation of $C3_a$ and $C4_a$ measured by radioimmunoassay, 5 min following protamine with maximal elevation at 10 min. $C4_d$/C4 ratios were also studied and increased to maximum 6h following the protamine dose. Parallel serological experiments demonstrated production of biologically active fragments $C4_a$, 3_a, and 5_a following serum incubation with heparin and protamine. Control studies, incubating serum with heparin or protamine alone, did not lead to frequent production. The failure to detect $C4_a$ generation during bypass in these studies fails to explain C4 depletion during perfusion and is at variance with the demonstration of $C4_a$ production during cardiopulmonary bypass by Tamiya *et al.* (1988). Bonser *et al.* (1990a) failed to detect a further significant rise in $C4_d$ or $C4_d$/C4 levels after protamine administration.

In association with the administration of protamine Kirklin *et al.* (1980) demonstrated transient thrombocytopenia. This has also been seen by other workers (Bjoracker and Ketchen, 1982) and is thought to be due to a transient hepatic sequestration of activated platelets and platelet aggregates. A clear relationship between exaggerated complement activation following protamine and circulatory disturbances has not been demonstrated in human studies (Best *et al.*, 1983; Cavarocchi *et al.*, 1985; Kirklin *et al.*, 1986). A progression from classical pathway activation to common pathway activation has not been well documented. *In vitro* activation of the classical pathway by protamine and heparin does not lead to completion of the complement cascade (Siegel *et al.*, 1974; Rent *et al.*, 1975). Minimal $C5_a$ generation was detected in the *in vitro* studies of Kirklin *et al.* (1986), and no $C5_a$ level changes in the clinical study following protamine. However, in animal experiments, using an ovine model, a relatively consistent relationship has been observed between the pulmonary vasoconstrictor response of protamine neutralization of heparin anticoagulation and the measured release of thromboxane B_2 (TXB_2), the stable metabolite of thromboxane A_2 (TXA_2), a potent platelet aggregator (Cooper *et al.*, 1980; McDonald *et al.*, 1983). This agent is also a powerful pulmonary vasoconstrictor and bronchoconstrictor and elevated levels have been demonstrated in several animal models of acute pulmonary hypertension induced by infusion of endotoxin, arachidonate, reactive oxygen metabolites, zymosan activated plasma and even after the institution of partial extracorporeal perfusion (Petersen *et al.*, 1982). Cyclo-oxygenase inhibition or thromboxane synthesis blockade abrogates the increases in thromboxane B_2 release and pulmonary vasoconstrictor responses in these models.

In a clinical study relating the pulmonary haemodynamic changes and bronchoconstrictor changes following cardiopulmonary bypass and protamine administration Morel *et al.* (1987) investigated 50 patients of which two developed sudden increases in airway pressure, pulmonary vascular resistance and systemic hypotension within minutes of protamine injection. The changes in these patients closely resembled those seen in animal models. When compared with the remaining 48 patients studied, the affected patients had markedly elevated levels of circulating $C5_a$ and thromboxane B_2. One patient, an insulin-dependent diabetic receiving an protamine–insulin suspension may have been presensitized. This report suggests a role of the thromboxanes in the clinical manifestations of excessive anaphylatoxin release following heparin–protamine interaction.

In conclusion it would appear that protamine administration following cardiopulmonary bypass is associated with a burst of complement activation via the classical pathway. Although this may not lead to common pathway activation and may be of no clinical consequence, occasional severe reactions occur which may be related to the release of a large number of mediators secondary to complement activation. Other inflammatory cascades activated during cardiopulmonary bypass may also be important in these effects. Polyanions are known to initiate autoactivation of coagulation factor XII (Taukersley, Alving and Finlayson, 1983). Once activated, factor XII is capable of triggering the classical pathway of complement (Ghebrehiwit, Silverberg and Kaplan, 1981). Heparin has minimal inhibitory effect on factor XII inhibition in plasma (Pixley, Schapira and Colman, 1985) and factor XII in the presence of heparin is capable of activating both prekallikrein and the first component of complement during cardiopulmonary bypass (Wachtfogel *et al*., 1986a). Potent neutrophil activators distinct from complement may be important in the context of cardiopulmonary bypass. Kallikrein is capable of aggregating neutrophils even in the presence of C5 depletion (Schapira *et al*., 1982). It also induces the release of neutrophil elastase (Wachtfogel *et al*., 1983) which is generated during cardiopulmonary bypass (Wachtfogel *et al*., 1987). The production of bradykinin from the action of kallikrein in kininogen could also contribute to systemic hypotension following protamine administration. Factor XIIa is additionally capable of producing neutrophil aggregation and degranulation (Wachtfogel *et al*., 1986b) and during plasma coagulation, neutrophil elastase release requires both factor XII and kallikrein but not C5. As neutrophil degranulation occurs during cardiopulmonary bypass it is possible that this may be due to kallikrein, XIIa, $C5_a$ or other mediators and the lack of specificity of complement activation as an index and predictor of postoperative morbidity may be explained.

The use of cyclo-oxygenase inhibitors has been suggested to prevent the adverse reactions to protamine if such responses are mediated by thromboxane release (Morel *et al*., 1987). The effects of their administration might also be beneficial in terms of reperfusion injury (Romson *et al*., 1982) and other mechanisms of lung injury (Brigham, 1982; Rinaldo and Rogers, 1982) but a possible aggravation of a haemorrhagic diathesis and disturbances in leucotriene synthesis which might also lead to vasoactive changes should be considered (Colman, 1987). The preoperative detection of patients who may be at high risk of protamine reaction by virtue of possible presensitization is also important and alternative methods of heparin neutralization considered (Castaneda, 1966; Sharath *et al*., 1985).

Modulation of complement activation during cardiopulmonary bypass

In view of the possible relationship between complement activation and postoperative morbidity, several workers have investigated systems in which the extent of complement activation might be reduced.

Membrane oxygenation carries certain advantages over bubble oxygenation in terms of red cell damage, haemoglobinuria, platelet activation and proteinuria (Wildevuur, 1980; Boers *et al*., 1983). In terms of complement activation any beneficial effects are less evident. Jones *et al*. (1982) were unable to detect any differences in complement activation in patients undergoing bubble or membrane perfusion. Hammerschmidt *et al*. (1981) randomly allocated patients to bubble oxygenation or membrane oxygenation groups, some of which received steroids. No difference in the decline in total haemolytic complement activity were detected but membrane oxygenation caused a significantly greater degree and duration of neutropenia during bypass. In a direct comparison of bubble oxygenators versus a hollow-fibre membrane oxygenator, van Oeveren *et al*. (1985) demonstrated beneficial effects of membrane oxygenation in terms of haemolysis, thrombocytopenia, and release of β-thromboglobulin. Polymorphonuclear neutrophils and monocytes taken from bubble oxygenation patients showed increased production of reactive oxygen species in both resting and stimulated states when compared with cells from the membrane oxygenation group. No differences between bubble and membrane oxygenation were demonstrable in the occurrence or intensity of leucopenia on cardiopulmonary bypass or post-bypass leucocytosis, or in the extent of complement activation as measured by $C3_a$ levels. In the membrane oxygenator group, complement activation appeared dependent upon the alternative pathway whereas significant C2 depletion suggesting classical pathway complement activation was found in the bubble oxygenator group. Concentrations of IgM but not IgG or IgA were found in both groups and tending to be lower after bubble oxygenation. Serum opsonizing capacity, dependent upon the alternative pathway was reduced in both groups and tended to be lower in bubble group. Although reduced, serum bactericidal activity to *Serratia marcescens*, requiring specific antibody and the proteins of the classical pathway, was not different between groups after correction for haemodilution. Similar findings were demonstrated by other workers (Mickleborough, Arnold and Chiu, 1986).

In contrast significant differences in complement activation between bubble and non-porous membrane oxygenator groups were demonstrated by Cavarocchi *et al.* (1986a), but these were only evident after the administration of protamine and not during cardiopulmonary bypass. No differences in postoperative morbidity were identified between groups. The use of a silicone membrane oxygenator, in which oxygen diffuses at a molecular level, may have contributed to these differences but this is unlikely as silicone polymers have been demonstrated to cause cardiopulmonary bypass complement activation *in vitro* (Jacob *et al.*, 1980). Membrane oxygenation was also associated with reduced transpulmonary leucocyte sequestration and postbypass leucocytosis in Cavarocchi's series, in contrast to the study by Hammerschmidt *et al.* (1981). Porous membrane oxygenators appear less efficient than non-porous membranes in reducing complement activation (Clancy *et al.*, 1985). Tamiya *et al.* (1988) found little difference in the extent of complement activation between membrane and bubble oxygenator groups. The rate of rise of $C3_a$ was however greater in the bubble group. Classical pathway activation was seen to be clearly related to the vigorous bubbling of oxygen through blood in this group.

Other workers have considered complement activation during *in vitro* perfusion with different oxygenator materials. Videm *et al.* (1989) detected fluid phase terminal complement complexes during perfusion with both membrane and bubble oxygenators. C3 activation was demonstrated in capillary, sheet and non-porous membranes and with hard shell bubblers but not in hollow-fibre membranes or soft shell bubble oxygenators. The reason for these differences is not clear but may be related to non-oxygenation in the *in vitro* studies. In haemodialysis, relevant clinical differences have been detected in the capacity of different dialyser membranes to induce complement activation (DeBacker *et al.*, 1984; Hakim *et al.*, 1984). It is likely that a number of factors influence the ability of an oxygenator to induce complement activation. These include the materials (Breillatt and Dorson, 1984; Videm *et al.*, 1989), the overall surface area of blood–material interaction, the influence of wetting agents and the degree of direct blood–gas interface (Chenoweth *et al.*, 1981; Tamiya *et al.*, 1988).

As corticosteroids in high concentration are capable of inhibiting complement activation (Packard and Weiler, 1983; Weiler and Packard, 1984), complement-induced granulocyte aggregation *in vitro* (O'Flaherty, Craddock and Jacob, 1977; Hammerschmidt *et al.*, 1979), and also reduce free radical release from leucocytes (Goldstein *et al.*, 1976), the possible beneficial effects of their use in cardiopulmonary bypass have been investigated. The evidence for a beneficial clinical effect is less compelling but despite this, some authors recommend the routine administration of high dose methylprednisolone before cardiopulmonary bypass (Maggart, 1987). Early studies with small sample sizes detected no differences in complement activation when steroids were used (Jones *et al.*, 1982; Haslam, Townsend and Branthwaite, 1980). Enderby, Boylett and Parker (1979) could find no differences in alveolar–arterial oxygen gradients or pulmonary shunt fractions in patients treated with a single dose of methylprednisolone 30 mg kg^{-1} administered intravenously before bypass. A similar dose of methylprednisolone protected against neutropenia but not complement activation in the study of Hammerschmidt *et al.* (1981), however, again only small numbers of patients were in each group. This dose of steroid may be insufficient to maintain plasma steroid levels sufficiently high during surgery (Thompson and Broadbent, 1980; Thompson, Broadbent and English, 1982). Boscoe *et al.* (1983) found a higher dose of steroid (methylprednisolone, total dose 60 mg kg^{-1}) ineffective in reducing complement activation during perfusion with bubble oxygenators despite apparently adequate plasma levels. The sensitivity of the complement immunoassay used in this study has been questioned (Collett *et al.*, 1984). In a larger study, Cavarocchi *et al.* (1986a) studied 91 patients, allocated to bubble oxygenator, bubble oxygenator with methylprednisolone 30 mg kg^{-1} and membrane oxygenator groups. The differences between bubble and membrane oxygenation have already been mentioned. In this study, corticosteroid administration was associated with significantly lower levels of $C3_a$ following the administration of protamine but not during cardiopulmonary bypass. These differences were not accompanied by any identifiable clinical benefit. Leucocyte sequestration was also reduced by steroid administration, findings confirmed by Tennenberg *et al.* (1986) who also could not detect any differences in $C3_a$ levels during cardiopulmonary bypass.

The composition of the solution used to prime the extracorporeal circuit may also influence complement activation (Gaspardone *et al.*, 1986). The use of citrated blood in the cardiopulmonary bypass prime may itself contaminate measurements because of in-storage complement activation (Haslam, Townsend and Branthwaite, 1980). Other workers have suggested that the addition of citrated blood and heparin may inhibit complement activation *in vitro* to some degree (Wegmüller, Kazatchkine and Nydegger, 1983). Boscoe *et al.* (1983) found no evidence of complement activation in over 50% of patients undergoing cardiopulmonary bypass with a bubble oxygenator in which the prime contained the urea-linked gelatin polygeline. In approximately half of the patients undergoing membrane oxygenation in the study by Cavarocchi *et al.* (1986a), in whom reduced complement activation was seen, the prime solution contained a significant quantity of albumin. Addonizio *et al.* (1979) have demonstrated that protein coating of the extracorporeal circuit polymers occurs and that this may be protective in preventing blood elements from foreign surface exposure. In a controlled study, reduced levels of the alternative pathway fragment, B_a, were demonstrated during and after cardiopulmonary bypass in patients undergoing bubble oxygenation with a prime containing polygeline (Bonser *et al.*, 1990b). Albumin priming has also been suggested to reduce complement activation (Tamiya *et al.*, 1988). Experimental agents including the protease inhibitor, natamstat mesilate (FUT-175), have been demonstrated to reduce *in vitro* complement activation induced by exposure of serum to oxygenator material, by blocking the classical pathway (Miyamoto *et al.*, 1985). Other studies have suggested that the avoidance of an oxygenator completely, by using a double reservoir bypass circuit using the patient's own lungs as an oxygenator, may reduce the inflammatory response to bypass (Glenville and Ross, 1986).

The role of complement activation in post-cardiopulmonary bypass morbidity and mortality

Activation of complement may be deleterious in two ways. Firstly consumption of factors may reduce the immunological competence of the patient and secondly generation of large amounts of biologically active fragments may be anticipated to lead to a generalized inflammatory response with haemodynamic changes, increasing capillary permeability and specific activation of neutrophils capable of causing host damage. Disturbances of organ function following cardiopulmonary bypass surgery are not uncommon. Cerebral, cardiac, renal and pulmonary function may decline following perfusion and in certain cases a syndrome of multiple organ failure may develop which cannot be attributed to a primary myocardial insufficiency. The terms 'postperfusion syndrome' and 'pump-lung' have been coined to describe generalized and specific organ failure following extracorporeal perfusion (Parker, 1975; Kirklin, 1983; Westaby, 1983). As an increase in pulmonary capillary permeability is a prominent feature in such cases it is attractive to hypothesize that complement activation and altered neutrophil function are fundamental to their pathogenesis (Till *et al.*, 1983). $C5_a$ is capable of inducing several neutrophil responses which may, at least in part, be responsible for an acute microvascular lung injury. These responses include increased neutrophil adherence and aggregation, altered neutrophil chemotactic activity, neutrophil degranulation and cytototoxic enzyme release and neutrophil free radical generation. In the context of cardiopulmonary bypass, production of $C3_a$ and $C5_a$ may lead to neutrophil adherence, aggregation and pulmonary leucocyte sequestration. Alterations in neutrophil chemotactic and oxidative responses after cardiopulmonary bypass are consistent with *in vivo* exposure to $C5_a$ (Hammerschmidt *et al.*, 1981; van Oeveren *et al.*, 1985) and elevated levels of circulating hydrogen peroxide, a byproduct of oxygen-derived free radical generation have been detected during and after cardiopulmonary bypass (Cavarocchi *et al.*, 1986b). Lysosomal enzyme release, a consequence of complement–neutrophil interactions, has also been demonstrated during cardiopulmonary bypass (Wachtfogel *et al.*, 1987). Histological and functional evidence of pulmonary injury after cardiopulmonary bypass compatible with injuries mediated by experimental complement activation give strength to the hypothesis of complement's role in postbypass morbidity (Ratliff *et al.*, 1972; Hasleton, 1982). What is less clear is whether such morbidity is predictable, avoidable or if knowledge of the extent of complement activation during cardiopulmonary bypass allows interventions to reduce the consequences of activation.

Although the hypothesis connecting the known biological effects of complement activation during bypass is attractive it does not exclude a significant role of other inflammatory cascades and mediators in the production of postoperative morbidity. In addition, a sufficiently close correlation between the extent of complement activation and morbidity has not been demonstrated to warrant measurement of complement fragments routinely. Lew *et al.* (1985) investigated 12 adult patients undergoing coronary surgery using a bubble oxygenator and compared a spectrum of indices of complement activation with those obtained from a control group of patients undergoing aortoiliac surgery. Cardiopulmonary bypass was associated with a statistically significant fall in the concentrations of C3, C4, factor B and $C1_q$. Significant perioperative elevation of $C3_d$ levels confirmed the presence of complement activation. Minor non-significant rises in $C3_d$ were observed in controls. Subsequently, two patients exhibiting low

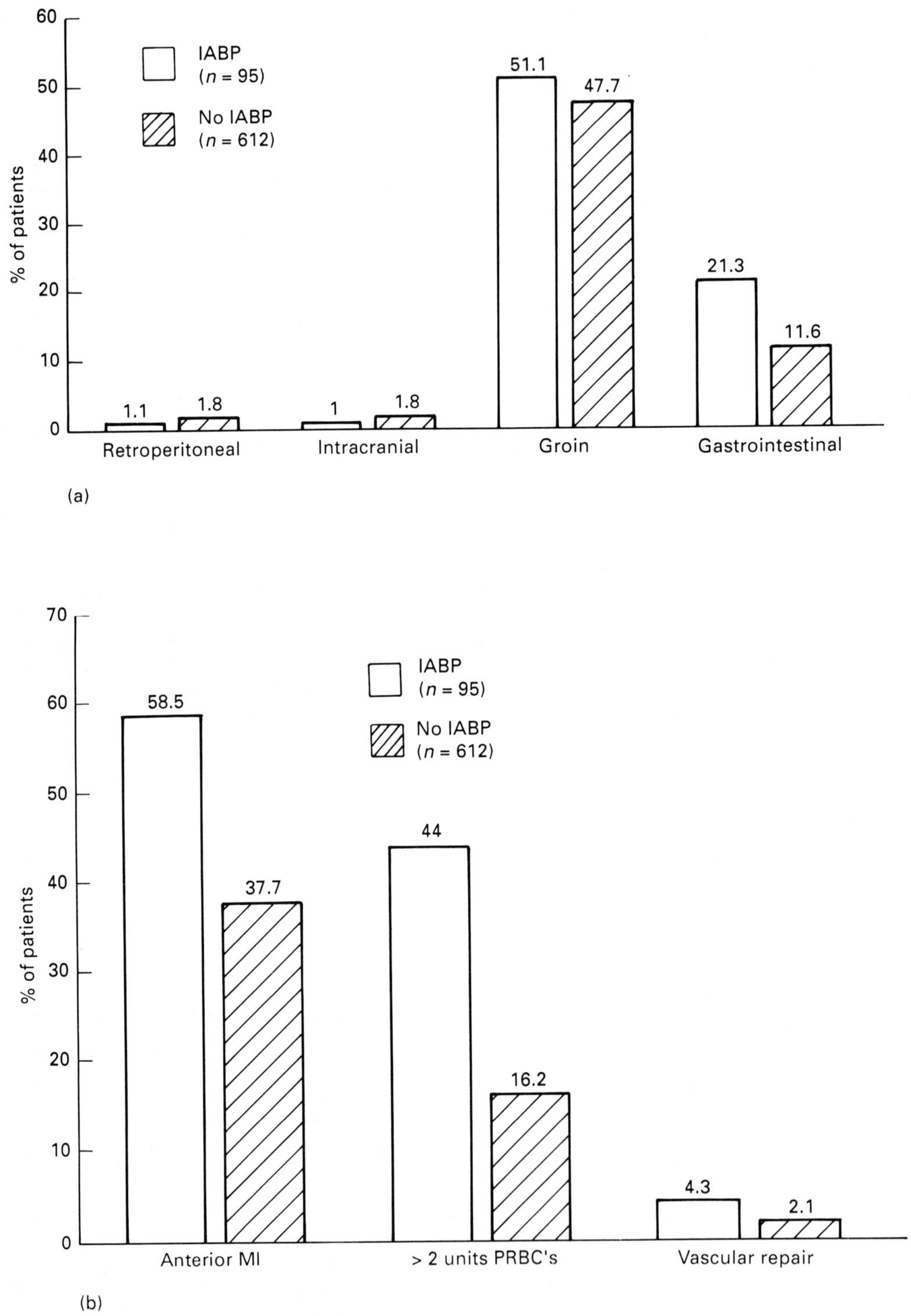

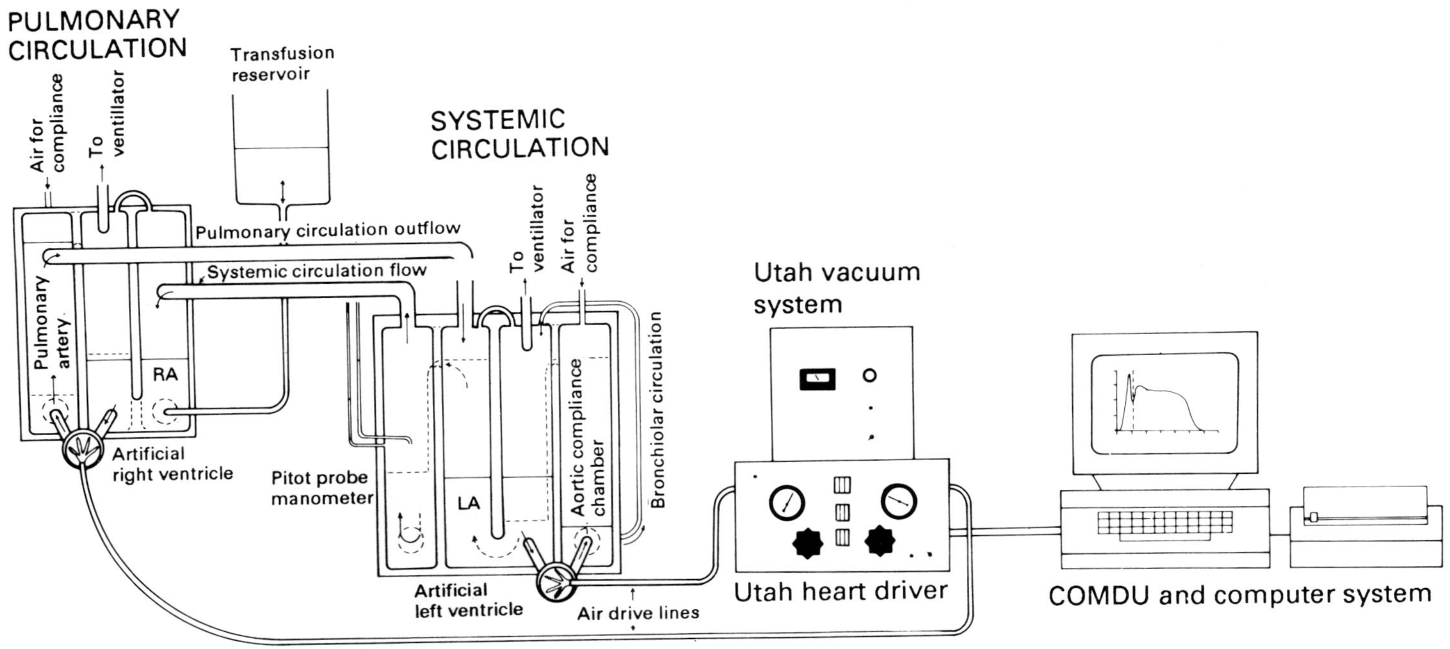

Figure 20.11 The Mock Circulatory System has two series of water cascades to represent the systemic and pulmonary circulations. They provide the typical physiological afterload pressures to the ejecting artificial ventricles. Air chambers in the cascade provide compliance. With its transparent walls, the mock circulatory system vividly displays the flow movement and balance of fluid volume between the lesser (pulmonary) and greater (systemic) circulation. Many of the circumstances that arose with the first human recipient, can be demonstrated with this system. Other pathologic states can also be created for the education of the physicians

wedge pressure, non-cardiogenic pulmonary oedema following cardiopulmonary bypass were demonstrated to have significantly higher levels of $C3_d$ and lower levels of $C1_q$ and CH50 compared with equivalently timed measurements in non-morbid bypass patients. C3 and C4 were also more depleted whereas factor B levels were not different. This anecdotal report supports the theory of a role for exaggerated complement activation in the development of lung injury. Interestingly, the classical pathway was most likely to be involved. Significant anaphylatoxin release occurs in almost all patients undergoing cardiopulmonary bypass surgery (Kirklin *et al.*, 1983). Although complement activation has been detected in non-bypass surgery it does not occur to the same extent (Hahn-Pedersen, Soresenson and Kahlet, 1978; Haslam, Townsend and Branthwaite, 1980; Hällgren, Samuellson and Modig, 1987; Loubser, 1987) and completion of the complement cascade does not occur (Fosse, Mollnes and Ingvaldsen, 1987). Kirklin *et al.* (1983) attempted to correlate the extent of complement activation during and after bypass with the likelihood and degree of postoperative organ dysfunction. $C3_a$ levels, 3h after surgery, correlated directly with the $C3_a$ level before and at the end of bypass, the duration of bypass, and with older age. Morbidity, measured on an ordinal scale, of cardiac, renal, pulmonary and haemostatic functions was assessed in 146 patients of whom 118 underwent open heart procedures. The occurrence and severity of any morbid event was then correlated with $C3_a$ levels, cardiopulmonary bypass time and age. Younger patients were at much greater risk of developing system dysfunction following cardiopulmonary bypass and this was associated with prolonged pump times and increasing levels of $C3_a$. Overall the risk of morbidity correlated with younger age, longer operations and rising $C3_a$ levels. The relationship of $C3_a$ levels and the risk and degree of morbidity appeared constant and increased in strength with younger age. However the risk of morbidity was considerably less in older patients and a separate effect of longer perfusion time and $C3_a$ levels less easy to define.

Complementary information can be obtained from studies of the role of complement activation in the development of the adult respiratory distress syndrome. Although the detection of complement activation correlates well with the potential risk of developing this condition, the measurement of circulating concentrations of complement split products cannot discriminate between those patients who will and those who will not subsequently progress to respiratory failure (Hammerschmidt *et al.*, 1980; Duchateau *et al.*, 1984; Weigelt *et al.*, 1987). It is likely that in cardiopulmonary bypass, complement activation is not the only biological process involved in the production of the 'whole body inflammatory reaction'. There is increasing evidence that other humoral amplification systems including the coagulation, fibrinolytic and kinin cascades also contribute.

References

Addonizio, V.P. Jnr., Macarak E.J., Nicolau, K.C., *et al.* (1979) Effects of prostacyclin and albumin on platelet loss during *in vitro* simulation of extracorporeal circulation. *Journal of the American Society of Hematology*, **53**, 1033–1037

Agnello, V. (1978) Complement deficiency states. *Medicine*, **57**, 1–23

Alper, C.A., Rawn, D., Awdeh, C.L., *et al.* (1980) Studies of hepatic synthesis *in vivo* of plasma proteins, including orosomucoid, transferrin, alpha-1-antitrypsin, C8 and factor B. *Clinical Immunology and Immunopathology*, **16**, 84–89

Bartlett, R.H. and Gazzaniga, A.B. (1981) Physiology and pathophysiology of extracorporeal circulation. In *Techniques of Extracorporeal Circulation*, 2nd edn, (ed. M.I. Ionescu), Butterworths, London, pp. 1–44

Best, N., Sinosich, M.J., Teisner, B., *et al.* (1984) Complement activation during by heparin-protamine interaction. *British Journal of Anaesthesia*, **56**, 339–343

Best, N., Teisner, B., Grudzinskas, J.G. and Fisher, M.M. (1983) Classical pathway activation during an adverse response to protamine sulphate. *British Journal of Anaesthesia*, **55**, 1149–1153

Biggar, W.D., Bohn, D. and Kent, G. (1983) Neutrophil circulation and release from bone marrow during hypothermia. *Infection and Immunity*, **5**, 708–712

Bjoracker, D.G. and Ketchen, T.R. (1982) *In vivo* platelet response to clinical protamine sulfate infusion. *Anaesthesiology*, **57**, A7

Blackstone, E.H., Kirklin, J.W., Stewart, R.W. and Chenoweth, D.E. (1981) In *Prostaglandins in Clinical Medicine*, (eds. K.K. Wu and E.C. Ross), Year Book, Chicago

Boers, M., van den Dungen, J.A.M., Karliczek, G.F., *et al.* (1983) Two membrane oxygenators and a bubbler: a clinical comparison. *Annals of Thoracic Surgery*, **35**, 455–462

Bonser, R.S., Dave, J.R., John, L., *et al.* (1990a) Complement activation before, during and after cardiopulmonary bypass. *European Journal of Cardiothoracic Surgery*, **4**, 291–296

Bonser, R.S., Dave, J.R., John, L., *et al.* (1990b) Reduction of complement activation during bypass by prime manipulation. *Annals of Thoracic Surgery*, **49**, 279–283

Bonser, R.S., Dave, J.R., Morgan, J., *et al.* (1991) Complement activation during bypass in acquired C1 esterase inhibitor deficiency. *Annals of Thoracic Surgery*, **52**, 541–543

Boscoe, M.J., Yewdall, V.M.A., Thompson, M.A. and Cameron, J.S. (1983) Complement activation during cardiopulmonary bypass: quantitative study of effects of methylprednisolone and pulsatile flow. *British Medical Journal*, **287**, 1747–1750

Boralessa, H., Shifferli, J.A., Zaimi, F., *et al.* (1982) Perioperative changes in complement associated with cardiopulmonary bypass. *British Journal of Anaesthesia*, **54**, 1047–1052

Breillatt, J. and Dorson, W.J. (1984) Quantification of serum complement activation by polymeric membranes and materials. *Journal of the American Society for Artificial Internal Organs*, **7**, 57–63

Brevard Haynes, J., Hyers, ThM, Giclas, P.C., *et al.* (1980) Elevated fibrin(ogen) degradation products in the adult respiratory distress syndrome. *American Review of Respiratory Diseases*, **122**, 841–847

Brigham, K.L. (1982) Mechanisms of lung injury. *Clinics in Chest Medicine*, **3**, 9–24

Castaneda, A.R. (1966) Must heparin always be neutralized following open heart operations. *Journal of Thoracic and Cardiovascular Surgery*

Cavarocchi, N.C., England, M.D., Schaff, H.V., *et al.* (1986b) Oxygen free radical generation during cardiopulmonary bypass: correlation with complement activation. *Circulation*, **74** (suppl. III) III-130–III-134

Cavarocchi, N.C., Pluth, J.R., Schaff, H.V., *et al.* (1986a) Complement activation during cardiopulmonary bypass: comparison of bubble and membrane oxygenators. *Journal of Thoracic and Cardiovascular Surgery*, **91**, 252–258

Cavarocchi, N.C., Schaff, H.V., Orszulack, T.A., *et al.* (1985) Evidence for complement activation by protamine–heparin interaction after cardiopulmonary bypass. *Surgery*, **98**, 525–531

Charlesworth, J.A., Gwyn-Williams, D., Sherington, E., *et al.* (1974) Metabolic studies of the third component of complement and the glycine rich beta glycoproteins in patients with hypocomplementaemia. *Journal of Clinical Investigation*, **53**, 1578–1582

Chenoworth, D.E. (1981) Reply to letter to the editor. *New England Journal of Medicine*, **305**, 51

Chenoweth, D.E., Cheung, A.K. and Henderson, L.W. (1983) Anaphylatoxin formation during hemodialysis: Effects of different dialyzer membranes. *Kidney International*, **24**, 764

Chenoweth, D.E., Cooper, S.W., Hugli, T.E., *et al.* (1981) Complement activation during cardiopulmonary bypass: evidence for generation of C3a and C5a anaphylatoxins. *New England Journal of Medicine*, **304**, 497–503

Chiu, R.C. and Samson, R. (1984) Complement (C3, C4) consumption in cardiopulmonary bypass, cardioplegia, and protamine administration. *Annals of Thoracic Surgery*, **37**, 229–232

Clancy, M., Brownstein, L., Cavarocchi, N.C., *et al.* (1985) Complement activation during cardiopulmonary bypass: a comparison of membrane oxygenators. *American Society for Extracorporeal Technology*

Claus, D.R., Siegel, J., Petras, K., *et al.* (1977) Complement activation by interaction of polyanions and polycations. III Complement activation by interaction of multiple polyanions and polycations in the presence of C-reactive protein. *Journal of Immunology*, **118**, 83–87

Collett, B., Alhaq, A., Abdullah, N.B., *et al.* (1984) Pathways to complement activation during cardiopulmonary bypass. *British Medical Journal*, **289**, 1251–1254

Colman, R.W. (1987) Humoral mediators of catastrophic reactions associated with protamine neutralization. *Anesthesiology*, **66**, 595–596

Colten, H.R. (1985) Complement biosynthesis. *Clinical Immunology*, **6**, 287–300

Conahan, T.S., Andrews, R.W. and McVaugh, H. (1981) Cardiovascular effects of protamine sulfate. *Anesthesia and Analgesia (Cleveland)*, **60**, 33

Cooper, J.D., McDonald, J.W.D., Ali, M., *et al.* (1980) Prostaglandin production associated with the pulmonary vascular response to complement activation. *Surgery*, **88**, 215–221

Cooper, N.R. (1985) C1–Inhibitor. *Advances in Immunology*, **37**, 178–183

Cooper, N.R. (1986) Assays for complement activation. *Clinical and Laboratory Medicine*, **6**, 139–155

Cooper, N.R. (1987) The complement system. In *Basic and Clinical Immunology*, 6th edn, (eds. D.P. Stiles, J.D. Stobo and V.J. Wells), Appleton and Lange, East Norwalk

Cooper, N.R., Nemerow, G.R. and Meyers, J.T. (1983) Methods to detect and quantitate complement activation. *Springer Seminars in Immunopathology*, **6**, 173–194

Craddock, P.R., Fehr, J., Dalmasso, A.P., *et al.* (1977a) Hemodialysis leukopenia: pulmonary vascular leukostasis resulting from complement activation by dialyzer cellophane membranes. *Journal of Clinical Investigation*, **59**, 879–888

Craddock, P.R., Hammerschmidt, D., White, J.G., *et al.* (1977b) Complement (C5a)-induced granulocyte aggregation *in vitro*. A possible mechanism of complement-mediated leukostasis and leukopenia. *Journal of Clinical Investigation*, **60**, 260–264

Craddock, P.R., Fehr, J., Brigham, K.L., *et al.* (1977c) Complement and leukocyte-mediated pulmonary dysfunction in hemodialysis. *New England Journal of Medicine*, **296**, 769–774

Davies, E.T., Nasaruddin, B.A., Alhaq, A., *et al.* (1988) Clinical application of a new technique that measures $C4_d$ for assessment of activation of the classical complement pathway. *Journal of Clinical Pathology*, **41**, 143–147

DeBacker, W.A., Verpooten, G.A., Borgonjou, D.S., *et al.* (1984) Hypoxemia during hemodialysis: effects of different membranes and dialysate composition. *Kidney International*, **23**, 738–743

De Leval, M.R., Hill, J.D. and Mielke, H. (1981) Haematological aspects of open heart surgery. In *Techniques in Extracorporeal Circulation*, 2nd edn (ed. M.I. Ionescu), Butterworths, London, pp. 369–390

Dennis, C., Spreng, D.S., Nelson, G.E., *et al.* (1951) Development of a pump oxygenator to replace the heart and lungs: an apparatus applicable to human patients and application to one case. *Annals of Surgery*, **134**, 709–712

Dodd, N.J., Vergani, D., Turney, J.H., *et al.* (1981)

Complement activation of $C1_q$ binding activity in haemodialysis. *Proceedings of the European Dialysis and Transplanation Association*, **18**, 300–304

Dowton, B.S. and Colten, H.R. (1988) Acute phase reactants in inflammation and infection. *Seminars in Haematology*, **25**, 84–90

Duchateau, J., Haas, M., Schreyen, H., *et al.* (1984) Complement activation in patients at risk of developing the adult respiratory distress syndrome. *American Review of Respiratory Diseases*, **130**, 1058–1064

Ecker, E. and Gross, P. (1929) Anticomplementary power of heparin. *Journal of Infectious Diseases*, **44**, 250–253

Ecker, E. and Pillemer, L. (1941) Anti-coagulants and complementary activity: an experimental study. *Journal of Immunology*, **40**, 73–80

Enderby, D.H., Boylett, A. and Parker, D.J. (1979) Methylprednisolone and lung function after cardiopulmonary bypass. *Thorax*, **34**, 720–725

Fauci, A., Haynes, B.F. and Katz, P. (1978) The spectrum of vasculitis. *Annals of Internal Medicine*, **89**, 660–676

Fehr, J. and Rohr, H. (1983) *In vivo* complement activation by polyanion-polycation complexes: evidence that $C5_a$ is generated intravascularly during heparin-protamine interaction. *Clinical Immunology and Immunopathology*, **29**, 7–14

Fiedel, B.B., Rent, R., Myhram, R. and Gewurz, H. (1976) Complement activation by interaction of polyanions and polycations. II. Precipitation and role of IgG, $C1_q$ and C1-Inh during heparin-protamine induced consumption of complement. *Immunology*, **30**, 161–169

Fosse, E., Mollnes, T.E. and Ingvaldsen, B. (1987) Complement activation during major operations with or without cardiopulmonary bypass. *Journal of Thoracic and Cardiovascular Surgery*, **93**, 860–866

Frank, M.M. (1987) Complement in the pathophysiology of human disease. *New England Journal of Medicine*, **316**, 1525–1530

Frater, R.W.M., Oka, Y., Hong, Y., *et al.* (1984) Protamine-induced circulatory changes. *Journal of Thoracic and Cardiovascular Surgery*, **87**, 687–692

Gandhi, J.G., Salm, T.V. and Szymanski, I.O. (1983) Effect of cardiopulmonary bypass of plasma fibronectin, IgG and C3. *Transfusion*, **23**, 476–479

Gans, H. and Krivit, W. (1962) Problems in hemostasis during open-heart surgery IV: on the changes in the blood clotting mechanisms during cardiopulmonary bypass procedures. *Annals of Surgery*, **135**, 353–359

Gaspardone, A., Ciavolella, M., Mercogliano, D., *et al.* (1986) Complement activation by different cardiopulmonary bypass priming solutions. *Perfusion*, **1**, 255–260

Ghebrehiwit, B., Silverberg, M. and Kaplan, A.P. (1981) Activation of the classical complement pathway by Hageman factor fragments. *Journal of Experimental Medicine*, **153**, 665–676

Ghoneim, A.T.M., McGoldrick, J. and Ionescu, M.I. (1982) Serial C-reactive protein measurements in infective complications following cardiac operations: evaluation and use in monitoring response to therapy. *Annals of Thoracic Surgery*, **34**, 166–171

Gibbon, J.H. Jnr. (1953) Application of a mechanical heart and lung apparatus to cardiac surgary. In *Recent Advances in Cardiovascular Physiology and Surgery*. University of Minnesota, Minneapolis, pp. 107–113

Glenville, B. and Ross, D. (1986) Coronary artery surgery with patients' lungs as the oxygenator. *Lancet*, **ii**, 1005–1006

Goldstein, I.M., Roos, D., Weissman, G. and Kaplan, H.B. (1976) Influence of corticosteroids on human polymorphonuclear leukocyte function *in vitro*. Reduction of lysosomal enzyme release and superoxide production. *Inflammation*, **1**, 305–315

Gomes, H.R. and McGoon, D.C. (1970) Bleeding patterns after open heart surgery. *Journal of Thoracic and Cardiovascular Surgery*, **60**, 87–97

Gorski, P.J. (1981) Quantitation of human complement fragment $C4_a$ in physiological fluids by competitive inhibition radioimmune assay. *Journal of Immunological Methods*, **47**, 61–65

Götze, O. and Müller-Eberhard, H.J. (1971) The C3-activator system: An alternative pathway of complement activation. *Journal of Experimental Medicine*, **134**, 90–108

Gross, P. and Ecker, E.E. (1928) Anticomplementary action of purified heparin. *Proceedings of the Society for Experimental Biology and Medicine*, **26**, 508–509

Hahn-Pedersen, J., Sorensen, H. and Kehlet, H. (1978) Complement activation during surgical procedures. *Surgery, Gynecology and Obstetrics*, **148**, 66–68

Hairston, P., Mann, J.P., Graber, C.P. and Lee, W.H.Jnr. (1969) Depression of immunologic surveillance by pump-oxygenator perfusion. *Journal of Surgical Research*, **9**, 587–590

Hakim, R.M., Breillatt, J., Lazarus, M. and Port, F.K. (1984) Complement activation and hypersensitivity reactions to dialysis membranes. *New England Journal of Medicine*, **311**, 878–882

Hällgren, G., Samuelson, T. and Modig, J. (1987) Complement activation and increased alveolar-capillary permeability after major surgery and in adult respiratory distress syndrome. *Critical Care Medicine*, **15**, 189–193

Hammerschmidt, D.E., White, J.G., Craddock, P.R. and Jacob, H.S. (1979) Corticosteroids inhibit complement induced granulocyte aggregation. *Journal of Clinical Investigation*, **63**, 798–803

Hammerschmidt, D.E., Weaver, L.J., Hudson, L.D., *et al.* (1980) Association of complement activation and elevated plasma-$C5_a$ with adult respiratory distress syndrone: pathophysiological relevance and posssible prognostic value. *Lancet*, **i**, 947–949

Hammerschmidt, D.E., Stroncek, D.F., Bowers, T.K., *et al.* (1981) Complement activation and neutropenia occurring during cardiopulmonary bypass. *Journal of Thoracic and Cardiovascular Surgery*, **81**, 370–377

Haslam, P.L., Townsend, P.J. and Branthwaite, M.A. (1980) Complement activation during cardiopulmonary bypass. *Anaesthesia*, **35**, 22–26

Hasleton, P.S. (1983) Adult respiratory distress syndrome–a review. *Histopathology*, **7**, 307–322

Hughli, T.E. (1979) Complement anaphylatoxins as plasma mediators, spasminogens and chemotaxins. In *Current Topics in Molecular Immunology*, (eds. B.A. Reisfled and W.J. Mandy), Plenum Press, New York, pp. 255–279

Hughli, T.E. (1984) Structure and function of the anaphylatoxins. *Springer Seminars in Immunopathology*, **7**, 193–219

Hughli, T.E. and Chenoweth, D.E. (1981) The anaphylatoxins. In *Immunoassays* (eds. R.M. Nakamura, W.R. Dito, and E.S. Tucker III), Alan R. Liss, New York, pp. 430–460

Hughli, T.E. and Müller-Eberhard, H.J. (1978) The anaphylatoxins C3a and C5a. *Advances in Immunology*, **26**, 1–34

Hyslop, N.E., Dowmashkis, R.R., Green, N.H. and Porter, R.R. (1970) The fixation of complement and the first activated component (C1) of complement by complexes formed between antibody and divalent hapten. *Journal of Experimental Medicine*, **131**, 783–802

Jacob, H.S. (1983) Complement mediated leucoembolization. A mechanism of tissue damage during extracorporeal perfusion, myocardial infarction and shock. *Quarterly Journal of Medicine*, **52**, 289–294

Jacob, H.S., Craddock, P.R., Hammerschmidt, D.E. and Moldow, C.F. (1980) Complement-induced granulocyte aggregation: an unsuspected mechanism of disease. *New England Journal of Medicine*, **302**, 789–794

Jastrzbebski, J., Sykes, M.K. and Woods, G.D. (1974) Cardiorespiratory effects of protamine after cardiopulmonary bypass in man. *Thorax*, **29**, 534

Jones, H.M., Matthews, N., Vaughan, R.S. and Stark, J.M. (1982) Cardiopulmonary bypass and complement activation: Involvement of classical and alternative pathways. *Anaesthesia*, **37**, 629–633

Kazatchkine, M.D. and Maillet, F. (1981) Modulation of the formation of the amplification C3 convertase of human complement by polycations. *Federation Proceedings*, **40**, 965

Kazatchkine, M.D. and Nydegger, U.E. (1982) The human alternative complement pathway: biology and immunopathology of activation and regulation. *Progress in Allergy*, **30**, 193–234

Kazatchkine, M.D., Fearon, D.T., Silbert, J.E. and Austen, K.F. (1979) Surface associated heparin inhibits zymosan induced activation of the human alternative complement pathway by augmenting the regulatory action of the control proteins on particle bound $C3_b$. *Journal of Experimental Medicine*, **150**, 1202–1208

Kazatchkine, M.D., Fearon, D.T., Metcalfe, D.D. *et al.* (1982) Structural determinants of the capacity of heparin to inhibit the formation of the human amplification C3 convertase. *Journal of Clinical Investigation*, **67**, 223–228

Kirklin, J.K. (1982) Discussion. *Journal of Thoracic and Cardiovascular Surgery*, **84**, 513

Kirklin, J.W. (1983) Cardiopulmonary bypass for cardiac surgery. In *Gibbon's Surgery of the Chest*, 4th edn (eds. D.C. Sabiston and F.C. Spencer), W.B. Saunders, Philadelphia, pp. 909–925

Kirklin, J.K., Chenoweth, D.E., Naftel, D.C., *et al.* (1986) Effects of protamine administration after cardiopulmonary bypass on complement, blood elements and the hemodynamic state. *Annals of Thoracic Surgery*, **41**, 193–199

Kirklin, J.K., Westaby, S., Blackstone, E.H., *et al.* (1983) Complement and the damaging effects of cardiopulmonary bypass. *Journal of Thoracic and Cardiovascular Surgery*, **86**, 845–857

Kouchoukos, N.T. and Karp, R.B. (1981) Functional disturbances following extracorporeal circulatory support in cardiac surgery. In *Techniques of Extracorporeal Circulation*, 2nd end (ed. M.I. Ionescu), Butterworths, London, pp. 295–344

Lachmann, P.J. (1966) Conglutinins and immunoconglutinins. *Advances in Immunology*, **6**, 479–485

Lachmann, P.J. and Peters, D.K. (1982) Complement. In *Clinical Aspects of Immunology* (eds. P.J. Lachmann and D.K. Peters), Blackwell, Oxford, pp. 18–49

Lachmann, P.J. and Hughes-Jones, N.C. (1985) In *Complement* (eds. H.J. Müller-Eberhard and P.A. Miescher), Springer-Verlag, Berlin, pp. 147–160

Lakin, J.D., Blocker, T.J., Strong, D.M. and Yocum, M.W. (1978) Anaphylaxis to protamine sulfate mediated by a complement dependent IgG antibody. *Journal of Allergy and Clinical Immunology*, **61**, 102–107

Law, S.K.A. and Reid, K.B.M. (1988) *Complement*, IRL Press, Oxford

Lew, P.D., Forster, A., Perrin, L.H., *et al.* (1985) Complement activation in the adult respiratory distress syndrome following cardiopulmonary bypass. *Bulletin of the European Society for the Physiopathology of Respiration*, **21**, 231–235

Loos, M. (1982) The classical complement pathway: mechanism of activation of the first component by antigen-antibody complexes. *Progress in Allergy*, **30**, 135–192

Loos, M., Raepple, E., Hadding, U. and Bitter-Suermann, D. (1974) Interaction of polyanions with the first and third component of complement. *Federation Proceedings*, **33**, 775

Loubser, P.G. (1987) Complement activation during cardiac and thoracic vascular operations. *Texas Heart Institute Journal*, **14**, 369–373

Lowenstein, E., Johnston, W.S., Lappan, O.G., *et al.* (1983) Catastrophic pulmonary vasoconstriction associated with protamine reversal of heparin. *Anesthesiology*, **59**, 470

McDonald, J.W.D., Ali, M., Morgan, E., Townsend, E.R. and Cooper, J.D. (1983) Thromboxane synthesis by sources other than platelets associated with complement induced pulmonary leukostasis and pulmonary hyertension in sheep. *Circulation Research*, **52**, 1–6

McLeod, B.C., Viernes, A. and Sassetti, R.J. (1983a) Complement metabolism during membrane plasma separation. *Artificial Organs*, **7**, 443–449

McLeod, B.C., Viernes, A. and Sassetti, R.J. (1983b)

Complement activation by plasma separator membranes. *Transfusion*, **23**, 143–147

Marcus, R.L., Shin, H.S. and Mayer, M.M. (1971) An alternative complement pathway. C3 cleaving activity not due to $C42_a$, on endotoxin lipopolysaccharide after treatment with guinea pig serum. *Proceedings of the National Academy of Sciences*, **68**, 1351–1360

Maggart, M. and Stewart, S. (1987) The mechanisms and management of non-cardiogenic pulmonary edema following cardiopulmonary bypass. *Annals of Thoracic Surgery*, **43**, 231–236

Mayer, M.M. (1961) Complement and complement fixation. In *Experimental Immunochemistry*, 2nd edn, (eds. E.A. Kabat and M.M. Mayer), Charles C. Thomas, Springfield, p. 133

Metzger, W.J., Grem, J., Halverson, P.C., *et al.* (1984) C1-INH deficiency and angioedema: a spectrum of disease. *Annals of Allergy*, **52**, 285–290

Michaels, P.A.L. and Barash, P.G. (1983) Hemodynamic changes during protamine administration. *Anesthesia and Analgesia (Cleveland)*, **62**, 831

Mickleborough, L.L., Arnold, G. and Chiu, R.C.J. (1986) Complement consumption during cardiopulmonary bypass: bubble versus membrane oxugenation. *Perfusion*, **1**, 261–269

Milgrom, H., Curd, J.G., Kaplan, R.A., *et al.* (1980) Activation of the fourth component of complement (C4): Assessment by rocket immunoelectrophoresis and correlation with metabolism of C4. *Journal of Immunology*, **124**, 2780–2785

Miyamoto, Y., Hirose, H., Matsuda, H., *et al.* (1985) Analysis of complement activation profile during cardiopulmonary bypass and its inhibition by FUT-175. *Transactions of the American Society for Artificial Internal Organs*, **31**, 508–511

Mollnes, T.E. (1985) Early and late phase activation of complement evaluated by plasma levels of C3dg and the terminal complement complex. *Complement*, **2**, 156–164

Mollnes, T.E., Lee, T. and Harboe, M. (1984) Detection and quantification of the terminal $C5_b$-9 complex of human complement by a sensitive enzyme-linked immunosorbent assay. *Scandinavian Journal of Immunology*, **20**, 157–166

Mollnes, T.E., Lee, T., Froland, S.S. and Harboe, M. (1985) Quantification of the terminal complement components in human plasma by an enzyme-linked immunosorbent assay based on monoclonal antibodies against a neoantigen of the complex. *Scandinavian Journal of Immunology*, **22**, 197–202

Morel, D.R., Zapol, W.M., Thomas, S.J., *et al.* (1987) $C5_a$ and thromboxane generation associated with pulmonary vaso- and broncho-constriction during protamine reversal of heparin. *Anesthesiology*, **66**, 597–604

Morse, J.H., Müller-Eberhard, H.J. and Kunkel, H.G. (1962) Antinuclear factors and serum complement in systemic lupus erythematosus. *Bulletin of the New York Academy of Medicine*, **38**, 641–651

Müller-Eberhard, H.J. (1984) The membrane attack complex. *Springer Seminars in Immunopathology*, **7**, 93–141

Müller-Eberhard, H.J. and Miescher, R.A. (eds.) (1985) *Complement*, Springer-Verlag, Berlin

Myhrman, R., Monckton, S. and Gewürz, H. (1973) *Clinical Research*, **21**, 877

Nordstrom, L., Fletcher, R. and Pavek, K. (1978) Shock of anaphylactoid type reaction induced by protamine: a continuous cardiopulmonary record. *Acta Anaesthesiologica Scandinavia*, **22**, 195

O'Flaherty, S., Craddock, P.R. and Jacob, H.S. (1977) Mechanism of anticomplentary activity of corticosteroids *in vivo*. Possible relevance in endotoxin shock (39638). *Proceedings of the Society for Experimental Biology and Medicine*, **154**, 206–209

Olinger, G.N., Becker, R.M. and Bonchek, L.I. (1980) Non-cardiogenic pulmonary oedema and peripheral vascular collapse following cardiopulmonary bypass. Rare protamine reaction? *Annals of Thoracic Surgery*, **29**, 20–25

Packard, B.D. and Wieler, J.M. (1983) Steroids inhibit activation of the alternate-amplification pathway of complement. *Infection and Immunity*, **40**, 1011–1014

Pangburn, M.K. (1986) In *Immunobiology of the Complement System* (ed. G.D. Ross), Academic Press, New York, p. 145

Pangburn, M.K. and Müller-Eberhard, H.J. (1984) The alternative pathway of complement. *Springer Seminar in Immunopathology*, **7**, 163–192

Parker, D.J. (1975) Some changes in the lungs associated with cardiopulmonary bypass. In *Lung Metabolism: Proteolysis and Anti-proteolysis, Biochemical Pharmacology, Handling of Bioactive Substances* (eds. A.F. Junod and R. De Haller), Academic Press, New York, pp. 459–479

Parker, D.J., Cantrell, J.W., Karp, R.B., *et al.* (1972) Changes in serum complement and immunoglobulins following cardiopulmonary bypass. *Surgery*, **71**, 824–827

Parker, D.J., Cook, S. and Turner-Warwick, M. (1975) Serum complement studies during and following cardiopulmonary bypass. In *Lung Metabolism: Proteolysis and Anti-proteolysis, Biochemical Pharmacology, Handling of Bioactive Substances* (eds A.F. Junod and R. De Haller), Academic Press, New York, pp. 481–487

Peakman, M., Lobo-Yeo, A., Senaldi, G., Nilsson, M., Tee, D.E.H. and Vergani, D. (1987) Quantification of C3d in biological fluids by a enzyme-linked immunosorbent assay. *Journal of Immunological Methods*, **104**, 51–56

Perrin, L.H., Lambert, P.H. and Miescher, P.A. (1975) Complement breakdown products in plasma from patients with membranoproliferative and other glomerulonephritides. *Journal of Clinical Investigation*, **56**, 165–176

Perrin, L.H., Shiraishi, S., Stroud, R.M. and Lambert, P.H. (1975) Detection and quantification in plasma and synovial fluids of a fragment of human C4 with a mobility generated during the activation of the complement system. *Journal of Immunology*, **115**, 32–35

Petersen, M.B., Huttemeier, P.C., Zapol, W.M., *et al.*

(1982) Thromboxane mediates acute pulmonary hypertension in sheep in extracorporeal perfusion. *American Journal of Physiology*, **243**, H471–479

Pillemer, L. (1943) Recent advances in the chemistry of complement. *Chemistry Reviews*, **33**, 1–26

Pillemer, L., Blum, L., Lepow, I.H., *et al.* (1954) The properdin system and immunity I. Demonstration and isolation of a new serum protein properdin and its role in immune phenomena. *Science*, **120**, 279

Pixley, R.A., Schapira, M. and Colman, R.W. (1985) Effect of heparin on the inactivation rate of human activated factor XII by antithrombin III. *Blood*, **66**, 192–203

Porter, R.R. and Reid, K.B.M. (1979) Activation of the complement system by antigen–antibody complexes. The classical pathway. *Advances in Protein Chemistry*, **33**, 1–71

Pruitt, K.M., Stroud, R.M. and Scottt, J.W. (1971) Blood damage in the heart–lung machine. *Proceedings of the Society for Experimental Biology and Medicine*, **137**, 714–718

Quiroga, M.M., Miyagishima, R., Haendchen, L.C., *et al.* (1985) The effect of body temperature on leukocyte kinetics during cardiopulmonary bypass. *Journal of Thoracic and Cardiovascular Surgery*, **90**, 91–96

Raepple, E., Hill, H-U. and Loos, M. (1976) Mode of interaction of different polyanions with the first (C1), second (C2) and the fourth (C4) components of complement. I. Effect on fluid phase C1 and on C1 bound to EA or to EAC4. *Immunology*, **13**, 251–255

Ratliff, N.B., Young, W.G., Hackel, D.B., *et al.* (1973) Pulmonary injury secondary to extracorporeal circulation: an ultrastructural study. *Journal of Thoracic and Cardiovascular Surgery*, **65**, 425–432

Reid, K.B.M. (1986) Activation and control of the complement system. *Essays in Biochemistry*, **22**, 27–68

Rent, R., Ertel, N., Eiesenstein, R. and Gewurz, H. (1975) Complement activation by interaction of polyanions and polycations. 1. Heparin-protamine induced consumption of complement. *Journal of Immunology*, **114**, 120–124

Rinaldo, J.E. and Rogers, R.M. (1982) Adult respiratory distress syndrome. *New England Journal of Medicine*, **206**, 900–909

Roitt, I., Brostoff, J. and Male, D. (1985) Complement. In *Immunology* (eds I. Roitt, J. Brostoff and D. Male), Gower Medical Publishing, London

Romson, J.L., Hook, B.G., Pigot, V.H., *et al.* (1982) The effect of ibuprofen on accumulation of indium labelled platelets and leukocytes in experimental myocardial infarction. *Circulation*, **66**, 1002–1011

Ross, G.D. (ed) (1986) *Immunology of the complement system. An introduction for research and clinical medicine*, Academic Press, New York

Roth, J.A., Golub, S.H., Cukingnan, R.A., *et al.* (1980) Cell mediated immunity is depressed following cardiopulmonary bypass. *Annals of Thoracic Surgery*, **31**, 350–356

Ruddy, S. and Austen, K.F. (1970) The complement system in rheumatoid arthritis. *Arthritis and Rheumatism*, **13**, 713–723

Ryan, U.S. and Ryan, J.W. (1983) Endothelial cells and inflammation. *Clinical and Laboratory Medicine*, **3**, 577–599

Salama, A., Hugo, F., Heinrich, D., *et al.* (1988) Deposition of terminal $C5_b$-9 complement complexes on erythrocytes and leukocytes during cardiopulmonary bypass. *New England Journal of Medicine*, **318**, 404–414

Schapira, M., Despland, E., Scott, C.E., *et al.* (1982) Purified human kallikrein aggregates human blood neutrophils. *Journal of Clinical Investigation*, **69**, 1199–1203

Schein, R.M.H., Bergman, R., Marcial, E.H., *et al.* (1987) Complement activation and corticosteroid therapy in the development of the adult respiratory distress syndrome. *Chest*, **91**, 850–854

Schirmer, W.J., Schirmer, J.M., Naff, G.B. and Fry, D.E. (1988) Systemic complement activation produces hemodynamic changes characteristic of sepsis. *Archives of Surgery*, **123**, 316–321

Senaldi, G., Peakman, M., Alhaq, A., *et al.* (1987) Activation of the alternative complement pathway: clinical application of a new technique to measure fragment Ba. *Journal of Clinical Pathology*, **40**, 1235–1239

Sharath, M.D., Metzger, W.J., Richerson, H.B., *et al.* (1985) Protamine-induced fatal anaphylaxis. *Journal of Thoracic and Cardiovascular Surgery*, **90**, 86–90

Shapira, N., Schaff, H.V., Piehler, J.M., *et al.* (1982) Cardiovascular effects of protamine sulfate in man. *Journal of Thoracic and Cardiovascular Surgery*, **84**, 505–514

Siegel, J., Rent, R. and Gewurz, H. (1974) Interactions of C-reactive protein with the complement system 1. Protamine-induced consumption of complement in acute phase sera. *Journal of Experimental Medicine*, **140**, 631–647

Stefaniszyn, H.J., Novick, R.J. and Salerno, T.A. (1984) Toward a better understanding of the hemodynamic effects of protamine and heparin interaction. *Journal of Thoracic and Cardiovascular Surgery*, **87**, 678–686

Stewart, W., McSweeney, S.M., Kellet, M.A., *et al.* (1984) Increased risk of severe protamine reaction in NPH insulin dependent diabetics undergoing cardiac catheterization. *Circulation*, **70**, 788–792

Subramanian, V., Laude, A.J., Gans, H. and Lowman, J.T. (1969) Depression of host defence mechanisms following extracorporeal circulation. *Transactions of the American Society for Artificial Internal Organs*, **15**, 165–168

Sundsmo, J.S. and Fair, D.S. (1983) Relationships among the complement, kinin, coagulation and fibrinolytic systems. *Springer Seminars in Immunopathology*, **6**, 231–258

Swaak, A.J.G., Van Rooyen, A., Vogelaar, C., *et al.* (1985) Complement C3 metabolism in systemic lupus erythematosus in relation to the disease course. *Rheumatology Interventions*, **6**, 221–226

Tamiya, T., Yamasaki, M., Maeo, Y., *et al.* (1988) Complement activation in cardiopulmonary bypass with special reference to anaphylatoxin production in membrane and bubble oxygenators. *Annals of Thoracic Surgery*, **46**, 47–57

Tankersley, D.L., Alving, P.M. and Finlayson, J.S. (1983) Activation of factor XII by dextran sulfate. The basis for an assay for factor Xii. *Blood*, **62**, 448–453

Tennenberg, S.D., Bailey, W.W., Cotta, L.A., *et al.* (1986) The effects of methylprednisolone on complement-mediated neutrophil activation during cardiopulmonary bypass. *Surgery*, **100**, 134–141

Thompson, M.A. and Broadbent, M.P. (1980) Methylprednisolone prior to cardiopulmonary bypass. *Anaesthesia*, **35**, 345–353

Thompson, M.A., Broadbent, M.P. and English, J. (1982) Plasma levels of methylprednisolone following administration during cardiac surgery. *Anaesthesia*, **37**, 405–407

Till, G.O., Johnson, K.J., Runkel, R. and Ward, P.A. (1982) Intravascular activation of complement and acute lung injury: dependency on neutrophils and toxic oxygen metabolites. *Journal of Clinical Investigation*, **69**, 1126–1135

Umebayashi, Y., Morishita, Y., Arikawa, K., *et al.* (1987) Hereditary angioneurotic oedema: report of a case undergoing open-heart surgery. *Vascular Surgery*, **21**, 138–1413

van Oeveren, W., Kazatchine, M.D., Descamps-Latscha, B., *et al.* (1985) Deleterious effects of cardiopulmonary bypass: a prospective study of bubble versus membrane oxygenators. *Journal of Thoracic and Cardiovascular Surgery*, **89**, 888–899

Vergani, D., Bevis, L., Nasaruddin, B.A., *et al.* (1983) Clinical application of a new nephelometric technique to measure complement activation. *Journal of Clinical Pathology*, **36**, 793–799

Videm, V., Fosse, E., Mollnes, T.E., *et al.* (1989) Different oxygenators for cardiopulmonary bypass lead to varying degress of human complement activation *in vitro*. *Journal of Thoracic and Cardiovascular Surgery*, **97**, 764–770

Wachtfogel, Y.T., Kucich, U., James, H.L., *et al.* (1983) Human plasma kallikrein release neutrophil elastase during blood coagulation. *Journal of Clinical Investigation*, **70**, 1672–1677

Wachtfogel, Y.T., Harpel, P.C., Edmunds, L.H.Jnr. and Colman, R.W. (1986a) Formation of C1–C1 inhibitor and kallikrein-C1 inhibitor complexes during cardiopulmonary bypass. *Blood*, **68**, 342a

Wachtfogel, Y.T., Pixley, R.A., Kucich, U., *et al.* (1986b) Purified factor XIIa aggregates human neutrophils and causes degranulation. *Blood*, **67**, 1731–1737

Wachtfogel, Y.T., Kucich, U., Greenplate, J., *et al.* (1987) Human neutrophil degranulation during extracorporeal circulation. *Blood*, **69**, 324–330

Wadsworth, A., Maltaner, F. and Maltaner, E. (1937) The inhibition of complementary activity by anticoagulants. *Journal of Immunology*, **33**, 297–303

Ward, P.A. (1971) Complement-derived leukotactic factors in pathological fluids. *Journal of Experimental Medicine*, **134**, 109–113

Weegmuller, E.W., Kazatchkine, M.D. and Nydegger, U.E. (1983) Complement activation during extracorporeal circulation. *Plasmatherapy and Transfusion Technology*, **4**, 361–371

Weigelt, J.A., Borman, K.R., Norcross, J.F. and Chenoweth, D.E. (1987) Complement and severity of pulmonary insufficiency. *Critical Care Medicine*, **15**, 407

Weiler, J.M. and Packard, B.D. (1982) Methylprednisolone inhibits the alternative and amplification pathways of complement. *Infection and Immunity*, **38**, 122–126

Westaby, S. (1983) Complement and the damaging effects of cardiopulmonary bypass. *Thorax*, **38**, 321–325

Westaby, S., Turner, M.W. and Stark, J. (1985) Complement activation and anaphylactoid response to protamine in a child after cardiopulmonary bypass. *British Heart Journal*, **53**, 574–576

Wildevuur, C.R.H. (1980) Towards safer cardiopulmonary bypass. In *Towards Safer Cardiac Surgery* (ed. D.B. Longmore), Internal Medical Publishers, Lancaster

Winkelstein, J.A. and Thonasz, A. (1978) Activation of the alternative complement pathway by pneumococcal cell wall teichoic acid. *Journal of Immunology*, **120**, 174–179

Williams, D.G. and Peters, D.K. (1982) The immunopathology of nephritis. In *Clinical Aspects of Immunology* (eds P.J. Lachmann and D.K. Peters), Blackwell, Oxford, pp. 853–877

Whaley, K. (ed.) (1970) *Complement in Health and Disease*, MTP Press, Lancaster

Whicher, J.T. (1978) The value of complement assays in clinical chemistry. *Clinical Chemistry*, **24**, 7–22

White, J.V. (1981) Complement activation during cardiopulmonary bypass. *New England Journal of Medicine*, **305**, 514

12

Changes in renal function associated with cardiopulmonary bypass

F.D. Thompson

The kidney, with its ability to control sodium and water excretion, eliminate hydrogen ions and secrete nitrogenous waste, is clearly central in maintaining the circulation in both its volume and biochemical content. The interdependence between the heart and kidney is obvious in physiological terms and important in clinical management as many diseases affect both: for example in left ventricular failure the glomerular filtration rate will fall simply because the energy required for ultrafiltration at the glomerulus is generated by the left ventricle as it pumps against a peripheral resistance, thus maintaining the arterial pressure. A low filtration rate is associated with cardiac failure and any procedure from the use of inotropes through to cardiac transplantation is capable of improving renal function. In low output states the kidney behaves as though the circulating volume is reduced and avid sodium and water retention is the result. This too is reversible when cardiac performance improves. Sub-acute bacterial endocarditis can lead not only to infected renal infarcts secondary to emboli but an immune complex glomerulonephritis produces haematuria, proteinuria and renal failure. The renal arteries can be involved in aortic dissection and both the coronary vessels and intrarenal vessels can be involved in a common vasculitic process, and finally the common example of the severe arteriopath is liable to have both myocardial and renal blood flow reduced by atheroma. These examples are cited to illustrate the common pathology that may involve both heart and kidney and to ensure that wherever possible a preoperative assessment of renal function is made, not only to help with clinical management but in order that the changes seen across bypass can be seen in perspective. A salutary reminder at this point is important. A normal blood urea does not mean that the glomerular filtration rate is normal, as significant nitrogen retention only occurs when the filtration rate has fallen below 30 ml min_{-1} and so a careful estimation of the glomerular filtration rate, examination of the urine deposit, a 24h estimate of protein excretion and if possible a radionucleide scan are essential. There are no short cuts!

Despite preoperative assessment and the subsequent careful management of the circulating volume during surgery, acute renal failure still occurs. Excluding aortic dissection involving the renal arteries, showers of cholesterol emboli and severe septicaemia, a minority of cases will develop acute renal failure during surgery and in order to prevent problems a better understanding of the pathophysiology of acute tubular dysfunction during bypass is beneficial. Advances have been made in our understanding during the last decade and these will now be reviewed with emphasis based on practical prevention.

Pathophysiological changes

One of the problems that has hindered our understanding is the absence of an animal model that mimics the changes seen in the human kidney when subject to periods of hypotension. However, hypotension produced experimentally can lead to acute renal failure, but it is clear that a reduced renal blood flow is not the sole answer – it may initiate the process but persistent acute tubular dysfunction, a better name than necrosis, depends on secondary factors, and some of these possible mechanisms are as follows.

Vascular events

When the renal perfusion pressure falls secondary to hypovolaemia or cardiac failure the renal vascular resistance increases due to sympathetic activity and activation of the renin–angiotensin system (Hollenberg, Wilkes and Shulman, 1983). The initial fall in renal blood flow is reflected in a reduction both in cortical and medullary flow, demonstrated radiographically by Lavender and Sherwood (1972). Initially glomerular perfusion diminished followed in order by blood flow through the arterioles and then the interlobular vessels. Persisting sodium depletion exacerbates these changes as demonstrated by Brenner, Zatz and Ichikawa (1986).

As a result of diminished cortical flow the glomerular filtration rate is reduced because of a fall in filtration pressure and a reduction in the surface area of the glomerular capillaries. The fall in filtration pressure is a combination of initial afferent arteriolar vasoconstriction, possibly mediated by angiotensin II and vasodilatory prostaglandins lowering the efferent arteriolar tone (Adams *et al.*, 1980). Mesangial cell contraction, possibly mediated by leukotrienes and angiotensin II, also reduces the capillary surface area. Long periods of ischaemia over 48h produce reduction in the glomerular filtration rate despite restoration of renal perfusion. Several factors may be responsible for perpetuating renal dysfunction. Firstly endothelial swelling and necrosis may impede the microcirculation which is affected by locally produced vasoconstrictors, e.g. thromboxane, leukotrienes and endothelin (endothelium derived constricting factor, EDCF). Autoregulation of blood flow is also impaired and Conger, Robinette and Schrier (1988) suggested that it is a lack of vasodilatory factors dependent upon an intact endothelium that is responsible. Various vasodilators, e.g. bradykinin and acetylcholine, depend on an intact, healthy endothelium for their action as these cells on stimulation release a relaxing factor thought to be nitric oxide (endothelial derived relaxing factor, EDRF). Damaged endothelium prevents relaxation and hence regulation of blood flow is lost. Adenosine is increased secondary to ischaemia and as this is a potent mediator of vasoconstriction it may well be another event which limits normal autoregulation, especially during the recovery phase from ischaemia.

Medullary blood flow is also reduced by up to 50% during periods of ischaemia and medullary flow may remain low, even when cortical blood flow is restored. Normally the oxygen content of the medulla is low and medullary tissue is virtually hypoxic. Minor reductions in blood flow will rapidly produce anoxia leading to abnormal sodium transport and concentrating ability (Brezis *et al.*, 1984).

Back leak of filtrate

Ischaemia is thought to disrupt the tubular epithelium, rendering it permeable so filtrate produced diffuses rapidly into the interstitium. Animal evidence exists but its relevance in man is not clear.

Tubular obstruction

The shedding of tubular cells which aggregate in the lumen may cause obstruction. In some experimental models micropuncture studies have confirmed a rise in intraluminal pressure – this however is not uniform and its clinical significance is again uncertain.

Possible additional contributing factors

1. Activation of the renin–angiotensin system. Elevated renal levels in acute renal failure have been reported. Whether the vascular events described above promote its release or whether it is a secondary event is still not clear. High renin levels are associated with aortic clamping required for aneurysmal repair but drugs which dampen down the renin response or block the effect of angiotensin II do not seem to alter the clinical outcome.
2. Haemolysis to a varying degree can occur during bypass. There is a release not only of free haemoglobin, which is known to be nephrotoxic, but also the red cell stroma may occlude the renal microvasculature. Unless haemolysis is severe it is unlikely to be important (Osborn *et al.*, 1982).
3. Non-pulsatile flow. Many investigators have examined the effect of non-pulsatile flow on renal perfusion and function. There is a continuing debate as to whether the absence of pulsatile flow has a deleterious effect on renal function. High levels of angiotensin II during non-pulsatile regimes may produce local vasoconstriction and a diminished perfusion (Porter *et al.*, 1966). The current conclusion is that in clinical terms the lack of pulsatile flow is not significant.

Prevention

With these pathophysiological events in mind, what can be done to prevent renal failure developing? Several vasoactive agents have been tried but as yet no 'magic' concoction has emerged. Two fundamental points are worth repeating.

1. It is important to assess the renal function preoperatively if at all possible and it is important to ensure that the patient remains well hydrated presurgery during bypass and postoperatively. It should be remembered that patients with chronic renal failure, i.e. clearances below 40 ml min^{-1}, are going to have a significant inability to concentrate and dilute urine. Therefore volume

control cannot be left to the kidney itself and the clinician in charge must, on clinical evidence, maintain the correct state of hydration.

2. During bypass the perfusion pressure should be maintained at approximately 40 mmHg and postoperatively every effort should be made to ensure an adequate cardiac output. This, by the nature of the underlying cardiac condition, may be difficult and it is the main reason why the incidence of renal failure has not fallen.

What constructive comments can be made on the various pharmacodynamic agents that theoretically at least could be beneficial during bypass or immediately postoperatively? Several agents have been studied in the experimental model and have either not been used in man or if they have their value has not been confirmed. Propranolol, which limits renin release and hence maintains renal perfusion, has been suggested but because of its negative inotropic action has not understandably been widely used in ill patients. Prostacyclin, which will increase renal blood flow, has been tried in man but found wanting: similarly imidazole which inhibits thromboxane synthesis has not found a place in clinical practice. The atrial natriuretic factor produces vasodilatation and an increase in glomerular filtration rate but to date no studies are available in the setting of acute renal failure prophylaxis. The increase of free hydroxyl radicals secondary to tissue ischaemia is thought to cause cellular injury and chelation with desferrioxamine remains a theoretical possibility. Bradykinin, acetylcholine and serotonin all increased renal blood flow but remain laboratory tools. In renal transplantation perfusion with adenosine nucleotides – a high energy source – limits ischaemia damage but they have to be perfused directly into the renal artery – not an impossible approach during bypass but as yet untried.

The following have been used during surgery as preventative measures and during the immediate postoperative period.

1. *Mannitol.* The osmotic effects of intravenous mannitol include the reduction of tubular swelling and the increased urine flow washes out damaged tubular cells, thereby limiting intraluminal obstruction. An increase in circulating volume may increase the cardiac output and reduce the haematocrit, both favouring renal perfusion (Schuster *et al.*, 1964).
2. *Frusemide* theoretically would increase the glomerular filtration rate by both limiting tubular glomerular feedback and by its vasodilating properties increasing cortical blood flow. There is little evidence that as a prophylactic measure it protects against renal failure but in the immediate postoperative period it may be helpful in promoting a diuresis. This may limit tubular obstruction by cellular debris and clinically may be beneficial in removing water and potassium. It is interesting that a constant intravenous infusion at the rate of 1–2 mg min^{-1} may be effective when bolus injections fail.
3. *Dopamine.* When administered in doses of 1–3 μg kg^{-1} min^{-1}, which have little effect on the systemic circulation, renal vasodilatation occurs. This vasodilatation may be beneficial both before and after the insult of hypotension. Its value is still open to question (Henderson, Beattie and Kennedy, 1980).
4. *Calcium channel blockers.* Healthy cells have a very low intracellular free calcium concentration but during ischaemia the calcium pumps are deprived of energy and there is a free influx of calcium ions which are taken up by the mitochondria. This high intracellular calcium is toxic, producing further cellular injury. The use of calcium channel blockers experimentally has proven beneficial in limiting both the degree and duration of renal failure and the results from clinical trials will soon be available (Schrier *et al.*, 1987).

In addition to mentioning drugs that may reduce renal damage it is important to recognize the potentially nephrotoxic agents commonly used in this field. The nephrotoxic effects of aminoglycosides, possibly made worse by the simultaneous use of loop diurectics, are well known. The interstitial nephritis caused by the non-steroidal anti-inflammatory drugs are a well recognized cause of acute renal failure in nephrological practice. The angiotension converting enzyme inhibitors are now established not only for the treatment of hypertension but also for patients with cardiac failure. In cases where there is a high efferent arteriolar tone produced by angiotensin II, the use of these agents may acutely reduce the filtration pressure and provoke renal failure. Fortunately in most instances this is reversible but nevertheless these drugs should be used with great care.

The recognition and treatment of acute renal failure in the postoperative period

Despite assiduous care, 5% of patients will develop acute renal failure following bypass. Some will require renal support but, despite the advances in haemodialysis and filtration, the mortality remains high at over 70%. What can be done to improve survival? Firstly the diagnosis should be made quickly. It is relatively easy in the oliguric patient. Here the differential diagnosis lies between a physiological oilguria because the patient had become dehydrated and that of acute renal failure. In the former the urine osmolarity is high, the urine: plasma ratio for urea is above 40:1 and there is relative sodium retention. In acute renal failure the position is reversed. The osmolarity is relatively fixed close to that of plasma, the U:P ratio is often below 10:1 in respect of urea and the urine sodium concentration is fixed at around 30 mmol l^{-1}. In both settings any hypovolaemia should be corrected with blood plasma or clear fluid and in cases of established renal failure diuretics and dopamine can be given as described in the previous section. In some patients the episode of renal failure would be transient and indeed can last a matter of hours but in others it will become established and supportive measures will be required. Some patients will have rising blood urea and creatinine despite an output of 2 l per 24h and these patients have polyuric renal failure. In these patients dialysis is rarely required for fluid overload or potassium but a rising urea and creatinine may demand renal support.

Peritoneal dialysis is excellent for removing fluid and potassium but surgical breaching of the diaphragm often limits its use. The main limitations are the risk of peritonitis and the low clearance of urea and creatinine. In children however the surface area of the peritoneum compared with the muscle mass is high and, unless the patient is very catabolic, adequate removal of nitrogenous waste is possible.

Conventional haemodialysis still has a place. The patient can be dialysed for 2–3h on a daily basis but an adequate blood pressure is required to produce flows through the dialyser for 200–300 ml min^{-1}, essential if adequate clearances are to be achieved. Haemodialysis is associated with hypotension and arrhythmias – possible hazards in the postoperative cardiac patient. These circulatory changes are often associated with fluid removal and shifts of potassium. The use of haemofiltration has reduced the frequency of these complications. In this technique blood is passed across a very permeable membrane which allows the removal of 1–1.5 l^{-1} of ultrafiltrate. This ultrafiltrate has the same composition as blood, minus red cells and protein, and if a physiological solution is returned in similar proportions then adequate clearances can be achieved. Clearances of up to 30 ml min^{-1} can be maintained if dialysate is run through the dialyser under the influence of gravity alone. This means that haemofiltration can be set up in the recovery area without the need of specialist dialysis personnel. In fact, with arterial cannulation, blood can be passed unpumped through a haemofilter and returned to a major vein without the use of expensive equipment. This unpumped filtration is useful in the early postoperative period if the services of an experienced nephrology unit cannot be called upon. Of course cardiac units are very experienced at gaining access to the circulation and many units can now manage acute renal failure in the first 2–3 days by performing haemofiltration with their own staff. It is only when the mixture of haemofiltration and haemodialysis is required that patients are referred to nephrology units. This means that they are often in a fitter state to travel and there is no doubt that with the advent of pumped or unpumped haemofiltration the management of the postoperative cardiac case is a great deal easier. A case can still be made for expert nephrological help as, as seen at the beginning of this chapter, many other causes of acute renal failure in the cardiac patient have to be considered. If the patient does not succumb because of their original problem then acute renal failure on the background of cardiopulmonary bypass is potentially reversible, and many patients who survive their initial insult fully regain renal function to a level that supports life without any form of dietary restriction or dialysis.

Renal function in the young person may return after 3–4 days of anuria but in the more elderly patient with generalized atheroma the recovery period may be up to 3 weeks. Normal renal function does not return swiftly and in the early diuretic phase the ability to conserve water and electrolytes is still impaired. It is important that fluid management is still carefully controlled and inappropriate losses of sodium and potassium replaced.

Just as in the opening paragraph the relationship between cardiac and renal function was outlined, it is hoped that the management of renal failure in the complex cardiac case will depend on a similar interdependence between cardiologist and nephrologist despite the advent of haemofiltration. It is only by close liaison between the two disciplines that the overall prognosis will improve.

References

Adams, P.L., Adams, F.F., Bell, P.D. and Navar, L.G. (1980) Impaired renal blood flow autoregulation in ischaemic acute renal failure. *Kidney International*, **18**, 68–76

Brenner, B.M., Zatz, R. and Ichikawa, I. (1986) The renal circulations. In *The Kidney*, 3rd edn, (eds. B.M. Brenner and J.M. Lazarus), W.B. Saunders, Philadelphia, pp. 93–123

Brezis, M., Rosen, S., Silva, P. and Epstein, F.H. (1984) Renal ischaemia: a new perspective. *Kidney International*, **26**, 375–383

Conger, J.D., Robinette, J.B. and Schrier, R.W. (1988) Smooth muscle calcium and endothelium derived relaxing factor in the abnormal vascular responses of acute renal failure. *Journal of Clinical Investigation*, **82**, 532–537

Henderson, I.S., Beattie, T.J. and Kennedy, A.C. (1980) Dopamine hydrochloride in oliguric states. *Lancet*, **ii**, 827–828

Hollenberg, N.K., Wilkes, B.M. and Shulman, G. (1983) The renin–angiotensin system in acute renal failure. In *Acute Renal Failure* (eds B.M. Brenner and J.M. Lazarus), W.B. Saunders, Philadelphia, pp. 137–156

Lavender, J.P. and Sherwood, T. (1972) The renal circulation in haemorrhagic hypotension. *British Medical Bulletin*, **28**, 241–246

Osborn, J.J., Cohn, K., Hait, M., *et al.* (1962) Haemolysis during perfusion. *Journal of Thoracic and Cardiovascular Surgery*, **43**, 459–464

Porter, G.A., Kolster, F.E., Herr, R.J., *et al.* (1966) Relationships between alterations in renal haemodynamics during cardiopulmonary bypass and post-operative renal function. *Circulation*, **34**, 1005–1021

Schrier, R.W., Arnold, P.E., Van Putten, V.J. and Burke, T.J. (1987) Cellular calcium in ischaemic acute renal failure: role of calcium entry blockers. *Kidney International*, **32**, 312–321

Schuster, S.R., Kakvan, M., Vawter, G.F. and Narter, N. (1964) An experimental study of the effect of mannitol during cardiopulmonary bypass. *Circulation*, **29** (Suppl), 72–76

13

The neurological sequelae of cardiopulmonary bypass

Peter Smith

The possible effect on cerebral function of operating on the heart has been paramount in the minds of cardiac surgeons ever since cardiac operations were first carried out. Sir Henry Souttar reported the first successful closed mitral valvotomy in the *British Medical Journal* of 3 October 1925. In his discussion of this paper he refers to the extreme danger to the brain from even the shortest check to its blood supply and notes that the operation itself caused a loss of blood pressure for a few seconds (Souttar, 1925). As cardiac surgery developed, checking of the blood supply in excess of a few seconds was needed for the more prolonged intracardiac operations. It was felt that cooling the patient to 30°C or more would offer an increased safe period of total circulatory arrest of perhaps up to 10 minutes, enabling more complex intracardiac operations to be carried out. Sir Thomas Holmes-Sellers reported 453 cases of ostium secundum atrial septal defect closures in his Bradshaw lecture to the Royal College of Surgeons in 1970 (Holmes-Sellers, 1970). However, it was not until the development of cardiopulmonary bypass in the early 1950s, enabling the surgeons to operate on a 'stilled quiet heart', that cardiac surgery could be carried out on a large scale. In the same year as Gibbon reported the use of cardiopulmonary bypass in the human (Gibbon, 1954), Fox, Risso and Gifford (1954) described neurological complications associated with cardiac surgery. Since this paper, reports have appeared in increasing numbers in the scientific literature defining and analysing the problem.

The cerebral consequences of cardiac surgery with cardiopulmonary bypass may be considered in terms of neurological, neuropsychological or psychiatric changes. Neurological studies have been particularly concerned with the postoperative incidence of stroke, visual disturbances, disturbances of conscious level and peripheral nerve lesions. Neuropsychological studies have investigated the postoperative incidences of intellectual deficit and tend to consist of a battery of well validated studies carried out pre- and postoperatively designed to investigate the cognitive abilities of the patient in a reproducible way. Within the battery of neuropsychological tests are usually found tests of memory, both verbal and non-verbal; concentration, reasoning and spatial orientation. Psychiatric examinations have studied the postoperative incidences of delirium, anxiety, depression and overt psychosis. In the following chapter it is proposed to consider the neurological and neuropsychological consequences of cardiopulmonary bypass in greater detail. Psychiatric consequences will not be discussed.

Neurological consequences of cardiopulmonary bypass

Early papers on the neurological consequences of cardiopulmonary bypass describe the sequelae following either operations for congenital heart disease or valve disease. Ehrenraft *et al.* (1961) reported the retrospective experience in the University of Iowa Cardiac Surgical Service, stating that 17 of 244 patients (7%) showed new generalized severe cerebral signs following cardiac surgery. Cerebral pathology tended to present on the first postoperative day and consisted of either epileptiform seizures, hemiparesis or visual field defects. In 1965, Gilman reported on a prospective study of a small group of 35 patients in terms of the neurological consequences of cardiac surgery. Severe early neurological complications were seen in 6 of 35 patients (17%), but the mortality in this group of patients was exceptionally high by today's standards.

A large scale prospective study of the neurological consequences of cardiac surgery was not reported until 1970 when Tufo *et al.* reported a prospective study of 100 patients who had undergone cardiac surgery for valve or congenital heart disease. Fifteen of these patients died, again, a very high number by contemporary standards. Of the 85 survivors, 37 (44%) had one or more abnormal neurological signs at first examination after recovery from anaesthesia. However many of these abnormal neurological signs were relatively unimportant consisting of the presence of a new primitive reflex, nystagmus, inequality of tendon reflexes or an extensor plantar response. Two patients had visual field defects. At discharge 12 patients (14%) still exhibited new abnormal neurological signs, namely, eight with extensor plantar responses, two with mild aphasia, one of whom had right hemiparesis, and two with visual field defects.

Stroke is a term used to describe the clinical results of acute focal ischaemia or infarction in the brain, the symptoms and signs of the cerebral ischaemia persisting beyond 30–60 min. It has been reported following coronary artery bypass surgery as occurring in 1–6% of all patients (Table 13.1).

Table 13.1 Recent reported incidences of stroke following coronary artery bypass surgery

Main author	*Year*	*Stroke rate*	
Retrospective studies			
Lee	1979	66/943	0.7%
Gonzales-Scarano	1981	18/1427	0.1%
Martin	1982	8/253	3.2%
Bojar	1983	32/3206	1.0%
Coffee	1983	13/1669	0.8%
Gardner	1985	56/3279	1.7%
Parker	1985	8/893	0.9%
Prospective studies			
Turnipseed	1980	8/170	4.7%
Breuer	1983	21/400	5.2%
Shaw	1985	15/320	4.8%

Retrospective series reported tend to give a lower incidence of this complication than prospective series reported by neurologists. The probability is that retrospective series consistently underestimate the occurrence of this complication. Stroke is usually reported as an acute hemiparesis or a visual field defect. Shaw *et al.* (1985), a neurologist, in her prospective analysis of 312 patients, reported 15 strokes following coronary artery bypass surgery.

A prolonged depression of the level of consciousness (in the absence of sedation) is seen postoperatively in a small number of patients following cardiac surgery. It is often associated with the signs of focal or multifocal neurological dysfunction. Widespread focal injury can be inferred perhaps due to large emboli or prolonged hypotension or hypoxia. Coma following cardiac surgery is known to carry with it a very high probability of death (Branthwaite, 1974; Sotaniemi, 1983). Shaw noted prolonged depression of the level of consciousness in ten of the 312 patients in her study reported in 1985.

Though not often clinically recognized, sensorineural hearing loss is probably relatively common following coronary artery bypass surgery. Shapiro, Prun and Raskin (1981), investigated 68 patients before and after cardiopulmonary bypass with pure tone audiometry. Nine of 68 patients had a loss in excess of 10 decibels and a further 36 patients, a loss of less than 10 decibels. Most importantly at follow-up none of these patients showed complete recovery. Sudden severe hearing loss was thought previous to this study to occur in approximately 1 of 1000 patients (Arenberg, Allen and Boer, 1972; Wright and Saunders, 1975; Plasse *et al.* 1980).

Neuropsychological consequences of cardiopulmonary bypass

Large studies of the effect of cardiac surgery using cardiopulmonary bypass on intellectual function were first published by Gilberstadt and Sako in 1967. In a short 3 week follow-up of 53 patients they showed significant deficit in perceptuomotor co-ordination, attention span and rote-memory. Similarly, both Tufo *et al.* in 1970 and Lee *et al.* in 1971 showed significant neuropsychological deficit following cardiopulmonary bypass. However the studies of Frank *et al.* published in 1972 on 98 patients confounded the previous results by showing improvement in all measured areas of intellectual function 6 months after cardiac surgery using cardiopulmonary bypass. Frank's co-workers used a very extensive test battery of verbal and non-verbal neuropsychological functioning in perceptual, motor and cognitive modalities in conjunction with an anxiety assessment. They found that the level of preoperative anxiety related significantly to postoperative intellectual gain. They also suggested that practice effects went much of the way to explaining improvement in postoperative performance scores. It is of interest that they showed that there was less intellectual gain with increasing bypass time. Intellectual gain was noted not to be enough to effect day to day intellectual integration or adjustment. The first definitive study of intellectual function following cardiac surgery using extracorporeal circulation was that of Aberg (1975). He studied 144 cardiac surgery patients, all of which were either valve or congenital heart disease patients. He also studied 46 control non-cardiopulmonary bypass general thoracic surgery patients. His extensive neuropsychological test battery consisted of tests of verbal comprehension, logical reasoning, visuospatial perception, perceptual speed, short-term memory and cognition. These tests were carried out preoperatively and at 1 week, 6 weeks and 1 year postoperatively. There were 144 patients in the cardiac group, only 113 completed tests at 8 weeks. The overall conclusions were that operations involving extracorporeal circulation bring about impairment in intellectual function unlike general surgical operations when intellectual functions remain unchanged and in fact show a small improvement due to practice effect. Changes were particularly common in tests reflecting visuospatial perception, perceptual speed and cognition, whereas tests of verbal comprehension, logical reasoning and short-term memory are relatively resistant to change. More recently Joulasmaa *et al.* (1981) reported the results of a 24 test neuropsychological examination in 60 patients undergoing cardiac valve replacement with cardiopulmonary bypass. He found that 5 months after surgery, up to 28% of patients showed some impairment in the ability to carry out neuropsychological tests. Of particular interest was the finding that the right cerebral hemisphere was more prone to damage as compared with the left. The most detailed studies of intellectual function following cardiac surgery have been in routine coronary artery bypass graft patients. Ellis *et al.* in 1980 showed 75% of 30 coronary artery bypass graft surgery patients developed intellectual impairment 1 week after surgery, 70% at 4 weeks and 0% at 6 months postoperatively. These results were also reflected in a similar small study of 31 patients by Raymond *et al.* (1984). Savageau *et al.* (1982a and b) reports findings in 227 cardiac surgery patients, of which 76% were coronary artery bypass surgery patients. The neuropsychological tests which she used preoperatively and at approximately 9 days and 6 months postoperatively were limited in the extent of their cognitive assessment. The trail making test and visual reproduction test of the Weschler Memory Scale was used in her early assessment paper and these two tests plus the logical memory test in her 6 month reassessment paper. With these tests she showed at 9 days postoperatively 30% of patients were significantly impaired in test performance. By 6 months postoperatively only 19% of patients showed a significant decrease in one or more test scores. However the patients showing deficit at 6 months were not necessarily the same as those showing a deficit at 9 days. In fact only 5% of patients showed consistent postoperative test score deterioration both at 9 days and at 6 months. From this study it is therefore concluded that it is inappropriate to attribute 6 month postoperative intellectual dysfunction to the surgical episode *per se*. The most extensive study of intellectual dysfunction following coronary artery bypass graft surgery has been that undertaken by Shaw and her colleagues in Newcastle (1986). She studied 298 patients, preoperatively and at 1 week postoperatively using 10 standard neuropsychological tests. These were the Weschler Adult Intelligence Scale (WAIS) vocabulary block design test, the Halstead–Reitan trail-making tests, the information, orientation, mental control, logical memory, digits total, visual reproduction and associate learning sub-sets of the Weschler Memory Scale. A significant deterioration in performance was judged to be present if the postoperative score was greater than one standard deviation below the patient's preoperative score. Of the patients studied, 235 of 298 (79%) deteriorated significantly in at least one sub-test, 143 of these in more than one sub-test. The deterioration was particularly noted in tests of psychomotor speed, attention and concentration, new learning ability and auditory short-term memory. A pattern of cognitive dysfunction which one might expect in organic cerebral injury. Of 235 patients 123 (52%) did not notice any cognitive dysfunction themselves. Moderate or severe deficit defined as significant deterioration in performance in three or more tests showed a significant correlation with prolonged depression of the level of consciousness postoperatively, stroke or the development of palmo-mental reflexes. Six month follow-up data is available in the study (Shaw *et al.*, 1987). Of the 259 patients remaining in the study, 147 (57%) showed deterioration in at least one test at 6 months postoperatively, but only 17 of 259 patients (7%) were significantly deteriorated in three or more tests. It is noteworthy that only 81 of 259 (31%) showed consistent impairment of the same test score at 7 days and 6 months postoperatively.

Smith (1988) carried out a prospective study of 79 coronary artery bypass graft surgery patients to determine the incidence of postoperative cerebral complications and the major factors associated with the cerebral morbidity. Surgery was rigidly standardized, both in terms of technique and anaesthesia. All patients underwent preoperatively and at 8 days, 8 weeks and 1 year postoperatively, detailed neuropsychological examinations. The neuropsychological test battery consisted of ten tests, some computer-administered. They were especially chosen to be sensitive to diffuse cortical damage and resistant to practice effects. The neuropsychological tests used were as follows:

1. Two computer-administered, non-verbal recognition tests
2. Computer-administered choice reaction time test

3 Computer-administered symbol digital replacement test
4. The trail-making tests A and B
5. A Purdue pegboard test for each and both hands
6. The block design test from the Weschler Adult Intelligence Scale, the WAIS
7. A letter cancellation task
8. The Rey Auditory verbal learning test for verbal memory.

Neuropsychological performance was considered in relation to the standard deviation of all preoperative scores on each test. An individual was considered to produce a significantly deteriorated performance in a test if they exhibited a drop from their preoperative performance greater than one standard deviation. A significant neuropsychological deficit was considered to have occurred in an individual who produced a significantly deteriorated performance in two or more tests. All drugs given with dosage during the operative stay in hospital were recorded. In addition physiological observation during operation and immediately postoperatively was extensive, including a recording of mean arterial pressure, blood gases and temperature. Significant neuropsychological deficit was found in 73% of patients 8 days after surgery, 37% 8 weeks after surgery and 35% 1 year after surgery. This was relatively similar to the incidence reported by Shaw previously. Increasing postoperative neuropsychological deficit appears to be associated with a longer bypass time and an increased age in the patient. No other factors could be found which were associated with the neuropsychological deficit demonstrated.

Aetiology of the cerebral complications of cardiopulmonary bypass

Peroperative stroke may potentially occur in any form of major surgery, particularly if the patient is older with preoperative hypertension and carotid artery disease. The stroke may be due to cerebral embolus or haemorrhage. Less severe neurological changes following general surgery have been demonstrated by Bedford and Leeds (1955) who showed that general surgery in the elderly often leads to noticeable diminution in mental faculties following the procedure. Many subsequent studies have confirmed this (Simpson *et al.*, 1961). It has been speculated that the increasing atherosclerotic disease found in the cerebral circulation of the elderly might be aetiologically implicated.

Several factors may lead to critical cerebral hypoperfusion peroperatively in the general surgical patient with the result that the patient exhibits a postoperative cerebral deficit. Sudden profound hypotension can result from torrential uncontrolled haemorrhage or from sudden left ventricular failure notably due to peroperative myocardial infarction. Peroperative dysrhythmias of the heart can lead to hypotension if uncontrolled and cardiac arrest if not promptly reversed may lead to a grossly brain damaged patient on eventual resuscitation. Though Sorenson and Lindeberg (1950) concluded that a properly administered anaesthetic did not cause subsequent changes in brain function measured by neuropsychological testing, many anaesthetic agents have more recently been shown to lead to a deficit in intellectual performance postoperatively e.g. halothane and nitrous oxide at a few hours postoperatively (Bruce, Bach and Arbit, 1974) or cyclopropane at 6 days following surgery (James, 1969).

Sleep deprivation and abnormal sensory stimulation, as experienced by the surgical patient in the intensive care unit, has been shown to lead to subsequent poor performance in neuropsychological testing as has the anxiety and emotional response which is an inevitable concomitant of the patient undergoing surgery (Sveinsson, 1975; Orr and Stahl, 1977). The manifestation or presentation of cerebral damage incurred at surgery may be profoundly affected by the psychological response of the patient to his illness and its management.

The aetiological factors associated with cerebral dysfunction following cardiac surgery are in many cases unique to cardiac surgery. Stroke presenting in the early postoperative period following cardiac surgery is likely to be due to a major cerebral embolic event. Large particles may be introduced into the circulation during aortic cannulation from dislodged atheromatous plaques or from dislodged clots from the mural surface of the left ventricle (Breuer *et al.*, 1981). Massive air embolus could occur through the aortic cannulation site, cardioplegic needle site or if the left ventricle is vented, through the left ventricle vent site (Utley and Stephens, 1986). In addition malfunction within the cardiopulmonary bypass circuit has also been implicated in massive air embolus, particularly if the cardiotomy reservoir blood level is allowed to become dangerously low.

The causes of neuropsychological deficit following cardiac surgery with cardiopulmonary bypass are probably similar to those observed in stroke but lesser in magnitude and extent. It is probable, for a proportion of patients, that during the period of cardiopulmonary bypass a degree of diffuse cortical damage takes place which can manifest itself in measurable neuropsychological impairment. The diffuse cortical damage is probably an expression of cerebral microemboli generated during the bypass and/or by relative cerebral hypoperfusion occurring at the same time. Pathological findings offer some evidence regarding the mechanism producing the deficit. Aguilar, Gerbode and Hill in 1971 reported the pathological findings of the brains of 206 patients who had died following cardiac surgery in the Pacific Medical Center in San Francisco. Of these patients 85% showed either fibrin–platelet, crystalline or fat emboli, acute petechial, perivascular or focal subarachnoid haemorrhages or acute ischaemic retinal damage. The microemboli are largely generated in the cardiopulmonary circuit (Kessler and Patterson, 1970) and may consist of air, platelet aggregates, fibrin or silicone (Lindeberg *et al.*, 1961; Orenstein *et al.*, 1982; Solis *et al.*, 1975). Many authorities have stressed the importance of fat as a cerebral microembolus (Miller *et al.*, 1962; Caguin and Carter, 1963). However, fibrin–platelet aggregates are of equal or greater importance (Dutton *et al.*, 1974). Microemboli have been measured with a transcranial doppler (Deverall *et al.*, 1988) and directly visualized in the retina during cardiopulmonary bypass by the use of retinal fluorescein angiography (Williams, 1971; Blauth *et al.*, 1986; Blauth *et al.*, 1988).

The mechanism whereby fibrin-platelet aggregates cause cerebral damage is probably both direct and indirect. Patterson, Rosenfeldt and Porro (1976) showed the presence of cerebral microvascular blockade with microparticles following cardiopulmonary bypass in dogs. This was transient in nature and he speculated that this form of damage might be the reason for the transient encephalopathy seen in patients after cardiac surgery with cardiopulmonary bypass. However Taylor (1986a) feels that the mechanism producing cerebral damage is not just a simple obstruction of flow, but may be alteration in the clotting lysis cascade with platelet activation at the site of the blockage and release of damaging vasoactive substances and free radicals. The dynamic balance between thromboxane and prostacyclin present in the normal circulation has been shown to orientate towards thromboxane during cardiopulmonary bypass (Watkins *et al.*, 1982). Cerebral microembolic insult undoubtedly occurs during cardiopulmonary bypass and many authorities would now consider it the major aetiological factor causing cerebral damage during cardiac surgery (Taylor, 1986b).

An alternative or additional aetiological factor is poor cerebral perfusion associated with low cerebral blood flow occurring during cardiopulmonary bypass. However several workers have shown that permanent cerebral damage is unlikely unless cerebral blood flow is less than 10 ml $100 g^{-1}$ min^{-1} (Astrup *et al.*, 1977). It is very rare for this to happen during routine cardiopulmonary bypass. Theoretically, if low perfusion has caused cerebral damage then it should appear maximally in the so-called watershed areas of the brain. These are boundary zones between areas of distribution of different cerebral arteries (Ross-Russell and Bharucha, 1978). There is little convincing evidence that this occurs.

It is likely that $P\text{CO}_2$ management during cardiopulmonary bypass is of importance as regards the degree of cerebral injury which takes place during cardiopulmonary bypass (Swan, 1984). Nevin *et al.* (1988) have shown a relationship between $P\text{CO}_2$ management and the extent of early postoperative neuropsychological deficit found in a study of 65 patients who had undergone coronary artery bypass graft surgery. $P\text{CO}_2$ management may be either pH-stat using temperature corrected data with the addition of $P\text{CO}_2$ to the oxygenator to maintain a $P\text{aCO}_2$ near 40 mmHg with a pH of approximately 7.4 or α-stat using temperature uncorrected data with a result that $P\text{aCO}_2$ falls reducing cerebral blood flow. It can be argued that α-stat $P\text{CO}_2$ management is more physiological, matching cerebral blood flow to demand, which is desirable when trying to minimize microembolic mediated cerebral damage.

A scrutiny of recent papers considering predictors of neuropsychological deficit following cardiac surgery presents evidence that increasing age of the patient at operation and increasing bypass time are the two major predictors of an increased neuropsychological deficit following surgery (Newman, 1989). Smith *et al.* (1986) have also shown that low mean arterial pressure on cardiopulmonary bypass may be implicated in the genesis of postoperative neuropsychological deficit. There is a risk of peroperative cerebral damage with all major surgery but especially with cardiac surgery using cardiopulmonary bypass.

Cerebral blood flow during cardiopulmonary bypass

For a resting adult with a presumed brain weight of 1.4 kg, normal cerebral blood flow is approximately 800 ml min^{-1} with an oxygen consumption of 52 ml min^{-1} and a glucose consumption of 0.45 mmol min^{-1} (Zilstra, 1981). Within these overall mean figures there is a wide variation of metabolism and blood flow to different areas of the brain at different times, enhanced activity in one part of the brain leading to enhanced metabolism and hence blood flow in that part of the brain (Oleson, 1971). In the normal person, energy metabolism, neuronal activity and cerebral blood flow are thought to be mutually dependent. However in many pathological conditions and possibly during cardiopulmonary bypass, cerebral blood flow metabolism can become uncoupled (Anderson *et al.*, 1985). In normal humans, autoregulation of cerebral blood flow occurs between approximately 60 and 150 mmHg (Zilstra, 1981). Cerebral autoregulation is due to a direct myogenic response of smooth muscle cells of the arterial wall to stretch caused by distending transmural pressure. Metabolic factors are the most important regulators of cerebral blood flow. Hypoxia and most importantly hypercapnia, increase cerebral blood flow (Larsen and Christensen, 1976). An increase in $Pa\text{CO}_2$ causes a cerebral vasodilatation and conversely a decrease in $Pa\text{CO}_2$ leads to vasoconstriction. Carbon dioxide reactivity is mediated by CSF pH variations. Cerebral lactic acidosis leads to abolition of cerebral blood flow autoregulation and often a 'luxury perfusion syndrome' (Larsen and Christensen, 1976). Nevin *et al.* (1988) stress the importance of the control of $P\text{CO}_2$ during cardiac surgery. In the previously quoted study of 65 coronary artery bypass graft surgery patients, they showed a reduction in both clinical, neurological and neuropsychological deficits measured 3 days after surgery in a sub-group of 30 patients who had a $Pa\text{CO}_2$ maintained at 35–45 mmHg as opposed to a subgroup of 35 patients who had not. The $Pa\text{CO}_2$ in this latter group was not altered by the anaesthetists, hypocarbia occurring immediately before the onset of cardiopulmonary bypass. The paper, as the authors state, is limited by the small number of patients entered, also and perhaps more seriously, there is the problem of interpretation of neuropsychological and, possibly, neurological tests so soon after major surgery.

Cerebral blood flow has been measured during cardiopulmonary bypass in both animals and man. Two major aims are apparent in these studies. The first being to determine the factors influencing cerebral blood flow during varying conditions of cardiopulmonary bypass. The second being to use the cerebral blood flow change peroperatively or from preoperative to postoperative, as an index of the degree of derangement of cerebral metabolism and possibly of neuronal damage resulting from the cardiac surgery. An early study was first reported by Halley, Reemstsma and Creech (1958) using non-pulsatile cardiopulmonary bypass in dogs. He concluded that cerebral blood flow during extracorporeal circulation was directly proportional to mean systemic blood pressure and can vary widely with perfusion flow rate. Autoregulation tended to be lost with ensuing pressure passivity at 55 mmHg. The bypass was not deliberately hypothermic. Santillan, Chemnitius and Bing (1985) have investigated cerebral blood flow during cardiopulmonary bypass in 51 cats using a method dependent on radioactive microspheres. His findings were of 'luxury perfusion' of cerebral blood flow during cardiopulmonary bypass.

Whereas invasive methods of measuring cerebral blood flow can be used in animal studies, in patients, methodology is more restricted. Woolman *et al.* (1966) estimated the cerebral blood flow using the arteriovenous oxygen difference in six patients undergoing cardiac surgery with cardiopulmonary bypass. He concluded that $Pa\text{CO}_2$ was the most important factor determining the level of cerebral blood flow during cardiopulmonary bypass. Branthwaite (1974), using a modified haemodilution method to investigate 30 patients, showed a reduction in cerebral blood flow at the onset of bypass in a large proportion of patients. This fall in cerebral blood flow occurred in association with a marked reduction in systemic blood pressure despite high blood flow. She argued that depression of the cerebral metabolism may be due to decreased oxygen availability because of haemodilution and hypotension and that this may lead to abnormal neurology and neuropsychology seen following cardiac surgery. However she also realized the severe limitations of the methodology she used to measure cerebral blood flow. More recently, Henriksen, Hjelms and Lindeberg (1983) investigated 29 patients undergoing cardiac surgery, measuring cerebral blood flow by intra-arterial injection of xenon^{133} with subsequent determination of the washout of the radioactive isotope from the brain. Only six of the patients underwent coronary artery bypass surgery, the rest underwent valve surgery or surgery for congenital heart disease. There was a normal and significant correlation between the level of cerebral blood flow, temperature and plasma $Pa\text{CO}_2$. Cerebral blood flow tended to decrease during the first minute of cardiopulmonary bypass supporting Branthwaite's observation of some 10 years earlier. Mean cerebral blood flow then increased during the steady state of hypothermic cardiopulmonary bypass. After rewarming during steady normothermic cardiopulmonary bypass, mean cerebral blood flow decreased again and remained at that level for 10–20 min after bypass ceased. Autoregulation was maintained to approximately a lower level of 55 mmHg systemic blood pressure. The perfusion pressure was significantly correlated with cerebral blood flow. $Pa\text{CO}_2$ was a significant regulation factor for the level of cerebral blood flow during cardiopulmonary bypass. As an overall conclusion, Henriksen felt that the results were suggestive of microembolism leading to cerebral damage caused during cardiopulmonary bypass for cardiac surgery.

These findings are at variance with many of those of Govier and a group from Birmingham, Alabama (1984). They investigated 67 patients undergoing coronary artery bypass surgery. Cerebral blood flow was measured with the intraarterial xenon^{133} clearance method. The principle finding was of a significant decrease in cerebral blood flow during hypothermic non-pulsatile cardiopulmonary bypass. It was felt that the mean 55% reduction in cerebral blood flow was related to the calculated 56% reduction in cerebral metabolism expected for the hypothermia achieved. Govier felt that these findings indicated a lack of important cerebral injury due to cardiopulmonary bypass. However there is a presumption that cerebral blood flow metabolism remained coupled during cardiopulmonary bypass. Subsequent work has suggested that this is not so, at least during non-pulsatile cardiopulmonary bypass in pigs (Anderson *et al.*, 1985), but may be so if pulsatile flow is used. Govier suggested the almost diametrically opposed results of her study compared with those of Henriksen may be due to important differences in anaesthetic techniques. It is known that many anaesthetic agents have profound effects on the limits of autoregulation of cerebral blood flow. Del Campo and Nicholls (1984), commenting on Henriksen's investigations, states that the change during the cardiac operation from enflurane (which increases cerebral blood flow) to profentanyl (which decreases cerebral blood flow) as well as the use of diazepam as a premedication, could largely explain many of the changes Henriksen reported. An alternative or additional explanation may be in the differing methods of measuring $P\text{CO}_2$ and $P\text{CO}_2$ management used by each group during the cardiac surgery. Govier did not correct her $P\text{aCO}_2$ samples for temperature and Henriksen did. In addition to his 1983 reported study, Henriksen also reported further studies in 1984 measuring cerebral blood flow in 37 patients using single photon emission computerized tomography after inhalation of xenon[133]. Investigations were preoperatively and within 10 days of cardiac surgery using cardiopulmonary bypass. Cardiac surgery was both for coronary artery and cardiac valve disease. A significant reduction in mean cerebral blood flow pre- to postoperatively was found. This reduction was significantly correlated in magnitude with increasing age, increased duration of extracorporeal circulation and low mean arterial pressure during cardiopulmonary bypass. He further showed a small but significant reduction in cerebral blood flow from preoperatively to 1 year postoperatively in 11 patients. A control group of 15 patients undergoing carotid endarterectomy or extracranial/intracranial shunts did not show this postoperative drop in mean cerebral blood flow. It was felt that these findings in the cardiac group were consistent with postoperative central nervous system dysfunction.

In summary studies to date of the changes in cerebral blood flow found during cardiopulmonary bypass and following cardiopulmonary bypass suggest that the management of the $P\text{CO}_2$ during the bypass is of paramount importance. It is likely that the change in cerebral blood flow seen during cardiopulmonary bypass does reflect a change in the metabolic requirement of the brain during hypothermia. Whether it also reflects a degree of cerebral damage occurring during cardiopulmonary bypass is more contentious. However Smith *et al.* (1986) duplicated the results of Henriksen in showing a significant drop in mean cerebral blood flow 8 days following cardiac surgery for routine coronary artery bypass graft surgery and the author feels that it is likely that this drop reflects at least early postoperative cerebral dysfunction. Both the significance and degree of this dysfunction in terms of patient well-being is arguable in most cases.

Interventions to reduce cerebral dysfunction occurring during cardiopulmonary bypass

The number, breadth and quality of the papers outlining many research groups' findings of brain dysfunction following cardiac surgery would now suggest that some form of cerebral deficit is not unusual during the immediate postoperative period following cardiopulmonary bypass. Whether this deficit can be found in terms of overt cognitive dysfunction some months after surgery is more contentious but it is not unlikely. Attention is being increasingly paid to possible interventions to reduce cerebral injury during cardiopulmonary bypass. They may be thought of in three categories:

Attention to anaesthetic and surgical technique

As previously stated neuropsychological deficit following cardiac surgery increases with increasing age of the patients at operation and increasing bypass time.

Probably the most important single factor in reducing cerebral injury during cardiac surgery is performing the surgery quickly, within the practical limitations of the procedure, particularly in the elderly.

The likelihood of major cerebral embolic insult is reduced by scrupulous attention to deairing at the end of the cardiac procedure, removal of all debris from valve excision or other cardiac manoeuvre and also by exercising care when clamping the aorta, particularly when it calcific and atheromatous. Many microemboli are generated in shed blood returned to the venous reservoir by the suckers during the cardiac operation. Every effort should be made to reduce suction of shed blood to a minimum. The acid–base management used during cardiopulmonary bypass is of great importance. It may be either pH-stat or α-stat. It can be argued that α-stat $P\text{CO}_2$ management is more physiological, matching cerebral blood flow to a demand which is desirable when trying to minimize microemboli mediated cerebral damage.

Attention to the cardiopulmonary bypass equipment

It is well known that bubble oxygenators produce greater damage to the formed elements of blood and greater denaturation of plasma proteins than membrane oxygenators (Mortensen, 1977). The damage is greatest at the blood–gas interface. Fewer microemboli are produced by membrane as opposed to bubble oxygenators (Carleson, Landé and Landis, 1973). In order to show whether a membrane oxygenator gives rise to less microembolism in the cerebral circulation with less postoperative neuropsychological deficit compared with a bubble oxygenator, a study was carried out at Hammersmith Hospital, London. Preliminary results of this study are now available in the first 40 patients entered (Blauth *et al.*, 1989). A Harvey H1700 bubble oxygenator (Bard Cardiopulmonary, Santa Ana, California) was compared with a Cobe CML flat sheet membrane oxygenator (Cobe Laboratories Inc, Lakewood, Colorado). The patients studied underwent elective uncomplicated routine coronary artery bypass surgery with a standardized anaesthetic and surgical technique. Cardiopulmonary bypass was carried out using a crystalloid Hartmann's solution prime, pulsatile perfusion during aortic cross clamping and a 40 μm arterial line filter. No left ventricular vent was used. Suction of shed blood was minimized and cold cardioplegic solution was used for myocardial protection.

Preoperatively and 5 min before the end of bypass, patients underwent retinal fluorescein angiography. The patients also underwent a battery of 10 neuropsychological tests preoperatively and at 8 days postoperatively. Twenty-three patients, with a mean age of 56 years (range 41–67 years) and a mean bypass time of 83.7 min (range 29–146 min), underwent cardiac surgery with a Harvey H1700 bubble oxygenator and 17 patients, with a mean age age of 55.6 years (range 44–67 years) and a mean bypass time of 88.4 min (range 57–118 min), with a Cobe CML flat sheet membrane oxygenator. All patients in the Harvey H1700 bubble oxygenator group had retinal microvascular occlusion consistent with microembolism compared with 8 of 17 (47%) in the Cobe CML flat sheet membrane oxygenator group ($P<0.001$, Fisher's exact test). The mean overall area of retinal non-perfusion per retina in the bubble group was 0.29 m^2 (range 0.041–1.23 m^2) compared with 0.05 m^2 (range 0–0.49 m^2) in the membrane group ($P<0.001$, Mann–Whitney *U*-test). If only those in the membrane group with occlusions are considered, the mean area of non-perfusion was 0.11 m^2 (range 0.01–0.49 m^2) and this was also significantly less than in the bubble group ($P<0.01$, Mann–Whitney *U*-test). Numbers in this preliminary report are too small to make useful comment on the neuropsychological test result, but early scrutiny suggests that there is a trend towards more severe neuropsychological postoperative deficit when the bubble oxygenator was used compared with the membrane oxygenator. Preliminary results of this study have shown there to be less microvascular occlusions in the cerebral microcirculation using a Cobe CML flat sheet membrane oxygenator compared with a Harvey H1700 bubble oxygenator with a suggestion that less neuropsychological deficit may also be seen in the former group of patients.

Several authors have shown arterial line filtration to be useful in reducing neuropsychological dysfunction following cardiac surgery. Taylor *et al.* (1980) have shown that a significant reduction of levels of creatine-kinase and creatine-kinase B isoenzyme in the cerebral spinal fluid occurred if an arterial line filter was used during conventional cardiopulmonary bypass in dogs compared to bypass without the filter. However Aris *et al.* (1986) in a study of 100 patients undergoing elective cardiac surgery showed no difference in the amount of postoperative neuropsychological deficit between two groups, one with a 20 μm filter in the circuit and one without. On balance the evidence for using a 40 μm main arterial line filter to reduce cerebral injury during routine cardiopulmonary bypass is, I think, very strong, particularly in view of the recent studies from the Middlesex Hospital London, research group, who showed that neuropsychological dysfunction following routine coronary artery bypass surgery is reduced when a 40 μm main arterial line filter is used compared with when it is not (Treasure, 1989).

Cerebroprotective drugs

Many types of drugs have been thought in the past to be cerebrally protective to the occurrence of cerebral damage during cardiopulmonary bypass, particularly high dose barbiturates such as Thiopentone and high dose steroids (Taylor, 1986b). Recently attention has been directed to lipid soluble calcium channel blockers, such as nimodipine, which has a potent dilating effect on the cerebral vasculature. Gelmers *et al.* (1988), in a controlled trial of acute ischaemic stroke patients, showed a reduced mortality and improved neurological status in those patients who had nimodipine. Similarly Allen *et al.* (1983) have shown the benefit of nimodipine in reducing cerebral arterial spasm in patients suffering from subarachnoid haemorrhage. Studies are now underway to evaluate whether nimodipine reduces the cerebral injury incurred during cardiopulmonary bypass.

Prostacyclins infused before and during the period of extracorporeal circulation have been shown to preserve platelet numbers and reduce the mass microaggregates produced during the bypass (Radegran, Ahren and Teyer-Nilsson, 1982). Consequently this has led to the hope that infusion of these substances may reduce the postoperative cerebral deficit following cardiac surgery. This has not been convincingly demonstrated.

Several new groups of possible cerebral protective drugs are currently being studied. Notably aspartate receptor antagonists. Glutamate is an excitatory transmitter in the brain. Its actions are mediated by three distinct types of receptor: quisqualate, kainate and *N*-methyl-*D*-aspartate (NMDA). Cerebral ischaemia results in a massive increase in extracellular glutamate concentration which is itself neurotoxic (Benveniste *et al.*, 1984). It has been shown that if the glutamate receptors are blocked, e.g. with an NMDA antagonist, less cerebral neuronal ischaemic damage results (Kochar *et al.*, 1988; Oyzurt *et al.*, 1988). The possible protective effect of NMDA antagonists in reducing the cerebral damage associated with cardiopulmonary bypass is currently being studied in dogs with plans to extend these studies to patients shortly.

At the present time evidence would suggest that the cardiac surgeon or perfusionist attempting to reduce cerebral injury in his patients to a minimum would carry out as quick a bypass as is practicably possible using a 40 μm main arterial line filter and membrane oxygenator, minimal suction of shed blood and α-stat $P\text{CO}_2$ management.

References

Aberg, T (1975) Effect of open heart surgery on intellectual function. *Scandinavian Journal of Thoracic and Cardiovascular Surgery*, **15** (suppl), 1–63

Aguilar, M.G., Gerbode, E.F. and Hill, J.D. (1971) Neuropathologic complications of cardiac surgery. *Journal of Thoracic and Cardiovascular Surgery*, **61**, 676–685

Allen, G.S., Ahn, H.S., Prezois, T.J., *et al.* (1983) Cerebral arterial spasm–a controlled trial of nimodipine in patients with subararchoid haemorrhage. *New England Journal of Medicine*, **308**, 619–624

Anderson, K., Waaben, J., Husum, B., *et al.* (1985) Non-pulsatile cardiopulmonary bypass disrupts the flow metabolism couple in the brain. *Journal of Thoracic and Cardiovascular Surgery*, **90**, 570–579

Arenberg, I.K., Allen, G.W. and De Boer, A. (1972) Sudden deafness immediately following cardiopulmonary bypass. *Journal of Laryngology and Otology*, **86**, 73–77

Aris, A., Solanes, H., Camara, M.L., *et al.* (1986) Arterial line filtration during cardiopulmonary bypass. Neurologic, neuropsychologic and haematologic studies. *Journal of Thoracic and Cardiovascular Surgery*, **91**, 526–533

Astrup, J., Symon, L., Branston, N.M. and Lassen, N.A. (1977) Cortisol evoked potential and extracellular K^+ and H^+ at critical levels of brain ischaemia. *Stroke*, **8**, 51–57

Bedford, P.O. and Leeds, M.D. (1955) Adverse effects of anaesthesia on old people. *Lancet*, **i**, 259–263

Benveniste, H., Drejer, J., Schousboe, A. and Diemer, N.H. (1984) Elevation of the extracellular concentrations of glutamate and aspartate in rat hippocampus during transient cerebral ischaemia monitored by intracerebral microdialysis. *Journal of Neurochemistry*, **43**, 1369–1374

Blauth, C., Arnold, J., Kohner, E.M. and Taylor, K.M. (1986) Retinal microembolism during cardiopulmonary bypass demonstrated by fluorescein angiography. *Lancet*, **ii**, 837–839

Blauth, C.I., Arnold, J.V., Schulenberg, W.E., *et al.* (1988) Cerebral microembolism during cardiopulmonary bypass. *Journal of Thoracic and Cardiovascular Surgery*, **95**, 668–676

Blauth, C., Smith, P.L., Newman, S.P., *et al.* (1989) Retinal microembolism and neuropsychological deficit following clinical cardiopulmonary bypass. A preliminary communication. *European Journal of Cardiothoracic Surgery*, **3**, 135–139

Bojar, R.M., Najafi, H., Delaria, G.A., *et al.* (1983) Neurological complications of coronary revascularization. *Annals of Thoracic Surgery*, **36**, 427–432

Branthwaite, M.A. (1974) Cerebral blood flow and metabolism during open heart surgery. *Thorax*, **29**, 633–638

Breuer, A.C., Furlan, A.J., Hanson, M.R. *et al.* (1981) Neurologic complications of open heart surgery. *Cleveland Clinic Quarterly*, **48**, 205–206

Bruce, D.L., Bach, M.J. and Arbit, J. (1974) Trace anaesthetic effects on perceptual, cognitive and motor skills. *Anesthesiology*, **40**, 453–458

Caguin, F. and Carter, M.G. (1963) Fat embolism with cardiotomy with the use of cardiopulmonary bypass. *Journal of Thoracic and Cardiovascular Surgery*, **46**, 665–672

Carleson, R.G., Landé, A.J., Landis, B., *et al.* (1973) The Landé–Edwards membrane oxygenator during heart surgery: oxygen transfer, microembolism counts and Beder–Gestalt visual motor scores. *Journal of Thoracic and Cardiovascular Surgery*, **66**, 896–905

Coffey, C.E., Massey, W., Roberts, K.B., *et al.* (1983) Natural history of arterial complications of coronary artery bypass surgery. *Neurology*, **33**, 1416–1421

Del Campo, C. and Nicholls, P.M.A. (1984) Cerebral blood flow during cardiac operations. *Journal of Thoracic and Cardiovascular Surgery*, **134**, 709–721

Deverall, P.B., Padayachee, T.S., Parsons, S., *et al.* (1988) Ultrasound detection of microemboli in the middle cerebral artery during cardiopulmonary bypass surgery. *European Journal of Cardiothoracic Surgery*, **2**, 256–260

Dutton, R.C., Edmunds, L.H.Jr, Hutchinson, J.C. and Roe, B.B. (1974) Platelet aggregate emboli produced by inpatients during cardiopulmonary bypass with membrane and bubble filters. *Journal of Thoracic and Cardiovascular Surgery*, **67**, 258–265

Ehrenraft, J.L., Claman, M.A., Layton, J.M. and Zimmerman, G.R. (1961) Cerebral complications of open heart surgery. *Journal of Thoracic and Cardiovascular Surgery*, **42**, 514–526

Ellis, R.J., Wisniewski, A., Potts, R., *et al.* (1980) Reduction of flow rate and arterial pressure at moderate hypothermia does not result in cerebral dysfunction. *Journal of Thoracic and Cardiovascular Surgery*, **79**, 173–180

Fox, H.M., Risso, N.D. and Gifford, S. (1954) Psychological observations of patients undergoing mitral surgery. *Psychosomatic Medicine*, **16**, 186–208

Frank, K.A., Heller, S.S., Kornfeld, D.S. and Malm, J.R. (1972) Long term effects of open heart surgery on intellectual functioning. *Journal of Thoracic and Cardiovascular Surgery*, **64**, 811–815

Gardner, T.J., Hormeffer, P.J., Manolio, T.A., *et al.* (1985) Stroke following coronary artery bypass grafting: a ten-year study. *Annals of Thoracic Surgery*, **40**, 574–581

Gelmers, H.J., Gorter, K., De Weerdt, C.J. and Wiezer, H.J. (1988) A controlled trial of nimodipine in acute ischemic stroke. *New England Journal of Medicine*, **318**, 203–207

Gibbon, J.H.Jr (1954) Artificial maintenance of circulation during experimental occlusion of the pulmonary artery. *Archives of Surgry*, **34**, 1105–1131

Gilberstadt, H. and Sako, Y. (1967) Intellectual and personality changes following open heart surgery. *Archives of General Psychiatry*, **16**, 210–215

Gilman, S. (1965) Cerebral disorders after open heart operations. *New England Journal of Medicine*, **272** 489–498

Gonzales-Scarano, S. and Hurtig, H.I. (1981) Neurlogic complications of coronary artery bypass grafting: case control study. *Neurology*, **31**, 1032–1035

Govier, A.V., Reves, J.G., McKay, R.D., *et al.* (1984) Factors and their influence on regional cerebral blood flow during non-pulsatile cardiopulmonary bypass. *Annals of Thoracic Surgery*, **38**, 592–600

Halley, M., Reemstsma, K. and Creech, O. (1958) Cerebral blood flow, metabolism and brain volume in extracorporeal circulation. *Journal of Thoracic and Cardiovascular Surgery*, **36**, 506–518

Henriksen, L. (1984) Evidence suggestive of difffuse brain damage following cardiac operations. *Lancet*, **i**, 816–820

Henriksen, L., Hjelms, E. and Lindeburgh, T. (1983) Cerebral blood flow measured in man by intraarterially injected 133 Xe: evidence suggestive of intraoperative microembolism. *Journal of Thoracic and Cardiovascular Surgery*, **86**, 202–208

Holmes-Sellers, T. (1970) Atrial septal defects. *Annals of the Royal College of Surgeons*, **46**, 1–19

James, F.M. (1969) The effects of cyclopropane anaesthesia without surgical operation on mental functions of normal man. *Anesthesiology*, **30**, 264–272

Joulasmaa, A., Outakoski, J., Hirvenoja, R., *et al.* (1981) Effect of open heart surgery on intellectual performance. *Journal of Clinical Neuropsychology*, **3**, 181–197

Kessler, J. and Patterson, R.H. (1970) The production of microemboli by various blood oxygenators. *Annals of Thoracic Surgery*, **9**, 221–228

Kochar, A., Zivin, J.A., Lyden, P.D. and Mazzarella, V. (1988) Glutamate antagonist therapy reduces neurologic deficits produced by focal central nervous system ischaemia. *Archives of Neurology*, **8**, 138–143

Larsen, N.A. and Christensen, M.S. (1976) Physiology of cerebral blood flow. *British Journal of Anaesthesia*, **48**, 719–734

Lee, M.C., Geiger, J., Nicoloff, D., *et al.* (1979) Cerebrovascular complications associated with coronary artery bypass (CAB) procedures. *Stroke*, **10**, 107–113

Lindeberg, D.A.B., Lucas, F.V., Sheagren, J. and Malm, J.R. (1961) Silicone embolisation during clinical and experimental heart surgery employing a bubble oxygenator. *American Journal of Pathology*, **39**, 129–135

Martin, W.R.W. and Hashimoto, S.A. (1982) Stroke in coronary bypass surgery. *Le Journal Canadien des Sciences Neurologiques*, **9**, 21–26

Miller, J.A., Fonkalsrud, E.W., Latta, H.L and Maroney, J.V. (1962) Fat embolism associated with extracorporeal circulation and blood transfusion. *Surgery*, **51**, 448–454

Mortensen, J.D. (1977) Evaluations of tests for blood damage produced by oxygenators. *Transactions of the American Society for Artificial Internal Organs*, **23**, 747–754

Nevin, M., Adams, S., Colchester, A.C.F. and Pepper, J.R. (1988) Evidence for involvement of hypocapnia and hypotension in aetiology of neurological deficit after cardiopulmonary bypass. *Lancet*, **ii**, 1943–1945

Newman, S.P. (1989) The incidence and nature of neuropsychological mobidity following cardiac surgery. *Perfusion*, **4**, 93–100

Oleson, J. (1971) Contralateral focal increase of cerebral blood flow in man during arm work. *Brain*, **94**, 635–646

Orenstein, J.M., Noriko, S., Aaron, B., *et al.* (1982) Microemboli observed in deaths following cardiopulmonary bypass surgery: silicone antifoam agents and polyvinyl chloride tubing as sources of emboli. *Human Pathology*, **13**, 1082–1090

Orr, W.C. and Stahl, M.L. (1977) Sleep disturbance after open heart surgery. *American Journal of Cardiology*, **39**, 196–201

Ozyurt, E., Graham, D.I., Woodruff, G.N. and McCulloch, J. (1988) Protective effect of glutamate antagonist, MK-801 in focal cerebral ischemia in the cat. *Journal of Cerebral Blood Flow and Metabolism*, **8**, 138–143

Parker, F.B., Marvasti, M.A. and Bare, E.L. (1985) Neurologic complications following coronary artery bypass. The role of atherosclerosis emboli. *Thorac. Cardiovasc. Surg.*, **33**, 736–741

Patterson, R.H., Rosenfeld, L. and Porro, R.S. (1976) Transitory cerebral microvascular blockade after cardiopulmonary bypass. *Thorax*, **31**, 736–741

Plasse, H.M., Spencer, F.C., Mittleman, M. and Frost, J.O. (1980) Unilateral sudden loss of hearing, an unusual complication of cardiac operation. *Journal of Thoracic and Cardiovascular Surgery*, **79**, 822–826

Radegran, K., Ahren, C. and Teger-Nilsson, A.C. (1982) Prostacyclin infusion during extracorporeal circulation for coronary bypass. *Journal of Thoracic and Cardiovascular Surgery*, **83**, 205–211

Raymond, M., Conklin, C., Schaeffer, J., *et al.* (1984) Coping with transient intellectual dysfunction after coronary bypass surgery. *Heart–Lung*, **13**, 531–539

Ross-Russell, R.W. and Bharucha, N. (1978) The recognition and prevention of border zone cerebral ischaemia during cardiac surgery. *Quarterly Journal of Medicine*, **47**, 303–323

Santillan, G.G., Chemnitius, J.M. and Bing, R.J. (1985) The effect of cardiopulmonary bypass on cerebral blood flow. *Brain Research*, **345**, 3–9

Savageau, J.A., Stanton, B.A., Jenkins, C.D. and Klein, M.D. (1982a) Neuropsychological dysfunction following elective cardiac operation. I. Early assessment. *Journal of Thoracic and Cardiovascular Surgery*, **84**, 585–594

Savageau, J.A., Stanton, B.A., Jenkins, C.D. and Frater, R.W.M. (1982b) Neuropsychological function following elective cardiac operation. II. A six-month assessment. *Journal of Thoracic and Cardiovascular Surgery*, **84**, 595–600

Shapiro, M.J., Prun, J.M. and Raskin, C. (1981) A study of the effects of cardiopulmonary bypass surgery on auditory function. *Laryngoscope*, **91**, 2046–2052

Shaw, P.J., Bates, D., Cartlidge, N.E.F., *et al.* (1985) Early neurological complications of coronary artery bypass surgery. *British Medical Journal*, **291**, 1384–1387

Shaw, P.J., Bates, D., Cartlidge, N.E.F., *et al.* (1986) Early intellectual dysfunction following coronary artery bypass surgery: a six-month follow-up study. *Quarterly Journal of Medicine*, **58**, 59–68

Shaw, P.J., Bates, D., Cartlidge, N.E.F., *et al.* (1987) Long term intellectual dysfunction following coronary artery bypass surgery: a six-month follow-up study. *Quarterly Journal of Medicine*, **62**, 259–268

Simpson, B.R., Williams, M., Scott, J.F. and Smith, A. (1961) The effects of anaesthesia and elective surgery on old people. *Lancet*, **ii**, 887–893

Smith, P.L.C. (1988) The cerebral complications of coronary artery bypass surgery. *Annals of the Royal College of Surgeons of England*, **70**, 212–216

Smith, P.L.C., Treasure, T., Newman, S.P., *et al.* (1986) Cerebral consequences of cardiopulmonary bypass. *Lancet*, **ii**, 823–825

Solis, R.T., Kennedy, P.S., Beall, A.C. Jr and Debakey, M.E. (1975) Cardiopulmonary bypass: microembolisation and platelet aggregation. *Circulation*, **52**, 103–108

Sorenson, H.R. and Lindeberg, J. (1950) Cerebral injury and cerebral function following anaesthesia. *Acta Chirurgica Scandinavica*, **99**, 40–50

Sotaneimi, K.A. (1983) Cerebral outcome after extracorporeal circulation. *Archives of Neurology*, **40**, 75–77

Souttar, H.S. (1925) The surgical treatment of mitral stenosis. *British Medical Journal*, 3rd October, 603–606

Sveinsson, I.S. (1975) Postoperative psychosis after open heart surgery. *Journal of Thoracic and Cardiovascular Surgery*, **70**, 717–726

Swan, H. (1984) The importance of acid–base management for cardiac and cerebral preservation during open heart operations. *Surgery, Gynecology and Obstetrics*, **158**, 391–413

Taylor, K.M. (1986a) Editorial: Brain damage after open heart surgery. *Lancet*, **ii**, 1161–1163

Taylor, K.M. (1986b) Pathophysiology of brain damage during open heart surgery. *Texas Heart Institute Journal*, **13**, 91–96

Taylor, K.M., Devlin, B.J., Mittra, S.M., *et al.* (1980) Assessment of cerebral damage during open heart surgery. A new experimental model. *Scandinavian Journal of Thoracic and Cardiovascular Surgery*, **14**, 197–203

Treasure, T. (1989) Interventions to reduce cerebral injury during cardiac surgery–the effect of arterial line filtration. *Perfusion*, **4**, 147–152

Tufo, H.M., Ostfeld, A.M. and Shekelle, R. (1970) Central nervous system dysfunction following open heart surgery. *JAMA*, **212**, 1333–1340

Turnipseed, W.D., Berkoff, H.A. and Beryer, F.O. (1980) Postoperative stroke in cardiac and peripheral vascular disease. *Annals of Surgery*, **192**, 365–368

Utley, J.R., Stephens, D.B., *et al.* (1986) Prevention of major perioperative neurological dysfunction: a personal perspective. *Perfusion*, **1**, 135–142

Watkins, W.D., Peterson, M.D., Kong, D.L., *et al.* (1982) Thromboxane and prostacyclin changes during cardiopulmonary bypass with and without pulsatile flow. *Journal of Thoracic and Cardiovascular Surgery*, **84**, 250–256

Williams, I.M. (1971) Intravascular changes in the retina during open heart surgery. *Lancet*, **ii**, 688–691

Woolman, H., Stephen, G.W., Clement, A.J. and Danielsen, G.K. (1966) Cerebral blood flow in man during extracorporeal circulation. *Journal of Thoracic and Cardiovascular Surgery*, **52**, 558–564

Wright, J.L.W. and Saunders, S.H. (1975) Sudden deafness following cardiopulmonary bypass surgery. *Journal of Laryngology and Otology*, **89**, 757–759

Zilstra, W.G. (1981) Physiology of the cerebral circulation. In *Cerebral Blood Flow, Basic Knowledge and Clinical Features* (ed. J.M. Minderhoud), Excerpta Medica, Amsterdam, Chapter III

14

Microbiological aspects of heart, heart–lung and lung transplant patients

Roger Freeman and Frances Kate Gould

Heart and heart–lung transplantation have come of age and are now regarded as part of the repertoire of cardiothoracic surgery. When units contemplate setting up heart and heart–lung transplantation programmes one of the most important considerations is the development of an adequate system for the prevention, control, diagnosis and treatment of the infective complications. These complications are responsible for up to half of the early deaths following transplantation. However, as the following account attempts to show, careful planning and attention to detail can do much to minimize infection in these patients.

Heart transplantation (and subsequently heart–lung and single lung transplantation) commenced at the Freeman Hospital in 1985. To date 100 heart transplants, 12 heart–lung transplants and eight single lung transplants have been carried out. We as microbiologists were heavily involved in the programme from the outset. Our account is, in part, a historical record of the evolution of the Freeman Hospital Unit, beginning with the planning that preceded the first operation. Although many problems were foreseen, several important changes have subsequently occurred in our methods as a result of experience. We have incorporated these in the belief that they will help others currently planning to introduce cardiac transplantation. Although this account concentrates on the needs of cardiac transplantation patients, the additional measures required for heart–lung and single lung transplant patients are dealt with at the end.

Planning

There are four essential components to the microbiological care of cardiac transplant patients:

Personnel

We think it essential for one or more microbiologists to be actively involved in the day-to-day management of these patients as well as being involved in the devising of protocols for their care. This involvement ensures that the correct specimens are obtained first time and that someone familiar with the laboratory processing of the specimens has an overview of the investigations. Additionally, knowledge on antibiotic and antifungal drugs and their metabolism is particularly important in transplant patients. In our Unit the transplant patients are routinely seen twice a day by a microbiologist.

Lung infection is the commonest early postoperative infection in cardiac transplantation and is of crucial importance in lung transplantation. It is a considerable advantage to have chest physicians involved in the programme, since the diagnosis of lung infection is greatly facilitated by the examination of invasive material. The obtaining of and analysis of bronchoalveolar lavage (BAL) and transbronchial lung biopsy (TBLB) specimens by co-operation between the chest physicians and the microbiologists is an enormous advantage in these patients (see later).

Laboratory facilities

The Microbiology Department can expect a considerable demand on its resources, time and ingenuity. Decisions will have to be made on which tests are best developed ‘in house’ and which tests demand access to local or distant Reference Laboratories. Again, the involvement of the microbiologist will greatly facilitate this process, ensure that laboratory time is not wasted and that co-operation of other laboratories is assured. Details of which tests are needed in addition to the standard repertoire of the conventional Microbiology Department are dealt with under specific items later.

Physical facilities

Microbiologists are often involved in the planning of accommodation for transplant patients. The need for isolation facilities, whether protective to the individual patient or, alternatively, to isolate infective patients from the rest of the susceptible pool, are often among the first considerations in setting up these Units. It was certainly the common view in the early days of cardiac transplantation that these patients required strict reverse-barrier isolation facilities. As will be seen in the subsequent description of our routine care of the early postoperative stage our experience has shown that these expensive and cumbersome precautions are unnecessary for the majority. This relaxation in the protective isolation facilities in the light of experience is a common feature of transplantation programmes. With the exception of bone-marrow transplantation with which we are not concerned here we would currently suggest the provision of cubicles with air-locks and ventilation systems capable of being either positive or negative pressure with respect to the main ward or unit. Nursing apparel should be similar to the ordinary (non-transplant) unit. No masks are needed and the patient should not be subjected to pre-sterilized meals, sterile bedding or sterilized drinks. One-to-one nursing with strict attention to hand washing with antiseptics remain fundamental to the nursing care of these patients as with all intensive care patients.

Protocols

In our view the early establishment of agreed protocols for the microbiological care and investigation of transplant patients is an essential prerequisite for a successful programme. Protocols have three benefits. They ensure that each patient has a complete programme of care, they minimize errors of commission as well as of omission and, if regularly audited, they provide the bases for logical developments in microbiological care. Protocols need to be set out for patients awaiting transplantation as well as those having undergone the operation. It is important that the surgical and nursing staff understand and agree to these protocols. Any suggestions for amendments should be encouraged but it should be accepted that no changes be made without adequate discussion and agreement. There are often constraints in the management of transplant patients which do not apply to other patients and which the well-meaning newcomer to the Unit will not appreciate. To give a simple example, the routine use of cyclosporin A in immunosuppression means that potential interactions between this drug and various antibiotics may influence selection of therapy for infection.

Operating the system

The simplest way to explain the system and to give details of the procedures involved is to follow a theoretical patient through the various stages.

Assessment and the preoperative stage

Patients offered for consideration for cardiac transplantation undergo rigorous examination. In purely microbiological terms there are two considerations:

Evaluation of current sepsis

Patients are carefully evaluated for current sepsis, which should include minor infections and dental infections. Transplantation across an active microbial infection or even an infection only very recently treated can be very hazardous. A cardinal principle of *postoperative* management is to try to detect developing infections at the earliest possible stage when the microbial 'load' is small and treatment is most likely to be effective. The imposition of massive immunosuppression on to an established infection, even one under appropriate treatment with evidence of control, is usually disastrous. On the two occasions that we tried to do this (one patient had active influenza A virus infection, the other had *Legionella* infection) we were unable to control the infection postoperatively. On the other hand we deprecate the idea that these patients should have swabs taken from everywhere. Transplant candidates should be checked for colonization with resistant organisms, especially in present times methicillin resistant *Staphylococcus aureus* (MRSA), but in this context they are really no different from other candidates for major surgery.

A variation on this theme is the patient with a recent history of any infection which tends to become dormant but can reactivate, the most common example being tuberculosis. Under such circumstances prophylactic therapy with isoniazid for the immediate postoperative period should be considered. Rarer infections meriting such considerations would include brucellosis, listeriosis, psittacosis and many parasitic diseases such as amoebiasis and trypanosomiasis.

Evaluation of immunity status

An evaluation is made of the patient's immunity status for several common infections that are known to persist in a permanent latent form and which may reactivate postoperatively or which, if the patient is susceptible may be transmitted by the graft if the donor has latent infection. These include:

1. Cytomegalovirus (CMV). This herpes virus remains latent in the T cells of persons recovering from the often subclinical infection which up to 40–50% of the normal population undergo. The fact that this is so can be detected by testing the serum for the presence of CMV-specific IgG using an enzyme-linked immunosorbent assay (ELISA) method. Previous methods of testing such as complement-fixation tests (CFT) have been found to be both non-specific and of insufficient sensitivity. More recently a passive latex agglutination method has become available. Despite its speed, convenience and low cost we have found it to be wanting in comparison to the ELISA test. The latex test in our hands produces occasional false negatives but, more importantly, appreciable numbers of false positives. False positives are much more commonly seen in donor sera (see later), but even in assessments we would still insist on the greater accuracy of the ELISA. As will be seen later, the antibody status of the patient at the time of transplantation has a considerable influence on management thereafter.
2. *Toxoplasma gondii*. This ubiquitous parasite again causes largely subclinical infections in the normal population and the permanent marker is a persisting antibody. The organism may persist in the body in the form of cysts, typically in muscle tissue. Again, reactivation may follow immunosuppression and again the donor heart may transmit the disease to a seronegative recipient. ELISA tests are carried out on the potential recipient to determine immune status.
3. Epstein–Barr virus (EBV). This is another herpes virus of man, this time found in latent form in the B cells. Although donor-transmitted disease is possible the importance of pretransplant testing for this antibody is predominantly because of the possible effects of massive T cell suppression in the postoperative period. Under these circumstances B cell proliferation is uninhibited and, if the proliferating B cells (in the patient) contain the EBV genome, malignant transformation can occur, leading to a form of lymphoma. The preoperative EBV IgG status (by ELISA tests or by indirect immunofluorescence test) will predict this possibility and facilitate later diagnosis.

Other latent infections are possible candidates for reactivation disease, for instance *Herpes simplex* virus and *Varicella zoster* virus (causing shingles or even disseminated zoster). We also routinely perform antibody tests for the most common viruses such as influenza A and B, adenovirus and other agents such as *Mycoplasma pneumoniae*, *Chlamydia psittaci* and *Coxiella burneti* to establish baseline data for subsequent use. In other countries it may be sensible to supplement this screen with tests for other local agents. All transplant candidates are, of course, tested for hepatitis B surface antigen (HBsAg) and antibody to human immunodeficiency virus (HIV). Although it used to be thought that the detection of HBsAg would preclude transplantation, modern testing allows a more sophisticated response. HBsAg +ve patients should be further tested for 'e' antigen (HBeAg) and 'e' antibody (anti-HBeAg). A minority of those tested (approximately 20%) will be found to be HbeAg +ve. Such patients continue to harbour hepatitis B virus (HBV) within the liver and after immunosuppression may well succumb to HBV infection. Although they should be referred for full liver examination, including a liver biopsy, they are highly likely to have progressive liver damage and cardiac transplantation may be disastrous.

Conversely, the remainder (approximately 80%) of HBsAg +ve carriers will prove to have anti-HBeAg in their serum. This combination of results usually implies the continued production of HBsAg *alone* as a residual marker of a post HBV infection. HBV is no longer present in the body and immunosuppression is not followed by any adverse effects. It is still advisable to seek expert assessment and even to proceed to liver biopsy, but transplantation need not be denied them on this basis alone.

Finally, we strongly commend the practice of always laying down a large sample of preoperative serum before transplantation. Once the operation has been performed it is impossible to return to preoperative specimens and the storage of preoperative serum has proven to be of value on several occasions, not all by any means for microbiological purposes.

Once the patient has been assessed and accepted for transplantation we advocate one further measure which will facilitate microbiological care immediately after transplantation. All our patients on the waiting list are given antifungal therapy so that at admission it is likely that colonization with yeasts is either absent or minimal. The patients are given the following regime:

Nystatin tablets, one per day orally
Nystatin suspension, 100 000 Units to be used as a mouthwash and then swallowed twice per day
Nystatin cream to be applied to any skin lesions such as eczema or psoriasis as needed
Patients with dentures are instructed to remove them at night and steep them in 2% chlorhexidine gluconate
Female patients are given nystatin pessaries to insert one daily

Whether because of this regime or not, we have yet to see a serious yeast infection in any cardiac transplant patient.

Admission, the operation and the immediate postoperative period

Once an offer of a potentially suitable donor has been made the patient is called into hospital and prepared for the operation. The opportunity should be taken to obtain a preoperative urine specimen and nose and throat swabs, although within the time frame of transplantation the results of these tests will not be available in time to influence the decision to transplant. Obviously, if on admission the patient is febrile and clinically thought to be infected the operation should be postponed. In practice many units admit more than one potential recipient in order that donated organs are not discarded. Since this is the last opportunity to obtain preoperative serum we advocate taking a sample for testing, especially if the patient has not been retested for CMV and *Toxoplasma* status for some time. There is a low but definite rate of antibody recruitment in the population and the occasional patient will have seroconverted while awaiting surgery. This specimen is the one used for immediate testing in parallel with donor serum (see below).

Perioperative antibiotic prophylaxis

The antibiotic(s) chosen for perioperative prophylaxis vary from unit to unit and represent custom and familiarity rather than being based upon any formal trial data. We have been convinced for many years that narrow spectrum prophylaxis with flucloxacillin is the method of choice for conventional cardiac surgery. We regard the transplant operation and the immediate postoperative period as a closely analogous situation and have continued to use this simple agent as our only form of routine antibiotic prophylaxis. Our experience to date appears to have justified this approach. In 100 consecutive cardiac transplants we have recorded only four cases of septicaemia, three cases of mediastinitis, no cases of sternal wound infection and, although early postoperative lung infection has occurred it has been due to relatively 'simple' organisms such as *Haemophilus influenzae*, *Streptococcus pneumoniae*, *Branhamella catarrhalis* and other upper respiratory tract streptococci. Our Unit did have a small number of lung infections due to *Legionella bozemannii* which were traced to an environmental source and control of the point source has prevented any further cases. We do not regard such occurrences as being relevant to the perioperative prophylaxis which exists to control infection related to the operative procedure. Most chest infection in the early postoperative phase is probably due to upper respiratory tract organisms gaining access to the susceptible lung parenchyma. Antibiotic administration *per se* will not prevent this process and the use of broad spectrum antibiotic prophylaxis will increase the likelihood that the descending flora will be Gram-negative bacilli ('coliforms') and yeasts. Lung infection due to coliform bacilli (*Escherichia coli*, *Proteus*, *Klebsiella*, *Pseudomonas* and so on) has been remarkably rare in our experience (only two cases to date) and we have seen no lung infection due to yeasts. We attribute this outcome to our use of a narrow spectrum agent. Flucloxacillin, 2 g intravenously, is commenced at induction and continued at a dose of 500 mg i.v. 6 hourly until all the central intravascular lines, apart from the triple lumen central venous line, are removed. This, in an uncomplicated patient, means a course of 2–3 days. With the exception of patients given prophylaxis against donor-transmitted toxoplasma infection (see later) no further antibiotics are given unless postoperative infection is detected.

Non-antibiotic prophylactic measures

All patients should continue with the antifungal measures described earlier. In addition, we have employed one further manoeuvre derived from our previous work on conventional cardiac surgical patients. It has been shown that the addition of 0.05% sodium metabisulphite (SMBS) to the dextrose–heparin solution used as a 'flush' on the left and right atrial and venous lines serves greatly to reduce colonization of the catheter tips with skin organisms, such as coagulase-negative staphylococci and diphtheroids. This measure is used in our transplant patients. It is extended beyond the routine for conventional patients being continued as a twice-daily bolus flush for the triple-lumen CVP line which transplant patients retain throughout their immediate postoperative stay for the purpose of emergency venous access. The triple-lumen lines are changed electively on a weekly basis. Despite the retention of such central lines for a week at a time we have yet to document a verified line-based bacteraemia in adult cardiac transplant patients. SMBS is not used in babies and small children and one instance of line-based bacteraemia occurred in a baby.

Antiviral prophylaxis with acyclovir

From the beginning of our transplant programme we adopted the practice of giving patients oral acyclovir for the first 3 months after operation, commencing as soon as a reliable oral route was established. The original rationale was the prevention of EBV-driven B-cell proliferation during the early period of high dose immunosuppression. Because of concerns at that time about the potential nephrotoxicity of acyclovir (since largely discounted) a regime of 200 mg three times a day, instead of the usual five times a day was adopted. It is difficult to say whether or not this has had any effect on B-cell proliferative disease, but it is noticeable that our patients have hardly been troubled at all by *Herpes simplex* infection and the associated 'mucositis'. Even patients rendered temporarily leucopenic by azathioprine have suffered few effects. Prophylactic acyclovir in other immunosuppression and neutropenic patients has been shown to significantly diminish mucosal breakdown and associated invasive infections. It has recently been claimed that post-transplant acyclovir, admittedly at a much higher dose, has a protective effect against infection and, if confirmed, this will be an additional indication.

Donor-transmitted diseases

Cytomegalovirus

As described earlier, the implantation of a heart (inevitably contaminated with donor blood) from a CMV antibody-positive donor into an antibody negative (i.e. susceptible) recipient carries a high risk of CMV transmission. Primary CMV infection, as opposed to the reactivation of the pre-existing latent disease in an antibody-positive recipient, is a serious disease with a substantial mortality and morbidity. It used to be thought that recipients with pre-existing antibodies were immune to donor-transmitted primary CMV infection, but recent work suggests that 'second primary' infections occur and, moreover, can be severe. It is, therefore, of great importance to define the CMV antibody status of both recipient and donor on specimens taken at the time of transplantation. Because of the methodological problems discussed earlier we recommend that both samples are tested in parallel by the ELISA method for CMV-specific IgG. ELISA tests will produce results within 4–6 h, allowing full assessment of the situation on they day of transplantation. The different patterns of possible results with the potential consequences are as shown in Table 14.1.

In Group A donor *graft*-transmitted CMV infection cannot occur but the patient remains at risk from *blood donation*. It has been well shown that CMV can be transmitted to susceptible patients by the infusion of blood or blood products from a seropositive donor. The strategy to be pursued for this group is to conduct the operation and all subsequent procedures with blood or blood products screened to be negative for CMV-specific antibody. We have adopted this strategy on 16 such occasions and none of the patients has yet developed primary CMV infection. It must, however, be realized that these patients remain susceptible to CMV thereafter and the usual 1% acquisition rate for general population can be expected to occur, albeit at a time well after transplantation when it will be better tolerated.

For Group B no action is required since the only possible CMV problem is reactivation of the latent infection in the recipient. Such infection ('secondary CMV') is almost always mild and in many cases is only diagnosed in retrospect on serial tests showing a rise in the previous antibody levels.

Group C patients have a very high risk of developing primary CMV infection within 4–6 weeks of transplantation. The severity of the disease varies and can range from a mild influenza-like illness to multiple organ failure involving the gut, kidneys, bone marrow and liver. It commonly terminates in a fatal pneumonitis.

More than one approach to this problem is possible.

Some units operate a policy whereby the possibility of implanting a graft from a seropositive donor into a seronegative patient is actively avoided. The limited donor pool and the limited ability to 'match' seropositive recipients to seropositive donors makes for potential wastage of donations with this approach. Additionally, it now seems certain (see below) that primary CMV infection is *not* completely avoidable by this means. We have now adopted this strategy.

A second approach is to accept that 'positive into negative' transplantation has occurred and to simply observe the patient. If primary CMV infection occurs treatment (currently with ganciclovir) is commenced. We have two reservations about this approach. Firstly, the diagnosis of primary CMV can take time to establish and requires a formidable commitment from the virology laboratories. Patients may become quite ill before the diagnosis is certain.

Secondly, ganciclovir is a toxic drug. Some of the toxic effects will be compounded by concurrent

Table 14.1 Results and consequences of ELISA tests for CMV-specific IgG

	Donor CMV status	*Recipient CMV status*	*Risk of primary CMV from graft*
A	IgG test negative	IgG test negative	Nil
B	IgG test negative	IgG test positive	Nil
C	IgG test positive	IgG test negative	High
D	IgG test positive	IgG test positive	?High

immunosuppressive therapy, particularly azathioprine. It seems logical to us to establish the fact of the 'mismatch' at the outset and then to undertake some form of prophylactic measure.

Our policy has been to commence prophylactic CMV-specific hyperimmune globulin as soon as the mismatch is diagnosed, usually on the day of transplantation. The globulin is administered at 100 mg Kg^{-1} i.v. on days 0, 7, 14, 21, 28 and 49. Each patient is then monitored both clinically and serologically. Since the globulin contains only IgG antibodies, serial testing for CMV-specific IgM allows the recognition of primary CMV infection. On eight consecutive occasions we have shown the appearance of CMV-specific IgM, accompanied by only very mild symptoms. In no instance was drug therapy even contemplated. Our experience strongly suggests that the use of CMV-specific hyperimmune globulin produces significant amelioration of primary CMV infection, allowing the safe management of 'positive into negative' transplantation. This method has the additional benefit of producing active immunity in the recipient. In several of our patients the successful amelioration of the primary CMV infection occurred despite several courses of augmented immunosuppression for rejection, even including two patients requiring OKT3 use.

It has already been mentioned that possession of CMV-specific IgG used to be thought to confer protection against second infections. We now know that this is not so and that 'second primary' infections can occur after implantation of a graft from a seropositive donor into a seropositive recipient. Naturally, this recent evidence also casts doubt on the avoidance policy described earlier under Group C. It also raises the question as to the strategy to be followed for Group D. One possibility is to extend the use of prophylactic globulin to all patients receiving a graft from a seropositive donor. Unfortunately, each course of prophylactic globulin costs several thousand pounds so that this would be an expensive option. Currently, our own strategy is to accept that second primary infection may occur and that the pre-existing antibodies will partially ameliorate the disease, thus allowing time for diagnosis and drug therapy. We accept that this is a less than ideal solution. In the future a logical approach would be to characterize the latent CMV DNA in the lymphocytes of both donor and recipient. Where a donor strain was sufficiently antigenically different from the recipient antibody that a second infection was likely, selective globulin prophylaxis could be offered.

Toxoplasmosis

In our experience this donor-transmitted disease has been a theoretical rather than a practical problem. There seems little doubt that primary toxoplasmosis has been transmitted by cardiac transplantation. Presumably dormant *T. gondii* in the cyst form is occasionally found in cardiac muscle and is engrafted. In patients without pre-existing antibody primary infection can follow. In the small number of such cases described the disease has been severe and has a mortality of up to 50%. Once developed the disease has seemed difficult to treat and even more difficult to eradicate. On the face of it this seems another situation calling for peritransplant testing of both donor and recipient sera, followed by some form of prophylaxis. We have followed this scheme, using an ELISA test for *T. gondii*-specific IgG and instituting prophylactic drug therapy with oral co-trimoxazole for 6 weeks after operation whenever a 'mismatch' has been detected. However, our experience of toxoplasmosis has differed from that of others in two ways.

First, we have found the incidence of toxoplasma antibody in both donors and recipients to be much lower than is generally thought to be the case (29% of patients; 8% of donors) so that the likelihood of a mismatch has been quite low (in fact seven occasions in 120 consecutive transplants). Second, despite serial monitoring for *T. gondii*-specific IgM and careful observation for any clinical signs of disease we have yet to show any evidence of donor-transmitted disease. Other units have used arguably more powerful prophylaxis with pyrimethamine and sulphonamides (a regime which is often poorly tolerated by the patient) and yet have still recorded instances of disease transmission.

For the moment we continue to recommend co-trimoxazole as a simple, cheap and relatively well-tolerated prophylactic measure if a mismatch is identified. However, we believe that this whole question needs to be re-examined. It may be that not all seropositive donors are capable of transmission (for instance, we may have been extraordinarily lucky in acquiring positive donors without myocardial cysts) and that some better testing strategy can be devised to identify only those donors likely to transmit the disease.

These measures comprise the microbiological care of an uneventful cardiac transplant. In such a case it can be expected that the patient will leave the intensive care unit within 1–3 days and thereafter remain on the convalescent ward for a further 10–14 days before first discharge. We do not advocate taking gratuitous microbiological specimens from well patients and our only additional specimens in such cases are the regular serum samples for virological and toxoplasma serology. We rely on intensive clinical and radiological observations to prompt appropriate investigations whenever necessary.

Complications

Early complications (before first discharge)

Postoperative transplant patients do not exhibit the commonly observed 'benign' febrile response to cardiopulmonary bypass seen after conventional cardiac surgery. Thus, any fever may be a sign of trouble and, if sustained and associated with any other untoward signs and symptoms (such as tachypnoea, sputum production, haemodynamic instability, and so on), is an indication for investigation. The intensive radiological surveillance (usually at this time patients are chest X-rayed twice per day) may indicate a lung infiltrate suggesting a pulmonary source. However, it is important to bear in mind that fever and haemodynamic instability are also the cardinal features of acute cardiac rejection. Both infection and rejection need to be looked for in any patient with sustained fever in the early days after cardiac transplantation. Rapid diagnosis is essential and a final important point is that on rare occasions the two processes may co-exist. Good management dictates a comprehensive response to the problem. We have adopted a simple but thorough protocol for this situation.

Procedure for investigating febrile episodes

1 Take blood cultures (NB *always* via a peripheral uncannulated vein, never through a line)
2. Obtain a mid stream or catheter specimen of urine for microscopy, including Gram stain, and culture.
3. Obtain material for Gram stain and culture from any other clinically suspicious site, e.g. the sternal wound. Although examination of any purulent expectorated sputum should also be performed initially, the demonstration of a pulmonary infiltrate may well dictate invasive specimens (see below).
4. Review the serial chest X-rays, supplemented by a new one. A developing infiltrate is often best recognized by comparison of serial films rather than one film.
5. Remove all intravascular lines, sending the severed tips for culture.
6. Take serum for the estimation of C-reactive protein (CRP) level. Using rapid semiquantitative methods CRP levels can be measured within a few minutes. Normal, or only slightly raised, levels suggest rejection or non-bacterial infection. Very high levels are almost always associated with a severe bacterial infection.
7. Perform an immediate endomyocardial biopsy for histological assessment of cardiac rejection.
8. If the chest X-ray reveals a pulmonary infiltrate, material from the affected area of lung should be obtained by bronchoalveolar lavage (BAL) or transthoracic lung biopsy. It is often helpful in cardiac transplant patients (and mandatory in heart–lung or lung transplant patients) to perform a transbronchial lung biopsy (TBLB) at the time of BAL. Material obtained by these methods is then examined for a comprehensive range of 'conventional' and opportunistic pathogens (see later).

The early results (microscopy, including fluorescent stains, CRP levels and endomyocardial biopsy) will be available within a few hours of initiating these investigations. Collation of these results will then allow a rational form of therapy. It is usually possible to await these early results but on rare occasions 'blind' therapy for either infection or rejection, or both, may need to be given.

Use of antibiotics

There are special constraints on the use of antibiotics in cardiac transplantation, but before discussing these in detail we emphasize that the most important constraint of all is that antibiotics must be used rationally and selectively. Familiarity with this very specialized field of infection may well lead the expert judiciously to anticipate laboratory results to the benefit of the patient. This is very different from indiscriminate use of antibiotics. Trials of antibiotics in an underinvestigated patient are foolish. Chief among the special constraints is the universal use of cyclosporin A (Cy A) in immunosuppression. Cy A is nephrotoxic and this toxicity can occur as an acute event when Cy A levels are too high and it is also manifest as a more insidious chronic phenomenon with continued use. Since these patients are also commonly given loop diurectics it is wise wherever possible to avoid the use of *aminoglycosides*. While it is essential that peak and trough assays are performed if aminoglycosides are being used, it should be realized that the cumulative nephrotoxicity of Cy A, diuretics and aminoglycosides mean that renal damage can still be sustained in the presence of immaculately controlled aminoglycoside levels.

A second problem is the effect of several antibiotics on the metabolism of Cy A. Some antibiotics, for instance rifampicin, induce liver mitochondrial enzyme systems and cause a precipitate fall in Cy A levels. Others, for instance erythromycin, block Cy A metabolism and produce unacceptably high levels. Whenever antibiotic selection is being made these effects must be borne in mind. Novel antibiotics must be introduced with great caution for these reasons. We believe that our adoption of a narrow spectrum prophylaxis has paid dividends in this context since most of the infections with which we have had to contend have been due to organisms sensitive to β-lactam antibiotics (penicillins and cephalosporins). β-lactams do not interact with Cy A. Where a very broad spectrum drug is required we have found that ciprofloxacin and aztreonam do not interfere with Cy A metabolism. The former has the additional merit of a useful action on Legionellae which would otherwise necessitate the use of both rifampicin and erythromycin. The latter has a purely 'Gram-negative' spectrum, including *Pseudomonas*, both would require the addition of metronidazole for activity against anaerobes.

A final general rule in antibiotic usage is that treatment should not be unduly prolonged just because the patient is immunosuppressed. Patients should be carefully monitored for an adequate response. When resolution has occurred treatment should be discontinued. Prolonged use of antibiotics will increase the risk of colonization with resistant bacteria and fungi.

Overall our experience has been that early infections after transplantation have been much more akin to our experience with conventional cardiac surgical patients than with immunosuppressed patients. Chest infection with 'conventional' organisms has been by far the commonest infective complication, followed by urinary tract infection, again with 'conventional' organisms such as *Escherichia coli*.

To date we have seen only one case of *P. carinii* infection (onset 6 weeks) after cardiac transplantation in a consecutive series of 100 patients. At the moment, therefore, we do not give routine post transplant prophylaxis with co-trimoxazole against this agent. Although co-trimoxazole will be given for the occasional patient with a toxoplasma 'mismatch' these patients have figured so rarely in our series (total number seven) that we do not believe that *P. carinii* infection is being inadvertently suppressed and therefore underdiagnosed.

Late complications (after first discharge)

In our small series of patients given globulin prophylaxis the mean time to the onset of the first referable sign or symptom of primary CMV infection was 29.6 days and the mean time to first detection of CMV-specific IgM was 52.2 days. In some patients with an uneventful course these problems may arise just after discharge. The possibility that patients susceptible to CMV infection may catch the virus by 'natural' routes should also be borne in mind, in which case the post-transplant 'incubation period' becomes irrelevant. CMV-specific IgM will persist in these patients for many months and it is important to perform regular testing in the immediate post-transplant period to document its first appearance. Failure to do this may cause diagnostic confusion in the patient many months after transplant with an unrelated febrile episode and the test is then performed for the first time.

These points apart, cardiac transplant patients require long-term surveillance for infection. With increasing time after transplantation the level of immunosuppression is usually reduced so that the risk of exotic opportunistic infection diminishes. Nonetheless continued vigilance is necessary. Although many of the intercurrent infections such as urinary tract infections can be managed on a simple basis the previous *caveats* on antibiotic usage should be recalled. If a transplant outpatient presents with a severe febrile episode and is clearly acutely ill the procedures outlined above for early infection are pursued. It is preferable that the unit which performed the transplant deals with such events, or at the very least is contacted for advice, since important information regarding the likelihood of individual infections will be most readily obtained on that basis.

The only common late-onset infection which we have seen in these patients (a total of nine episodes to date) is pneumococcal lobar pneumonia. Interestingly, two of these patients presented initially with mild fevers and purulent sputum but clear chest X-rays. In both cases a pulmonary infiltrate appeared within 2 days accompanied by rapid deterioration. They and the other seven patients who presented with obvious pneumonia from the outset, were successfully diagnosed by BAL or lung biopsy. All responded promptly to intravenous ampicillin. It may be that pneumococcal vaccination while awaiting transplantation merits consideration.

Lung and heart–lung transplantation

The management of lung and heart–lung transplant patients shares many common principles with that of cardiac transplantation, but there are a number of features pertaining to lung transplantation which require particular attention:

Donor selection

Since the consequences of primary CMV disease, especially pneumonitis, are particularly severe in lung transplantation, where possible CMV-negative recipients should be matched with CMV-negative donors. However, in centres where the waiting list is too short and the donor pool too small to accommodate this policy, organs from CMV-positive donors can be used in CMV-negative recipients if a full course of CMV hyperimmune globulin is administered (see above).

Patients, especially those who have been ventilated for some time, whose airways are known to be colonized with antibiotic-resistant Gram-negative organisms should be rejected as potential lung donors. Similarly potential donors with any history of chronic lung infection or tuberculosis would be unsuitable.

Antibiotic prophylaxis

Preoperative

Recipients should be commenced on antifungal prophylaxis when accepted for transplantation in the same way as cardiac transplants. Patients with chronic bronchial sepsis should be monitored closely, with sputum collected for bacterial and fungal culture at least weekly. Similarly, if antibiotic therapy for any intercurrent infection is indicated, this should be noted. If these guidelines are followed, when the patient comes for transplantation there will be a recent assessment of the antibiotic sensitivity of their flora available, upon which logical decisions about prophylaxis can be made. Under certain circumstances, for example patients with cystic fibrosis, continuous therapy may be indicated before transplantation. In these cases the systemic antibiotic regime should be kept to as narrow a spectrum as possible, and any broad spectrum agents administered locally. For example, orally administered flucloxacillin with nebulized colomycin will adequately cover methicillin-sensitive strains of staphylococci and all strains of *Pseudomonas* with minimal risk of inducing resistant organisms.

Perioperative

Routine administration of antibiotics to donors before retrieval is not necessary in lung transplantation, but transplantation of other organs, especially liver, requires a loading dose of antibiotics before transplantation. It is important that a full antibiotic history of the donor, including any 'prophylactic' agent used should be carefully noted in the recipient's records.

Patients without a history of chronic lung sepsis should receive prophylactic flucloxacillin in the same manner as cardiac transplant patients. In addition, since the normal commensal flora of the mouth is largely anaerobic, we recommend prophylactic metronidazole, 400 mg 12 hourly, to protect the tracheal/bronchial anastomosis. This is usually continued for 7 days.

Patients with longstanding bronchial sepsis are given additional anti-Gram-negative cover according to the result of their most recent sputum culture. Again, the agent with the narrowest spectrum is preferred. In our hands this is usually aztreonam 2 g at induction followed by 2 g 8-hourly, continued for 48 h postoperatively in the first instance.

Donor lungs should be lavaged at the time of transplantation. The fluid is examined by Gram staining, and then cultured for aerobic, anaerobic and microaerophilic bacteria and *Candida*. If large numbers of organisms are seen, consideration should be given to adding to or amending the prophylactic regime.

Postoperatively, antifungal, antiviral and toxoplasma prophylaxis should be continued as in cardiac transplants. Additionally, since the incidence of *Pneumocystis carinii* pneumonia is purported to be greater following lung transplantation, we recommend prophylactic co-trimoxazole, 960 mg b.d. to be taken 3 days per week and to be continued indefinitely. Some patients, unfortunately, cannot tolerate co-trimoxazole, and in these cases dapsone, Fansidar or nebulized pentamidine can be used as an alternative.

Postoperative care

There is no evidence to suggest that any additional precautions, over and above those outlined in the management of cardiac transplantation are necessary following lung and heart–lung transplantation. Hospitals known to have a high incidence of *Aspergillus* infections in their other immunosuppressed patients should consider the possibility of nursing their patients in cubicles supplied with filtered air, especially during augmented immunosuppression.

As in cardiac transplantation, collection of 'routine' specimens of sputum, urine etc. is not only time-consuming for nursing and laboratory staff, but unhelpful in patient management. It is, however, a useful practice to collect serum specimens from transplant patients (storage space permitting) on a regular basis. This allows easy back-reference for virus serology.

Early infective complications

Any pyrexial episode should be investigated thoroughly by following the guidelines described for cardiac transplants. C-reactive protein levels appear to remain elevated for longer following lung transplantation. This limits the usefulness as an indicator of bacterial infection, certainly in the first postoperative week.

Chest X-ray changes, pyrexia, deterioration in lung infection, alone or in combination, can indicate infection in lung transplantation. They can, however, also be the presenting features of implantation injury, adult respiratory distress syndrome and, more particularly, graft rejection.

It is of prime importance in these patients that appropriate specific treatment is commenced without delay, and it is well accepted that in these circumstances urgent bronchoalveolar lavage (BAL) with transbronchial lung biopsy (TBLB) should be performed in every case.

In order that the specimens are processed with minimal delay the laboratory should be forewarned that a diagnostic BAL is planned, and the case discussed with a microbiologist. Where possible, at least 30 ml of lavage fluid should be obtained for microbiological examination, and a full screen should include each of the following:

1. Gram staining and culture for bacterial pathogens including *Legionella* sp., *Mycoplasma*, *Nocardia* and *Mycobacterium* spp.
2. Direct microscopy and culture for fungi.
3. Microscopy for *Pneumocystis carinii*, either by conventional silver staining techniques (Grocott's stain) or by fluoroscein-labelled monoclonal antibody.
4. Direct examination and culture for respiratory viruses.
5. Direct examination and culture for CMV, including direct early antigen fluorescent focus (DEAFF) test where practicable.

Results obtained from BAL should be interpreted in the light of the patient's clinical condition and with the histological report of the transbronchial biopsy. The temptation to treat colonizing or commensal organisms with broad spectrum antibiotics in the absence of clinical evidence of infection should be resisted. It may result in superinfection with resistant organisms or yeasts and may mask the presence of an underlying transplantation. This is particularly important in cystic fibrosis patients, who often remain colonized with Gram-negative organisms post-transplantation, presumably as a result of extensive colonization of the nasal sinuses. In our experience, if the use of broad spectrum antibiotics can be avoided or minimized, the flora of these latter patients will become more sensitive, and, eventually, we hope return to normal. The only situation where it may be appropriate to treat a colonizing organism is when a potential pathogen, particularly *Aspergillus* sp. or *Candida* is isolated in large numbers from a patient about to undergo augmented immunosuppression for a rejection episode. In these cases we usually cover the period of such therapy with one of the new oral, less toxic antifungal agents.

As mentioned previously, primary CMV pneumonitis is a potentially lethal, but often preventable, complication of lung transplantation. Careful matching of donors and the use of CMV-negative blood products will minimize the risk of donor-transmitted disease. If a CMV mismatch is unavoidable, a course of prophylactic hyperimmune globulin should be given. Although our experience of CMV 'mismatches' in lung transplantation is small, to date we have successfully managed two such patients with minimal morbidity. As in the cardiac transplant patients, seroconversion, usually at 6–8 weeks post-transplantation, is accompanied by a transient fever and malaise, and it is usually possible to isolate the virus from urine and bronchial secretions.

CMV pneumonitis can also occur in seropositive recipients receiving organs from seropositive donors. This so-called 'second primary' infection is probably due to different serotype of CMV. Diagnosis can be difficult if based on BAL results alone, since any seropositive individual, if immunosuppressed, may excrete large numbers of virus particles from the kidney and lungs with little, if any, clinical symptoms of infection. The appearance in the serum of CMV specific IgM, together with the classical appearances of CMV pneumonitis on TBLB will confirm the diagnosis. The decision to commence antiviral therapy in such cases should be based on each individual patient's clinical condition with the results of all relevant investigations to hand.

The role of CMV pneumonitis in the subsequent development of chronic rejection, fibrosis and obliterative bronchiolitis is still unclear, but experience in other centres suggests that it is equally associated with both primary and 'second primary' CMV disease.

Late infective complications

Late complications of lung transplantation should be investigated and managed in a similar manner to cardiac transplants, with particular emphasis on the early, invasive investigation of any pulmonary infiltrate.

Transplantation in children

The general principles of management are similar in both adults and children, but there are a small number of additional considerations which should not be overlooked.

Preoperative assessment

The screening procedures suggested for adults should be followed, but it must be remembered that any IgG antibodies detected in babies up to the age of one year could be maternal. Consequently, unless the positive IgG test is backed up by the presence of IgM, the child should be regarded as seronegative.

Details of previous immunization should be documented, and, where possible, courses completed before transplantation. Parents should be asked about any history of childhood infectious diseases and, if there is no clinical history of chickenpox, serum should be tested for *Varicella zoster* antibodies. If this proves negative, vaccination should be considered, time permitting.

Perioperative management

Babies and children should be nursed under the same conditions as adult patients and there should be no additional barrier nursing requirements. Prophylactic antibiotic protocols should be the same as in adults, with the appropriate dosages calculated according to the child's weight.

Postoperative complications

Again, the guidelines for the investigation of febrile episodes in adults should be followed, with special reference to viral infections. Diarrhoea can be a particular problem in young babies. It is often associated with the presence of rotavirus in the faeces. This form of diarrhoea can be protracted, but often resolves when lactose-free feeds are introduced.

Later febrile illnesses can often be attributable to upper respiratory viral infections, e.g. adenovirus and parainfluenza. These episodes are usually self-limiting and chemotherapy is usually only indicated when there is a proven bacterial superinfection. Antiviral therapy may be appropriate in serious respiratory syncitial virus (RSV) or influenza in children under the age of 2 years. Since the complications of *Varicella zoster* virus infection in immunosuppressed patients can be life-threatening, any seronegative patient who has been in contact with shingles or chickenpox should be immediately commenced on a prophylactic course of acyclovir.

The use of LIVE vaccines is contraindicated in immunosuppressed patients. Killed vaccines can, and should, be used to complete a course of immunization.

Conclusions

We conclude this brief account with two observations. First, we have found our involvement in the cardiothoracic transplantation service to be challenging, interesting and rewarding. We recommend the experience to our microbiological colleagues.

Second, we wish to record or appreciation of the co-operation and enthusiasm of our surgical, medical, nursing and other colleagues in this team approach. A particular word of thanks goes to our own laboratory staff who have all responded magnificently to every challenge.

Addendum

Although the basic outline and planning of the protocols of microbiological care set out in this chapter in relation to cardiac and pulmonary transplantation remain valid, the rapid progression of transplantation in general and of cardiothoracic transplantation in particular in recent years leads us to caution the reader to supplement this outline account with specific details from recent journal publications.

RF
FKG

15

Blood conservation following cardiovascular surgery

Altagracia M. Chavez and Delos M. Cosgrove III

The development of cardiopulmonary bypass technology permitted the evolution of operative approaches to a wide range of cardiac pathology. As the volume of cardiac operations increased, a tremendous demand was placed on blood banks to ensure an adequate supply of safe homologous blood. Advances in blood banking technology have not, however, achieved a risk-free product. In the past few years, the possible transmission of infectious agents with blood transfusion has been a focus of increased attention from both patients and physicians. This attention has centred particularly on the viruses responsible for the autoimmune deficiency syndrome and hepatitis. Concern about transfusion associated risks, together with the escalating costs of banked blood products and limitations in the availability of donor blood, has inspired a renewed interest in blood substitutes and measures to conserve blood.

In cardiac surgery, efforts to minimize use of banked blood involve preoperative, intraoperative, and postoperative measures to conserve and recycle the patient's own blood.

Preoperatively, patients are screened for pertinent history including anaemia, coagulation abnormalities, and use of medications which interfere with normal coagulation pathways. Under optimal conditions, predeposit of autologous blood is a useful option.

Commonly used intraoperative blood conservation techniques include utilization of crystalloid oxygenator prime, acceptance of normovolaemic anaemia, transfusion of all oxygenator contents, and salvage of shed blood.

Postoperatively, the use of non-blood volume expanders and acceptance of normovolaemic anaemia are both recognized as safe measures that help minimize the use of homologous blood products. Autotransfusion of shed mediastinal and/or pleural blood is also an important adjunct in the care of cardiac surgical patients.

Historical background

In 1883 Halstead reported the first therapeutic autotransfusion used to treat a case of carbon monoxide poisoning. Intraoperative blood salvage and autotransfusion were first reported by Duncan in 1886 when he reinfused blood during an amputation. Thies, in 1914, reported reinfusion of salvaged blood in three patients each with ectopic pregnancy. Lockwood (1917) was the first in the United States to advocate autotransfusion. In Germany, Elmendorf (1917) reported reinfusion of blood collected from a haemothorax. Such blood did not clot and so required no anticoagulation. In the subsequent decades, more experience with autotransfusion was reported (Coley, 1928; May, 1930; Brown and Debenham, 1931; Rumbaugh, 1931; Davis and Cushing, 1925). However, as improvements in blood banking in the 1940s and 1950s made homologous blood safer and simpler to use, interest in autotransfusion waned.

In the 1960s reports of intraoperative blood salvage reappeared and Dyer (1966) and Klebanoff (1970) developed an autotransfusion device for intraoperative use which consisted of a cardiotomy reservoir and a roller pump. After initial good results, Bentley Laboratories made the device available commercially. Despite early enthusiasm, cases of air embolization with this device were reported in 1974 by Duncan, Klebanoff and Rogers, and interest diminished.

New methodology developed in the 1970s rekindled interest in autotransfusion systems. In 1976

Noon published the first reported clinical use of the Sorenson Autotransfusion System. Methods were also developed for collecting, washing and reinfusing shed blood during operations (Wilson and Taswell, 1968; Gilcher and Orr, 1975; Watson-Williams *et al.*, 1975). In 1977 Hauer described use of a modified Sorenson system for postoperative cardiac surgery patients. Further developments followed and in 1980 Weniger *et al.* described a system for autotransfusion after cardiac surgery which utilized the cardiotomy reservoir used during cardiopulmonary bypass. The system was modified by Cosgrove (1985) to overcome the problem of a clotted filter impeding chest tube drainage.

All of these developments evolved because of interest in methods to salvage and reinfuse shed blood. An important underlying assumption was that such blood would be safe to use.

Characteristics of shed blood

Blood collected from pleural and mediastinal surfaces shows alterations in the quantity and quality of both formed elements and coagulation factors. Cardiopulmonary bypass, *per se*, also causes changes in factors responsible for normal haemostasis by exposing blood to a non-endothelial surface (Table 15.1). After bypass, mild to moderate elevations in prothrombin time (PT), partial thromboplastin time (PTT) and thrombin time (TT) are commonly seen while platelet counts and platelet function are usually depressed. A reduction in the number of normally functioning platelets is not an infrequent cause of postoperative bleeding in cardiac surgery patients. This factor has led to interest in drugs, such as desmopressin acetate, that would enhance platelet function and thereby reduce blood loss after cardiopulmonary bypass (Salzman *et al.*, 1986).

Table 15.1 Haematologic values in control group before and after cardiopulmonary bypass (From Thurer *et al.*, 1979)

	Preoperative	*Immediate postoperative*
Haematocrit (%)	43.9	30.9
Platelets ($\times 10^3$ mm^{-3})	252	152
PT (s)	12.5	15.8
PTT (s)	26.9	33.0
TT (s)	10.4	12.2
Free plasma haemoglobin (mg 100 ml)	18.4	52.4

Various authors have examined the changes in blood aspirated from the mediastinum. Table 15.2 shows some of these data summarized and compared with banked whole blood. Shed blood consistently showed lower values for haematocrit and fibrinogen content but higher platelet counts. Blood collected from the mediastinum had a higher free haemoglobin content than banked whole blood. The question was whether or not these alterations had clinical significance. Before autotransfusion of blood from pleural or mediastinal cavities could be widely accepted, safety had to be demonstrated.

Table 15.2 Characteristics of shed mediastinal blood

	Stored whole blood	*Mediastinal blood*			
		Adan et al. (1988)	*Hartz et al. (1988)*	*Bennett (1982)*	*Thurer et al. (1979)*
Haematocrit (%)	38	21	25.0	18.0	19.9
Platelets ($\times 10^3$ mm^{-3})	0	132	60.0	15.0	67.8
Free plasma haemoglobin (mg 100 ml^{-1})	14	224	—	72.6	315
Fibrinogen	155	<100	19	0	—

Blood collected from the pleural cavity does not clot. This is due to defibrination of the blood both by contact with the functioning heart and lungs and by biochemical alterations brought about through contact with serosa lined surfaces (Broadie *et al.*, 1981). Some authors have presented evidence consistent with the idea that there is clot formation and subsequent fibrinolysis before the blood drains from the chest cavity (Broadie *et al.*, 1981; Adan *et al.*, 1988; Hartz, Smith and Green, 1988). Schaff, Haver and Brawley (1978) demonstrated that reinfusion of blood collected after cardiac surgery does not adversely affect clinical haemostasis. These authors found that fibrinogen rose within 4 h and returned to control levels within 24 h after surgery in patients who were autotransfused. Some authors have shown normal levels of factors VIII and IX in mediastinal blood (Bell, 1981). Hartz, Smith and Green (1988) found markedly decreased factor VIII levels in shed blood, but demonstrated no adverse effects on clinical coagulation due to the reinfusion of blood salvaged postoperatively.

Although salvaged blood has a higher platelet count than banked blood, the salvaged platelets have abnormal aggregation responses *in vitro* and probably contribute little to haemostasis (Carter, McArdle, Morrit, 1981; Bennett, 1982). There is no evidence, however, that patients bleed more after reinfusion of shed blood.

Glover *et al.* (1976) addressed the possibility of renal failure from the increased free haemoglobin levels seen in shed mediastinal blood. While patients who are autotransfused may have elevations of plasma haemoglobin and haemoglobinuria, haemoglobinaemia is sometimes seen after otherwise uncomplicated cardiopulmonary bypass. Thurer and his colleagues (1979) showed that the free haemoglobin levels in both the control group and the autotransfused group returned to normal by the first postoperative day. The additional haemoglobin from autotransfusion is probably without clinical significance. In experimental work using infusions of stroma-free haemoglobin, there were no detrimental effects on renal function in animals which were not acidotic and in whom an adequate output of alkaline urine was maintained (Relihan, Olsen, Litwin, 1972).

Devices

Cell washing systems

Blood lost before systemic heparinization or after administration of protamine can be retrieved via a system which adds an anticoagulant. The resulting mixture can then be rid of contaminants by a device which washes, filters, and packs the remaining red cells. The final product can be administered to the patient using standard blood administration sets.

The Haemonetics Cell Saver is a free-standing unit which can be used in the operating room. Newer models are easier to use and fully automated. Multiple washing cycles can be run during the course of an operation but the unit is available for only one patient at a time.

An alternative system is the Cobe Blood Cell Processor. For this device also, blood is collected from the operative field in a manner that adds an anticoagulant. The collection bag is carefully labelled with the patient's name, removed from the operating room, and taken to a central location for processing. The Blood Cell Processor washes, filters, and packs the retrieved erythrocytes. Unlike the Haemonetics Cells Saver, this system is available for more than one patient at a time. Both these devices are useful for the intraoperative salvage of blood shed while the patient is not systemically heparinized. Each, however, suffers from limitations imposed by high costs and the need for a certain amount of technical intervention for the processing steps.

Sorenson autotransfusion system

The Sorenson system was originally designed for intraoperative blood collection (Noon, Solis, Natelson, 1976; Noon, 1978). The device consisted of a rigid reusable canister containing two disposable plastic bags connected in series. A special connector allowed suction to be applied to both canister and bag. Blood was filtered on entry into the collection bag while the lower bag served as a reservoir. A modification allowed one large bag of approximately 1800 ml to be used in place of the double bag.

In intraoperative use, blood collected from the field is anticoagulated with a specially designed suction wand. In postoperative applications, the unit can be attached directly to chest tubes to collect shed mediastinal or pleural blood. With either configuration, when a sufficient volume of blood is collected, the plastic bag can be removed from the canister and replaced. Blood which contains particulate matter can be washed in one of the cell-washing devices. Alternatively, the filled lower reservoir bag can be detached from the filter bag and administered directly to the patient via a filtered blood administration set.

Schaff and his colleagues (1979) demonstrated a 50% reduction in homologous blood utilization when this system was applied to cardiac surgical patients. Thurer *et al.* (1979), in a similar patient population, showed no adverse haematologic, pulmonary, renal, hepatic, or systemic sequelae associated with use of this system.

The basic Sorenson concept has been adapted by most manufacturers of chest tube drainage systems. A wide variety of collection devices with autotransfusion capability is currently available.

Cardiotomy system

In 1980 Weniger and associates described conversion of the cardiotomy reservoir for use in a postoperative autotransfusion system. At the completion of cardiopulmonary bypass the cardiotomy was converted into a receptacle for mediastinal and pleural drainage by removing bypass tubings from the inlet ports and sealing these ports until chest tubes were attached at the completion of the operation. The cardiotomy outlet port was capped with a connector which transformed the 9.5 mm port to standard intravenous tubing. Blood drained through the chest tubes and into the cardiotomy reservoir via a 20 μm filter. Negative suction could be applied to the reservoir. A standard infusion pump was used to return collected filtered blood to the patient. Each hour's collection could be measured and that amount delivered over the subsequent hour. This closed system could be used for as long as substantial drainage continued or a maximum of 12 h. After that period, the cardiotomy could function as a chest bottle until the tubes were removed.

If the cardiotomy filter became obstructed with clot, the chest tubes could not drain satisfactorily. For this reason, Cosgrove described a modification of the system which introduced a shunt between the non-filtered rapid prime port and the filtered portion of the cardiotomy (Cosgrove, Amiot, Meserko, 1985). By this means, constant negative pressure could be maintained on the chest tubes

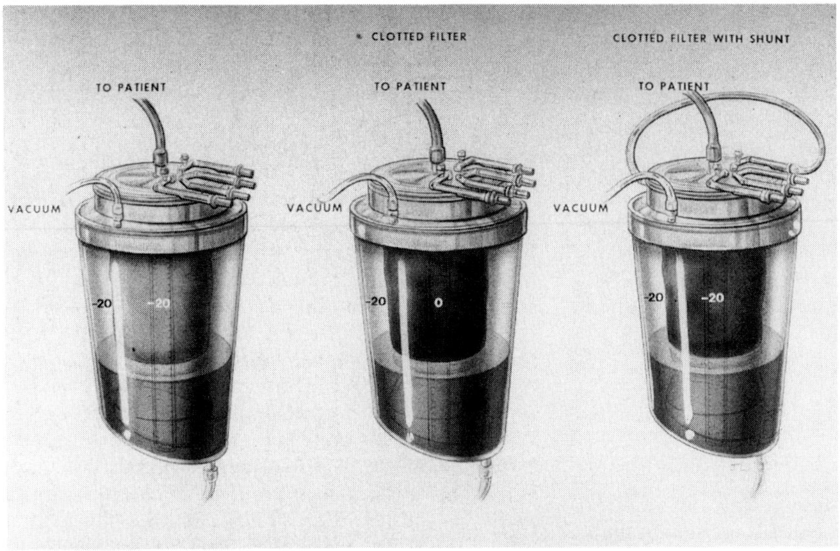

Figure 15.1 Modified cardiotomy system

even if the filter was no longer functional (Figure 15.1).

There are several advantages of the cardiotomy system. First, the risk of contamination is decreased by maintenance of a closed system. Second, the integral 20 μm filter provides improved filtration and precludes the need for additional filters. Third, greater haemodynamic stability is achieved by continuous reinfusion of shed blood. Fourth, the system is cost effective since the cost of the reservoir is already included in the set-up of the cardiopulmonary circuit. Fifth, the device is readily accepted by nursing personnel because it is easy to use and requires minimal additional labour. Finally, the continuous closed nature of the system makes it applicable for use in patients who are Jehovah's Witnesses.

Other postoperative considerations

After cardiac surgery patients are monitored for cardiorespiratory stability and for excessive bleeding. Efforts to minimize the use of banked blood during this period include acceptance of normovolaemic anaemia, use of non-blood volume expanders, control of hypertension, as well as salvage and reinfusion of shed mediastinal blood.

Intravascular volume deficits are common in patients after cardiopulmonary bypass. These patients usually tolerate normovolaemic anaemia without detrimental effect. Haemoglobin levels as low as 7–8 g 100 ml^{-1} pose no additional risk to wound healing or early hospital discharge. The use of banked red cells can be individualized and used to achieve specific clinical goals rather than to achieve an arbitrary haematocrit level. In the absence of very severe anaemia or active bleeding, red cells should not be the first choice for treating intravascular volume deficits. Likewise, the use of fresh frozen plasma for volume repletion alone is to be condemned. For postoperative volume expansion, salt poor albumin or hetastarch solutions are useful options which do not carry the same risks as banked blood, are less expensive than banked blood, and are retained in the vascular compartment better than crystalloid solutions.

Control of hypertension is another important consideration in the postoperative patient. Transient hypertension is common in this setting and potentially detrimental both because it increases myocardial work and because it can cause increased bleeding from, or disruption of, cardiac suture lines. Sodium nitroprusside is the most frequently used drug in the treatment of postoperative hypertension. The onset and duration of action for sodium nitroprusside are both short and the drug can be titrated for optimal blood pressure control. An automated system for nitroprusside delivery was recently made available by IVAC, Corp.: The Titrator Model 10K. The system consists of a sensor which monitors the patient's arterial blood pressure every 0.01 s and a microprocessor which calculates a nitroprusside infusion rate. This rate is derived from a user selected target blood pressure, the current blood pressure, and algorithms that determine the patient's nitroprusside sensitivity. The infusion rate is updated every 10 s and transmitted to a standard infusion pump. In clinical trials this closed loop system was superior to manual titration of nitroprusside. For patients in the titrator group, blood pressure in the desired range was more frequently and more quickly attained, nursing time for interventions related to blood pressure control was reduced, and there was less bleeding from chest tubes. This system is potentially a very useful tool in the postoperative management of the cardiac surgical patient.

Conclusion

Use of banked blood products in cardiac surgery can best be minimized by an integrated programme which begins with preoperative patient screening and is carried through into the postoperative period. Certainly, salvage and reinfusion of shed blood, both intra- and postoperatively, are important components of any such scheme. Multiple studies exist documenting a reduction in banked blood usage among patients autotransfused after cardiac operations (Schaff *et al.*, 1979; Cordell, Lavender, 1981; Johnson *et al.*, 1983; Breyer *et al.*, 1987; Giordano *et al.*, 1988). Such reduction in the use of banked blood decreases risks for patients.

The issue of whether costs are also reduced may be harder to assess. While blood bank costs are saved, the additional expenses for equipment and supplies involved in typical salvage programmes must be taken into account. Breyer and his associates (1987) found that the costs associated with use of intra- and postoperative blood salvage devices were offset by the savings from the reduction in use of homologous blood. This group used the Haemonetics Cell Saver intraoperatively and the Sorenson system postoperatively. It is possible further to reduce costs associated with autotransfusion by judicious choice of equipment. For example, conversion of the cardiotomy reservoir for autotransfusion costs about $35 and eliminates the added expense of a separate chest drainage system for use in the period after operation. A more important consideration is that the expense associated with morbidity and mortality related to complications of homologous transfusion cannot be estimated. Such risks are best decreased by efforts which result in a minimal utilization of banked blood products.

Today, the cardiac surgical community is under increasing pressure to provide safer operations at lower costs. Integrated programmes which result in decreased use of banked blood are important means to help accomplish both these goals. Techniques for salvage and recycling of autologous blood are important components of such programmes in the cardiac surgical patient.

References

Adan, A.J., Brutel de la Riviere, A., Haas, F., van Zalk, A. and de Nooij, E. (1988) Autotransfusion of drained mediastinal blood after cardiac surgery: a reappraisal. *Journal of Thoracic and Cardiovascular Surgery*, **36**, 10–14

Bell, W.R. (1981) Hematologic aspects of autotransfusion. In *Autotransfusion* (ed J.M. Hauer *et al.*) Elsevier/North-Holland, New York, pp. 1–9

Bennett, J.G. (1982) Autotransfusion of drained mediastinal blood. *Thoracic and Cardiovascular Surgeon*, **30**, 28–30

Breyer, R.H., Engleman, R.M., Rousou, J.A. and Lemeshow, S. (1987) Blood conservation for myocardial revascularization–is it cost effective? *Journal of Thoracic and Cardiovascular Surgery*, **93**, 512–522

Broadie, T.A., Glover, J.L., Bang, N., *et al.* (1981) Clotting competence of intracavitary blood in trauma victims. *Annals of Emergency Medicine*, **10**, 127–130

Brown, A.L., Debenham, M.W. (1931) Autotransfusion: use of blood from hemothorax. *Journal of the American Medical Association*, **96**, 1223–1225

Carter, R.F., McArdle, B. and Morritt, G.M. (1981) Autologous transfusion of mediastinal drainage blood: a report of its use following open-heart surgery. *Anesthesia*, **36**, 54–59

Coley, B.L. (1928) Traumatic rupture of spleen, splenectomy: autotransfusion. *American Journal of Surgery*, **4**, 334–335

Cordell, A.R. and Lavender, S.W. (1981) An appraisal of blood salvage techniques in vascular and cardiac operations. *Annals of Thoracic Surgery*, **31**, 421–425

Cosgrove, D.M., Amiot, D.M. and Meserko, J.J. (1985) An improved technique for autotransfusion of shed mediastinal blood. *Annals of Thoracic Surgery*, **40**, 519–520

Davis, L.E. and Cushing, H. (1925) Experiences with blood replacement during or after major intracranial operations. *Surgery, Gynecology and Obstetrics*, **40**, 310–322

Duncan, J. (1886) On reinfusion of blood in primary and other amputations. *British Medical Journal*, **1**, 192–193

Duncan, S.E., Klebanoff, G. and Rogers, W. (1974) Patient experience with intraoperative autotransfusion. *Review of Surgery*, **31**, 121–124

Dyer, R.H. (1966) Intraoperative autotransfusion: A preliminary report and new method. *American Journal of Surgery*, **112**, 874–878

Elmendorf, A. (1917) Ueber Widerinfusion mach punkiton elnes firschen hamathorax. *Muchener Medizinische Wochenschrift*, **64**, 36

Gilcher, R.D. and Orr, M.D. (1975) Intraoperative autotransfusion. *Transfusion*, **15**, 520 (abstract)

Giordano, G.F., Goldman, D.S., Mammana, R.B., *et al.* (1988) Intraoperative autotransfusion in cardiac operations–effect on intraoperative and postoperative transfusion requirements. *Journal of Thoracic and Cardiovascular Surgery*, **96**, 382–386

Glover, J.L., Smith, R., Yaw, P., *et al.* (1976) Intraoperative autotransfusion: an underutilized technique. *Surgery*, **80**, 474–479

Halstead, W.S. (1883) Refusion of carbonic oxide poisoning. *New York Medical Journal*, 625

Hartz, R.S., Smith, J.A., Green, D. (1988) Autotransfusion after cardiac operation. Assessment of hemostatic factors. *Journal of Thoracic and Cardiovascular Surgery*, **96**, 178–182

Hauer, J.M., Schaff, H.V., Bell, W.R., *et al.* (1977) Reinfusion of shed mediastinal blood following cardiac surgery: a prospective study. *Circulation*, **56**, (Suppl. III) 250 (abstract)

Johnson, R.G., Rosenkrantz, K.R., Preston, R.A., *et al.* (1983) The efficacy of postoperative autotransfusion in patients undergoing cardiac operations. *Annals of Thoracic Surgery*, **36**, 173–179

Klebanoff, G. (1970) Early clinical experience with a disposable unit for the intraoperative salvage and reinfusion of blood loss (intraoperative autotransfusion). *American Journal of Surgery*, **120**, 718

Lockwood, C.D. (1917) Surgical treatment of Banti's disease. Report of 3 cases. *Surgery, Gynecology and Obstetrics*, **25**, 188–191

May, G.E. (1930) Auto blood transfusion. *New England Journal of Medicine*, **203**, 1197–1198

Noon, G.P. (1978) Intraoperative autotransfusion. *Surgery*, **84**, 719–721

Noon, G.P., Solis, R.T. and Natelson, E.A. (1976) A simple method of intraoperative autotransfusion. *Surgery, Gynecology and Obstetrics*, **143**, 65–70

Rumbaugh, M.C. (1931) Ruptured tubal pregnancy: report of a case in which life was saved by autotransfusion of blood. *Pennsylvania Medical Journal*, **34**, 710–711

Relihan, M., Olsen, R., Litwin, M.S. (1972) Clearance rate and effect on renal function of stroma-free hemoglobin following renal ischemia. *Annals of Surgery*, **176**, 700–704

Salzman, E.W., Weinstein, M.J., Weintraub, R.M., *et al.* (1986) Treatment with desmopressin acetate to reduce blood loss after cardiac surgery: a double-blind randomized trial. *New England Journal of Medicine*, **314**, 1402–1406

Schaff, H.V., Hauer, J.M. and Brawley, R.K. (1978) Autotransfusion in cardiac surgical patients after operation. *Surgery*, **84**, 713–719

Schaff, H.V., Hauer, J., Gardner, T.J., *et al.* (1979) Routine use of autotransfusion: experience in 700 patients. *Annals of Thoracic Surgery*, **27**, 493–499

Thies, H.J. (1914) Bur Behandlung der extrauteringraviditat. *Zentralblattl Fuer Gynaekologie*, **38**, 1191

Thurer, R.L., Lytle, B.W., Cosgrove, D.M. and Loop, F.D. (1979) Autotransfusion following cardiac surgery: a randomized, prospective study. *Annals of Thoracic Surgery*, **27**, 500–506

Watson-Williams, E.J., Kelly, P.B., Smeloff, E.A., *et al.* (1975) A simple program to conserve isologous blood used for open-heart surgery. *Transfusion*, **15**, 520 (abstract)

Weniger, J., von der Emde, J., Schricker, K.T. and Blechschmidt, J. (1980) Retransfusion von drainageblut nach herzchirugischen eingriffen. *Langenbecks Archiv fur Chirurgie*, **351**, 229–241

Wilson, J.D. and Taswell, H.F. (1968) Autotransfusion: Historical review and preliminary report of a new method. *Mayo Clinic Proceedings*, **43**, 26–35

16

Pulsatile flow during cardiopulmonary bypass

David Bregman, Michael Kesselbrenner and Jeffrey B. Sack

And now I see with eye serene
The very pulse of the machine;
A being breathing thoughtful breath,
A traveller between life and death

William Wordsworth

Since the second rewriting of this chapter in 1981, much has been said about the role of pulsatile perfusion during cardiopulmonary bypass. However, there remains much controversy over the advantages and disadvantages of pulsatile perfusion to that of non-pulsatile perfusion. Recent technical advances and an improved understanding of the physiology of pulsatile flow have led to a greater appreciation of its importance. No longer is non-pulsatile perfusion the standard means of extracorporeal circulatory support.

The purpose of this chapter is to review the development of pulsatile perfusion, its physiology, technology and the role of new circulatory assist devices. The results of our own clinical experience with the pulsatile assist device at the Columbia Presbyterian Medical Center will be presented.

Evolution of pulsatile perfusion

The earliest systems for the artificial perfusion of organs were designed by physiologists for use in research laboratories. They attempted to reproduce normal circulatory physiology as closely as possible. The importance of fluctuations in perfusion pressure was first realized as long ago as 1868 by Ludwig and Schmidt, using a syringe injection technique. In 1888 Hamel described a perfusion apparatus which delivered intermittent flow by means of a pendulum.

Carl Jacobj may properly be described as the 'father' of pulsatile perfusion in extracorporeal circulation. In 1890 he reported the use of a perfusion apparatus which delivered pulsatile flow by means of intermittent compression of a rubber balloon in the arterial end of the circuit.

In 1910 Hooker compared the effects of pulsatile and non-pulsatile perfusion on the isolated kidney. The pump that he used was capable of producing pulsatile flow by means of a cam, and the amplitude of the pulse pressure could be varied. He found that reducing the amplitude of the pulse pressure during perfusion of the isolated kidney lowered both the blood flow and urinary output. Although Gesell (1913) was unable to confirm Hooker's observations concerning renal blood flow *in vivo*, he reported that lowering the pulse pressure caused a decrease in urinary output and in chloride excretion.

The pump oxygenators which were used during the early days of extracorporeal circulation were capable of producing pulsatile flow, but, because of the problems with excessive haemolysis, this feature was not routinely employed. The use of non-pulsatile flow for perfusion of short duration did not appear to be deleterious and the problem of haemolysis was much less obvious.

In 1955 Wesolowski, Sauvage and Pine reported a series of experiments in which they compared the effects of pulsatile and non-pulsatile perfusion and they wrote that '...the entire systemic circulation appears to be maintained equally well by the use of pulsatile and non-pulsatile flows for periods up to six hours'. Pulsatile perfusion reached its nadir, and non-pulsatile perfusion had become the standard technique of extracorporeal circulation used during cardiopulmonary bypass in most cardiac surgical centres.

Since 1955 significant improvements have been made in the design of pumps for extracorporeal circulation. In 1961 Clauss *et al.* introduced the concept of counterpulsation, but the early arterio-arterial counterpulsators were cumbersome and haemolysis was a major problem. In 1962 Moulopoulos, Topaz and Kolff developed the concept of an intra-aortic balloon which could act as an arterial counterpulsator without the need for withdrawal and reinfusion of blood. This resulted in minimal haemolysis.

However, it was not until 1968 that Kantrowitz *et al.* reported the first successful clinical use of intra-aortic balloon pumping. The development of tough, flexible plastics that are biologically inert, combined with the rapid advances made in cardiology and cardiac surgery, ultimately led to the widespread and enthusiastic acceptance of intra-aortic balloon pumping.

In 1972 Berger and Saini reported the clinical use of an intra-aortic balloon to create pulsatile cardiopulmonary bypass, and others soon reported similar experiences (Pappas *et al.*, 1975). The potential morbidity from the use of the intra-aortic balloon, however, obviated its routine use of the creation of pulsatile perfusion (Alpert *et al.*, 1976; Biddle, Stewart and Stuard, 1976; Beckman *et al.*, 1977; Lefemine *et al.*, 1977; Pace *et al.*, 1977; McCabe *et al.*, 1978; Tyras and Williams, 1978).

In 1975 a pulsatile assist device (PAD^R) was introduced by Bregman *et al.* It applied the balloon concept externally in the cardiopulmonary bypass circuit. The device made it possible to use pulsatile perfusion routinely during cardiopulmonary bypass without the problems of haemolysis or the complications associated with the insertion of an intra-aortic balloon.

Pump technology and pulsatile flow

The pumps used for perfusion during cardiopulmonary bypass may be divided into two broad groups:

1. *The positive displacement pumps*
   (a) Rotary pumps, in which a bolus of blood is trapped in a segment of tubing by rotating members and 'milked' towards the output. The *roller pump*, which is the most widely used of any of the pumps for routine extracorporeal circulation, is an example of this type.
   (b) Reciprocating pumps, in which blood is allowed to collect in a valved cavity, from which it is ejected by the reciprocating action of a piston, diaphragm or similar device. This group includes the 'ventricle' pumps.
2. *The kinetic pumps*
   In these the velocity of the blood at the inlet is increased by the forced rotation of an impeller and then decreased at the outlet by a diffuser. The result is an increase in the kinetic energy (pressure head) of the blood at the outlet of the pump. The principal advantage of this concept is that the output is directly related to the input pressure and is inversely related to the pressure head against which it works. Because the amount of kinetic energy imparted to the blood is directly proportional to the revolutions per minute (r.p.m.) of the impeller, a given perfusion pressure can be maintained over a wide range of flow rates. Thus, the greater the inflow, the greater the output, and, similarly, the greater the resistance to flow, the smaller the output. The centrifugal force-vortex pump is an example of this type. Improvements in the design of such 'load sensitive' pumps have led to a reduction in haemolysis, which had been a problem in earlier models, and they are now considered the most suitable for use in artificial hearts (Kolff and Lawson, 1975).

Pulsatile flow may be defined as flow which is subject to periodic variations in velocity.

This, roller pumps actually deliver pulsatile flow but the pulses are of low amplitude and high frequency, depending upon the degree of occlusion, the number of rollers on the pump head and the number of revolutions per minute. The pulsatile flow produced by standard roller pumps has aptly been described as 'ripple flow' as the pulses are rapidly eliminated by damping within the arterial tree.

The reciprocating pumps produce pulse waves analogous to those of the normal circulation.

Only the kinetic pumps produce truly non-pulsatile flow.

In the present discussion however, the flow produced by roller pumps will be considered non-pulsatile, and the terms 'non-pulsatile' and 'continuous' will be used synonymously.

In addition to the combination of intra-aortic balloon pumping with otherwise non-pulsatile cardiopulmonary bypass circuits, three systems for pulsatile perfusion are available at present:

1. The pulsatile assist device (PAD^R)*
This is installed in the arterial line of the bypass circuit, and may be used with any of the pumps commonly used for extracorporeal circulation, including the centrifugal force-vortex type (Figures 16.1, 16.2 and 16.3). It consists of a valveless, flexible inner blood conduit surrounded by a rigid plastic shell. Air is pumped in and out of the chamber between conduit and housing, resulting in compression and expansion

*Datascope Corporation, Paramus, New Jersey, USA

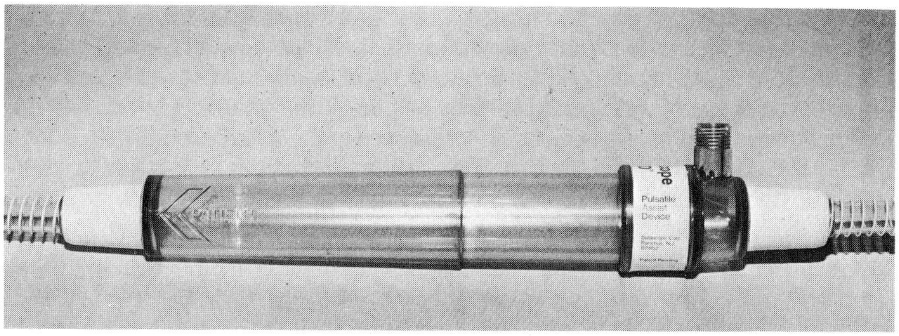

Figure 16.1 The pulsatile assist device (PAD[R]). Maximum displacement of the balloon conduit is 80 ml

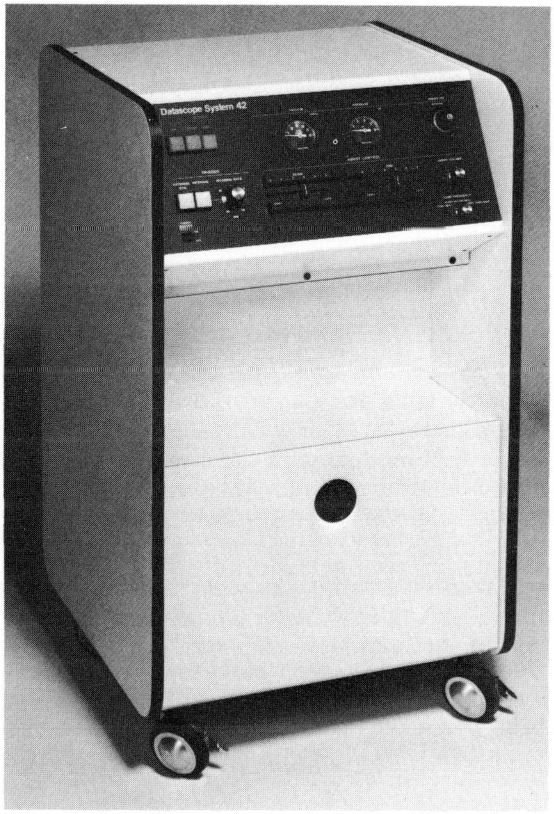

Figure 16.2 The System 42 console. This console was especially designed to create pulsatile cardiopulmonary bypass using any of the standard pumps in conjunction with the pulsatile assist device. However, the PAD can also be used with the standard intra-aortic balloon pumping console (system 80 or 82)

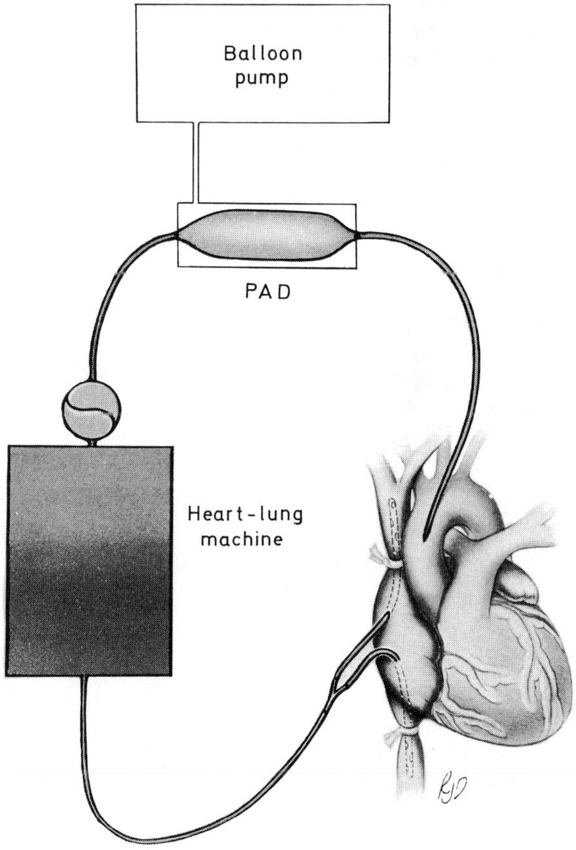

Figure 16.3 Schematic view of the pulsatile assist device in the cardiopulmonary bypass circuit. The PAD may also be used to produce either synchronous counter-pulsation through the arterial cannula or pulsatile cardiopulmonary bypass

of the balloon conduit. Synchronization with the R wave of the ECG is achieved by the electronic logic in the pumping console. During induced cardiac arrest or ventricular fibrillation the rate of pulsation may be controlled by using an internal trigger from the console.

Other devices based upon the same concept have also been developed (Tamari *et al.*, 1976).

2. *The 'bubble tube' system*
This incorporates an especially dilated segment of tubing used in conjunction with a roller pump (Eguchi and Asano, 1968). As the roller passes over the 'bubble' the stroke volume of the pump is increased. In this way pulsatile flow is created, but the frequency is dependent upon the number of rollers and the RPM of the pump head. The pulse pressure is fixed by the dimensions of the bubble used.
Both the PAD and the 'bubble tube' are versions of the 'ventricle' pump, the difference being that no valves are used.
3. *The 'stepping' motor pump* (Hoffman *et al.*, 1970)
This is a modification of the standard roller pump with a motor capable of producing rapid acceleration and deceleration of the rollers. The system may be triggered either from the ECG or internally. The amplitude, frequency and duration of the pulse wave can be varied from the control console. A similar modification of the motor of the centrifugal force-vortex pump is also available.

Haemodynamic aspects of pulsatile flow

There have been many attempts to derive an equation to describe blood flow based on Poiseuille's Equation:

$$Q = \frac{dp \times \pi \times r^4}{8 \times \eta \times 1}$$

where Q = volume flow rate; dp = pressure drop along the tube; r = radius of the tube; η = coefficient of viscosity of the liquid; and l = length of the tube.

However, the equation does not apply to the circulation of the blood for several reasons:

1. Blood is not a Newtonian fluid*
2. The radius of the blood vessels is not constant throughout their length, and the cross-sectional area of the vascular tree increases every time a vessel branches. Smooth muscle fibres in the vascular wall may also vary the calibre of the vessel.
3. The walls of the blood vessels are elastic rather than rigid, and the elasticity is not uniformly disturbed. Larger arteries tend to be more elastic than small ones, and the vessels become progressively less distensible the further they are from the heart in the arterial tree.
4. The flow of blood is not laminar.

It would therefore be difficult to describe blood flow in mathematical terms even if the velocity of blood flow were constant (i.e. continuous blood flow). In the normal circulation, flow is pulsatile, however, and the flow is dependent upon the elasticity of the blood vessels as well as their calibre. The vascular elasticity determines the velocity at which the pressure and flow waves travel. The less elastic the vascular wall, the greater the velocity of the pressure and the flow waves and therefore the less the pressure gradient and the less the flow.

The elastic recoil has the effect of amplifying the pulse wave as it travels toward the periphery, therefore the pulse pressure is greater in the terminal aorta than in the ascending aorta. As the elastic properties of the vessel wall decrease with age the amplification diminishes and finally disappears so that the pulse pressure becomes the same throughout the aorta. It must be kept in mind, however that the viscosity of blood tends to reduce the amplitude of the pulse wave. Recent clinical studies have shown that patients with coronary artery disease or recent myocardial infarction have a higher degree of 'stiffness' of the descending and terminal aorta (Hirai *et al.*, 1989). It would be expected, therefore that these patients, regardless of age, would experience similar haemodynamic characteristics. Because of the changes in the calibre and elasticity of the blood vessels, the pressure and flow waves are reflected within the arterial system at each branching so that the pressure and flow waves at any given point represent the summation of the incident waves (travelling towards the periphery) and reflected waves (from the periphery).

The arterial tree may therefore be considered as being in a steady state of oscillation. The concept of mean flow is based upon continuous flow; in order to describe oscillatory flow it is necessary to introduce the concept of vascular impedance, which is the ratio of the pulsatile pressure to the pulsatile flow. The peripheral resistance depends upon the calibre of the blood vessels, but the vascular impedance depends upon both their calibre and their elasticity.

If it is assumed that the heart rate is regular, the wave forms of pulsatile pressure and flow may be

*The coefficient of viscosity *n*, is the ratio of the shear stress (which is proportional to the pressure drop along the tube) to the shear rate (the velocity gradient *across* the tube). For a Newtonian fluid, viscosity is independent of shear rate. However, the viscosity of blood varies greatly depending upon the shear rate.

mathematically reduced by harmonic analysis to a Fourier series. The pulse wave is represented by describing the true mean flow in terms of a sinusoidal wave at a frequency of the heart rate (fundamental or first harmonic) and in terms describing sinusoidal waves, whose frequencies are multiples of the heart rate (second, third, fourth, etc. harmonics). Harmonic analysis is a useful tool with which to study and compare the properties of the normal circulation with those of either the abnormal circulation, on the one hand, or of an extracorporeal perfusion system on the other.

The importance of comparing the wave forms in this way has been pointed out (Min *et al.*, 1978; Wright, Sanderson and Furness, 1978). The frequency and amplitude of the pulse wave are obviously most important in any consideration of pulsatile flow. If the characteristics of the pulse wave are not similar to those of the normal circulation it is doubtful whether such pulsatile flow is physiologically superior to non-pulsatile flow. Therefore pulsatile *flow* cannot be equated with pulsatile *perfusion*.

Hydraulic energy

Normally the arterial circulation is maintained by two pumps which are out of phase with one another. The first is the left ventricle and the second is the elastic walls of the larger arteries. Similarly the venous circulation is maintained by two pumps, skeletal muscle and the thoracoabdominal pump, as well as by *vis a tergo*. Pulsatile blood flow therefore requires more energy to move a given volume of blood in a given time than continuous flow. Hydraulic energy is of two kinds:

1. Kinetic energy which can be calculated from the mass of the blood (stroke volume) and the square of its velocity*.
2. Potential energy which is stored in the walls of the arteries and retransformed into kinetic energy by elastic recoil.

In this context, calculations of stroke work based upon multiplying the mean pressure by the mean flow will clearly underestimate the true values, which can be more closely approximated in terms of the vascular impedance (the ratio of the pulsatile pressure to the pulsatile flow) calculated by using harmonic analysis. It has been estimated in this way that the energy required to deliver pulsatile flow is twice that required for non-pulsatile flow at the same mean arterial pressure (Shepard, Simpson and Sharp, 1966). Other investigators have quantified the additional energy required for pulsatile flow by subtracting hydraulic energy calculated using mean values from the hydraulic energy using instantaneous values (Milnor, Bergel and Bargainer, 1966; Shepard, Simpson and Sharp, 1966; Milnor, 1972). In healthy animals, the extra energy required for pulsatile flow ranges from as much as 30% of the total energy in the pulmonary artery to 10% of the total energy in the aorta (Shepard, Simpson and Sharp, 1966). It is postulated that, as most of the dissipation of energy occurs at or beyond the arteriolar level in the circulation, the importance of the additional energy lies in maintaining perfusion by keeping capillary beds open and promoting lymphatic flow. This is merely an updated version of the concept of 'vascular shocks' introduced in 1913 by Gesell. In other words, the concept of a 'critical closing pressure' should be applied to pulsatile as well as to mean flow.

For a more detailed discussion of pulsatile flow the reader is referred to McDonald's monograph (1960).

Experimental aspects of pulsatile perfusion

There have been several excellent reviews on the evidence in favour of and against pulsatile, as opposed to non-pulsatile perfusion (Mavroudis, 1978; Hickey, Buckley and Philbin, 1983).

The published studies, especially the earlier ones, comparing the effects of pulsatile and non-pulsatile perfusion are confusing. There are several reasons that have been given to explain the difference in results that have been obtained. One of the simplest explanations is that different investigators employ different methods of pulsatile perfusion, only some of which are effective. In an effort to overcome this difficulty, Grossi *et al.*, 1985 derived a pulsatility and pulse power index (PI and PPI respectively) from harmonic analysis of pulsatile waveforms. Using the PI and serum lactate levels as a measure of perfusion, they compared the effectiveness of various types of pulsatile and non-pulsatile perfusion. They were able to demonstrate that various combinations of pulse shape and a minimum pulse rate are required to avoid the adverse effects in the circulation associated with non-pulsatile cardiopulmonary bypass. However, both a standard roller pump and pulsatile pump for cardiopulmonary bypass resulted in significant decreases in both the PI and PPI as compared with baseline pre-bypass values. It would seem then, that the same mean flow can have very different physiological effects depending on how it is delivered.

Unfortunately, although there is a large growing body of evidence to support its routine use, we still have no conclusive studies regarding the effective-

$$*e = \frac{m \times v^2}{2}$$

ness of various types of pulsatile perfusion. We will see later on, however, that the results using the pulsatile assist device[R] (Datascope) have been extremely encouraging and have shown an improvement over standard non-pulsatile perfusion.

Another extremely important consideration that makes comparisons between different studies difficult is the flow rate used during the period of assisted circulation. It must be kept in mind that flows in the range of 50–100 ml kg^{-1} min^{-1} are routinely used in clinical cardiopulmonary bypass. Normal blood flow is about 110 ml kg^{-1} min^{-1} with a pulse pressure of 30–40 mmHg. Wesolowski, Sauvage and Pinc (1955), for example, used flow rates of 130 ml kg^{-1} min^{-1} and other workers have used flows as high as 200 ml kg^{-1} min^{-1} (Rudy, Heyman and Edmunds, 1973; Boucher, Rudy and Edmunds, 1974; Harken, 1975). Ogata *et al.* (1960) pointed out that the differences between the effects of pulsatile and non-pulsatile flow only become obvious at flows less than 100 ml kg^{-1} min^{-1}, and it was only in the studies in which flow rates in this range were used that the differences between pulsatile and non-pulsatile perfusion were demonstrated in experimental animals (Replogle *et al.*, 1962; Shepard and Kirklin, 1969; Sanderson, Wright and Sims, 1972; Dunn *et al.*, 1974; Watanabe *et al.*, 1989) and in humans (Trinkle *et al.*, 1969).

Clinical aspects of pulsatile perfusion

Although non-pulsatile perfusion had proved to be fairly satisfactory for short periods of cardiopulmonary bypass, it is well established that certain characteristic changes occur as a consequence of longer periods of non-pulsatile perfusion.

There are disturbances of vasomotor control with alterations in the distribution of blood flow, arteriovenous shunting, and venous pooling. Cardiopulmonary bypass leads to accumulation of extracellular fluid causing interstitial oedema and further interference with blood flow. We routinely see increases in both systemic and pulmonary vascular resistance. This may lead to inadequate perfusion of the peripheral tissues, as well as place an undue burden on the left ventricle in the post-bypass period. Metabolic changes with anaerobic cellular metabolism manifested by metabolic acidosis, accumulation of lactate, and reduced oxygen utilization are seen. Progressive dysfunction of various organs, notably the brain, kidneys, lung and heart is seen to some extent with all types of cardiopulmonary bypass, as well as abnormalities of the endocrine system.

Metabolic effects

Ogata *et al.* (1960) observed increased oxygen consumption, more physiological pH, and increased buffer base levels with pulsatile cardiopulmonary bypass (CPB) in dogs at flow rates in the 60–70 ml kg^{-1} m^{-2} range compared with non-pulsatile cardiopulmonary bypass. At flow rates greater than 100 ml kg^{-1} m^{-2}, no difference was observed. Geha *et al.* (1972) noted lower lactate levels with pulsatile CPB in animals. Trinkle *et al.* (1969) found lower lactate levels and increased pH with pulsatile flow. Pappas (1974), using the intra-aortic balloon pump to produce pulsatile perfusion, found patients to have decreased lactate levels and lower serum LDH levels with pulsatile cardiopulmonary bypass.

Shepard and Kirklin (1969) measured whole-body oxygen consumption as an index of tissue perfusion during pulsatile and non-pulsatile perfusion in calves. They reported higher oxygen and lactate extraction and a decreased tendency to acidosis in the animals subjected to pulsatile perfusion. Other investigators (Ogata *et al.*, 1960; Jacobs *et al.*, 1969; Trinkle *et al.*, 1969; Angell James and de Burgh Daly, 1970; German *et al.*, 1972) have confirmed that the findings of reduced oxygen consumption and metabolic acidosis during non-pulsatile perfusion are absent during pulsatile perfusion, or, if present, are reserved by it.

Another widely considered indicator of tissue perfusion is the speed of cooling and re-warming during cardiopulmonary bypass and the thermal gradients established in the body. Williams *et al.*, (1979a and b), using the pulsatile assist device to deliver pulsatile cardiopulmonary bypass, noted decreased cooling and re-warming times in infants compared with non-pulsatile cardiopulmonary bypass. However, other investigators (Nieminen *et al.*, 1983; Singh, Barrett-Boyes and Harris, 1989) have failed to show a difference in cooling and re-warming times with hypothermic pulsatile cardiopulmonary bypass in adults.

The data would support the fact that pulsatile perfusion is associated with improved metabolism as manifested by increased oxygen consumption, higher blood pH, and lower lactate levels.

Haemodynamic effects

As alluded to before, there are conflicting reports regarding the effects of pulsatile and non-pulsatile perfusion on haemodynamics during cardiopulmonary bypass. In general, peripheral vascular resistance decreases with pulsatile perfusion and increases with non-pulsatile perfusion. The majority of animal and human studies confirms this (Ead, Green and Neil, 1952; Halley, Reemtsma and Creech, 1958; Trank and Visscher, 1962; Wilkens, Regelson and Hoffmeister, 1962; Nakayama *et al.*, 1963; Mandelbaum and Burns, 1965; Giron *et al.*, 1966; Spickler and Kezdi, 1967; Jacobs *et al.*, 1969; Koushanapour and McGee, 1969; Trinkle *et al.*, 1969; Angell James and de Burgh Daly, 1970;

Angell James, 1971a; Angell James, 1971b; Angell James and de Burgh Daly, 1971; Berger and Saini, 1972; Dunn *et al.*, 1974).

Nakayama *et al.* (1963) showed a significant improvement in venous return during pulsatile perfusion, thereby improving loading conditions on the myocardium.

Similar responses have been reported in the pulmonary circulation (Lee and DuBois, 1955; Clarke *et al.*, 1968; Mandelbaum and Burns, 1965). Because the pulmonary circulation is really two different sets of vascular beds, the pulmonary and bronchial circulation, the effects on each must be looked at individually.

Increases in mean arterial pressure are seen during non-pulsatile perfusion. The cause of the increase in pressure is not well understood. Elegantly designed experiments by Angell James and de Burgh Daly (Angell James 1971a and b; Angell James and de Burgh Daly 1970 and 1971) involving recordings from the aortic arch and carotid sinus baroreceptors with simultaneous recordings of pressure in the carotid artery and in the femoral artery have led to the suggestion that pulsatile flow, by stimulating the baroreceptors, plays an important role in normal reflex vasomotor control. Other investigators have observed similar findings (Ead, Green and Neil, 1952; Douglas, Ritchie and Schaumann, 1956; Giron *et al.*, 1966; Spickler and Kezdi, 1967; Koushanapour and McGee, 1969). Mandelbaum and Burns, on the basis of equally impressive studies (Mandelbaum and Burns 1956), have suggested that the pulse wave serves the more direct purpose of keeping the capillary beds open, and that non-pulsatile perfusion fails to perform this function, leading to precapillary shunting and an increase in peripheral resistance. This hypothesis is consistent with the finding that more energy is required to maintain pulsatile perfusion at a given mean arterial pressure (Shepard, Simpson and Sharp, 1966).

The normal microcirculation is dependent on pulsatile flow. Ssentjurin (1927), in experiments on the isolated rabbit ear, observed that pulsatile perfusion produced a greater rate of flow than non-pulsatile perfusion, a finding confirmed more recently in humans by Trinkle *et al.* (1969). Similarly Long (1960) and Ogata (1960) reported that non-pulsatile perfusion caused sluggish movement of erythrocytes and a tendency to intravascular aggregation, with marked impairment of capillary blood flow. Ogata *et al.* (1960) studied the microcirculation of the omentum and demonstrated that capillary perfusion ceased after 20 min of non-pulsatile perfusion, as arteriolar flow was diverted by shunting. By contrast, pulsatile flow produced constant and more evenly distributed capillary perfusion.

Parsons and McMaster (1938a and b; McMaster and Parsons, 1938) demonstrated that dye injected into the tissue of rabbit ears cleared faster with pulsatile than with non-pulsatile flow and noted that oedema occurred more commonly during non-pulsatile flow. They also reported that the flow of lymph, which was quite rapid during pulsatile flow, was almost abolished by non-pulsatile flow. Dunn *et al.* (1974) and Jacobs *et al.* (1969) provide indirect evidence that suggests more oedema results from non-pulsatile bypass. Matsumoto, Wolferth and Perlman (1971) noted vasodilation of venules, microcirculation sludging, and oedema formation with non-pulsatile flow that was not seen with pulsatile flow.

Other authors have remarked on the increased tendency towards the formation of oedema and the greater fluid requirements of experimental animals (Nakayama, 1963; Dalton *et al.*, 1965; Jacob *et al.*, 1969; Matsumoto, Wolferth and Perlman, 1971) and humans (Trinkle *et al.*, 1969) during non-pulsatile cardiopulmonary bypass.

Gross lymph flow in the thoracic duct initially increases during non-pulsatile cardiopulmonary bypass, and then returns to prebypass levels (Baue *et al.*, 1965; Anabtawi, Womack and Ellison, 1966).

Capillary exchange depends not only on the mean capillary pressure and the pulsations, but also on the pressure gradient across the capillary wall. If the tissue pressure rises because of fluid accumulation in the extracellular space, whether due to protein leakage from damaged capillary endothelium or to the failure of lymphatic and venous drainage, the resulting interference with capillary exchange may initiate a vicious cycle of progressively increasing ischaemia and injury.

Haematological effects

Most of the earlier systems used in cardiopulmonary bypass produced significant amounts of destruction of blood elements. Notably, we saw haemolysis and destruction of platelets. With recent cardiopulmonary bypass systems, this has been much less of a significant factor. More recent studies with current technology regarding haemolysis and platelet destruction vary.

Pulsatile perfusion systems were initially thought to increase the amount of haemolysis and platelet destruction. However, pulsatile perfusion generated with the pulsatile assist device (PAD^R, Datascope) has been shown to not increase haemolysis and platelets (Bregman *et al.*, 1977a; Williams *et al.*, 1979a). The effects on blood element function, including the white cell series has not been extensively studied.

It would appear then that some forms of pulsatile cardiopulmonary bypass are more damaging to red cells and platelets than non-pulsatile bypass. More work regarding the function of blood elements is needed.

Hormonal responses to extracorporeal circulation

Many investigators have shown that pulsatile perfusion prevents or reduces the circulating levels of catecholamines (Replogle *et al.*, 1962; Harrison *et al.*, 1970; Harrison and Seaton, 1973; Dunn *et al.*, 1974). Other studies (Shepard and Kirklin, 1969; Landymore *et al.*, 1979; Philbin *et al.*, 1981) have failed to show any differences in catecholamine response to cardiopulmonary bypass with pulsatile or non-pulsatile perfusion. Similar increases in both epinephrine and norepinephrine levels have been observed during pulsatile and non-pulsatile perfusion. However, one investigator (Philbin *et al.*, 1981) noted a significantly higher level of both these catecholamines in the post-bypass period in patients who underwent non-pulsatile cardiopulmonary bypass.

Pulsatile perfusion has been shown to prevent or reduce the increases in circulating levels of plasma renin seen with non-pulsatile perfusion (Brull, 1931; Corcoran and Page, 1938; Kohlstaedt and Page 1940; Corcoran and Page, 1942; Hawthorne, Perry and Pogue, 1953; Skinner, McCubbin and Page, 1963; Many *et al.*, 1968a and b; Many *et al.*, 1969; Goodman *et al.*, 1976; Watkins *et al.*, 1979). Evaluation of studies concerning plasma renin levels during pulsatile and non-pulsatile cardiopulmonary bypass must take into account whether or not the patients were preoperatively taken off of beta-blockers. Beta-blockers are known inhibitors of renin release. Studies that have failed to show a difference in plasma renin levels with pulsatile and non-pulsatile cardiopulmonary bypass did not take their patients off beta-blockers preoperatively. Landymore *et al.* (1979) demonstrated lower plasma renin levels after cardiopulmonary bypass in patients with pulsatile perfusion who had been taken off beta-blockers preoperatively.

Angiotensin II levels have also been demonstrated to be significantly lower during pulsatile cardiopulmonary bypass (Taylor *et al.*, 1979; Watkins *et al.*, 1979). However, it is not clear if these patients were taken off beta-blockers pre-bypass. In a recent study by Nagaoka, Innami and Arai (1988) all patients were taken off beta-blockers. They found that pulsatile cardiopulmonary bypass offers significant advantages in terms of lower plasma angiotensin II and serum aldosterone levels, when compared with non-pulsatile cardiopulmonary bypass soon after open-heart surgery requiring total cardiopulmonary bypass for more than 60 min.

The importance of plasma renin activity in the maintenance of both salt and water homoeostasis is well known. Angiotensin II is an extremely potent vasoconstrictor. Furthermore, since renin is the stimulator of angiotensin II release, both renin and angiotensin II play a significant role in peripheral vascular resistance.

Thus, the reported increases in the levels of catecholamines, plasma renin activity, and angiotensin II levels during and after non-pulsatile cardiopulmonary bypass have been attenuated by pulsatile bypass. All of these elevate the peripheral vascular resistance, and it is precisely the studies in which these hormonal agents were significantly lower with pulsatile cardiopulmonary bypass that lower peripheral vascular resistance during bypass (Taylor *et al.*, 1979; Watkins *et al.*, 1979) was seen. We will discuss later on the fact that increased peripheral vascular resistance in the immediate post-bypass setting is manifest by an undue increase in afterload of the left ventricle.

Anti-diuretic hormone (ADH) levels have been reported to increase with non-pulsatile perfusion (Philbin *et al.*, 1977 and 1979; Simpson and Forsling, 1977). It has been shown that this increase is attenuated by pulsatile bypass (Philbin *et al.*, 1977 and 1981). Because vasopressin is a known potent vasoconstrictor, the increased levels observed during non-pulsatile flow cardiopulmonary bypass might also contribute to the increased peripheral vascular resistance and hypertension seen post-operatively with non-pulsatile bypass.

As part of the normal response to stress, plasma ACTH and cortisol levels rise following major surgery (Taylor *et al.*, 1975, 1976a and b). Although such increases have been demonstrated after closed cardiac surgery not involving the use of cardiopulmonary bypass, such as closed mitral valvotomy (Carveth *et al.*, 1965; Taylor *et al.*, 1976b), both adrenal and anterior pituitary function have been shown to be abnormal (Brenner *et al.*, 1978) following non-pulsatile cardiopulmonary bypass. The serum ACTH and cortisol levels are low and the pituitary fails to respond normally to thyrotropin-releasing hormone.

Although the studies are mixed on the findings, several investigators have found that plasma cortisol levels decrease during non-pulsatile cardiopulmonary bypass (Britt *et al.*, 1961; Taylor *et al.*, 1975), and that the initial decline in plasma cortisol levels can be reversed in patients at normothermia with pulsatile cardiopulmonary bypass (Taylor *et al.*, 1978b). Taylor's group noted suboptimal anterior pituitary function in response to thyrotropin-releasing hormone with non-pulsatile cardiopulmonary bypass and have demonstrated a rise in plasma cortisol levels (i.e. normal stress response) (Taylor *et al.*, 1978b) and a normal anterior pituitary response to thyrotropin-releasing hormone in humans during pulsatile cardiopulmonary bypass (Taylor *et al.*, 1978a). However, other investigators have not observed these effects (Frater *et al.*, 1979 and 1980; Pollock *et al.*, 1988).

Effects of pulsatile perfusion on various organ systems

Central nervous system

Although disturbances of cerebral function following cardiopulmonary bypass have been related to embolic phenomena, the use of filters has failed to entirely eliminate the problem (Branthwaite, 1973; Heimbecker, Robert and McKenzie, 1976). Unfortunately, the effects of the various types of perfusion systems on cerebral function have not been extensively studied. Surely, inadequate perfusion is related to cerebral dysfunction post-cardiopulmonary bypass.

It was observed long ago that the cerebrospinal fluid pulsates with the heart beat (Ryder *et al.*, 1952) and de Langen (1959) has shown that these pulsations can be increased or decreased in response to similar changes in the amplitude of the pulse in the carotid artery.

The brain is very vulnerable to inadequate perfusion and hypoxia. Halley, Reemtsma, and Creech (1958) reported decreased cerebral oxygen consumption following non-pulsatile perfusion, and Sanderson and Wright found no evidence of diffuse nerve cell ischaemic injury after non-pulsatile perfusion which was not present following pulsatile cardiopulmonary bypass (Sanderson, Wright and Sims, 1972; Wright and Sanderson, 1972). Matsumoto reported improved cerebral and conjunctival perfusion in dogs during pulsatile flow, by comparison with non-pulsatile flow (Matsumoto, Wolferth and Perlman, 1971). Recently, in an experiment designed to compare the differences in pulsatile and non-pulsatile blood flow in the treatment of cerebral ischaemia, Tranner *et al.* (1986) found that pulsatile flow increased local cerebral blood flow in ischaemic and non-ischaemic brain 19% and 55% respectively, as compared with non-pulsatile flow.

The kidney

The effects of pulsatile blood flow on the function of the kidney has been the subject of many investigations. It is well established that non-pulsatile flow is associated with abnormalities of renal function which do not occur during pulsatile perfusion (Senning *et al.*, 1960; Many *et al.*, 1967; Agishi, Peirce and Kent, 1969; Paquet, 1969). Changes in total renal blood flow have been cited as the causes of altered renal function. In general, pulsatile and non-pulsatile perfusion at fixed mean pressures have not resulted in any differences in total renal blood flow (Gesell *et al.*, 1913; Clauss *et al.*, 1961; Mandelbaum *et al.*, 1965; Boucher, Rudy and Edmunds, 1974). However, shifts in the distribution of intrarenal blood flow with non-pulsatile perfusion have been documented. Many and associates (1967b) found evidence of shunting of flow from the outer cortex to juxtaglomerular areas with non-pulsatile renal perfusion. By comparison with non-pulsatile flow, pulsatile flow has been shown to improve the volume (Moores *et al.*, 1977) and distribution (Finsterbusch *et al.*, 1961; Habal *et al.*, 1976; Many *et al.*, 1968b) of renal blood flow, increase renal oxygen consumption (Mukhgerjee, 1973), urine output (Hooker, 1910; Gesell *et al.*, 1913; Judson and Rausch, 1957; Jacobs *et al.*, 1969; Paquet, 1969; Berger and Saini, 1972; Boucher, Rudy and Edmunds, 1974; Levine *et al.*, 1978), creatine clearance (Jacobs *et al.*, 1969) and resorption of water and electrolytes (Paquet, 1969; Hoffman *et al.*, 1970; Levine *et al.*, 1978). Judson and Rausch (1957) confirmed the findings of earlier investigators that urine volume was related to the pulse pressure amplitude in situ. Thus, it is the pulse itself, rather than the mean pressure in the renal artery which is the critical factor.

Studies by Agishi, Peirce and Kent (1969) and Beltzer *et al.* (1968) drew attention to the importance of pulsatile perfusion in the maintenance of renal structure and function with the result that most centres now preserve cadaveric donor kidneys with pulsatile pumps until transplantation.

The evidence to date clearly shows that pulsatile perfusion better preserves renal function, maintains more normal renal metabolism, preserves outer cortical renal blood flow, and prevents ischaemic changes in the kidneys, especially during longer periods of perfusion.

The lungs

When we consider the effects of different types of perfusion systems on the lungs, we must keep in mind that there are two separate circulations, the bronchial and pulmonary circuits. Conventional cardiopulmonary bypass perfuses only the bronchial circulation. Right heart bypass perfuses the pulmonary circulation. Lee and Du Bois (1955) demonstrated that the pulmonary capillary bed has pulsatile flow under normal conditions.

Clarke *et al.* (1968) reported thickening of the alveolar walls and increased pulmonary vascular resistance following non-pulsatile blood flow. Mandelbaum and Burns (1965), using normothermic right heart bypass in dogs, demonstrated that pulmonary vascular resistance with non-pulsatile flow was 127% that of pulsatile flow. Furthermore, this difference was observed with pharmacologic adrenergic and chlorinergic blockade.

A significant amount of arteriovenous shunting is common after cardiopulmonary bypass, but, as similar changes occur following any major surgical procedure because of alveolar collapse, this phenomenon cannot be attributed to the effects of non-pulsatile perfusion alone. Hauge and Nicolaysen (1980) recently showed no difference in oxygen transfer in normal lungs with either pulsatile or non-pulsatile flow, however, they noted improved oxygenation using pulsatile flow in abnormal oedematous lungs with high pulmonary venous pressures.

The phenomenon of 'pump lung' was frequently a problem during the early days of cardiac surgery and several authors have reported reduced pulmonary compliance and alterations in the alveolar–capillary oxygen exchange. Although the 'pump lung' has been attributed to microemboli of damaged blood cells or platelets, denatured plasma proteins and fat emboli, the use of filters in the extracorporeal circuit has failed to prevent its occurrence (Lesage *et al.*, 1966). Improved understanding of the pathophysiology of shock lung, the use of haemodilution with colloids as well as crystalloids in the heart–lung machine prime, and shorter durations of extracorporeal circulation have played a major role in reducing such complications. However, no studies have so far been published on the effect of pulsatile perfusion in relation to these abnormalities.

In summary than, it would appear that pulsatile perfusion leads to lower pulmonary vascular resistance, but there is no consistent effect on gas exchange. Pulsatile flow in the pulmonary circuit does not appear to be necessary for normal gas exchange. There is little data regarding the effect of pulsatile flow on embolic phenomena, and even less data looking at pulmonary function after cardiopulmonary bypass in patients who have undergone either pulsatile or non-pulsatile flow.

The pancreas

Conventional non-pulsatile cardiopulmonary bypass is associated with elevated serum amylase and urinary amylase clearance (Hennings and Jacobson, 1974; Moores *et al.*, 1977; Traverso *et al.*, 1977; Murray *et al.*, 1981). Acute pancreatitis following cardiopulmonary bypass has been well documented (Horton, Murthy and Seal, 1968; Peterson, Collins and Wibon, 1968). Post-mortem examinations have revealed a 16% incidence of unexplained (no clinical symptoms) pancreatitis in patients who had undergone cardiopulmonary bypass (Feiner, 1976). Evidence from Feiner (1976) and Warshaw (Warshaw and O'Hara, 1978) suggests that ischaemia may be an important factor in the development of pancreatitis post-bypass. Recent clinical studies (Moores *et al.*, 1977; Philbin *et al.*, 1979) have shown that non-pulsatile cardiopulmonary bypass causes a significantly higher serum amylase and amylase clearance than pulsatile cardiopulmonary bypass. The percentage of cardiac flow to the pancreas has been shown to be no different with pulsatile and non-pulsatile perfusion.

The evidence would suggest that pulsatile flow causes less damage to the pancreas than non-pulsatile perfusion as assessed by changes in serum amylase and urinary amylase clearance. Similar observations have been made regarding the effect of pulsatile and non-pulsatile perfusion on the liver (Pappas *et al.*, 1975).

Pulsatile flow and the heart

The effects of intra-aortic balloon pumping on the myocardium are discussed in Chapter 18.

There are conflicting reports concerning the effects of pulsatile perfusion on the heart itself. Since the last rewriting of this chapter, there has been much work done regarding the effects of pulsatile perfusion on the myocardium and coronary blood flow. However, the number of reports is still small, and different methods have been used to achieve pulsatile flow by different groups. other variables, such as temperature, perfusion pressure, and the duration of heart–lung bypass make it still more difficult to interpret the findings.

Unlike other organs, the beating heart provides its own pulsatile flow regardless of the type of perfusion used during cardiopulmonary bypass. Moores *et al.* (1977) found that flow in the left anterior descending (LAD) coronary artery is pulsatile (in the beating heart) whether continuous or pulsatile perfusion is used during extracorporeal circulation. However, in the fibrillating heart, LAD flow is continuous with non-pulsatile perfusion and pulsatile with pulsatile perfusion.

Habel *et al.* (1976) demonstrated that during prolonged ventricular fibrillation in dogs, pulsatile flow produced better subendocardial perfusion than non-pulsatile flow, a finding confirmed by Steed *et al.* (1978), but not by other investigators (Hewitt and Weichert, 1970; Moores *et al.*, 1971; Grover *et al.*, 1979; Wakabayshi *et al.*, 1981). Furthermore, Habel reported higher coronary vascular resistance and relatively lower coronary blood flow to the left ventricle (indicating more effective perfusion) during pulsatile flow, as well as increased myocardial oxygen utilization and lactate extraction (implying less anaerobic metabolism), confirming the earlier clinical findings of Pappas *et al.* (1975).

Schaff and colleagues (1977a) noted significantly higher myocardial blood flow in the region supplied by a critically stenosed LAD coronary artery in fibrillating hearts with pulsatile bypass as compared with non-pulsatile bypass. However, no change was noted in flow with the two modes of bypass in the region supplied by an unstenosed circumflex coronary artery. Bregman *et al.* (1977b) reported a 21% increase in coronary graft flow in patients with pulsatile cardiopulmonary bypass using the pulsatile assist device. Bixler and co-workers (1979) looking at the hypertrophied heart during ventricular fibrillation, found that the blood flow to all layers of the myocardium was improved with pulsatile flow.

Thus, it is suggested by experimental and clinical studies of patients with left ventricular hypertrophy or coronary stenosis, that endocardial flow may be better maintained in fibrillating hearts with pulsatile cardiopulmonary bypass. There is no study in the literature demonstrating improvement in total coronary blood flow or subendocardial perfusion with pulsatile perfusion in the beating heart.

Similar studies have shown that the left ventricular ejection fraction in the early postoperative period is higher in patients undergoing aortocoronary bypass grafting with pulsatile perfusion, when compared with a similar group of patients undergoing non-pulsatile cardiopulmonary bypass (Habal *et al.*, 1976; Maddoux *et al.*, 1976). Other investigators have also reported a lower incidence of perioperative myocardial infarction in patients subjected to pulsatile cardiopulmonary bypass (Pappas *et al.*, 1975; Bregman *et al.*, 1977), and less necessity for use of the intra-aortic balloon postoperatively (Bregman *et al.*, 1977b).

Laboratory studies by Dunn, Peterson and Kirsh (1978) have shown that pulsatile flow is superior to non-pulsatile perfusion of the fibrillating heart in terms of maintenance of left ventricular contractility, compliance, and reduced water content, while Schaff and his colleagues have demonstrated that pulsatile perfusion reduces the regional myocardial ischaemia which occurs with non-pulsatile perfusion in the presence of a critical stenosis of the LAD coronary artery in the fibrillating ventricle (Schaff *et al.*, 1977a and b). Laschinger *et al.* (1983), using pulsatile left atrial–femoral artery bypass in dogs, demonstrated that the addition of pulsatile diastolic counterpulsation led to significant reductions in the limitations of myocardial infarct size as compared with non-pulsatile bypass.

Although there is not yet any conclusive evidence of the superiority of pulsatile perfusion of the beating heart, several investigators have reported improvement in coronary blood flow and subendocardial perfusion, perfusion to areas of myocardium in the region of significant coronary stenosis, and a significant increase in coronary venous graft flow during pulsatile cardiopulmonary bypass in the fibrillating heart. Furthermore, it is suggested (Habal *et al.*, 1976; Maddoux *et al.*, 1976) that left ventricular ejection fraction in the early post-bypass period improved with pulsatile perfusion. There are reports of lower incidence of perioperative myocardial infarction (Pappas *et al.*, 1975; Bregman *et al.*, 1977) and limitation of infarct size (Laschinger *et al.*, 1983) with the use of pulsatile perfusion during cardiopulmonary bypass. Clearly, more work in this area is needed.

Table 16.1 Summary of the results of preliminary evaluation of the pulsatile assist device in the laboratory

Counterpulsation	
Cardiac output	62% (25–95%)
Diastolic augmentation	90% (35–140%)
Systolic pressure	10% (0–50%)
Haemolysis (2 h) =	4–12 mg/100ml
Pulsation	
Pulse pressure	40–50 mmHg
Haemolysis (2 h) =	10.5–17.5 mg/100ml

Experience with the pulsatile assist device at the Columbia Presbyterian Medical Center

The PAD was first evaluated in the laboratory by inducing cardiogenic shock to 12 dogs with intravenous injections of propanolol (3 mg kg^{-1} of body weight). Representative tracings illustrating the efficacy of the PAD for counterpulsation and for providing pulsatile total cardiopulmonary bypass are represented in Figures 16.4 and 16.5, and the overall results obtained are summarized in Table 16.1.

Technical aspects

We routinely use roller pumps and bubble-type oxygenators for cardiopulmonary bypass. A No. 24 Bardic (U.S.C.I. Division of C.R. Bard Incorporated, Billerica, Massachusetts, USA) arterial cannula is inserted in the ascending aorta. The tip of the cannula is directed towards the descending thoracic aorta at the beginning of the operation. However, turning the tip towards the aortic valve will maximize the effect of aortic root counterpulsation. During the insertion of the venous cannulae the triggering of the PAD is adjusted to alternate beats because of the frequency of premature atrial contractions.

The PAD is switched off during the initiation of cardiopulmonary bypass until the patient's bypass flow is stable.

It is important to switch off the PAD for a moment whenever the cross-clamp or partial occlusion clamp is applied to, or removed from, the ascending aorta.

While the heart–lung bypass is being discontinued at the end of the operation, PAD counterpulsation can be used with the advantage to increase coronary blood flow, to stabilize the patient with ventricular arrhythmias, and to reduce the work of a functionally depressed left ventricle.

The PAD should be used with caution, if at all, in patients with significant disease of the aorta such as aneurysms, cystic medial necrosis, etc. and in patients with significant aortic valvular insufficiency, in whom the PAD may tend to increase the work load of the left ventricle.

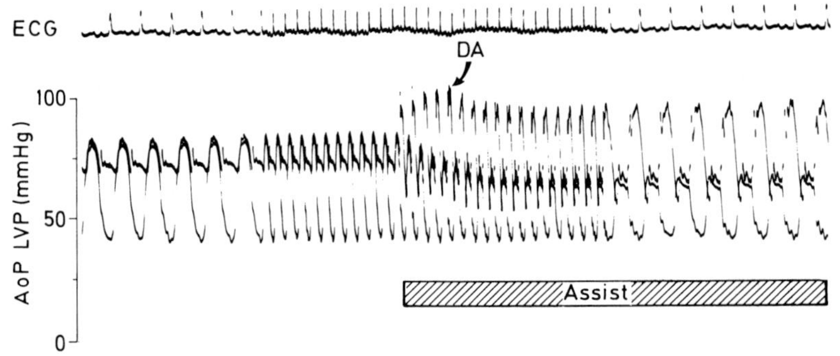

Figure 16.4 Counterpulsation of the aortic root of the dog with a pulsatile assist device. AoP = aortic pressure; LVP = left ventricular pressure. DA denotes diastolic augmentation of the aortic pressure. Note the systolic unloading and diastolic augmentation which is comparable to that achieved with intra-aortic balloon pumping

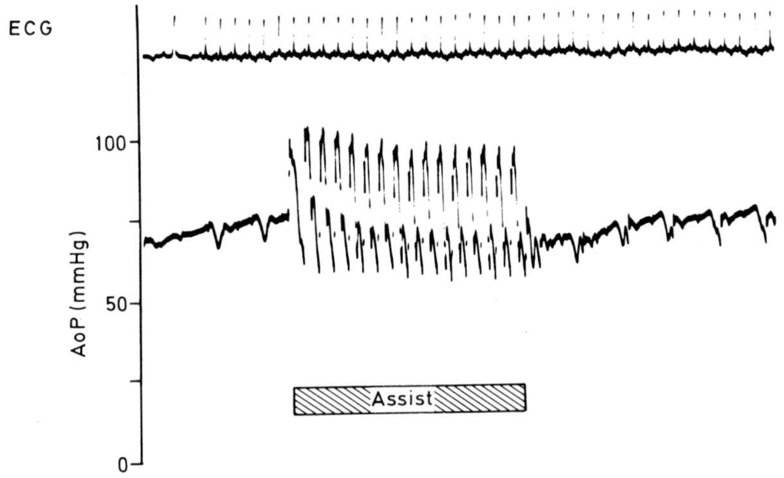

Figure 16.5 Pulsatile total cardiopulmonary bypass in the dog. AoP = aortic pressure. Pulse pressures of 40–50 mmHg are easily achieved

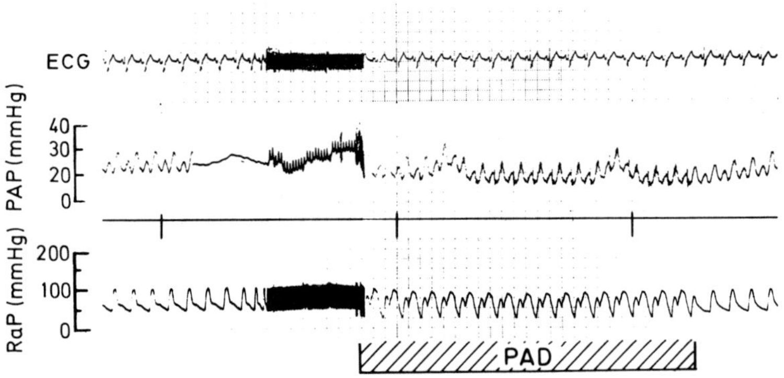

Figure 16.6 Aortic root counterpulsation with the PAD in the adult. The tracings were obtained before the institution of cardiopulmonary bypass in a patient undergoing coronary artery bypass grafting for ischaemic discharge. PAP = pulmonary artery pressure; RaP = radial artery pressure. Note the systolic unloading and the diastolic augmentation of the arterial pressure and the reduction in pulmonary artery end-diastolic pressure produced by the pulsatile assist device

Since 1975, when it was introduced for clinical use, and 1979, the PAD has been employed in thousands of patients undergoing cardiopulmonary bypass at our institution. An analysis of the first 1000 patients has been detailed (Bregman, 1978) and outlined here.

The haemodynamic effectiveness of the PAD for counterpulsation of the aortic root may be readily appreciated from the recording illustrated in Figure 16.6.

Figure 16.7 shows the effect of PAD counterpulsation on the flow in an aortocoronary bypass graft. The blood flow in the vein grafts was measured while the PAD was being used in a group of 17 consecutive patients undergoing coronary bypass grafting and it was found that the PAD produced an average increase flow of 21.4 ± 6.1% (Bregman *et al.*, 1977b).

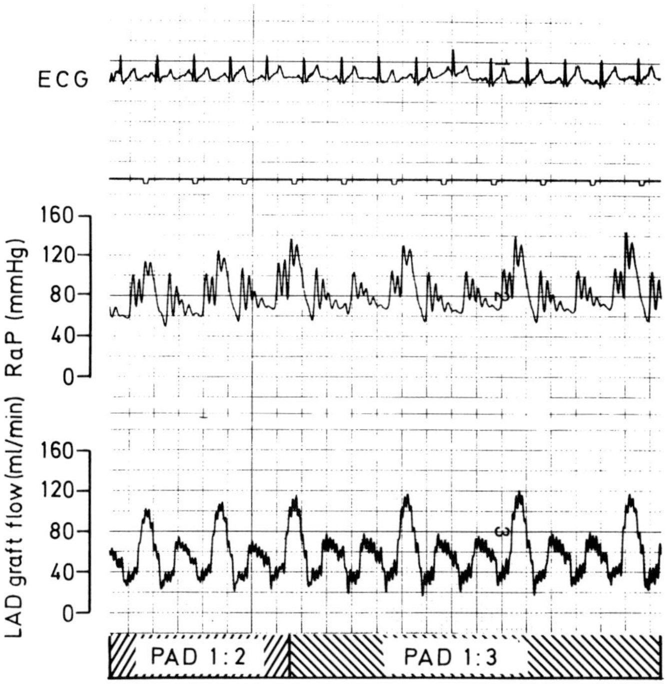

Figure 16.7 Flow augmentation by the PAD in a coronary bypass graft. This tracing was obtained in the same patient as in Figure 16.6, after termination of cardiopulmonary bypass. LAD graft = bypass graft to the left anterior descending coronary artery. The effect of the PAD on the graft flow is shown with triggering on alternate (1:2) and on every third (1:3) heartbeat

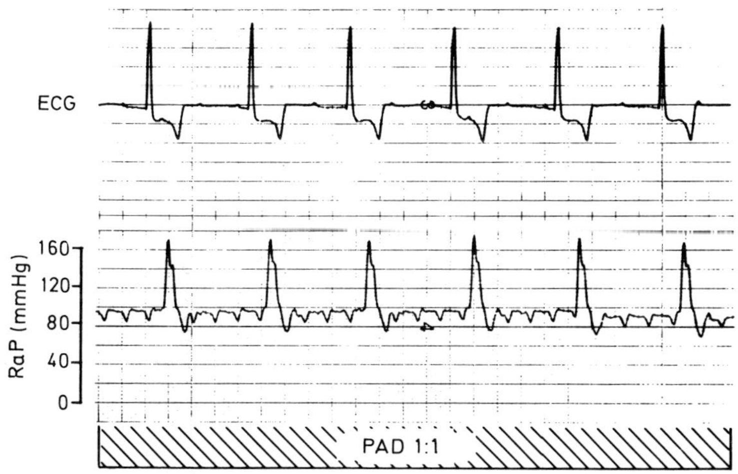

Figure 16.8 Pulsatile cardiopulmonary bypass with the PAD in children. This tracing was obtained during the repair of a ventricular septal defect in a 5-year-old child on total cardiopulmonary bypass. RaP = radial artery pressure

The urinary output during cardiopulmonary bypass was measured in another group of 100 patients. The PAD group had a mean urine output of 9.18 ± 0.68 ml min^{-1}, whereas the output of the group treated with non-pulsatile cardiopulmonary bypass was only 3.90 ± 0.35 ml min^{-1} (P<0.001).

Table 16.2 summarizes our experience with the first 1000 patients. We have been particularly impressed by the reduction in the number of patients who require intra-aortic balloon pumping postoperatively (Bregman *et al.*, 1977a). At this institution the advent of the PAD had markedly reduced the incidence of postoperative low cardiac-output syndrome, and the great majority of patients can be weaned smoothly and uneventfully from cardiopulmonary bypass. The results are particularly impressive for those patients with severe or unstable ischaemic heart disease. The data from the subset of patients with critical left mainstem coronary artery disease are presented in Table 16.3.

Figures 16.8 and 16.9 show the effective use of the PAD in a 5-year-old child. Our experience with

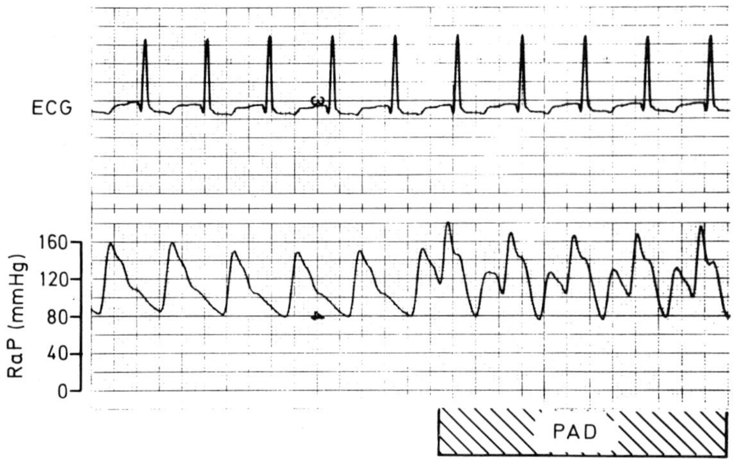

Figure 16.9 Aortic root counterpulsation with the PAD in children. This tracing was obtained from the same patient as in Figure 16.8 after termination of cardiopulmonary bypass. RaP = radial artery pressure

Table 16.2 Summary of the experience using the pulsatile assist device in 1000 patients at the Columbia Presbyterian Medical Center (1975–1979)

Patients	
Age: 18–82 (average = 59)	
Sex: 735 males	
265 females	
(A) 776 patients NYHA Class III or IV	
Ejection fraction less than 0.3	
LVEDP more than 18 mmHg	
(B) 207 patients left main (or equivalent) coronary lesion	
(158 in A)	
(C) 51 patients crescendo angina	
(47 in A)	
Operations	
Coronary bypass alone	519
Valve replacement alone	341
Ventricular aneurysm resection alone	12
Combined coronary bypass and valve replacement	105
Combined coronary bypass and ventricular aneurysm resection	23
Results	
Number weaned from CPB	993 (99.3%)
(with PAD alone = 987)	
(with PAD + IABP = 6)	
Need for postoperative IABP	7 (0.7%)
Intraoperative myocardial infarction	15 (1.5%)
Postoperative hospital deaths (< 4 weeks)	12 (1.2%)

Table 16.3 Summary of the experience using the pulsatile assist device with left main coronary artery disease at the Columbia Presbyterian Medical Center (1975–1979)

Number of patients: 50	
Age: 39–71 (average = 58)	
Sex: 44 males	
6 females	
Previous transmural myocardial infarction	25 (50%)
Crescendo angina	6 (12%)
NYHA Class II	12 (24%)
Class III	24 (48%)
Class IV	14 (28%)
Preoperative LVEDP ≥ 18 mmHg	13 (26%)
Preoperative E.F. ≤ 40%	15 (30%)
Surgical results	
Number of patients	50
Preoperative left ventricular dysfunction	39 (78%)
Preoperative use of IABP	0
Number of patients weaned from CPB with PAD	50 (100%)
Need for postoperative IABP	0
Perioperative myocardial infarctions	1 (2%)
Postoperative hospital deaths	1 (2%)

the PAD in children has been limited but encouraging. The use of profound hypothermia and circulatory arrest for cardiac surgery in infants has obviated the need for the PAD, although it has been suggested that more efficient cooling and rewarming of such patients could be achieved by pulsatile perfusion (Williams *et al.*, 1979a).

Conclusions

Although much work has been done on the physiology of pulsatile perfusion and the clinical benefits of using pulsatile flow systems during cardiopulmonary bypass, it is evident that more information is needed. Hopefully, as more and more centres use pulsatile cardiopulmonary bypass, the benefits of pulsatile perfusion will be more clearly delineated. However, certain conclusion can be drawn from the present data.

1. Pulsatile flow is desirable for the preservation of normal function of various organs and systems of the body.
2. The PAD safely creates pulsatile cardiopulmonary bypass.
3. The PAD is effective when used for aortic root counterpulsation.
4. The PAD is a simple alternative to intra-aortic balloon pumping for patients undergoing cardiac surgery.

References

Addetia, A.M. and Callaghan, J.C. (1981) Intramyocardial arteriovenous shunting of blood with non-pulsatile perfusion. *Journal of Thoracic and Cardiovascular Surgery*, **81**, 219

Agishi, T., Peirce, E.C. II and Kent, B.B. (1969) A comparison of pulsatile and non-pulsatile pumping for *ex vivo* renal perfusion. *Journal of Surgical Research*, **9**, 623

Alpert, J., Bhaktan, E.K., Gielchinsky, I., *et al.* (1976) Vascular complications of intra-aortic balloon pumping. *Archives of Surgery*, **111**, 1190

Anabtawi, I.M., Womack, C.E. and Ellison, R.G. (1966) Thoracic duct lymph flow during pulsatile and non-pulsatile extracorporeal circulation. *Annals of Thoracic Surgery*, **2**, 38

Angell James, J.E. (1971a) The effects of altering mean pressure, pulse pressure and pulse frequency on the impulse activity in baroreceptor fibers from the aortic arch and right subclavin artery in the rabbit. *Journal of Physiology (London)*, **214**, 65

Angell James, J.E. (1971b) The responses of aortic arch and right subclavin baroreceptors to changes of nonpulsatile pressure and their modification by hypothermia. *Journal of Physiology (London)*, **214**, 201

Angell James, J.E. and de Burgh Daly, M. (1970) Comparison of the reflex vasomotor responses to separate and combined stimulation of the carotid sinus and aortic arch baroreceptors by pulsatile and nonpulsatile pressures in the dog. *Journal of Physiology (London)*, **209**, 257

Angell James, J.E. and de Burgh Daly, M. (1971) Effects of graded pulsatile pressure on the reflex vasomotor responses elicited by changes of mean pressure in the perfused carotid sinus-aortic arch regions of the dog. *Journal of Physiology (London)*, **214**, 51

Baue, A.S., Nussbaum, M., Amstadt, G. and Blackmore, W.S. (1965) The pattern of lymphatic flow during extracorporeal circulation. *Journal of Thoracic and Cardiovascular Surgery*, **50**, 648

Beckman, C.B., Geha, A.S., Hammond, G.L. and Baue, A.E. (1977) Results and complications of intra-aortic balloon counterpulsation. *Annals of Thoracic Surgery*, **24**, 550

Belzer, F.O., Ashby, B.S., Huang, J.S. and Dunphy, J.E. (1968) Etiology of rising perfusion pressure in isolated organ perfusion. *Annals of Thoracic Surgery*, **168**, 382

Berger, R.L. and Saini, V.K. (1972) Conversion of non-pulsatile cardiopulmonary bypass to pulsatile flow by intra-aortic balloon pumping during myocardial revascularization for cardiogenic shock. (Abstr). *Circulation*, **45** and **46** (**Suppl. II**), 130

Biddle, T.L., Stewart, S. and Stuard, I.D. (1976) Dissection of the aorta complicating intra-aortic balloon counterpulsation. *American Heart Journal*, **92**, 781

Bixler, T.J., Magee, P.G., Flaherty, J.T., *et al.* (1979) Beneficial effects of pulsatile perfusion in the hypertrophied ventricle during ventricular fibrillation. *Circulation*, **60** (*Suppl. I*), 141

Boucher, J.K., Rudy, L.W., Jr. and Edmunds, L.H., Jr. (1974) Organ blood flow during pulsatile cardiopulmonary bypass. *Journal of Applied Physiology*, **36**, 86

Branthwaite, M.A. (1973) Detection of neurological damage during open-heart surgery. *Thorax*, **28**, 464

Bregman, D. (1978) Clinical exprience with a new pulsatile assist device (PAD) during open-heart surgery. *Artificial Organs*, **2**, 244

Bregman, D., Bailin, M., Bowman, F.O., Jr., *et al.* (1977a) A pulsatile assist device (PAD) for use during cardiopulmonary bypass. *Annals of Thoracic Surgery*, **24**, 574

Bregman, D., Bowman, F.O. Jr., Parodi, E.N., *et al.* (1977b) An improved method of myocardial protection with pulsation during cardiopulmonary bypass. *Circulation*, **56** (*Suppl. II*), 157

Bregman, D., Parodi, E.N., Bowman, F.O. Jr., *et al.* (1976) Clinical experience with a new cardiac assist device-the pulsatile assist device (PAD). (Abstr.) *Clinical Research*, **24**, 211A

Bremner, W.F., Taylor, K.M., Baird, S., *et al.* (1978) Hypothalamo-pituitary-thyroid axis function during cardiopulmonary bypass. *Journal of Thoracic and Cardiovascular Surgery*, **75**, 392

Britt, C.I., Hoyd, J.R., Blizzard, R.M., *et al.* (1961) Adrenocortical response to total body perfusion. *Archives of Surgery*, **82**, 584

Brull, L. (1973) Nouvelle methode pour l'etude des fonctions du rein: l'anastomose simultanee de la circulation renale avec la circulation carotid-jugulaire de deux donneurs. *Comptes Rendus des Seances de la Societe de Biologie et de ses Filiales (Paris)*, **107**, 248

Carveth, S.W., McGoon, D.C., Mattox, V.R. and Moffitt, E.A. (1965) Effect of surgery with and without whole body perfusion on plasma 17-hydroxy corticosteroids in man. *Annals of Surgery*, **161**, 105

Clarke, C.P., Kahn, D.R., Dufek, J.H. and Sloan, H. (1968) The effects of non-pulsatile blood flow on canine lungs. *Annals of Thoracic Surgery*, **6**, 450

Clauss, R.H., Birtwell, W.C., Albertal, G., *et al.* (1961) Asssisted circulation. 1. The arterial counterpulsator. *Journal of Thoracic and Cardiovascular Surgery*, **41**, 447

Corcoran, A.C. and Page, I.H. (1938) Observaions on relation of experimental hypertension to renal clearance and renal ischaemia. *American Journal of Physiology*, **123**, 43

Corcoran, A.C. and Page, I.H. (1942) Renal blood flow in experimental renal hypertension. *American Journal of Physiology*, **135**, 361

Dalton, M.L., Mosley, E.C., Woodward, K.E. and Barila, T.G. (1965) The effect of pulsatile flow on renal blood flow during extracorporeal circulation. *Journal of Surgical Research*, **5**, 127

de Langen, C.D. (1959) Die klinische Bedeuytung der Pulsdruckamplitude. *Muchener Medizinische Wochenschrift*, **101**, 2132

Douglas, W.W., Ritchie, J.M. and Schaumann, W. (1956) A study of the effect of the pattern of electrical stimulation of the aortic nerve on the reflex depressor responses. *Journal of Physiology (London)*, **133**, 232

Dunn, J., Kirsh, M.M., Harness, J., *et al.* (1974) Haemodynamic, metabolic and haemotological effects of pulsatile cardiopulmonary bypass. *Journal of Thoracic and Cardiovascular Surgery*, **68**, 138

Dunn, J., Peterson, A. and Kirsh, M.M. (1978) Effects of pulsatile perfusion upon left ventricular function. *Journal of Surgical Research*, **25**, 211

Ead, H.W., Green, J.H. and Neil, E. (1952) A comparison of the effects of pulsatile and non-pulsatile blood flow through the carotid sinus on the reflexogenic activity of the sinus baroreceptors in the cat. *Journal of Physiology (London)*, **118**, 509

Eguchi, S. and Asano, K. (1968) A new pulsatile pump controlled by a roller system. *Surgery*, **63**, 490

Feiner, H. (1976) Pancreatitis after cardiac surgery: a morphological study. *American Journal of Surgery*, **131**, 684

Finterbusch, W., Long, D.M., Sellers, R.D., *et al.* (1961) Renal arteriography during extracorporeal circulation in dogs, with preliminary report upon the effects of low molecular weight dextran. *Journal of Thoracic and Cardiovascular Surgery*, **41**, 252

Frater, R.W.M., Wakayama, S., Oka, Y., *et al.* (1979) Pulsatile cardiopulmonary bypass: failure to influence hemodynamics or hormones. *Circulation*, (Abstracts) (*Suppl II*) **60**, 34

Frater, R.W.M., Wakayama, S., Oka, Y., *et al.* (1980) Pulsatile cardiopulmonary bypass: failure to influence hemodynamics or hormones. *Circulation*, **62** (**Suppl 1**), 19

Geha, A.S., Salaymeh, M.T., Abe, T. and Baue, A. (1972) Effect of pulsatile cardiopulmonary bypass on cerebral metabolism. *Journal of Surgical Research*, **12**, 381

German, J.C., Chalmers, G.S., Hirai, J., *et al.* (1972) Comparison of nonpulsatile and pulsatile extracorporeal circulation on renal tissue perfusion. *Chest*, **61**, 65

Gesell, R.A. (1913) On the relation of pulse pressure to renal secretion. *American Journal of Physiology*, **32**, 70

Giron, F., Birtwell, W.C., Soroff, H.S. and Deterling, R.A. (1966) Hemodynamic effects of pulsatile and nonpulsatile flow. *Archives of Surgery*, **93**, 802

Goodman, T.A., Gerard, D.F., Bernstein, E.F. and Dilley, R.B. (1976) The effects of pulseless perfusion on the distribution of renal cortical blood flow and on renin release. *Surgery*, **80**, 31

Grossi, E.E., Connolly, M.W., Krieger, K.H., *et al.* (1985) Quantification of pulse flow during cardiopulmonary bypass to permit direct comparison of the effectiveness of various types of pulsatile and nonpulsatile flow. *Surgery*, **98**, 547

Grover, F.L., Fewel, J.G., Vinas, J., *et al.* (1979) Effects of aortic balloon pumping during cardiopulmonary bypass on myocardial perfusion, metabolism and contractility. *Chest*, **75**, 37

Habal, S.M., Weiss, M.B., Spontiz, H.M., *et al.* (1976) Effects of pulsatile and nonpulsatile coronary perfusion on performance of the canine left ventricle. *Journal of Thoracic and Cardiovascular Surgery*, **72**, 742

Halley, M.M., Reemtsma, K. and Creech, O., Jr. (1958) Cerebral blood flow, metabolism and brain volume in extracorporeal circulation. *Journal of Thoracic Surgery*, **36**, 506

Hamel, G. (1898) Die Bedeutung des Pulses fur den Blutstrom. *Zeitschrift fur Biologie (Munich)*, **25**, 474

Harken, A.H. (1975) The influence of pulsatile perfusion on oxygen uptake by the isolated canine hind limb. *Journal of Thoracic and Cardiovascular Surgery*, **70**, 237

Harrison, T.S., Chawla, R.C., Seaton, J.F. and Robinson, B.H. (1970) Carotid sinus origin of adrenergic responses compromising the effectiveness of artificial circulatory support. *Surgery*, **68**, 20

Harrison, T.S. and Seaton, J.F. (1973) An analysis of pulse frequency as an adrenergic excitant in pulsatile circulatory support. *Surgery*, **73**, 868

Hauge, A. and Nicolaysen, G. (1980) Pulmonary O_2 transfer during pulsatile and non-pulsatile perfusion. *Acta Physiologica Scandinavica*, **109**, 325

Hawthorne, E.W., Perry, S.L.C. and Pogue, W.G. (1953) Development of experimental renal hypertension in the dog following reduction of renal artery pulse pressure without reducing mean pressure. *American Journal of Physiology*, **174**, 393

Heimbecker, R., Robert, A. and Mckenzie, F.N. (1976) The extracorporeal pump filter–Saint or sinner? *Annals of Thoracic Surgery*, **21**, 55

Hennings, B. and Jacobson, G. (1974) Postoperative amylase excretion: a study following thoracic surgery with and without extracorporeal circulation. *Annals of Clinical Research*, **6**, 215

Hewitt, R.L. and Weichert, R.F. (1970) Diastolic augmentation during heart bypass. *Journal of Thoracic and Cardiovascular Surgery*, **60**, 123

Hickey, P.R., Buckley, M.J. and Philbin, D.M. (1983) Pulsatile and nonpulsatile cardiopulmonary bypass: Review of a counterproductive controversy. *Annals of Thoracic Surgery*, **36**, 720

Hirai, T., Sasayama, S., Kawasaki, T. and Yagi, S. (1989) Stiffness of systemic arteries in patients with myocardial infarction: a non-invasive method to predict severity of coronary atherosclerosis. *Circulation*, **80**, 78

Hoffman, B.F., Klopp, E.H., Jacobs, L.A., *et al.* (1970) A pulsatile roller pump for cardiac bypass. *IEEE Transactions on Bio-medical Engineering*, **17**, 78

Hooker, D.R. (1910) A study of the isolated kidney: the

influence of pulse pressure upon renal function. *American Journal of Physiology*, **27**, 24

Horton, E.H., Murthy, S.K. and Seal, R.M.E. (1968) Haemorrhagic necrosis of small intestine and acute pancreatitis following open heart surgery. *Thorax*, **23**, 438

Jacobj, C. (1890) Apparat zur Durchblutung isolirter uberlebender Organe. *Archiv fur experimentalle Pathologie und Pharmakologie (Leipzig)*, **26**, 388

Jocobs, L.A., Klopp, E.H., Seamone, W., *et al.* (1969) Improved organ function during cardiac bypass with a roller pump modified to deliver pulsatile flow. *Journal of Thoracic and Cardiovascular Surgery*, **58**, 703

Judson, W.E. and Rausch, N.H. (1957) Effects of acute reduction of renal artery blood pressure on renal haemodynamics and excretion of electrolytes and water. *Journal of Laboratory and Clinical Medicine*, **50**, 923

Kantrowitz, A., TjOnneland, S., Freed, P.S., *et al.* (1968) Initial clinical experience with intra-aortic balloon pumping in cardiogenic shock. *Journal of the American Medical Association*, **203**, 135

Kohlstaedt, K.G. and Page, I.H. (1940) The liberation of renin by perfusion of kidneys following reduction in pulse pressure. *Journal of Experimental Medicine*, **72**, 201

Kolff, W.J. and Lawson, J. (1975) Status of the artificial heart and cardiac assist device in the United States. *Transactions of the American Society for Artificial Internal Organs*, **21**, 160

Koushanapour, E. and McGee, J.P. (1969) Effect of mean pressure on carotid sinus baroreceptor response to pulsatile pressure. *American Journal of Physiology*, **216**, 599

Landymore, R.W., Murphy, D.A., Kinley, C.E., *et al.* (1979) Does pulsatile flow influence the incidence of postoperative hypertension? *Annals of Thoracic Surgery*, **28**, 261

Laschinger, J.C., Cunningham, J.N., Catinella, F.P., *et al.* (1983) Pulsatile left atrial-femoral artery bypass: a new method of preventing extension of myocardial infarction. *Archives of Surgery*, **118**, 965

Lee, G.J. and DuBois, A.B. (1955) Pulmonary capillary blood flow in man. *Journal of Clinical Investigation*, **34**, 1380

Lefemine, A.A., Kosowsky, B., Madoff, I., *et al.* (1977) Results and complications of intra-aortic balloon pumping in surgical and medical patients. *American Journal of Cardiology*, **40**, 416

Lesage, A.M., Tsuchioka, H., Young, W.G., Jr. and Sealy, W.C. (1966) Pathogenesis of pulmonary damage during extracorporeal perfusion. *Archives of Surgery*, **93**, 1002

Levine, F.H., Grotte, G.J., Fallon, J.T., *et al.* (1980) Effects of pulsatile and nonpulsatile reperfusion on the post ischaemic myocardium. *American Journal of Cardiology* (Abstract), **45**, 394

Levine, F.H., Philbin, D.M., Coggins, C.H., *et al.* (1978) Plasma vasopressin and urinary sodium ion excretion during cardiopulmonary bypass: a comparison of pulsatile and nonpulsatile flow. *Surgical Forum*, **29**, 320

Levine, F.H., Phillips, H.R., Carter, J.E., *et al.* (1981) The effect of pulsatile perfusion on preservation of left ventricular function after aortocoronary bypass grafting. *Circulation*, **64 (Suppl. 2)**, 40

Long, D. (1960) Discussion of: Sanger, P.W., Robicsek, F., Taylor, F.H., *et al.* Vasomotor regulation during extracorporeal circulation and open-heart surgery. *Journal of Thoracic and Cardiovascular Surgery*, **40**, 355

Ludwig, C. and Schmidt, A. (1868) Das Verhalten der Gase, welche mit dem Blut durch den reizbaren Saugethiermuskel stromen. *Arbeiten aus der Physiologischen Anstalt zu Leipzig*, **3**, 1

McCabe, J.C., Abel, R.M., Subramanian, V.A. and Guy, W.A., Jr. (1978) Complications of intra-aortic balloon insertion and counterpulsation. *Circulation*, **57**, 769

McDonald, D.A. (1960) *Blood Flow in Arteries*. Williams and Wilkins Company, Baltimore

McMaster, P.D. and Parsons, R.J. (1938) Effect of pulse pressure on spread of substances through tissues. *Journal of Experimental Medicine*, **68**, 377

Maddoux, G., Pappas, G., Jenkins, M., *et al.* (1976) Effect of pulsatile and nonpulsatile flow during cardiopulmonary bypass on left ventricular ejection fraction early after aortocoronary bypass surgery. *American Journal of Cardiology*, **37**, 1000

Mandelbaum, I. and Burns, W.H. (1965) Pulsatile and nonpulsatile blood flow. *Journal of the American Medical Association*, **191**, 657

Mandelbaum, I., Berry, J., Silbert, M., *et al.* (1965) Haemodynamic effects of pulsatile and nonpulsatile flow. *Archives of Surgery*, **9**, 771

Many, M., Birtwell, W.C., Giron, F., *et al.* (1967a) The effects of pulse wave pattern on renal function. *Transactions of the Amrican Society for Artificial Internal Organs*, **13**, 157

Many, M., Soroff, H.S., Birtwell, W.C., *et al.* (1967b) The physiologic role of pulsatile and nonpulsatile blood flow: II. Effects on renal function. *Archives of Surgery*, **95**, 762

Many, M., Soroff, H.S., Birtwell, W.C. and Deterling, R.A., Jr. (1968a) Effects of bilateral renal artery depulsation on renin levels. *Surgical Forum*, **19**, 387

Many, M., Soroff, H.S., Birtwell, W.C., *et al.* (1968b) The physiologic role of pulsatile and nonpulsatile blood flow. III. Effects of unilateral renal artery depulsation. *Archives of Surgery*, **97**, 917

Many, M., Giron, F., Birtwell, W.C., (1969) Effects of depulsation of renal blood flow on renal function and renin secretion. *Surgery*, **66**, 242

Matsumoto, T., Wolferth, C.C., Jr. and Perlman, M.H. (1971) Effects of pulsatile and non-pulsatile perfusion upon cerebral and conjunctival microcirculation in dogs. *American Surgeon*, **37**, 61

Mavroudis, C. (1978) To pulse or not to pulse. *Annals of Surgery*, **25**, 259

Milnor, W.R. (1972) Pulsatile blood flow. *New England Journal of Medicine*, **287**, 27

Milnor, W.R., Bergel, D.H. and Bargainer, J.D. (1966) Hydraulic power associated with pulmonary blood flow and its relation to the heart. *Circulation Research*, **17**, 467

Min, B.G., Abbassi, M.Z., Welkowitz, W., *et al.* (1978) Significance of left ventricular power waveform on changes in stroke work during pulsatile left ventricular bypass. *Journal of Surgical Research*, **24**, 544

Moores, W.Y., Kahn, D.R., Kirsh, M.M., *et al.* (1971) Mechanical support of the circulation by a modified pulsatile roller pump. *Annals of Thoracic Surgery*, **12**, 262

Moores, W.Y., Gago, O., Morris, J.D. and Peck, C.C. (1977) Serum and urinary amylase levels following pulsatile and continuous cardiopulmonary bypass. *Journal of Thoracic and Cardiovascular Surgery*, **74**, 73

Moores, W.Y., Hannon, J.P., Crum, J., *et al.* (1977) Coronary flow distribution and dynamics during continuous and pulsatile extracorporeal circulation in pigs. *Annals of Thoracic Surgery*, **24**, 582

Moulopoulos, S.D., Topaz, S. and Wolff, W.J. (1962) Diastolic balloon pumping (with carbon dioxide) in the aorta–a mechanical assistance to the failing circulation. *American Heart Journal*, **63**, 669

Mukhgerjee, N.D., Beran, A.V., Hirai, J., *et al.* (1973) *In vivo* determination of renal tissue oxygenation during pulsatile and nonpulsatile left heart bypass. *Annals of Thoracic Surgery*, **15**, 354

Murray, W.R., Mittra, S., Mittra, D., *et al.* (1981) The amylase-creatine clearance ratio following cardiopulmonary bypass. *Journal of Thoracic and Cardiovascular Surgery*, **82**, 248

Nagaoka, H., Innami, R. and Arai, H. (1988) Effects of pulsatile cardiopulmonary bypass on the renin-angiotensin-aldosterone system following open heart surgery. *Japanese Journal of Surgery*, **4**, 390

Nakayama, K., Tamiya, T., Yamamoto, K., *et al.* (1963) High-amplitude pulsatile pump in extracorporeal circulation with particular reference to haemodynamics. *Surgery*, **54**, 798

Nieminen, M.T., Philbin, D.M., Roscow, C.E., *et al.* (1983) Temperature gradients and rewarming time during hypothermic cardiopulmonary bypass with and without pulsatile flow. *Annals of Thoracic Surgery*, **35**, 488

Ninomiya, I. and Irisawa, H. (1967) Aortic nervous activities in response to pulsatile and non-pulsatile pressure. *American Journal of Physiology*, **213**, 1504

Ogata, T., Ida, Y., Nonoyama, A., *et al.* (1960) A comparative study of the effectiveness of pulsatile and nonpulsatile blood flow in extracorporeal circulation. *Nippon Geka Hokan (Kyoto)*, **29**, 59

Pace, P.D., Tilney, N.L., Lesch, M. and Couch, N.P. (1977) Peripheral arterial complications of intra-aortic balloon counterpulsation. *Surgery*, **82**, 685

Pappas, G. (1974) A simple method of producing pulsatile flow during clinical cardiopulmonary bypass. *Annals of Thoracic Surgery*, **17**, 405

Pappas, G., Winter, S.D., Kopriva, C.J. and Steel, P.P. (1975) Improvement of myocardial and other vital organ functions and metabolism with a simple method of pulsatile flow (IABP) during clinical cardiopulmonary bypass. *Surgery*, 34

Paquet, K.J. (1969) Haemodynamic studies on normothermic perfusion of the isolated pig kidney with pulsatile and non-pulsatile flows. *Journal of Cardiovascular Surgery*, **1**, 45

Parsons, R.J. and McMaster, P.D. (1938a) Effect of pulse upon formation and flow of lymph. *Journal of Experimental Medicine*, **68**, 353

Parsons, R.J. and McMaster, P.D. (1938b) Normal and pathological factors influencing the spread of vital dye in connective tissue. *Journal of Experimental Medicine*, **68**, 869

Peterson, L.M., Collins, J.J. and Wibon, R.E. (1968) Acute pancreatitis occurring after operation. *Surgery, Gynecolocy and Obstetrics*, **128**, 23

Philbin, D.M., Coggins, C.H., Wilson, N. and Sokoloski, J. (1977) Anti-diuretic hormone levels during cardiopulmonary bypass. *Journal of Thoracic and Cardiovascular Surgery*, **73**, 145

Philbin, D.M., Coggins, C.H., Emerson, C.W., *et al.* (1979) Plasma vasopressin levels and urinary sodium excretion during cardiopulmonary bypass: comparison of halothane and morphine anesthesia. *Journal of Thoracic and Cardiovascular Surgery*, **77**, 582

Philbin, D.M., Levine, F.H., Emerson, C.W., *et al.* (1979) Plasma vasopressin levels and urinary sodium excretion during cardiopulmonary bypass in patients with valvular heart disease: Effect of pulsatile flow. *Journal of Thoracic and Cardiovascular Surgery*, **78**, 779

Philbin, D.M., Levine, F.H., Kono, K., *et al.* (1981) Attenuation of the stress response to cardiopulmonary bypass by the addition of pulsatile flow. *Circulation*, **64**, 808

Pollock, E.M.M., Pollock, J.C.S., Jamieson, M.P.G., *et al.* (1988) Adrenocortical hormone concentrations in children during cardiopulmonary bypass with and without pulsatile flow. *British Journal of Anaesthesia*, **60**, 536

Replogle, R., Levy, M., Dewall, R.A. and Lillehei, R.C. (1962) Catecholamine and serotonin response to cardiopulmonary bypass. *Journal of Thoracic and Cardiovascular Surgery*, **44**, 638

Rudy, L.W., Heyman, M.A. and Edmunds, L.H. (1973) Distribution of systemic blood flow during cardiopulmonary bypass. *Journal of Applied Physiology*, **34**, 194

Ryder, H.W., Epsey, F.F., Kimbell, F.D., *et al.* (1952) Modification of effect of cerebral blood flow on cerebrospinal fluid pressure by variations in craniospinal blood volume. *Archives of Neurology and Psychiatry*, **68**, 170

Salerno, T.A., Shizgae, H.M. and Dobell, A.R.C. (1979) Pulsatile perfusion: its effects on blood flow distribution in hypertrophied hearts. *Annals of Thoracic Surgery*, **27**, 559

Sanderson, J.M., Wright, G. and Sims, F.W. (1972) Brain damage in dogs immediately following pulsatile and non-pulsatile blood flows in extracorporeal circulation. *Thorax*, **27**, 275

Schaff, H.V., Ciardullo, R.C., Flaherty, J.T., (1977a) Regional ischaemia distal to a critical coronary stenosis during prolonged fibrillation–improvement with pulsatile perfusion. *Circulation*, **56 (Suppl. II)**, 25

Schaff, H.V., Flaherty, J.T., Ciardullo, R. and Gott, V.L. (1977b) Effects of a critical coronary stenosis on regional myocardial blood flows in a fibrillating heart. *Journal of Thoracic and Cardiovascular Surgery*, **73**, 746

Senning, A., Andres, J., Bornstein, P., *et al.* (1960) Renal function during extracorporeal circulation at high and low flow rates in dogs. *Annals of Surgery*, **151**, 63

Shepard, R.B. and Kirklin, J.W. (1969) Relation of pulsatile flow to oxygen consumptions and other variables during cardiopulmonary bypass. *Journal of Thoracic and Cardiovascular Surgery*, **58**, 694

Shepard, R.C., Simpson, D.C. and Sharp, J.F. (1966) Energy equivalent pressure. *Archives of Surgery*, **93**, 730

Skinner, S.L., McCubbin, J.W. and Page, I.H. (1963) Renal baroreceptor control of renin secretion. *Science*, **141**, 814

Simpson, P. and Forsling, M. (1977) The effects of halothane on plasma vasopressin during cardiopulmonary bypass. *Clinical Endocrinology (Oxford)*, **7**, 33

Singh, R.K.K., Barrett-Boyes, B.G. and Harris, E.A. (1989) Does pulsatile flow improve perfusion during hypothermic cardiopulmonary bypass? *Journal of Thoracic and Cardiovascular Surgery*, **79**, 827

Spickler, J.W. and Kezdi, P. (1967) Dynamic response characteristics of carotid sinus baroreceptors. *American Journal of Physiology*, **212**, 472

Sentjurin, B.S. (1927) Ueber die Wirkung von Giften auf die Gefasse des isolierten Ohrs bei konstantem und pulsierendem Flussigkeitsstrom. *Pfulger's Archiv fur die gesamte Physiologie des Menschen und der Tiere (Bonn)*, **215**, 683

Steed, D.L., Follette, D.M., Foglia, R., *et al.* (1978) Effects of pulsatile assistance and non-pulsatile flow on subendocardial perfusion during cardiopulmonary bypass. *Annals of Thoracic Surgery*, **26**, 133

Tamari, Y., Frantz, S.L., Vagnini, F.J., *et al.* (1976) Experimental evaluation and clinical application of intraoperative counterpulsation without balloon pumping. *Journal of Cardiovascular Surgery*, **17**, 398

Taylor, K.M., Bain, W.H., Jones, J.V. and Walker, M.S. (1976a) The effect of haemodilution on plasma levels of cortisol and free cortisol. *Journal of Thoracic and Cardiovascular Surgery*, **72**, 57

Taylor, K.M., Bain, W.H., Russell, M., *et al.* (1979) Peripheral vascular resistance and angiotensin II levels during pulsatile and nonpulsatile cardiopulmonary bypass. *Thorax*, **34**, 594

Taylor, K.M., Jones, J.V., Walker, M.S., *et al.* (1976b) The cortisol response during heart-lung bypass. *Circulation*, **54**, 20

Taylor, K.M., Walker, M.S., Rao, L.G.S., *et al.* (1975) Plasma levels of cortisol, free cortisol and corticotrophin during cardiopulmonary bypass. *Journal of Endocrinology*, **67**, 29

Taylor, K.M., Wright, G.S., Bain, W.H., (1978a) Comparative studies of pulsatile and non-pulsatile flow during cardiopulmonary bypass: III. Response of anterior pituitary gland to thyrotropin-releasing hormone. *Journal of Thoracic and Cardiovascular Surgery*, **75**, 579

Taylor, K.M., Wright, G.S., Reid, J.M., (1978b) Comparative studies of pulsatile and non-pulsatile flow during cardiopulmonary bypass: II. The effects of adrenal secretion of cortisol. *Journal of Thoracic and Cardiovascular Surgery*, **75**, 574

Trammer, B.I., Gross, C.E., Kinat, G.W. and Adey, G.R. (1986) Pulsatile v. nonpulsatile blood flow in the treatment of acute cerebral ischaemia. *Neurosurgery*, **19**, 724

Trank, J.W. and Visscher, M.B. (1962) Carotid sinus baroreceptor modification associated with endotoxin shock. *Journal of Physiology (London)*, **202**, 971

Traverso, L.W., Ferrari, B.T., Buckberg, G.D. and Tompkins, R.K. (1977) Elevated postoperative renal clearance of amylase without pancreatitis after cardiopulmonary bypass. *American Journal of Surgery*, **133**, 298

Trinkle, J.K., Helton, N.E., Wood, R.E. and Bryant, L.R. (1969) Metabolic comparison of a new pulsatile pump and roller pump for cardiopulmonary bypass. *Journal of Thoracic and Cardiovascular Surgery*, **58**, 562

Tyras, D.H. and Williams, V.L. (1978) Paraplegia following intra-aortic balloon assistance. *Annals of Thoracic Surgery*, **25**, 164

Wakabayashi, A., Kubo, T., Gilman, P., *et al.* (1981) Pulsatile pressure-regulated coronary perfusion during ventricular fibrillation. *Archives of Surgery*, **105**, 36

Warshaw, A.L. and O'Hara, P.J. (1978) Susceptibility of the pancreas to ischaemic injury in shock. *Annals of Surgery*, **188**, 197

Watanabe, T., Orita, H., Kobayashi, M. and Washio, M. (1989) Brain tissue pH, oxygen tension and carbon dioxide tension in profoundly hypothermic cardiopulmonary bypass. *Journal of Thoracic and Cardiovascular Surgery*, **97**, 396

Watkins, L., Jr., Lucas, S.K., Gardner, T.J., *et al.* (1979) Angiotensin II levels during cardiopulmonary bypass: a comparison of pulsatile and nonpulsatile flow. *Surgical Forum*, **30**, 229

Wesolowski, S.A., Sauvage, L.R. and Pinc, R.D. (1955) Extracorporeal circulation: the role of the pulse in maintenance of the systemic circulation during heart-lung bypass. *Surgery*, **37**, 663

Wilkens, H., Regelson, W. and Hoffmeister, F.S. (1962) The physiologic importance of pulsatile blood flow. *New England Journal of Medicine*, **267**, 443

Williams, G.D., Callaway, J.K., Seifen, A.B., *et al.* (1979a) Repair of Swiss cheese ventricular septal defect utilizing core cooling with pulsatile bypass and hypothermic arrest. *Fifteenth Annual Meeting of the Society of Thoracic Surgeons*, Phoenix, Arizona

Williams, G.D., Seifen, A.B., Lawson, N.W., *et al.* (1979b) Pulsatile perfusion v. conventional high flow non-pulsatile perfusion for rapid core cooling and rewarming of infants for circulatory arrest in cardiac operation. *Journal of Thoracic and Cardiovascular Surgery*, **78**, 667

Wright, G. and Sanderson, J.M. (1972) Brain damage and mortality in dogs following pulsatile and non-pulsatile blood flow in extracorporeal circulation. *Thorax*, **27**, 738

Wright, G., Sanderson, J.M. and Furness, A. (1978) Pulsatile pumps for open-heart surgery. *Lancet*, **i**, 217

17

Low flow and circulatory arrest

P.H. Kay

Cardiopulmonary bypass is a technique employed by surgical teams with their attendant anaesthetist and perfusionists to allow the surgeon to operate safely on the heart. During the periods of the operation when the heart is not ejecting normally the perfusionist uses the heart–lung machine to take over the role of these two vital organs in providing an adequate supply of oxygenated blood to the tissues of the body.

A perfusion flow rate of 2.4 l min^{-1} m^{-2} is maintained at the commencement and completion of cardiopulmonary bypass when the temperature is in the normal range (Jynge *et al.*, 1978). However during the cardiac procedure the flow rate may be reduced to improve operating conditions for the surgeon.

Low flow cardiopulmonary bypass

Michenfelder and Theyer (1968) found that moderate hypothermia to 28°C reduced tissue oxygen requirements by 50%. Further reduction in core temperature to 25°C in turn reduced tissue oxygen consumption to 33% of normal. Anaesthesia, muscle relaxation, and positive pressure ventilation further reduce oxygen requirements. In addition, the coronary circulation, which normally takes 6–8% of the cardiac output is excluded from the circulation provided by the heart–lung machine during the period of aortic cross clamping. Thus, it has been argued by Belcher and Lennox (1985) that it should be possible to reduce the flow on cardiopulmonary bypass by up to 50% at 28°C and still maintain an adequate safety margin. This concept was supported by Fox and co-workers (1982) who found that a flow of 1.2 l min^{-1} m^{-2} at 20°C was adequate for short periods in man, but cautioned against its use because of limited reserves. The main advantage of this manipulation in flow is a reduction in flow through the bronchial coronary collaterals, warming the heart and washing out the cardioplegia (Conti *et al.*, 1978).

Adequacy of cardiopulmonary bypass

During periods of low flow cardiopulmonary bypass it is essential to assess whether or not the prescribed flow is adequate to meet tissue requirements.

In terms of overall function metabolic indices are probably the most valuable. As the fundamental role of cardiopulmonary bypass is to provide oxygenated blood to the tissues Kirklin and Kirklin (1981) studied mixed venous oxygen levels during cardiopulmonary bypass. They found that a mixed venous oxygen level of 30 mmHg, corresponding to a saturation of 60%, was consistent with a normal convalescence. Techniques of monitoring this have now improved with the introduction of continuous in-line monitoring of blood gases in both the arterial (reflecting provision) and venous (reflecting uptake) lines throughout the period of cardiopulmonary bypass.

However safety relying on adequate metabolic indices assumes a uniformity of blood flow to the tissues. To be sure that a given organ is receiving an adequate blood supply it is necessary to study the function of that organ during cardiopulmonary bypass. In general the brain is regarded as the most sensitive organ and therefore at most risk from inadequate perfusion. Two problems however emerge: there is no adequate diagnostic tool continuously to monitor cerebral function during cardiopulmonary bypass; multiple factors are involved in the aetiology of cerebral injury which may become apparent after cardiopulmonary bypass.

Branthwaite (1973) recommended the use of the cerebral function monitor to assess adequacy of the cerebral perfusion. Bolsin (1986) founds its derivative, the cerebral function analysis monitor (CFAM) to be useful in detecting major problems with cerebral blood flow, e.g. those arising from inadequate placement of the aortic cannula. However there is no evidence regarding the benefit of the CFAM in more subtle situations. Furthermore Salerno and colleagues (1978) highlighted the problems of cerebral assessment in the presence of anaesthesia, hypothermia and haemodilution.

Experimental studies

Thus the safety of cerebral perfusion, and therefore it is assumed the perfusion of all other organs, relies principally on experience gleaned from animal and human studies.

Paneth (1957) working with dogs at normothermia showed that cerebral oxygen consumption was uniform at flows above 1.2 l min^{-1} m^{-2}. Fox, Blackstone and Kirklin (1984) performed an elegant series of experiments on cynomolous monkeys, chosen because they have the same circle of Willis cerebral circulation as man. He found that cerebral perfusion continued to all areas of the brain with the flow reduced to 0.25 l min^{-1} m^{-2}. This autoregulation resulted from an increase in systemic vascular resistance while the cerebral vascular resistance remained unchanged, with proportionate increase in the brain:body flow ratio. Furthermore, cerebral oxygen extraction increased as the flow was reduced from 2.4 l min^{-1} m^{-2} to 1.2 l min^{-1} m^{-2}, with the result that the cerebral oxygen consumption remained unchanged.

With these experimental studies in mind further workers have determined safe limits for various perfusion parameters during periods of low flow. Govier and colleagues (1984) measuring cerebral blood flow with xenon-133 clearance showed that temperature and arterial carbon dioxide concentrations were the only significant factors affecting the cerebral circulation in man at flows in the range of 1.0–2.0 l min^{-1} m^{-2}. Both Govier (1984) and Wollman *et al.* (1966) found no correlation between cerebral blood flow and mean arterial pressure. However Hendricksen, Hjelms and Lindeburgh (1983) suggested that this autoregulation was only effective at mean arterial pressures greater than 55 mmHg.

Low flow technique

Thus, there is much evidence to support the safe reduction of perfusion flow rate during periods of moderate hypothermia (25–28°C) to a level of 1.2 l min^{-1} m^{-2} providing that attention is paid to perfusion pressure and metabolic indices. In our patients mean arterial pressure is maintained at 60 mmHg with use of vasoconstrictors (0.5 mg aliquots of phenylephrine) or vasodilators (0.5 mg aliquots of phentolamine). Arterial partial pressure of carbon dioxide is maintained in the range 4.2–5.6 kPa by adjusting the flow of the sweep gas (100% oxygen). Fall in mixed venous oxygen saturation below 60% is immediately followed by an increase in flow rate until mixed venous oxygen rises above 30 mmHg (4 kPa).

This technique provides excellent operating conditions and myocardial protection but must be used with caution in patients with known impairment of the cerebral circulation.

Total circulatory arrest

As a logical extension to the concept of low flow during periods of hypothermia it is both theoretically and practically possible to achieve safe periods of total circulatory arrest during relatively short periods of profound hypothermia. This technique is particularly applicable to neonates and young infants undergoing repair of congenital heart defects requiring cardiopulmonary bypass.

History

In 1950 Bigelow, Lindsay and Greenwood reported full recovery of dogs undergoing 15 min of total circulatory arrest at 20°C by surface cooling. Three years later Lewis and Taufic (1953) successfully repaired an atrioseptal defect in a 5-year-old child using surface cooling. In 1958 this technique was successfully combined with cardiopulmonary bypass (Sealy, Brown and Young, 1958). In 1961 Kirklin *et al.* reported excellent results from the Mayo Clinic in 52 patients using profound hypothermia and circulatory arrest. Subsequently this technique has been widely accepted for infants requiring cardiopulmonary bypass for the correction of congenital heart defects. In infants the profound hypothermia may be achieved either by a combination of surface cooling followed by a short period of cardiopulmonary bypass (Barrett-Boyes *et al.*, 1976) or simply cardiopulmonary bypass alone.

Technique of circulatory arrest in paediatric cardiac surgery

At the Brompton Hospital surface cooling with circulatory arrest is the method of choice for the majority of infants under the weight of 8 kg undergoing intracardiac repair of congenital heart defects. Following introduction of anaesthesia the infant is placed on a water mattress insulated at this stage by a dry towel. Because of the sluggish nature of the circulation it is essential to give the heparin before the cooling phase is induced. Water at 1°C is circulated through the mattress. Bags of ice are then placed over the chest and flanks and around the head. The patient's temperature is reduced to 25°C (nasopharyngeal) by this method. The chest is then opened routinely through a median sternotomy incision and cardiopulmonary bypass is established between a single atrial cannula and the ascending aorta. There is a small risk of ventricular fibrillation during the cooling phase. In such event cardiopulmonary bypass should be rapidly but unhurriedly established. Following the onset of cardiopulmonary bypass further cooling to 15°C is achieved. At this stage the circulation is stopped and the patient drained of blood. The venous cannula is then removed from the right atrium and the intracardiac repair performed. It has generally been assumed that a period of 35–40 min of circulatory arrest is safe using this technique (Ekroth *et al.*, 1989). This is satisfactory for operations such as the correction of ventricular septal defect, tetralogy of Fallot, and atrioventricular canal. However for more complex procedures such as arterial switch operations or correction of truncus arteriosus cardiopulmonary bypass is established with two caval cannulae and periods of circulatory arrest are interspersed with low flow cardiopulmonary bypass (Rossi *et al.*, 1989).

Following completion of the intracardiac repair the patient is re-warmed. The temperature of fluid in the water mattress is increased from 15°C to 40°C. The heat exchanger is adjusted to maintain a 10°C gradient between the temperature of the blood leaving the heat exchanger and the nasopharyngeal temperature until the temperature of the blood leaving the heat exchanger is at 38°C. After an interval of 20–30 min when the nasopharyngeal temperature has reached 35°C and the rectal temperature 28°C bypass is discontinued providing the heart action is satisfactory.

Safe duration of circulatory arrest

A safe period of total circulatory arrest is one in which there is no subsequent detectable loss of organ structure or function during postoperative period. This safe period is related to the degree of hypothermia during the arrest period. The aim is to reduce metabolic activity within the cells to permit cellular metabolism without complete exhaustion of cellular reserves. These have not been measured directly but oxygen consumption has been used as a marker of metabolic activity. At physiological temperatures biochemical systems obey van't Hoffs law. This relates the logarithm of the rate of chemical reaction directly to the temperature. Bigelow *et al.* (1950) working with animals showed that increase in temperature of 10°C (Q_{10}) increased the reaction rate by a power of between two and three. Similarly Harris (1973) estimated Q_{10} to lie between 1.9 and 4.2 in ten surface cooled infants. Even at 15°C, the usual temperature chosen for circulatory arrest, metabolic activity continues and therefore the safe period of circulatory arrest must be finite.

Damaging effects of total circulatory arrest

Again the brain is the most critical organ and therefore has the shortest 'safe' circulatory arrest time. Clearly other organs such as the kidneys and liver may suffer from periods of prolonged circulatory arrest but their 'safe' times appear to be generally longer than those of the brain.

Animal studies

Folkerth and colleagues (1975) showed no functional or structural brain abnormalities in dogs undergoing 30 min of total circulatory arrest at 20°C. Kramer *et al.* (1968) showed that adenosine triphosphate (ATP) concentrations in the brain fell to 34% of control values after 30 min of total circulatory arrest at an oesophageal temperature of 5°C (cerebral cortical temperature 13°C) produced by 50 min of cooling on cardiopulmonary bypass. The concentrations rapidly returned to normal after restoration of the circulation. This concept of a 30 min safe period is also supported by Treasure *et al.* (1983) who found no evidence of structural or cerebral damage in gerbils undergoing circulatory arrest at 18°C. However damage was detected when circulatory periods were extended beyond 45 min. Furthermore the probability of cerebral damage appeared to increase with increasing circulatory arrest time.

Little work has been done to establish whether hypothermia alone is damaging to the brain. However Wolin, Massopust and White (1973) showed that a 30 min period of continuous cold perfusion at 15°C in trained rhesus monkeys had no effect on intellectual performance.

EEG studies

Electroenchephalographic (EEG) studies in humans show that during cooling there is a gradual disappearance in the fast component of the EEG and an increase in slow components. When circulatory arrest is established EEG activity disappears within 2 min. On re-warming using cardiopulmonary bypass EEG activity remains absent for several minutes but gradually returns to normal after a period of 20–30 min of re-warming. This initial latent period varies with the duration of the arrest period and the temperature and almost certainly relates to repayment of the oxygen debt (Weiss *et al.*, 1960).

Human studies

There is a small but definite incidence of cerebral damage following the use of profound hypothermia circulatory arrest in infants. At the most severe end of the spectrum Stewart, Blackstone and Kirklin (1981) reported severe brain damage in 1% of infants undergoing repair of common types of congenital heart disease with profound hypothermia and circulatory arrest. In all these cases the circulatory arrest time was greater than 45 minutes and core cooling alone was used.

The more common neurological complications of circulatory arrest are choreoathetosis or epileptic fits. Choreoathetosis has been reported as occurring in between 2% (Stewart, Blackstone and Kirklin, 1981) and 15% (Bergouignan *et al.*, 1961) of children using this technique. The choreiform movements normally develop 2–3 days post operatively and have varying degrees of resolution.

Epileptic fits occur in 5–10% of patients undergoing total circulatory arrest. In the majority of cases these are transient and followed by an uneventful recovery. Their aetiology is complex. In addition to the circulatory arrest disturbances in thermoregulation, fluid balance and metabolic disorders may play a role particularly in infants who are already prone to seizures as a result of underlying cerebral pathology.

Intellectual impairment

Though the above major problems appear to occur in only a relatively small percentage of patients undergoing hypothermic circulatory arrest more sophisticated changes involving intellectual impairment may be more widespread. Clarkson *et al.* (1980) reporting the Green Lane Hospital, Auckland, experience showed a mean IQ of 93 in 72 patients undergoing profoundly hypothermic total circulatory arrest compared with an IQ of 106 in a control group. However the study group was weighted by a group of infants with low birthweight or important preoperative neurological problems. Once these had been removed from the circulatory arrest group there were no differences from the controls. Similarly, both Haka-Ikse, Blackwood and Steward (1980) and Messmer and colleagues (1976) found no evidence of long term psychomotor problems.

However, Wells *et al.* (1983) at the Brompton Hospital studying intellectual and psychological development in infants who had undergone total circulatory arrest with profound hypothermia found that their siblings, without congenital heart disease, had a higher intelligence quotient that that of the patient group. Furthermore there was an an inverse relationship between arrest time and intelligence quotient.

Though the above figures suggest a low incidence of cerebral dysfunction after total circulatory arrest we should not be too complacent in our acceptance of this particular technique. Studies from Newcastle show that even patients undergoing straightforward adult coronary artery surgery without opening the heart, have a high incidence of dysfunction in the immediate postoperative period (Shaw, Bates and Cartlidge, 1986). The brain is a highly sensitive organ with a large amount of spare capacity. The incidence of damage will almost certainly reflect how hard damage is looked for. Fortunately the brain's large spare capacity appears to compensate well for the neuronal damage sustained and much of the intellectual deficit recovers (Smith, Treasure and Newman, 1986).

Aetiology of cerebral damage

The causes of cerebral damage in patients undergoing open heart surgery are myriad. These have been fully explored in Chapter 13. However certain specific causes relate to the technique of profound hypothermia and circulatory arrest.

It is apparent that uniform cooling is important. Weiss and colleagues (1960) have shown persisting EEG activity in the white matter and cerebellum producing choreoathetosis in patients who have undergone uneven cooling. This in turn almost certainly reflects a high level of continuing metabolic activity and is thought to be the principle cause of choreoathetosis (Reilly, Brunberg and Doty, 1974). The incidence of this complication may be reduced by the use of surface cooling followed by a short period of final core cooling. This appears to produce a far more even cooling of the cerebral structures than when cooling is done on bypass alone.

A second important concept is the loss of cerebral pressure–flow autoregulation with deep hypothermia (Greely *et al.*, 1989). Cerebral reperfusion after deep hypothermia and circulatory arrest is impaired compared with patients in whom the circulation has been maintained throughout. This may be due to sludging and occlusion of cerebral capillaries in certain areas.

Finally biochemical disturbances appear to have an important role in the aetiology of cerebral damage. Ekroth and co-workers (1989) using creatinine kinase BB concentrations in jugular venous blood as an indicator of cerebral damage showed that there was a strong positive correlation between creatinine kinase BB release and arrest time, pH and blood glucose level. This in turn suggests that improved control of hyperglycaemia may improve cerebral protection.

Circulatory arrest in adults

Crawford (1989) has successfully used the technique of circulatory arrest in adults undergoing replacement of the ascending aorta and/or aortic arch. In such cases the aetiology is either acute dissection or chronic aneurysm formation.

Cardiopulmonary bypass is established between the right atrium and a femoral artery. The patients are cooled on cardiopulmonary bypass to a temperature 3°C below that at which the EEG becomes isoelectric (Coselli *et al.*, 1988). The heart is then protected with cold cardioplegia. Due to extreme friability of the tissues the most difficult part of the operation is normally the completion of the distal anastomosis. Bypass is discontinued and the venous line left open. With the distal aorta left unclamped (Cooley and Livesay, 1981) the distal anastomosis and arch repair are completed as the first procedure. In Crawford's series this required a median circulatory arrest time of 31 min. A clamp is then placed on the graft and the circulation re-established allowing the head vessels to be perfused. The proximal anastomosis is then completed. Using this technique in 401 patients between 1980 and 1989 Crawford has been able to achieve the remarkable figures of a 10% mortality and 63% 5-year survival.

Summary

Clearly circulatory arrest is a most useful technique in cardiac surgery providing optimal conditions for the surgeon in the difficult circumstances of complex intracardiac repair of congenital heart defects in small children or repair of friable aortic tissue in adults. With greater understanding of its limitations, particularly the safe arrest period, and improved cerebral protection with drugs such as propofol it has become an important part of the armamentarium of the cardiac surgeon, anaesthetist and perfusionist.

References

Barratt-Boyes, R.G., Neutz, J.M., Clarkson, P., *et al.* (1976) Repair of ventricular septal defect in the first two years of life using profound hypothermic circulatory arrest techniques. *Annals of Surgery*, **184**, 376

Belcher, P. and Lennox, S.C. (1985) The effects of low flow, low pressure pulsatile bypass. *Journal of Cardiovascular Surgery*, **26**, 223–227

Bergouignan, M., Fontan, F., Trarieux, M. and Julien, J. (1961) Syndromes choreiformes de l'enfant au decours d'interventions cardiochirugicals sans hypothermie profonde. *Revue Neurologique*, (Paris) **105**, 48*

Bigelow, W.G., Lindsay, W.K. and Greenwood, W.F. (1950) Hypothermia–its possible role in cardiac surgery: an investigation of factors governing survival in dogs at low body temperatures. *Annals of Surgery*, **132**, 849

Bolsin, S. (1986) Detention of neurological damage during cardiopulmonary bypass. *Anaesthesia*, **41**, 61–66

Branthwaite, M.A. (1973) Detection of neurological damage during open heart surgery. *Thorax*, **28**, 464–472

Brunberg, J.A., Reilly, E.L. and Doty, D.B. (1973) Central nervous system consequences in infants of cardiac surgery using deep hypothermia and circulatory arrest. *Circulation*, **49 50** (Suppl 2), 11

Clarkson, P.M., MacArthur, B.A., Barratt-Boyes, B.G. *et al.* (1980) Developmenta; progress following cardiac surgery in infancy using profound hypothermia and circulatory arrest. *Circulation*, **62**, 855

Conti, V., Bertranou, E., Blackstone, E., *et al.* (1978) Cold cardioplegia versus hypothermia for myocardial protection. *Journal of Thoracic and Cardiovascular Surgery*, **76**, 577–589

Cooley, D.A. and Livesay, J.J. (1981) Technique of open distal anastomosis for ascending and transverse arch resection. *Bulletin of the Texas Heart Institute*, **198**, 421–426

Coselli, J.S., Crawford, E.S., Beall, A.C., *et al.* (1988) Determination of brain temperatures for safe circulatory arrest during cardiovascular operation. *Annals of Thoracic Surgery*, **45**, 638–642

Crawford, E.S., Svensson, L.G., Coselli, J.S., *et al.* (1989) Surgical treatment of aneurysm and/or dissection of the ascending aorta, transverse aortic arch, and descending aorta and transverse aortic arch. Factors influencing survival in 717 patients. *Journal of Thoracic and Cardiovascular Surgery*, **98**, 659–674

Ekroth, R., Thompson, R.J., Lincoln, C., *et al.* (1989) Elective deep hypothermia with total circulatory arrest changes in creatinine kinase BB, blood glucose and clinical variables. *Journal of Thoracic and Cardiovascular Surgery*, **97**, 30–35

Folkerth, T.L., Angell, W.W., Fosburg, R.G. and Oury, J.H. (1975) Effect of deep hypothermia, limited cardiopulmonary bypass and total arrest on growing puppies. In *Recent Advances in Studies on Cardiac Structure and Metabolism*, **10**, 411–421, Baltimore: University Park

Fox, L., Blackstone, E. and Kirklin, J. (1984) Relationship of brain blood flow and oxygen consumption to perfusion flow rate during profoundly hypothermic cardiopulmonary bypass: an experimental study. *Journal of Thoracic and Cardiovascular Surgery*, **87**, 658–664

Fox, L., Blackstone, E., Kirklin, J., *et al.* (1982) Relationship of whole body oxygen consumption to perfusion flow rate during hypothermic cardiopulmonary bypass. *Journal of Thoracic and Cardiovascular Surgery*, **83**, 239–248

Govier, A., Reves, J., McKay, R., *et al.* (1984) Factors and their influence on regional cerebral blood flow during non-pulsatile cardiopulmonary bypass. *Annals of Thoracic Surgery*, **38**, 592–600

Greely, W.J., Ungerleder, R.M., Smith, L.R. and Reves, J.G. (1989) The effects of deep hypothermic cardiopulmonary bypass and total circulatory arrest on cerebral blood flow in infants and children. *Journal of Thoracic and Cardiovascular Surgery*, **97**, 737–745

Haka-Ikse, K., Blackwood, M.J.A. and Steward, D.J. (1980) Psychomotor development of infants and children after profound hypothermia during surgery for congenital heart disease. *Developments in Medical Child Neurology*, **20**, 62

Harris, E.A. (1973) Metabolic effects of profound hypothermia. In *Heart Disease in Infancy* (eds B. Barratt-Boyes, J.M. Neutz and E.A. Harris), Williams and Wilkins, Baltimore, p. 65.

Hendricksen, L., Hjelms, E. and Lindeburgh, T. (1983) Brain hyperfusion during cardiac operations. *Journal of Thoracic and Cardiovascular Surgery*, **86**, 202–206

Jynge, P., Hearse, D., de Leiris, J., *et al.* (1978) Protection of the ischaemic myocardium. *Journal of Thoracic and Cardiovascular Surgery*, **76**, 2–15

Kirklin, J.W., Dawson, B., Devloo, Ra and Theye, R.A. (1961) Open intracardiac operations in the use of circulatory arrest during hypothermia induced by blood cooling. *Annals of Surgery*, **154**, 769

Kirklin, J.K. and Kirklin, J.W. (1981) Management of the cardiovascular system after cardiac surgery. *Annals of Thoracic Surgery*, **32**, 311–319

Kramer, R.S., Saunders, A.P., Lesage, A.M., *et al.* (1968) The effect of profound hypothermia on preservation of cerebral ATP content during circulatory arrest. *Journal of Thoracic and Cardiovascular Surgery*, **56**, 699

Lewis, F.S. and Taufic, M. (1953) Closure of atrial septal defects with the aid of hypothermia. Experimental accomplishments and the report of one successful case. *Surgery*, **33**, 52

Messmer, B.J., Schallberger, U., Gattiker, R. and Senning, A. (1976) Psychomotor and intellectual development after deep hypothermia and circulatory arrest in infancy. *Journal of Thoracic and Cardiovascular Surgery*, **72**, 495

Michenfelder, J. and Theye, R. (1968) Hypothermia: effect on canine brain and whole body metabolism. *Anaesthesiology*, **29**, 1107–1112

Panneth, M., Sellers, R., Gott, V., *et al.* (1957) Physiologic studies upon prolonged cardiopulmonary bypass with the pump oxygenator with particular reference to (1) acid base balance (2) siphon caval drainage. *Journal of Thoracic and Cardiovascular Surgery*, **34**, 570–579

Reilly, E.L., Brunberg, J.A. and Doty, D.B. (1974) The effect of deep hypothermia and total circulatory arrest on the encephalogram in children. *Clinical Neurophysiology*, **36**, 661

Rossi, R., Linden, J., Ekroth, R., *et al.* (1989) No flow or low flow? A study of the ischaemic marker creatinine kinase BB after deep hypothermic procedures. *Journal of Thoracic and Cardiovascular Surgery*, **98**, 193–199

Salerno, T.A., Linc, D.P., White, D.N., *et al.* (1978) Monitoring of the electroencephalogram during open heart surgery. *Journal of Thoracic and Cardiovascular Surgery*, **76**, 97–100

Sealy, W.C., Brown, I.W. and Young, W.G. (1958) A report on the use of both extracorporeal circulation and hypothermia for open heart surgery. *Annals of Surgery*, **147**, 603

Shaw, P.J., Bates, D. and Cartlidge, N.E. (1986) Early intellectual dysfunction following coronary bypass surgery. *Quarterly Journal of Medicine*, **58**, 59–68

Smith, P.L., Treasure, T. and Newman, S.P. (1986) Cerebral consequences of cardiopulmonary bypass. *Lancet*, **i**, 823–825

Stewart, R.W., Blackstone, E.H. and Kirklin, J.W. (1981) Neurological dysfunction after cardiac surgery. In *Congenital Heart Disease in the first three months of life. Medical and Surgical Aspects.* (eds L. Parenzan, G. Grupi and G. Graham), Patron Editore, Bologna, Italy, p. 431

Treasure, T., Naftel, D.C., Conger, K.A., *et al.* (1983) The effect of hypothermic circulatory arrest time on cerebral function, morphology and biochemistry. *Journal of Thoracic and Cardiovascular Surgery*, **86**, 761

Weiss, M., Piwnica, A., Lenfant, C., *et al.* (1960) Deep hypothermia with total circulatory arrest. *Transactions of the American Society for Artificial Internal Organs*, **6**, 227

Wells, F.C., Coghill, S., Caplan, H.L., *et al.* (1983) Duration of circulatory arrest does influence the psychological development of children after cardiac operation in early life. *Journal of Thoracic and Cardiovascular Surgery*, **86**, 823

Wolin, L.R., Massopust, L.C. and White, R.J. (1973) Behavioural effects of autocerebral perfusion hypothermia and arrest of cerebral blood flow in the rhesus monkey. *Experiments in Neurology*, **39**, 336

Wollman, H., Stephen, G., Clement, A. and Danileson, G. (1966) Cerebral blood flow in man during extracorporeal circulation. *Journal of Thoracic and Cardiovascular Surgery*, **52**, 558–564

18

Intra-aortic balloon counterpulsation

Michael Kesselbrenner, Jeffrey B. Sack, Robert A. Saporito, Jr and David Bregman

Introduction and historical background

The intra-aortic balloon pump (IABP) is currently the most widely used temporary circulatory assist device. The concept of counterpulsation, which is the basic physiological principle underlying intra-aortic balloon pumping, was first described by Harken in 1958, and, as originally proposed, involved the removal of blood via the femoral route from the arterial tree during ventricular systole and the rapid reinfusion of the same blood during diastole to increase coronary perfusion pressure. By this method, in the normotensive preparation, one could decrease the work of the left ventricle and increase coronary blood flow (Braunwald *et al.*, 1969). Further pioneering work was done by Kantrowitz (Kantrowitz and McKinnon, 1958; Kantrowitz, 1969), who surmised that poor left ventricle indices could be improved by retarding the diastolic pressure.

The initial concept was well received and several investigators reported some success with its clinical application (Jacoby *et al.*, 1963; Jacoby *et al.*, 1968; Rosenweig, Chatterjee and Merino, 1970; Sugg *et al.*, 1970). However, the initial devices used for counterpulsation had several drawbacks: (1) the excessive turbulence caused by rapid withdrawal and reinfusion of the blood caused appreciable haemolysis and therefore limited the duration of clinical applicability; (2) either bilateral femoral arteriotomies or a subclavain arteriotomy was required for the procedure; (3) it had been shown by Dormandy, Goetz and Kripke (1965) that counterpulsation via the femoral route in the hypotensive state does not increase coronary blood flow. Because of these drawbacks, other investigators chose to apply the principle of counterpulsation in another, unique fashion.

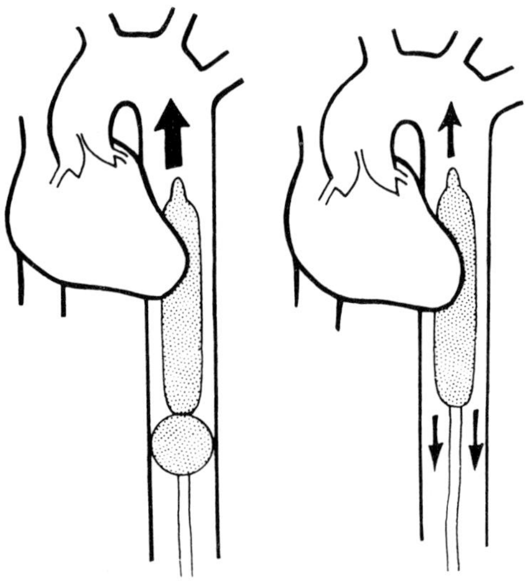

Figure 18.1 Intra-aortic balloon pumping action of omnidirectional (single-chambered) versus unidirectional (dual-chambered) balloons

Moulopoulos, Topas and Kolff in 1962 (a and b), suggested the use of a single-chambered intra-aortic balloon positioned in the descending thoracic aorta to accomplish the same purpose of counterpulsation, but without the drawbacks of earlier methods used. The balloon is inflated in diastole concurrent with closure of the aortic valve, and is held in inflation until the onset of ventricular systole. With the onset of ventricular systole, the balloon is rapidly deflated. The inflation of the balloon displaces blood in the aorta (by an amount equal to the volume of the balloon) towards the coronary tree, thereby augmenting coronary perfusion pressure and blood flow. The collapse of the balloon creates a reduction in impedance to left ventricular ejection (i.e. decreased afterload), and consequently reduces left ventricular work (Corday *et al.*, 1970).

In 1968, Adrian Kantrowitz introduced the intra-aortic balloon pump to the clinical setting of cardiogenic shock. Careful follow-up of such patients showed that mortality remained largely unaltered (Bregman *et al.*, 1977). However, the findings that counterpulsation decreases the extent and severity of ischaemic injury (Nachlas and Sieband, 1967; Feola, Limet and Glick, 1971; Weber and Janicki, 1974; Gold *et al.*, 1976; Johnson *et al.*, 1977b) and opens dormant coronary vessels (Gold *et al.*, 1976), suggested that perhaps counterpulsation ought to be applied in patients sustaining uncomplicated myocardial infarction. This then could minimize the quantity of myocardium that ultimately became necrotic (Maroko *et al.*, 1972), theoretically preserving left ventricular function.

The applications and indications for intra-aortic balloon pumping have come a long way since the early days of counterpulsation. At present, the intra-aortic balloon pump is widely used for circulatory support with post-operative left ventricular failure, unstable angina pectoris refractory to medical treatment, recurring myocardial ischaemia in the setting of acute myocardial infarction, as well as refractory congestive heart failure and recurrent ventricular arrhythmia. We have seen increasing use of intra-aortic balloon counterpulsation in the paediatric population, as a bridge to cardiac transplantation, and for prophylactic use during high-risk percutaneous transluminal coronary angioplasty. The intra-aortic balloon is now also used at times once thought relatively contraindicated, such as patients with acute myocardial infarction who have received thrombolytic therapy.

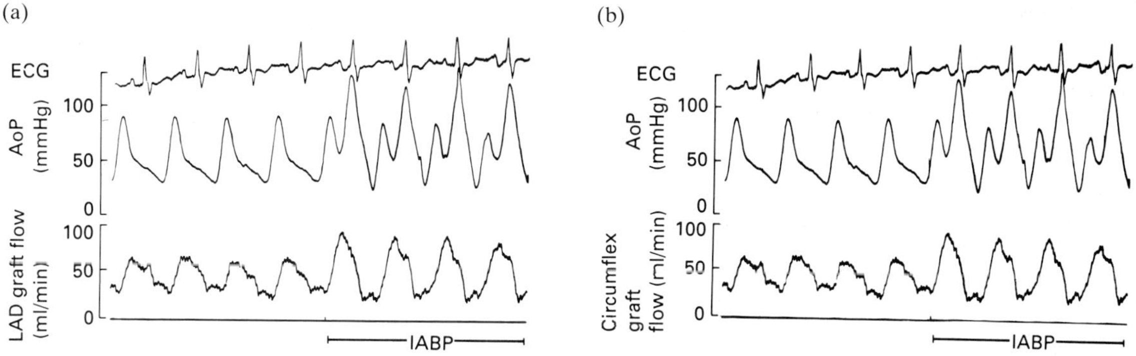

Figures 18.2a and b Dual chambered IABP assistance in a patient after aortocoronary bypass graft surgery. AoP = aortic artery pressure; DA = diastolic augmentation; LAD = left anterior descending coronary artery; RCA = right coronary artery; IABP = periods of IABP assist. Flows were measured with a square-wave electromagnetic flowmeter. With patient assisted every other beat, note the 100% increase in (a) LAD and (b) circumflex graft flows during diastole. Tracing speed: 25 mm^{-1}

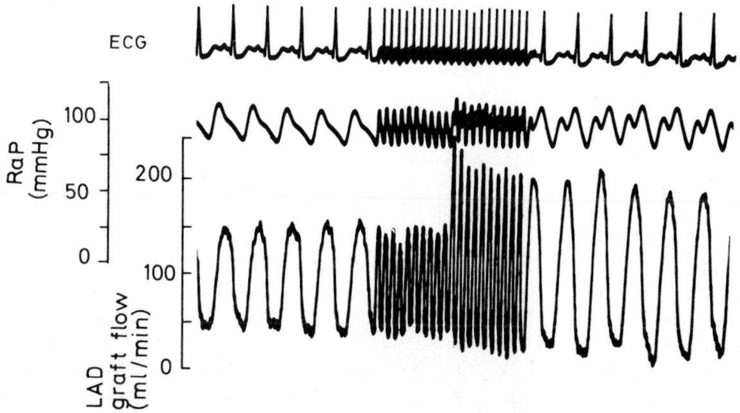

Figure 18.3 Note doubling of LAD graft flow during the period of assistance with the dual-chambered IABP in a patient after coronary reconstructive surgery. Tracing speeds: 25 mm s^{-1} and 10 mm s^{-1}. See legend for Figure 18.2

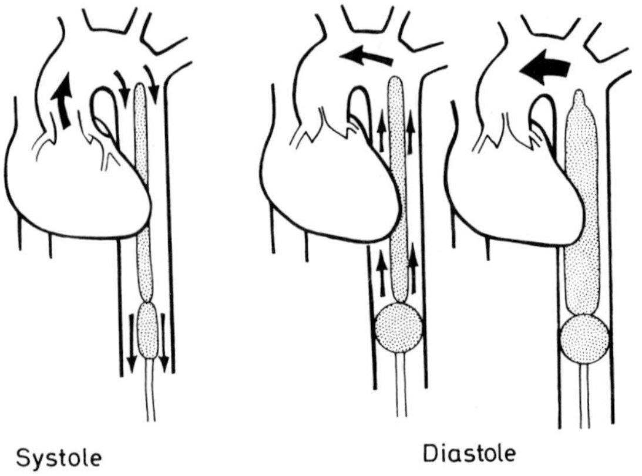

Figure 18.4 Mechanism of action of the dual-chambered intra-aortic balloon. The distal spherical balloon inflates slightly earlier in diastole and phasically obstructs aortic flow. The larger cylindrical proximal balloon then directs blood flow unidirectionally towards the aortic root. Both balloons are then completely deflated by an active vacuum just before ventricular ejection, markedly reducing the afterload against which the left ventricle must work.

Principles

The principle of counterpulsation is based upon the assumption that the reduction of end-diastolic pressure will improve left ventricular function. This is accomplished with improved stroke volume as created by the balloon. The balloon is positioned in the proximal descending thoracic aorta (*see* Figure 18.4). During diastole, it is rapidly inflated concurrent with closure of the aortic valve. At the onset of systole, initiated via a sensing electrocardiogram, the balloon is then rapidly deflated. This creates a 'vacuum' effect, decreasing the afterload, thereby augmenting ventricular outflow.

The mechanism of improved haemodynamics is therefore twofold. First, by raising diastolic pressures within the proximal aorta at balloon expansion, coronary perfusion pressure is increased, generating an increased myocardial oxygen supply, with concomitant bolstering of myocardial contractility. Then, with rapid balloon deflation, there is a sudden volume loss within the aorta (proportional to the volume of the balloon), effectively reducing the afterload by which the left ventricle must work against. This decreases myocardial oxygen demand, and at the same time, increases cardiac output at any given level of filling pressure (Berger *et al.*, 1973).

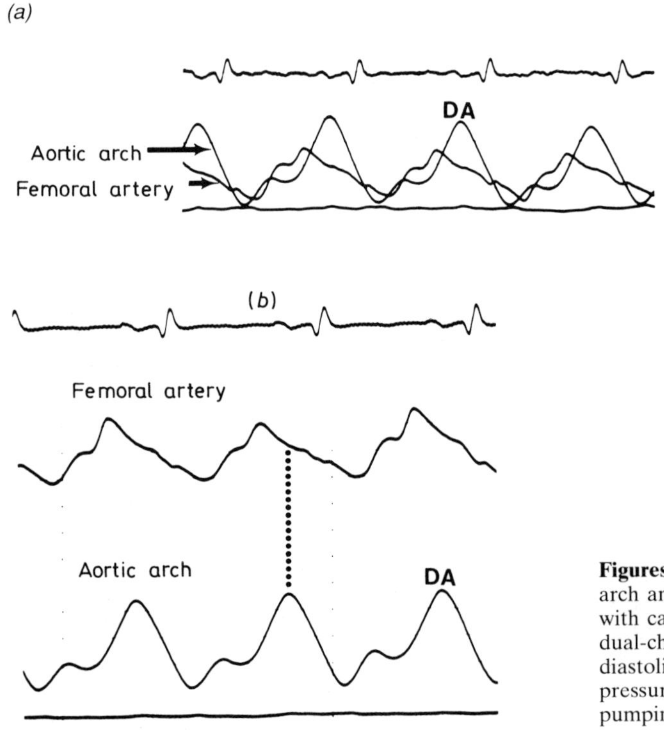

Figures 18.5a and b Simultaneous recordings of aortic arch and femoral artery pressure tracings in a patient with cardiogenic shock undergoing assistance with a dual-chambered IABP. Note the large augmentation of diastolic pressure (DA) obtained in the aortic arch pressure tracing due to unidirectional intra-aortic balloon pumping

The main advantage of the intra-aortic balloon pump over conventional aterioarterial counterpulsation are: (1) circulatory assistance may be maintained at prolonged periods of time without clinically significant haemolysis; (2) a single arterial puncture is required; (3) coronary blood flow is augmented even in the hypotensive state (Talpins, Kripke and Goetz, 1968).

Two additional advantages result from the use of either counterpulsation or intra-aortic balloon pumping: (1) it has been demonstrated by Jacoby *et al.* (1968) that after a short period of counterpulsation, dormant intercoronary collateral beds are opened; and these channels remain open after termination of counterpulsation; (2) it has been demonstrated by several investigators (Cox *et al.*, 1968; Nachlas and Sieband, 1967; Sugg, Webb and Ecker, 1969; Maroko *et al.*, 1972) that early institution of intra-aortic balloon pumping decreases the size of the potential infarction after coronary occlusion.

There is clinical and experimental evidence to demonstrate that the critical factor which improves the performance of the heart suffering from an acute myocardial infarction and power failure is an increase in coronary blood flow (Kuhn, 1970; Kuhn *et al.*, 1970; Kralios *et al.*, 1972; Clayman *et al.*, 1973; Reemtsma *et al.*, 1974). It has also been shown that a major determinant of improved retrograde coronary blood flow is an elevation in the mean aortic diastolic pressure (Brown *et al.*, 1972; Weber, Janicki and Walker, 1972; Gill *et al.*, 1973; Weber and Janicki, 1973; Watson *et al.*, 1973). Under conditions of hypoxaemia, cardiac performance is coronary-flow dependent, and unloading of the left ventricle does not in itself improve myocardial efficiency. Therefore, any method of mechanical assistance should be aimed at maximally increasing coronary blood flow. Years of early work confirmed that this assistance to circulatory performance would decrease the extent and severity of ischaemic injury (Kantrowitz *et al.*, 1968; Nachlas and Sieband, 1967) as well as perfused dormant coronary vessels (Feola, Limet and Glick, 1971) during left ventricular power failure.

Mechanism of balloon action

Our classic device is a unidirectional dual-chambered intra-aortic balloon (Figure 18.1). The balloon has a spherical distal chamber which inflates early in diastole and occludes the aorta. This is sequentially followed by the inflation of a narrower, cylindrical, proximal pumping chamber in the same diastolic interval, which displaces intra-aortic blood entirely (unidirectional) towards the aortic root. Both chambers are completely deflated by an active vacuum just before ventricular ejection.

The action of the dual-chambered balloon in a patient is illustrated in Figure 18.5a. With the onset of inflation of the occluding balloon, a small pressure wave is transmitted to the femoral artery. However, when the occluding balloon is maximally inflated, pumping is entirely unidirectional towards the aortic root. The diastolic augmentation is seen only in the aortic arch tracing and not in the femoral artery tracing. Figure 18.5b illustrates the same physiological principle in another patient.

Effect of intra-aortic balloon pumping on right heart haemodynamics

The haemodynamic effect of intra-aortic balloon pumping on left ventricular performance is well known. Intra-aortic balloon pump support immediately decreases heart rate, left ventricular end-diastolic pressure, and mean left atrial pressure. It

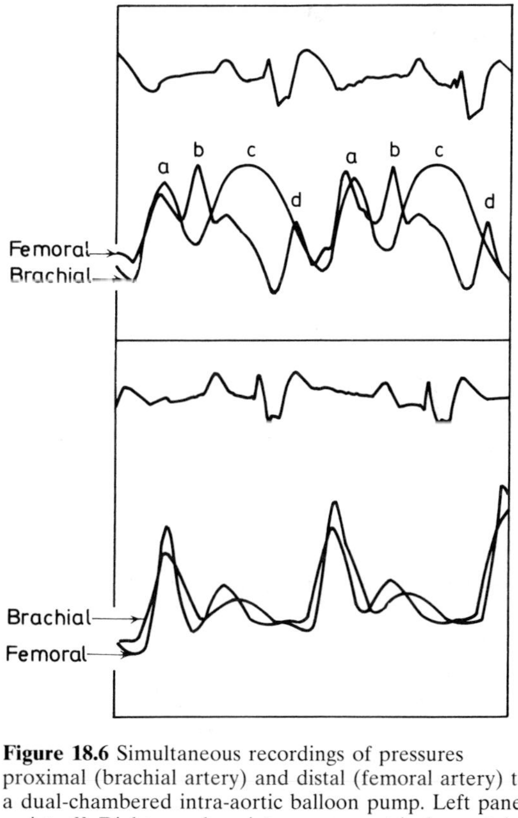

Figure 18.6 Simultaneous recordings of pressures proximal (brachial artery) and distal (femoral artery) to a dual-chambered intra-aortic balloon pump. Left panel: assist off. Right panel: assist on. a = ventricular systole; b = deflection resulting from inflation of occluding balloon in femoral artery tracing–note its absence in brachial artery tracing; c = diastolic augmentation produced by pumping balloon–observe its absence in femoral artery tracing; d = equilibration of brachial and femoral artery pressures with deflation of balloons

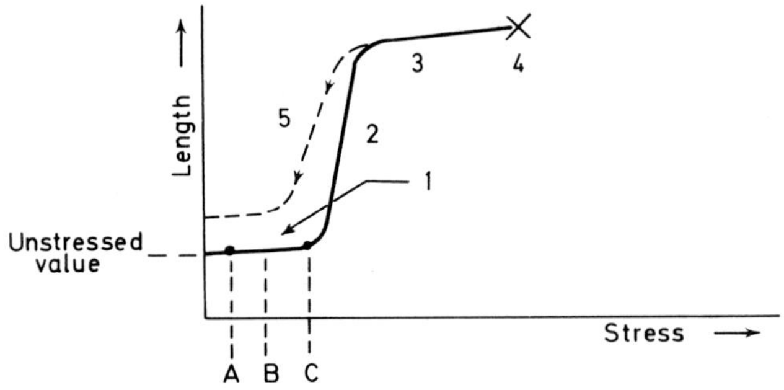

Figure 18.7 Stress/strain characteristics of polyurethane formula in dual-chambered intra-aortic balloon (see text)

also causes a modest increase in cardiac output. Johnson *et al.* (1977) have looked at the effects of intra-aortic balloon pumping on right heart haemodynamics. Implementation of intra-aortic balloon pumping was consistently found to produce an instantaneous decrease in right atrial pressure averaging 11%, reflecting a decrease in preload. In addition, the major determinants of right ventricular afterload were found to decrease significantly. Pulmonary artery pressure decreased 12% on average, and pulmonary vascular resistance decreased 19%. These haemodynamic changes all occurred without a significant change in mean aortic pressure.

Balloon construction and safety

Balloon membrane

The basic dual-chambered balloon is a single-cast tubular membrane of a specially formulated polyurethane polymer. Wall thickness is generally 4–5 mils* and, for a given balloon, is consistent within 0.5 mil over the major wall section. Tapered end sections are slightly thicker to counter additional end stresses. The polyurethane formula utilized has a very non-linear stress characteristic peculiar to the needs of the intra-aortic balloon. Figure 18.7 shows the behaviour of a 4 ml cast of this polyurethane film subjected to increasing stress. In region 1, length changes very little with stress. Region 2 is an elastic zone; the molecular chains, normally folded and entangled, begin to straighten after the stress reaches the threshold value and the material stretches similar to a rubber band. When the chains are fully straightened, the curve then enters a saturation region, 3, and 'locks' at its ultimate length. Sufficient force, at region 4, will break the chain and then cause rupture. The dual-chambered balloon is operated totally within region 1 for several reasons. The obvious reason is that we make use of a safety chamber and utilize only enough gas to 'fill', but not to 'distend', the intra-aortic balloon. Since work equals force times distance, one can see that cyclic forces within region 1 cause very little distance change and, consequently, very little work is expended on the balloon material, resulting in minimal fatigue.

Balloons operated in region 2 will exhibit fatigue as evidenced by the fact that once stretched, the material takes a different return path. In physics, this can be recognized as a rudimentary hysteresis loop in which the energy dissipated is proportional to the loop area. The minor loop in region 1 is virtually non-measurable.

The stretched molecular chains do not fully return to their folded state.

The linkages are weakened, and ultimately they will fail. The stress required to reach point C (all other factors remaining equal) will depend upon the thickness of the polyurethane. The film thickness used, therefore, is determined by the size of the folded balloon when inserted, and by the stress range to keep it within region 1. With a 4 ml film in a typical human dual-chambered balloon, point C is reached at 8–12 p.s.i. (400–600 mmHg) of differential pressure.

Each balloon manufactured is statically and dynamically tested to point B, and the exact value is marked on a quality control sheet accompanying the balloon. For example, a typical value might be 4 p.s.i. (200 mmHg). When the balloon is used with a safety chamber, the peak pressure only reaches point A, usually 1–2 p.s.i. or 50–100 mmHg. The polyurethane formula chosen is a prudent compromise between good folding properties and a low degree of initial distensibility. Over the test range, this formula stretches about 1%. Since the balloon volume varies with the square of the radius (axial stress being less significant in an elongated balloon than radial stress), this is equivalent to 2% variation in volume.

* 1 mil = 0.001 inches (25.4 μm)

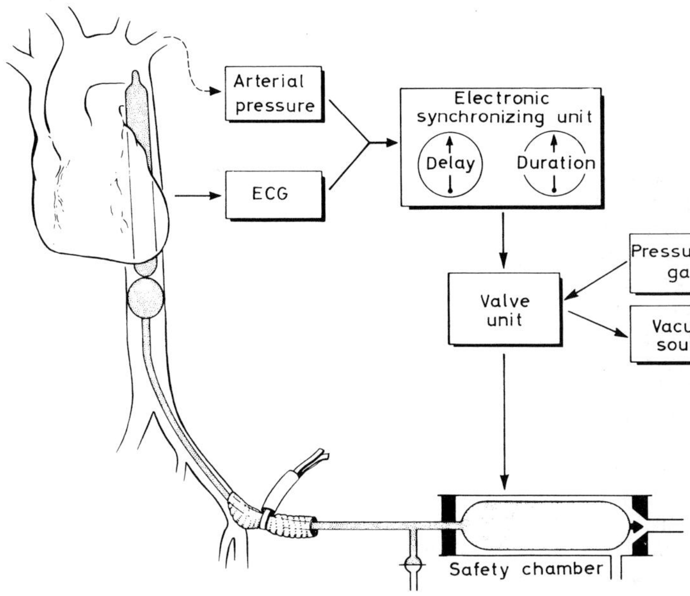

Figure 18.8 Schematic representation of clinical dual-chambered IABP

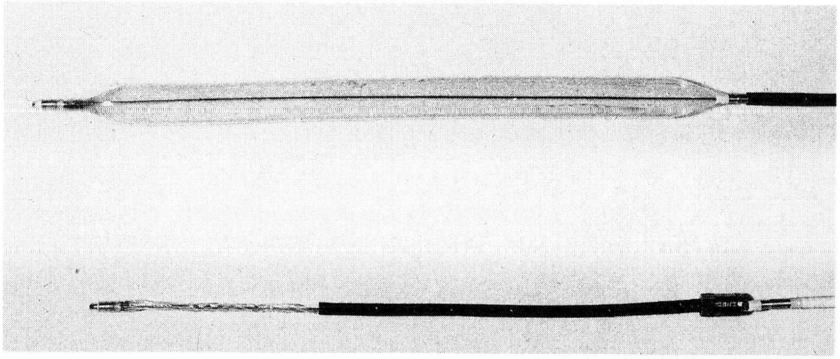

Figure 18.9 Percutaneous balloon (PERCOR[R]) wrapped and unwrapped

Balloon catheter

A one-piece polyurethane catheter is utilized with a 10% radio-opaque filler. Hence the entire catheter is radio-opaque, which aids in proper intra-aortic balloon positioning. In addition, a flexible stainless steel strut has been built into the proximal balloon section to facilitate insertion and to prevent the balloon from folding over upon itself after it has been inserted into the aorta. The basic stiffness of the catheter is such that a stylet is not required for insertion, but the balloon cannot be forced so as to initiate an aortic dissection as has been reported with a more rigid balloon catheter design (Caulfield, Dunkman and Leinbach, 1972).

In the late model percutaneous balloons, the catheter section is replaced by a straight wire that swivels inside the balloon catheter and the balloon membrane. The balloon membrane may be compactly wrapped around the wire enabling easy insertion through a number No. 12 Fr sheath (*see* Figure 18.9). The driving gas enters the balloon at the junction of the catheter and the balloon membrane through a port of entry that is slightly less than No. 12 Fr in size. The balloon membrane is constructed of polyurethane similar to that used in the standard single- and dual-chambered Datascope intra-aortic balloons. The new balloon is currently available in a 40 ml size mounted on a 12 Fr catheter.

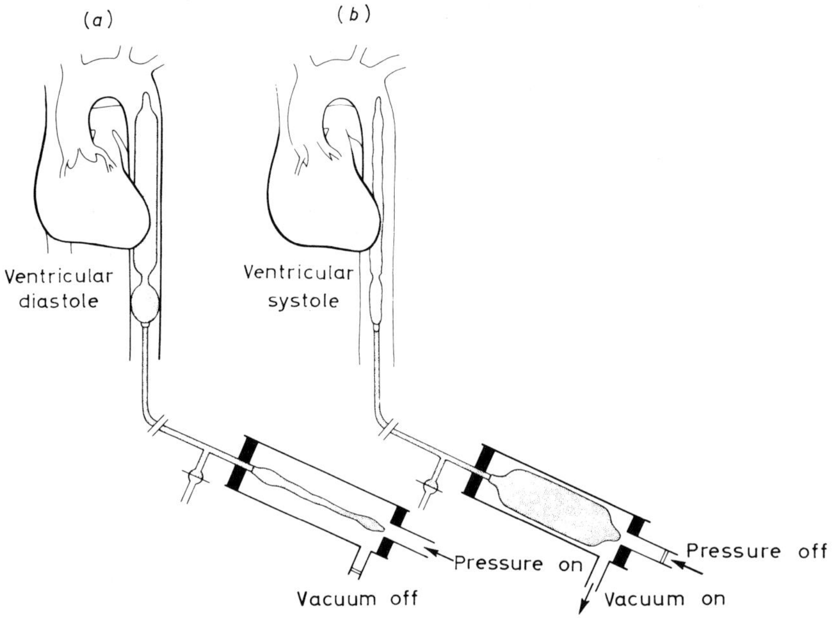

Figure 18.10 Dual-chambered balloon acting in tandem with slave balloon in safety chamber. (a) Transfer of CO_2 during diastole from the slave balloon in safety chamber to intra-aortic balloon. (b) Complete deflation of intra-aortic balloon asssisted by vacuum acting on slave balloon

Seals

The dual-chambered balloon is chemically welded to the polyurethane catheter so that a polyurethane seal is obtained. In addition, the proximal and distal ends of the balloon are overcoated with additional polyurethane layers to complete the seal.

Arterial grafts

As will be described subsequently, a Dacron graft is sutured on to the common femoral artery and the dual-chambered balloon is inserted through the graft and is then positioned just distal to the left subclavain artery in the descending thoracic aorta. When the graft and the catheter are snared, this allows distal perfusion of the extremity during the period of cardiac arrest.

The clinical system for intra-aortic balloon pumping

In order for the intra-aortic balloon pump to perform its function of cardiac assistance, the timing of balloon inflation and deflation must be extremely accurate and responsive to changes in heart rate. The intra-aortic balloon console therefore had to undergo evolution along with the development of balloons with improved design (Wolvek, 1989).

In its original concept, the console processed the patient ECG signal into an electrical output which commanded a solenoid valve to open, permitting the driving gas to inflate the balloon. At first, gas was supplied directly to the solenoid from the tank regulator. Balloon deflation was accomplished by closing the solenoid valve and permitting the balloon to vent to atmosphere. The console controlled only the point of balloon inflation, expressed as the delay after the R wave of the ECG (which served as an electronic triggering event) and the duration of inflation over a given period of the cardiac cycle. Manual triggering was provided for use during cardiac resuscitation. While the system worked well enough to introduce intra-aortic balloon pumping to the scientific community, it responded only to the basic needs of the balloon pump console.

In 1970, the Datascope system 80 was introduced. The system addressed the safety requirements by incorporating the safety chamber concept, which guards against balloon rupture. This system also introduced a fail-safe design which automatically placed the balloon in a deflate mode in the event of system failure. Another safety feature prevented the balloon from inflating during cardiac systole.

The Datascope system 80 was continuously refined over the next 15 years, eventually incorporating automatic pacemaker ejection, an auto-filling mechanism and offering the user a choice of helium or carbon dioxide as a gas fill. Electrical surgical interference suppression (ESIS) was also built into the system to permit intra-operative balloon pump triggering in the presence of electronic cautery or cutting.

As the console developed into the Datascope system 90, the units became more automatic. Fully-automated prefilling of the safety chamber system, as well as alarms to signal a loss of trigger, gas, augmentation or of a kinked catheter became incorporated into the late model systems. In 1987, the Datascope system 90T was designed to allow continuous use of the balloon pump both at the community hospital and during transport to a tertiary care centre.

Although we currently are using the system 90T, the majority of our clinical experience has been with the Datascope System 82*. The Datascope system 82 has incorporated several significant improvements over its predecessor, the Datascope system 80, as described in previous editions of this chapter. Particular attention has now been devoted to redesigning and simplifying the operating controls, since, with greater frequency, nursing staff and other paramedical personnel are in actual fact running the balloon pump console. As a result, the setting of two prominent slide controls is essentially all that is needed for proper operation of the balloon pump. The System 82 utilizes a non-fade physiological monitor, which gives excellent viewing of all pertinent data. In addition, it has the advantage of being able to freeze the tracing so that the pumping waves may be critically analysed. Furthermore, the System 82 incorporates the above mentioned ESIS, which virtually eliminates interference from electrocautery during surgery. The result is an ECG signal essentially free of noise and a reliable triggering of the balloon pump console even during use of an electrosurgical unit. The balloon pump console is also considerably quieter than its predecessor. The System 82 has built in battery power, which can easily enable transport of the patient, although the newer System 90T is more compact and specifically designed for transport of patients on the intra-aortic balloon pump.

Inflation and deflation of the balloon is accomplished by alternately applying pressure and vacuum to a closed circuit consisting of the intra-aortic balloon and a slave balloon within a safety chamber. This circuit is precharged with a fixed amount of carbon dioxide. Consequently, the System 82 is safe under virtually any conditions.

* Manufactured by the Datascope Corp., Paramus, New Jersey, USA

Safety chamber

Use of a fixed volume of CO_2 (closed system)

The slave balloon in the safety chamber is precharged with an effective volume of CO_2 equal to the volume of the intra-aortic balloon selected for clinical use (Figure 18.10). Because this is basically a closed system, the patient can never be exposed to more than 1 bolus of the driving gas. Lethal sequelae from the intra-aortic balloon rupture with helium, both in animals (Furman *et al.*, 1971) and in humans (Mueller *et al.*, 1970; Mueller *et al.*, 1971; Mueller *et al.*, 1972) have further convinced us that the use of CO_2 is a prudent choice as the driving gas for clinical intra-aortic balloon pumping. To our knowledge, there has only been one patient death as a result of a ruptured intra-aortic balloon when CO_2 was used.

Overdistension

Because the effective pumping volume of CO_2 introduced into the slave balloon in the safety chamber is never more than the displacement volume of the actual intra-aortic balloon, the intra-aortic balloon can never be overdistended. If the balloon is connected to a cylinder of the driving gas and inflation is then judged by the pressure build-up in the balloon, the intra-aortic balloon may become distended with each inflation cycle leading to eventual fatigue and balloon herniation and with subsequent weakness and eventual rupture.

Gas diffusion from balloon

Because of ambient CO_2 tension in the arterial tree, there is minimal diffusion of CO_2 between the intra-aortic balloon and the patient's blood. However, a small amount of CO_2 is lost from the slave balloon in the safety chamber to the ambient external air under normal line-operated circumstances, since compressed air is the positive driving force within the safety chamber external to the slave balloon. This loss may account to 1–2 ml h^{-1}. The loss would be accenuated if helium were used, since helium is a smaller molecule than CO_2 and because the arterial tension of helium is zero.

Vacuum

Not only is the intra-aortic balloon actively inflated, but it is actively deflated as well (*see* Figure 18.11). By actively deflating the intra-aortic balloon, one has the advantage of precise timing of deflation and of a more completely deflated intra-aortic balloon which can never act as a partial intra-aortic obstruction.

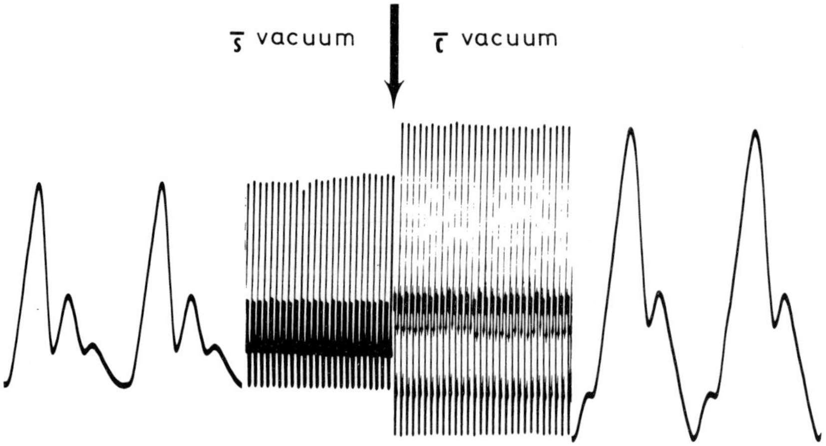

Figure 18.11 Advantage of using vacuum during IABP. Note completeness of deflation with vacuum (on right) and resultant greater pumping effectiveness of the balloon as demonstrated in a mock circulatory system

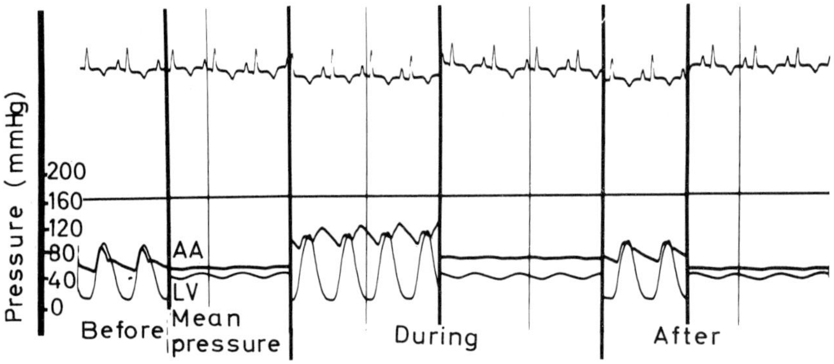

Figure 18.12 With systemic hypotension, complete collapse of the intra-aortic balloon just before ventricular systole cannot be asssured if deflation is not uniformly assisted. In this animal experiment without vacuum assist, partial obstruction of the aorta, as evidenced by the rise in aortic and left ventricular systolic pressures during the assist, resulted from incomplete collapse of the balloon. A vacuum should be used at all times during IABP to assure total and complete balloon deflation

Visual control and flexibility

Finally, the safety chamber provides accurate visual control of the intra-aortic balloon's performance by observing the slave balloon in the safety chamber. This feature has been found to be a useful adjunct in addition to monitoring the patient's ECG and blood pressure. It is particularly useful when initiating balloon pumping so that only the smallest augmentation can at first be applied to the patient to ensure that balloon pumping begins in the appropriate diastolic interval.

The safety chamber, which is supported by a flexible stainless steel arm, can be extended several inches beyond the pumping unit towards the patient's groin. Thus, the pumping unit itself does not necessarily require close proximity to the operating table or patient's bedside. This is particularly important during sterile surgical procedures where adequate draping of a large console next to the patient would be cumbersome.

Battery operation

In light of the present clinical experience with intra-aortic balloon pump which shows that quite frequently it is necessary to move a patient on assistance, and the cardiac assist console, from one part of the hospital to another it is necessary, therefore, to have a system which is mobile and which can be readily battery operated. To initiate battery operation with the System 82, one need only turn on one

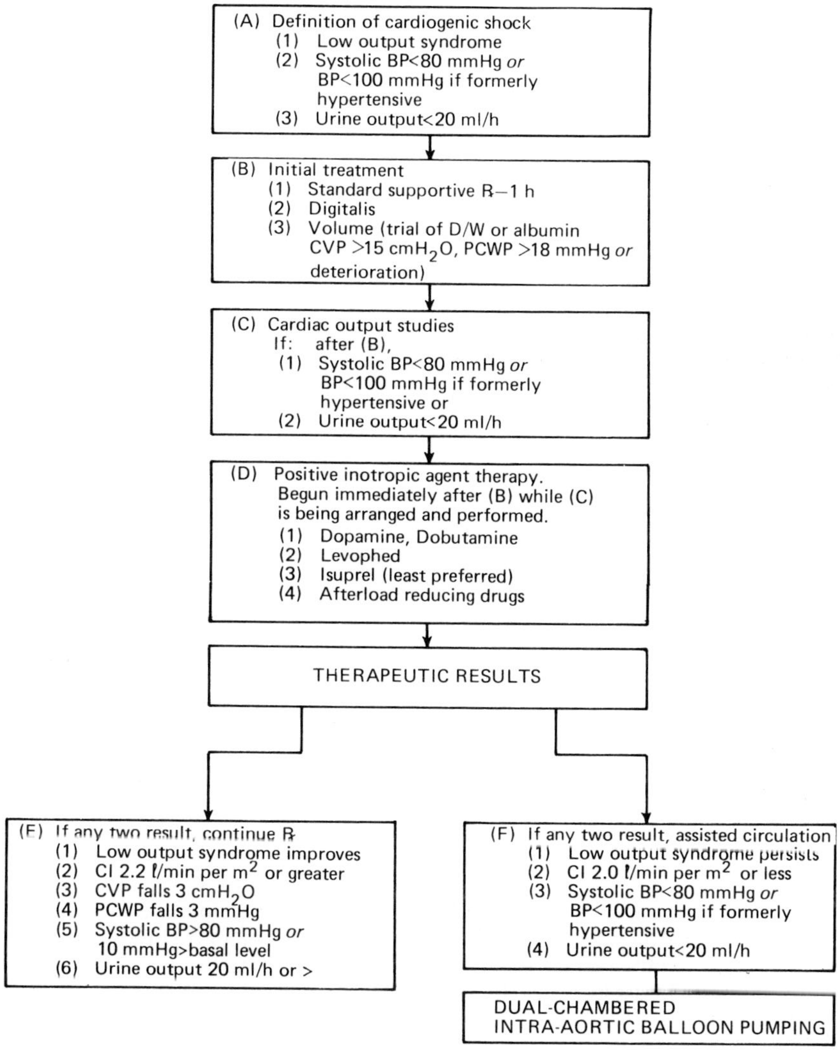

Figure 18.13 Management of cardiogenic shock

of the two CO_2 cylinders on the rear of the cart. Once this is done, the unit can be immediately unplugged from the wall outlet and the entire system will automatically be battery operated without any lapse in circulatory assistance. No further adjustments are necessary to maintain the same diastolic augmentation. The System 90 and System 90T are equally easily battery operated. At a heart rate of 70 beats min^{-1}, each of the two cylinders on the System 82 will function for approximately 45 min.

Weaning feature

After the patient has become haemodynamically stable during balloon pumping, it may be desirable to wean him from the assist device. This can be easily accomplished with the System 82, 90 and 90T, because not only can the balloon volume be gradually decreased, but the assist can also operate in the 1:1, 1:2 and 1:3 modes so that the patient is assisted with every beat, every other beat and every third beat respectively. Hence, by a combination of these features, the balloon volume and assist frequency can be gradually and synchronously (Bernstein and Murphy, 1973) decreased until assist has been discontinued.

Experience with intra-aortic balloon pumping

The indications for IABP are changing almost daily. We will discuss initially the patient in cardiogenic

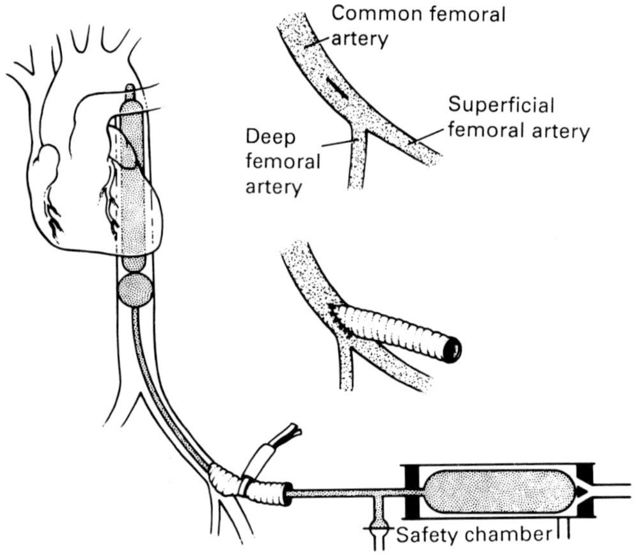

Figure 18.14 Artist's rendering of clinical dual-chambered IABP

shock whose management is summarized in Figure 18.13.

All patients with an acute myocardial infarction diagnosed by the clinical picture, the ECG and enzyme studies should be admitted to the coronary care unit (Bregman, 1974). Those patients who demonstrate systolic hypotension (systolic blood pressure <80 mmHg or systolic blood pressure <100 mmHg if formerly hypertensive) or, even without hypotension, a low output syndrome resulting in diminished tissue perfusion, peripheral cyanosis, cold clammy skin, oliguria (urine output < than 20 ml h^{-1}, low sodium) and mental confusion or agitation are then evaluated for the possible effects of:

1. Drug depression
2. Arrhythmias
3. Metabolic disturbances
4. Volume depletion
5. Gram-negative sepsis

If the hypotensive or low-output state is not related to any of these disturbances or persists after one or more of the disturbances have been corrected, then the patient is described as suffering from *cardiogenic shock as a result of myocardial infarction or ongoing myocardial ischaemia.*

Whether or not the patient is a candidate for thrombolytic therapy or emergency revascularization, initially, patients should receive standard supportive therapy including medications for pain and cardiac failure, as well as oxygen and the correction of acidosis. A central venous catheter should be inserted, a Swan–Ganz catheter positioned to monitor pulmonary artery wedge pressures, and a Foley catheter inserted. If the initial central venous pressure is less than 15 cmH_2O or the pulmonary capillary wedge pressure (PCWP) as measured with a Swan–Ganz catheter is less than 16 mmHg, a volume infusion should be started and given in increments of 100 ml of either normal saline or dextrose in water, with or without salt poor albumin added. If after a trial of volume expansion, the systolic arterial pressure remains below 80 mmHg or is less than 100 mmHg in a formerly hypertensive patient or if the urine output remains below 20 ml h^{-1}, then initial cardiac-output studies should be undertaken. While these are being arranged and performed, the patient should be given a therapeutic trial of inotropic agents, including dobutamine, amrinone or dopamine. Isoproterenol should not be used in the setting of myocardial ischaemia or infarction unless extreme bradycardia is present and is unresponsive to atropine. In this case, a temporary pacemaker should be strongly considered. In addition, afterload reduction with sodium nitroprusside can be used alone or in combination with the above inotropic agents.

Therapy should be considered temporarily successful and continued if any of two of the following measurements result from any agents:

1. There is improvement in the low output syndrome.
2. The cardiac index is 2.2 l min^{-1} m^{-2} or greater.
3. The central venous pressure is lowered by 3 cmH_2O) or more.

4. The pulmonary capillary wedge pressure falls by 3 mmHg or more.
5. The systolic arterial blood pressure is greater than 80 mmHg or shows an increase of 10 mmHg from the prior basal level.
6. The urinary output is 20 ml h^{-1} or greater.

However, if any two of the following measurements apply, proceeding to IABP should be strongly considered:

1. The low output syndrome clinically persists.
2. The cardiac index remains below 2.2 l min^{-1} m^{-2}.
3. The systolic blood pressure remains below 80 mmHg (or less than 100 mmHg in a previously hypertensive patient).
4. The urinary output persists at less than 20 ml h^{-1} (less than 0.5 ml kg^{-1} h^{-1}).

This entire diagnostic and therapeutic scheme can be performed in 2–3 h.

Once the diagnosis of cardiogenic shock is established, these routine therapeutic procedures should be instituted as rapidly as possible, since the earlier the patient is referred for circulatory assistance, the better the result will be. Surrounding the actual area of the infarct, or the area of frank myocardial necrosis, there is a significant area of marginal myocardial ischaemia. It is this area of diminished myocardial perfusion that can be restored to viability by the early institution of IABP. Hence, more patients will survive from the circulatory assist alone, the earlier they are referred for treatment.

Metabolic effects of IABP

The metabolic effects of intra-aortic balloon pumping are now well described. Feola *et al.* (1977) have examined myocardial lactate metabolism with pacing-induced tachycardia in seven patients. They found that lactate production changed from 0.24 ± 0.07 extraction at rest to 0.94 ± 0.01 production after pacing ($P \leqslant 0.001$) without intra-aortic balloon pump and from 0.10 ± 0.003 extraction at rest to 0.57 ± 0.001 production after pacing ($P \leqslant 0.001$) with intra-aortic balloon pumping. The difference between lactate production levels occurring with and without intra-aortic balloon counterpulsation was statistically significant ($P<0.005$).

Previous studies have demonstrated that intra-aortic balloon pumping or arterial counterpulsation reduces MVO_2 in the normal circulation by diminishing heart rate, peak left ventricular systolic wall stress, and possibly, contractility (Spotnitz *et al.*, 1969; Summers *et al.*, 1969). Wall stress in the left ventricle, the major determinant of myocardial oxygen demand, can be decreased through a reduction of either peak systolic pressure or a reduction in left ventricular end-diastolic pressure and heart size (American Heart Association, 1981). Decreases in heart rate and a reduction in the frequency of ventricular ectopic beats suggest that intra-aortic balloon counterpulsation may reduce sympathetic tone and cardiac contractility through baroreceptor-mediated reflexes. This impression has been strengthened by observations of peripheral vasodilatation (Feola, Limet and Glick, 1971) and increased frequency of discharge of the carotid sinus nerve (Norman and Kennedy, 1971) during intra-aortic balloon pumping. The postulated reduction of sympathetic tone during intra-aortic balloon pumping is further supported in the present study by observation of a decrease in circulating arterial epinephrine and norepinephrine during intra-aortic balloon counterpulsation.

Contraindications to IABP

There is an ever expanding list of uses for the intra-aortic balloon pump. However, there remain only two absolute contraindications to its implementation. These include gross aortic insufficiency and acute aortic dissection. Minor aortic insufficiency should not be a deterrent (Yellin, Levy and Bregman, 1978). The presence of an aortic aneurysm or the history of prior aortic surgery are only relative contraindications, their significance to be judged in light of the entire clinical picture.

The use of the intra-aortic balloon pump with cardiac standstill, especially in the setting of open-heart surgery, remains controversial (Bregman, 1971), however, it never impairs survival when continued with closed chest cardiopulmonary resuscitation.

Techniques of IABP insertion

The initial description of intra-aortic balloon pump insertion was first outlined by Kantrowitz (*see* Figure 18.14). The common femoral artery is exposed through a vertical incision beginning high in the groin over the inguinal ligament. The vessel is then encircled by tapes for control. A 10 mm woven dacron sidearm graft is sutured on to the arterial site. Using bulldog clamps to control the blood flow above and below the arteriotomy site, the balloon catheter is inserted through the graft into the artery. An umbilical snare is used to secure the balloon catheter within the graft. The balloon catheter can now be advanced up into the descending and thoracic aorta (Bregman, Bolooki and Malm, 1973).

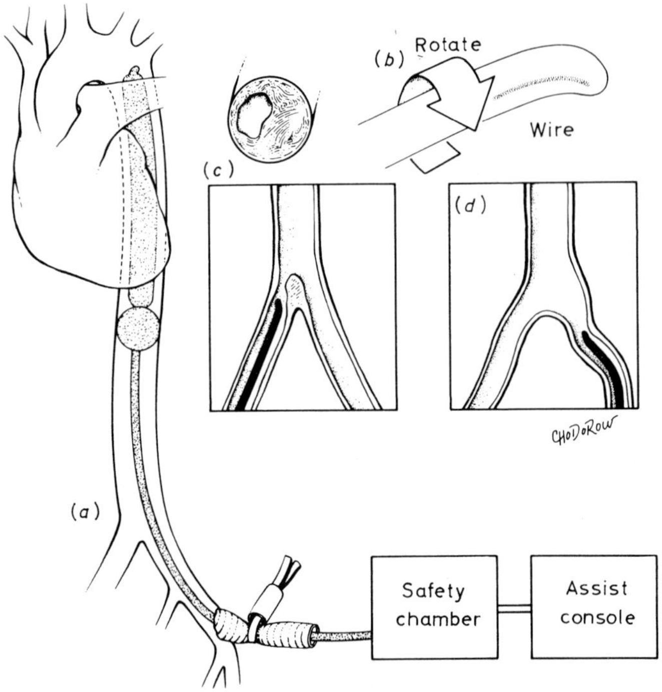

Figure 18.15 (a) A proper position of dual-chambered intra-aortic balloon just distal to left subclavian artery. Note that the balloon is inserted through a Dacron prosthesis that is snared, permitting perfusion of the distal extremity during the period of cardiac assist. (b) Technique of bending and rotating distal balloon catheter during insertion. (c) Balloon negotiating eccentric arteriosclerotic stenosis. (d) Balloon passing through an arterial tortuosity

Transiliac artery insertion

Using the same technique, the balloon can be inserted into the common iliac artery. Exposure is obtained with a retroperitoneal approach using an oblique incision above the left inguinal ligament (Lambert, Cohen and Collins, 1974).

Transaxillary insertion

In the event of severe diffuse aorto-iliac disease, tortuosity, or some other contraindication to femoro-iliac insertion, the intra-aortic balloon pump catheter may be placed from the left subclavian artery. Surgical isolation of the vessel through the axilla allows advancement to the descending aorta. Although rarely required, this method may be ideal for the patient with an acute aortic dissection or aneurysm, when retrograde insertion of the intra-aortic balloon pump catheter may be possible.

Transthoracic insertion

Yet another approach to circumvent peripheral vascular disease or anomalies, is the transthoracic insertion. This is also advantageous if recent prior exposure to the aortic arch expedites access (Pappas, 1974; Gueldner, 1975; Shirley, Loughridge and Lain, 1976). Purse string sutures are embedded into the ascending aortic wall, lateral to the cannulation site, for catheter retention. The balloon may then be inserted and directed downward just below the left subclavian artery. Leaving the sternum unanchored, the catheter may exit at the inferior aspect of the midline incision. When balloon support is no longer necessary, the patient is returned to the operating room for balloon removal and aortic and sternal closure.

Ogogi, Turner and McGee (1980) reviewed data on 28 patients requiring aortic arch intra-aortic balloon pump insertion. Of these, five of 21 males

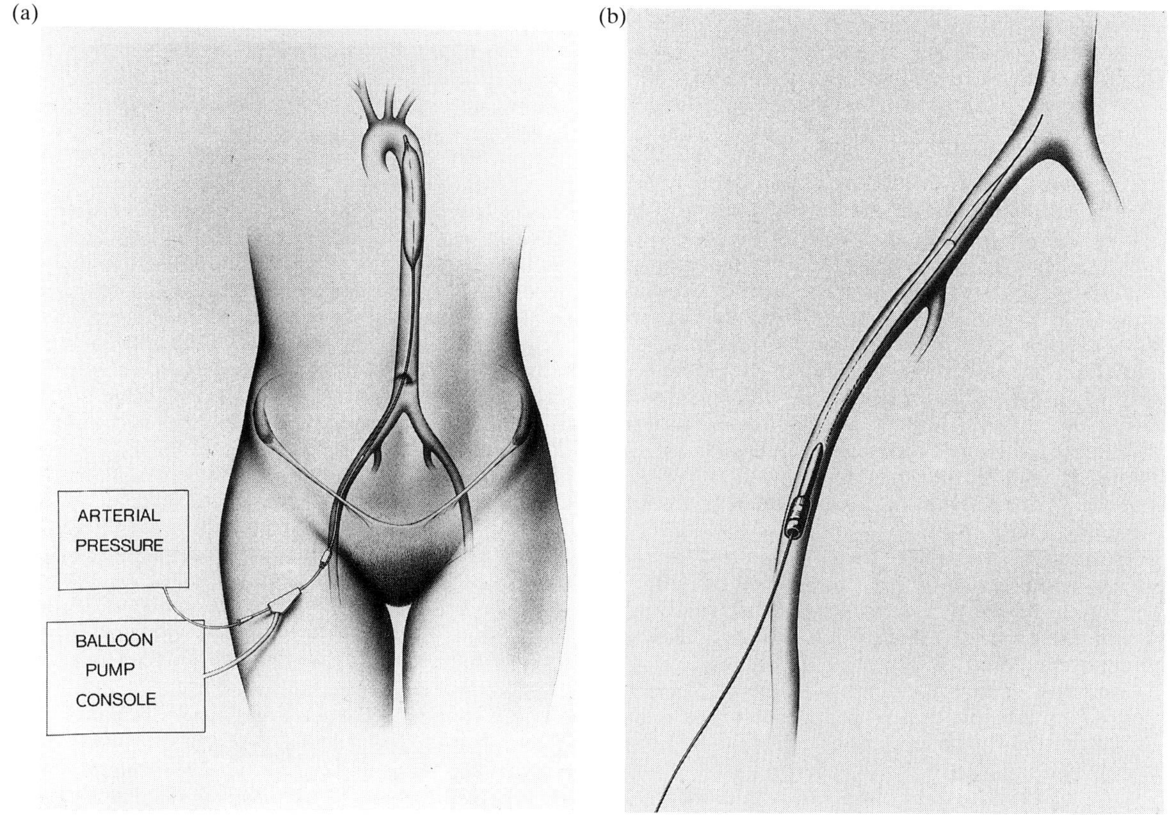

Figure 18.16a and b (a) Dual chambered IABP passing through the right iliac artery into the aorta. (b) Proper position of the intra-aortic balloon in the descending thoracic aorta

and three of seven females survived. No complications could be directly referred to the site of insertion. Snow and Harrigan (1986) reported on 23 patients undergoing the transthoracic approach. Twenty-one had insertion in the operating room, while two were placed postoperatively in the intensive care unit. Sixteen (69%) of these patients were eventually discharged.

Although the method of arteriotomy is still widely used during cardiac surgery, and is currently the procedure required during intra-aortic balloon pump insertion in infants and children, the most common insertion technique used today is the percutaneous method adapted by Bregman and Casarella (1979).

The percutaneous intra-aortic balloon pump

In 1979 a single chambered 40 ml percutaneous intra-aortic balloon (IAB) was constructed around a central wire (Bregman, 1980a and b; Bregman *et al.*, 1980). The intra-aortic balloon was wrapped manually about the wire, which then allowed for percutaneous insertion into the femoral artery. A No 12 Fr sheath-dilator assembly was previously inserted into the artery using the modified Seldinger technique (Seldinger, 1953) (*see* Figure 18.15). Percutaneous balloon insertion requires approximately 5–10 min, and has been successfully performed in the cardiac catheterization laboratory, coronary care unit, and operating suite. Although under extreme circumstances the intra-aortic balloon can be inserted without fluoroscopic guidance, it is recommended that the procedure be done under fluoroscopy, and that abdominal aortography can frequently be helpful in deciding which femoral artery be used for insertion (Vignok, Swaye and Gosselin, 1981). Difficulties with percutaneous insertion were sometimes encountered during the following circumstances:

1. tortuous vessels preventing IAB insertion
2. a small femoral pulse; a difficult to find pulse
3. balloons failing to unfurl due to overwrapping
4. dislodging of atherosclerosis plaque or thrombus.

Isner *et al.* (1980), in their post-mortem study of intra-aortic balloon pumping complications, found that most complications appear related to the insertion of the balloon catheter. This information coupled with the clinical experience gained through the use of the first percutaneous balloon (Nachlas and Sieband, 1968), resulted in a redesigning of the earlier percutaneous balloons.

In 1981, the second generation of percutaneous intra-aortic balloons were introduced, featuring a dual-lumen catheter (Leinbach *et al.*, 1982; Bedderman, 1985). This dual-lumen intra-aortic balloon has a flexible inner lumen incorporated inside the catheter that allows the balloon to be advanced over the 0.038" J-tipped guide-wire; the guide wire having already been inserted into the femoral artery and advanced into the descending thoracic aorta. Access to this central lumen is achieved by removing the central stylet, which is attached to the 'wrapping-knob' assembly. After the balloon has been advanced over the 0.038" J-tip guide-wire, the wire is removed, and the central lumen can either be closed with a male luer lock cap, or alternatively, it can be used to monitor aortic arch pressure (Reemtsma *et al.*, 1974). The ability quickly to establish an arterial line along with the rapid insertion of the balloon, makes the percutaneous dual-lumen intra-aortic balloon a powerful adjunct in an emergency situation.

One of the early problems identified with the original percutaneous intra-aortic balloon occurred while manually wrapping it. Under tense circumstances accompanying intra-aortic balloon pump insertion, too often, the balloon was either overwrapped or not wrapped uniformly. To circumvent this problem, a 'wrapping knob' was incorporated into the base of the catheter, which takes all the guess work out of wrapping the balloon membrane. This knob rotates the inner lumen a mechanically fixed number of turns and causes the balloon membrane to wrap around the inner-lumen. A threaded screw assembly inside the knob prevents either the over wrapping or under wrapping of the IAB. The sterile IAB package is designed to act as a passive guide, and facilitates the balloon wrapping procedure.

In another approach to ameliorate the difficulties with wrapping the IAB, the Datascope Percor® Star* has been introduced. This is a specially designed package that contains a pre-wrapped dual-lumen intra-aortic balloon.

Using this system, the balloon does not have to leave the sterile package until after the sheath-dilator assembly has been introduced into the femoral artery. Once the IAB has been advanced into the aorta, the balloon is unfurled rotating the wrapping knob counterclockwise. Because the balloon is pre-wrapped, the problems associated with the improper wrapping of the IAB are eliminated.

There are four new adult balloons included in the second generation of IABs: the 40 ml dual-lumen IAB available on a No. 10.5 Fr catheter; the 50 ml dual-lumen IAB which is also available on a No. 10.5 Fr catheter; a No. 9.5 Fr single-lumen balloon, that can use either carbon dioxide or helium; and finally a very narrow No 8.5 Fr 40 ml single-lumen balloon which can only be operated with helium as the shuttle gas. All four balloons incorporate the 'wrapping-knob' assembly into the base of the catheter. The 50 ml dual-lumen balloon was specifically developed for the patient with a large aortic diameter. By increasing the cross-sectional diameter of the 40 ml balloon (an increase of 1.25 mm), balloon volume is enlarged to 50 ml, and blood volume displacement is increased by 25%.

The Nos. 8.5 and 9.5 Fr single-lumen IAB were designed for patients with severe peripheral vascular disease or small tortuous femoral arteries. The greatly reduced catheter diameters will allow more blood flow distal to the balloon insertion site, thereby reducing the potential for limb ischaemia.

Although the first patient to receive the balloon pump was female (Feola, Limet and Glick, 1971), it has been recognized that the survival of women is much less than of men. Bedderman *et al.* (1985), in their study of this trend, believe that it is due to the smaller aortoiliac arteries in women necessitating a smaller balloon; a smaller balloon produces less diastolic augmentation. The new Nos. 8.5 and 9.5 Fr IABs are ideally suited to address this problem.

The pumping mechanism, System 90® and System 90T® (which is only used for transport) are semi-computerized mobile units with advanced rhythm monitoring capability.

Technique of percutaneous insertion of the IABP

Employing the modified Seldinger technique (Nachlas and Sieband, 1968), the No. 9.5 Fr Percor Stat® DL percutaneous IAB is inserted in the following manner: first, the inguinal region is prepared and draped, the common femoral artery is then punctured with a standard 18-gauge arterial needle (care is taken so that the posterior wall of the artery is not punctured), and a 0.030 inch (0.097 cm) tip guidewire is introduced through the needle. The needle is now removed, and a No. 8 Fr dilator is passed over the guidewire to predilate the subcutaneous tissues and the arterial puncture site. Then a No. 10 Fr sheath-dilator combination is advanced over the guidewire into the puncture site. It is

* Datascope Corp. Paramus, New Jersey

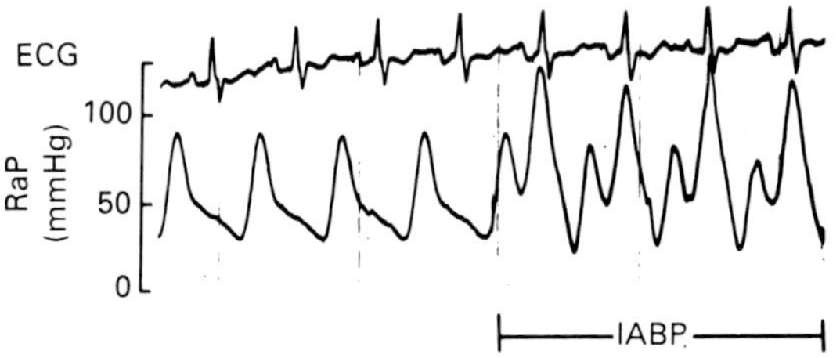

Figure 18.17 Unidirectional dual-chambered IABP in a patient with cardiogenic shock. S = systole; D = diastolic augmentation. Note the fall in systolic pressure, large diastolic augmentation, and fall in end diastolic presssure

important to leave approximately 2.5 cm of sheath exposed to control bleeding.

The percutaneous balloon should be prepared as follows: after removing the balloon from its sterile package under aseptic technique, connect the one-way valve to the IAB luer lock connector and aspirate with a 50 ml syringe to remove any residual air in the furled balloon. Using a large bowl, moisten the balloon membrane in a sterile saline solution. To estimate the length of the catheter, place the catheter on the patient's chest with the balloon tip 1 cm below the angle of Louis. Note the marking on the catheter.

If wrapping is required, while holding the balloon package firmly, rotate the wrapping knob clockwise in a smooth motion. The wrapping knob will stop turning when the balloon is completely wrapped. Inspect the balloon membrane, observing that the membrane is evenly wrapped over its entire length.

After balloon preparation, IAB insertion should be carried out in the following sequence: Remove the guidewire and dilator, leaving the No. 10 Fr sheath in place. Control bleeding by carefully yet firmly pinching the exposed 2.5 cm sheath stem. The moistened balloon is then inserted into the sheath and watched with fluoroscopy as the catheter is advanced up into the descending thoracic aorta (Figure 18.16a). The balloon tip should be distal to the left subclavian artery (Figure 18.16b). Pull back the sheath before initiating intra-aortic balloon pumping so that only a few inches of sheath remain *in vivo*. Release the vacuum by detaching the one-way valve and unwrap the IAB by rotating the wrapping knob counterclockwise until rotation is mechanically stopped. Now, the balloon catheter can be attached to the balloon pump console for initiation of pumping. While it is preferable to insert the IAB under fluoroscopic guidance, it is not mandatory. We have successfully inserted the IAB 'blindly' using the estimates above for catheter length without any major complications.

If a difficult insertion is anticipated because of tortuosity of the aorta or from difficulty in advancing the initial guidewire (as happens with severe calcific disease), the IAB can be advanced over the guidewire directly from the onset (without use of the dilator). Under these circumstances, advance the initial guidewire up into the thoracic aorta. For balloons that are not of the pre-wrapped type, wrap the balloon next as previously described. Remove the inner stylet from the balloon while holding with both hands. Submerge the IAB in sterile saline solution while maintaining the vacuum. Remove the dilator from the dilator-sheath assembly. Do not remove either the sheath or the guidewire. Control any bleeding by pinching the sheath. Insert the tip of the balloon into the sheath and rotate the balloon counterclockwise; this will tighten the balloon wrapping. Advance the balloon up into the thoracic aorta over the guidewire. When the IAB is positioned properly, remove the vacuum and initiate pumping.

If during the conventional insertion sequence there is resistance as the balloon passes through the sheath or the femoral artery, do not force the balloon. This is to prevent arterial dissection. Instead, with the balloon still in the artery, remove the inner stylet from the wrapping knob and insert the guidewire through the inner lumen. The DL balloon is flexible and will follow the tortuous path of the guidewire. Sometimes, as the balloon is advanced, the tip may be felt against the aortic arch. Should this occur, withdraw the catheter approximately 2.5 cm so that the tip will lie immediately below the left subclavian artery.

Correct inflation and deflation of the balloon may be confirmed with fluoroscopic visualization. Be sure to feel the pulse in the left arm so that the tip of the balloon is not in the subclavian orifice and occluding the left subclavian inflow. In all cases, it is necessary to confirm catheter tip position with a chest roentegram. The sheath and balloon catheter are ligated with umbilical tape to prevent bleeding around the catheter, and a sterile dressing is applied to the sheath and catheter assembly. Suture the sheath seal to the skin so that the catheter position is secure.

In high-risk cardiac surgical patients undergoing open-heart surgery, and in whom an intra-aortic balloon pump was not inserted before anaesthetic induction, we recommend preparing for a potential intra-aortic balloon pump insertion. Using an arterial needle, obtain femoral artery access and insert the guidewire. Should intra-aortic balloon pumping be required for separation from cardiopulmonary bypass, arterial access is then already established for the intra-aortic balloon pump insertion.

Long sheath insertion

A newer technique for percutaneous insertion of the intra-aortic balloon in patients with tortuous or narrowed external iliac arteries was described by Nicols, Weiss and Bregman (1981). This method uses a long (45 cm) No. 12 Fr sheath-dilator combination which extends up to the descending thoracic aorta and protects the iliac artery and aorta from injury during insertion of the balloon catheter. In patients with severe acute myocardial ischaemia in whom insertion of the IAB catheters is not possible by the conventional percutaneous technique, use of the long sheath approach permits rapid institution of circulatory support (Wolvek, 1989).

Placement of the IAB using the long sheath technique is performed in a manner similar to conventional percutaneous balloon insertion. However, following proper positioning of the balloon and catheter in the descending thoracic aorta, the long sheath is withdrawn into the iliac artery to allow complete unfurling of the balloon membrane.

In patients whom percutaneous techniques fail, surgical insertion of the IAB is necessary.

Insertion during acute myocardial infarction

These improved techniques for insertion of the intra-aortic balloon pump have curtailed major vascular complications, especially extensive blood loss. This is critical in the new age of thrombolysis. At Riverside Methodist Hospital, investigators in the TAMI co-operative trials (George, 1988) have used the single wall technique. Their data suggest that no significant increase in bleeding related to thrombolysis is seen. In fact, there were no reports of groin bleeding requiring surgical evacuation or repair.

Ideal balloon function

The primary goals of intra-aortic balloon pumping are to implement the maximal increase in coronary blood flow during diastole and at the same time effect a decrease in left ventricular work (Corday *et al.*, 1970). Realization that these two beneficial effects are dependent upon one another permits maximal benefit to be obtained from each factor in the following fashion: the diastolic augmentation ordinarily begins at the dicrotic notch (Figure 18.17), using an initial sequence of 1:3, whereby every third ventricular beat is augmented by the intra-aortic balloon. One can encroach upon the dicrotic notch to begin balloon inflation slightly earlier in diastole. Provided the patient does not have premature ventricular contractions from this manipulation, it can be performed in patients who appear to be responding poorly to intra-aortic balloon pumping to give them additional benefit. The right-hand side or downslope of the augmentation is the part most intimately involved with the

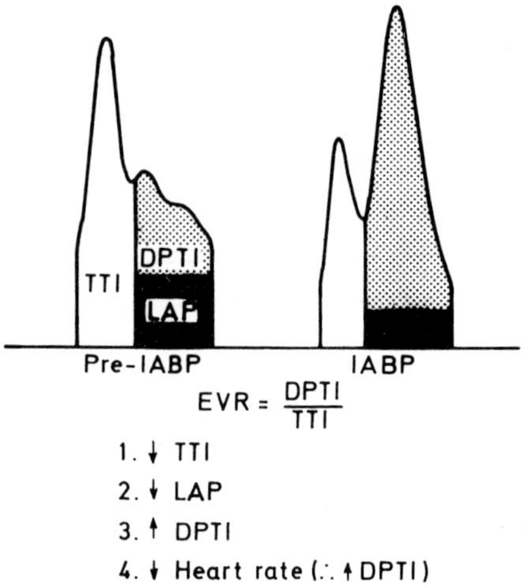

Figure 18.18 Effects of unidirectional IABP on the endocardial viability ratio (EVR). DPTI = diastolic pressure-time index; TTI = tension-time index; LAP = left atrial pressure

ventricular unloading aspect of intra-aortic balloon pumping. If the fall in left ventricular end-diastolic pressure is too great, the following sequence of events occurs: excessive fall in left ventricular end-diastolic pressure essentially means that the balloon has collapsed too soon before the aortic valve has opened. Since blood must flow to occupy the space of the formerly expanded balloon, it flows retrograde from all branches of the aorta, including the coronary arteries (if the fall in left ventricular end-diastolic pressure is excessive) (Corday *et al.*, 1970). Therefore, one must effect a compromise and have some fall in left ventricular end-diastolic pressure, but not an excessive decrease. Recent experimental and clinical work has indicated that this fall in left ventricular end-diastolic pressure should not exceed 10 mmHg.

As far as the position of the balloon is concerned, we initially place the balloon as far proximally in the aorta as possible (that is, with the tip of the balloon just distal to the left subclavian artery). Be sure to feel the pulse in the left arm so that the tip of the balloon is not in the subclavian orifice and is not occluding the left subclavian inflow.

At rapid heart rates, there is more dead space in the safety chamber balloon. Therefore, one could increase the volume of carbon dioxide in the safety chamber balloon (e.g. to 45 ml with a 30 ml balloon) at heart rates over 120 beats min^{-1}. This will improve intra-aortic balloon function (Bregman, 1976).

In this clinical setting, heart rates of up to 140 beats min^{-1} can usually be followed with the smaller

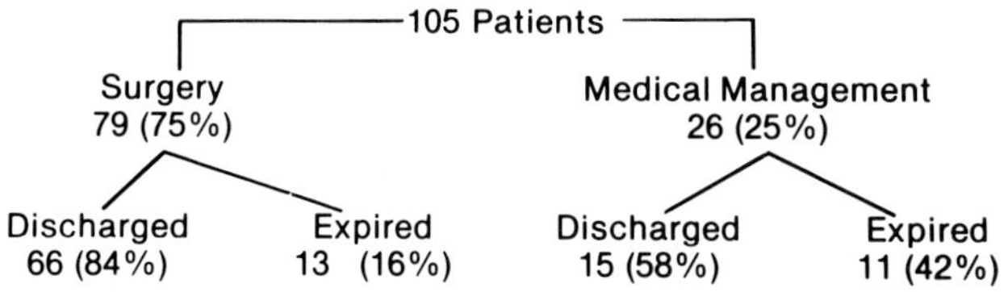

Figure 18.19 Use of percutaneous intra-aortic balloon pumping for medical indications at the Columbia–Presbyterian Medical Center 1979–1985

size balloon. If the rate is higher, it may be necessary to assist on 1:2 (every other beat) in order to achieve effective diastolic augmentation, until the rate slows, when 1:1 assistance can be instituted.

If weaning a patient from intra-aortic balloon assistance is undertaken by changing from a 1:1 to a 1:2 or 1:3 assisting sequence, additional time will be present for the vacuum to build up, and augmentation may demonstrate a deep 'sink'; the end-diastolic point may need elevation by a minor adjustment on the console.

Paramount for effective counterpulsation is the timing of balloon inflation and deflation. A pulse contour recorder within the central lumen, or radial arterial monitor, will display a pressure waveform on to the console screen. An electronic signal, which may be manually manoeuvred within the cardiac cycle, then indicates balloon inflation and deflation.

For optimal augmentation of haemodynamics, the balloon should be deflated just before left ventricular ejection (i.e. at the QRS complex). Delay would present the ventricle with an obstruction to outflow. If deflated too early, the 'vacuum' effect to enhance cardiac output is not only compromised, but may actually hinder left ventricular ejection, thereby markedly decreasing cardiac output.

Inflation should take place during the dicrotic notch of the arterial pressure wave, corresponding to the peak of the T-wave on the electrocardiogram. Early expansion creates increased afterload for the contracting ventricle. Delayed expansion will decrease coronary perfusion and create less diastolic augmentation. Most consoles will automatically collapse the balloon in case of timing errors.

Obviously, cardiac arrhythmias will also alter the efficiency of intra-aortic balloon counterpulsation, owing to the reliance of timing of balloon inflation and deflation on the surface electrocardiogram. Therefore, every effort should be made to suppress cardiac arrhythmias while the patient is on intra-aortic balloon support. Atrial arrhythmias, especially atrial fibrillation with a rapid ventricular response, may also lead to inadequate augmentation.

Removal of the percutaneous IABP

The principal problem associated with removal of the percutaneous balloon catheter is release of thrombi as the sheath-catheter assembly is withdrawn. These thrombi form around the catheter at the insertion site where blood flow is reduced (Martin *et al.*, 1983). Complications associated with distal embolization have been well documented (Cogbill and Gunderson, 1985; Rodigas and Bridges, 1986; Inverson *et al.*, 1987). The initial experience with the use of the percutaneous IAB at the Columbia University–Presbyterian Medical Center has resulted in a protocol that greatly reduces the likelihood of distal embolization (Bregman, 1982).

Before removal of the balloon catheter, completely collapse the balloon by aspiration with a 50 ml syringe and a stopcock. Pull the balloon down to (but not into) the sheath. Compress the femoral artery distal to the insertion site and remove the balloon and sheath as a single unit. Blood is allowed to spurt from the artery for a few seconds so that any thrombus material is removed. Now, shift compression of the femoral artery over the puncture site for 30 min. Distal pulses are monitored with Doppler apparatus, and manual compression is adjusted so that an audible pulse is registered. A compression dressing is applied to the puncture site for a 24 h period.

Rodigas and Finnegan (1985) reported good results with a variation of this procedure; after flushing out any proximal thrombi from the artery, the pressure applied to the insertion site was reversed to allow back-bleeding and the removal of any distal thrombi.

Investigators in the TAMI trials similarly applied pressure above the insertion site while subsequently 'milking' the thigh to extrude distal clots. Again, the safety record was not adversely affected by the use of thrombolysis (George, 1988).

Percutaneous clinical experience

Percutaneous intra-aortic balloon insertion was attempted in 202 patients from February 1979 to

Table 18.1 Use of percutaneous intra-aortic balloon pumping at the Columbia–Presbyterian Medical Center 1979–1985

Successful insertions	*CCU*	*Cath Lab*
Preop		
Unstable angina with general surgery	1	—
Unstable angina with cardiac surgery	18 (3)	13 (2)
Unstable angina – treated with medication	4 (1)	1
Postinfarction angina – treated with medication	4 (2)	4 (1)
Postinfarction angina with surgery	10 (1)	3
Cardiogenic shock – treated with medication	2	4 (3)
Cardiogenic shock with surgery	2	5 (2)
Cardiac arrest	4 (3)	1
Recurrent ventricular tachycardia – medication	1	—
Failed Gruntzig procedure with emergency surgery	—	6 (2)
Acute VSD with surgery	1	2 (1)
Acute VSD without surgery	—	1 (1)
Anaesthesia support for open heart surgery	6 (1)	12 (1)
Periop		
Low output – OR	71 (44)	
Postop		
Low output	16 (9)	
Cardiac arrest	4 (3)	
Total number assisted	196	
Total number discharged	116 (60%)	

Parentheses indicate number of deaths

January 1985 at the Columbia–Presbyterian Medical Center (Table 18.1). Successful insertion was accomplished in 196 of 202 patients (97%). In ten patients, the initial insertion attempt failed, however, four of the ten patients eventually underwent successful intra-aortic balloon pump implantation when the 28 cm sheath-dilator was employed.

Indications in these patients were broadly divided among medical and surgical groups. Of the 196 patients, 91 received the IAB for a surgical indication. Surgical indications included intraoperative low cardiac output in 71, postoperative low output syndrome in 16, and cardiac arrest in four. Medical indications for counterpulsation with the IAB included unstable angina refractory to medical management in 36, post-infarction angina in 21, cardiogenic shock in 13, acute ventricular septal defect complicating myocardial infarction in four, recurrent ventricular tachycardia in one, and six patients received the IAB when haemodynamic decompensation occurred during transluminal coronary angioplasty. All six patients required emergent surgical coronary revascularization. Only one patient received the IAB prophylactically for unstable angina before a general surgical procedure. This patient survived and the balloon was removed in the immediate postoperative period.

The location of intra-aortic balloon pump insertion varied. Seventy-one patients had the balloon implanted in the operating room, 20 in the open-heart recovery room, 52 in the cardiac catheterization laboratory, and 53 in the cardiac intensive care unit.

Of the 105 patients in whom the intra-aortic balloon pump was successfully inserted for a medical indication (Figure 18.19), 79 (75%) eventually underwent a cardiac surgical procedure, whereas, 26 (25%) were treated medically. Only 13 of the 79 patients (16%) undergoing preoperative IAB support combined with a definitive surgical procedure died. In contrast, 56 of the 91 patients (61%) requiring intraoperative and postoperative IAB expired.

Complications associated with IABs

The nature of intra-aortic balloon insertion and function, as well as the critical status of those patients requiring its use, presents potential for major complications. Alcan *et al.* (1984) collected data on 321 patients from 1974 to 1982 requiring intra-aortic balloon counterpulsation for a variety of reasons, under both emergent and controlled situations. They reported major complications in 9% of patients who had undergone intra-aortic balloon counterpulsation. Complications ranged from thrombosis and embolization, accounting for greater than half of these, to aortic dissection in one case. If the contingency exists, however, it is felt

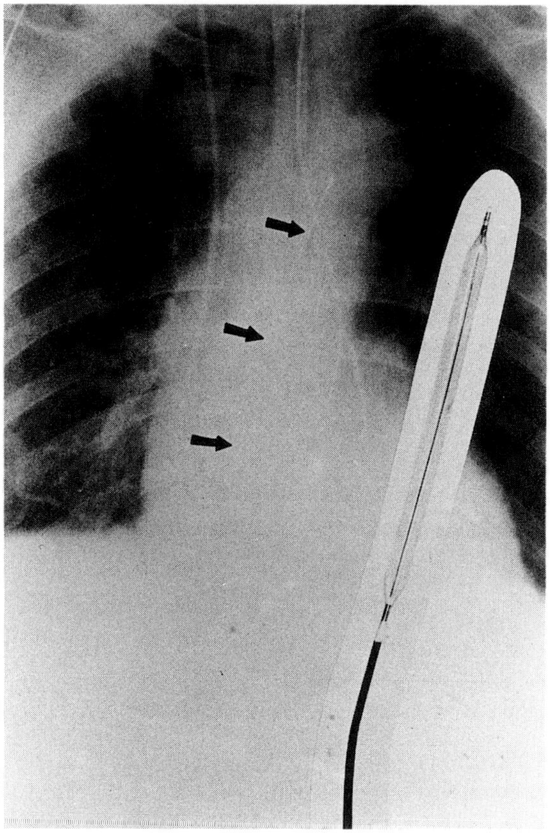

Figure 18.20 Chest roentgenogram showing proper positioning of the intra-aortic balloon pump in the descending thoracic aorta. Note positioning of the tip of the balloon

that risk factors include severity of peripheral vascular disease, extent of myocardial failure, significant long-standing hypertension, female sex, and duration of use.

The principle complications associated with intra-aortic balloon pumping fall into three main categories:

1. Trauma to the arterial wall incurred while inserting and advancing the guidewire or balloon.
2. Limb ischaemia associated with the position of the balloon catheter, and which disappears with catheter removal.
3. Dislodged thrombus created during balloon removal resulting in distal embolization.

Isner and associates found that 60% of the complications of the IAB appear to result from trauma associated with insertion of the catheter. These included aortoiliac dissection, arterial perforation, and dislodged atherosclerotic plaque. In addition, it was noted that the older the patient, the more likely that atherosclerotic disease will diminish the arterial lumen diameter, resulting in a greater potential for insertion damage. Along with these more common types of complications, several notable ones have appeared, including a patient with an improperly positioned IAB which intermittently occluded the origin of the superior mesenteric artery. The resulting abdominal pain was relieved upon advancing the balloon to its 'correct position' (Karlson *et al.*, 1981). Rodigas reports an occlusion of the left internal mammary artery by an improperly positioned balloon catheter. A splenic infarction precipitated by IAB placement was reported by Busch (Busch, Cogbill and Gunderson, 1985). And there have been several instances of paraplegia related to balloon pumping, including the report by Rose and colleagues.

We reviewed the first 113 consecutive patients undergoing percutaneous IAB insertion at the Columbia–Presbyterian Medical Center (Todd *et al.*, 1983). Complications of percutaneous IAB insertion occurred in seven of the 113 patients. Included in these seven complications is one guidewire perforation of the aorta, which was a result of IAB insertion. Complications related to the maintenance and removal of the IAB included four patients requiring embolectomy for femoral thrombi, one asymptomatic occlusion of the iliac artery, and one patient with persistently diminished dorsalis pedis pulses. There were no false aneurysms, aortic dissections or septic complications noted resulting from the percutaneous balloon in our series. However, it should be noted that extensive necropsy examinations were not performed.

Four patients, in whom percutaneous IAB insertion by conventional approach was unsuccessful underwent successful balloon implantation by the long-catheter technique. There were no insertion related complications in these four patients.

More recently, though, improved technique has curtailed major vascular complications, especially extensive blood loss. This is of major importance in the new age of thrombolysis in acute myocardial infarction.

Percutaneous *v.* surgical insertion

The rapidly changing designs and sizes of intra-aortic balloons, including the new percutaneous designs, have made their comparison problematic. In addition, indications for insertion have been widened and many investigators now favour early institution of intra-aortic balloon pumping. Several recent reports address these variables while comparing the surgical and percutaneous approaches to balloon pumping. Collier and associates (1986), in reviewing their records report a

Table 18.2 Uses of dual-chambered intra-aortic balloon pumping

1. As an aid in enabling the cardiovascular surgeon to remove a refractory patient from total cardiopulmonary bypass.
2. As a support during emergency coronary arteriography or ventriculography in a haemodynamically unstable patient or in a patient with crescendo angina.
3. As a preoperative, intraoperative, or postoperative aid in conjunction with open heart surgery or myocardial irevascularization procedures.
4. In selected cases of cardiogenic shock secondary to myocardial infarction.

similar complication rate of both surgical and percutaneous balloons. The ischaemic complications were higher in the percutaneous balloon insertion group than the surgical balloon insertion group (26.8% *v.* 19.2%, respectively). However, when only major ischaemic complications are calculated, the ischaemic complication rate for percutaneous insertion of IAB is 18.6% as compared with 16.4% for the surgically inserted IAB group (difference is not statistically significant). Martin and associates, in their review of 100 percutaneous IAB insertions, found that 12 out of 95 (12.6%) who received the IAB required surgical correction of a major complication.

Clinical literature review

Myocardial infarction with shock

Initially, it was believed that the intra-aortic balloon pump would be the physicians' salvation in the management of patients with acute myocardial infarction and shock. In fact, when a given patient who was in shock syndrome secondary to acute myocardial infarction was placed on intra-aortic balloon pump support, the patient invariably showed some clinical improvement. However, as the major experience has evolved throughout the world with support of cardiogenic shock patients on the intra-aortic balloon pump (Cohn, 1975; Mundth *et al.*, 1975; Willerson *et al.*, 1975; Baron and O'Rouke, 1976; Kveim *et al.*, 1976; Bardet *et al.*, 1977; Ehrich *et al.*, 1977; Jackson *et al.*, 1977; Johnson *et al.*, 1977), certain basic and consistent observations have been made. Offering balloon support to patients who have been in cardiogenic shock for extended periods of time is not practical (Scheidt *et al.*, 1973). Although frequently there is improvement in the patients' haemodynamics, organ function has often reached irreversible deterioration, and the ultimate outcome of these patients is uniformly fatal. Therefore, it appears more advisable to try to insert the intra-aortic balloon pump early in the course of cardiogenic shock.

A report by Hagemaijer *et al.* (1977) involved 25 patients with NYHA class III or IV acute myocardial infarction who were treated with intra-aortic balloon pumping during a 4-year period. Twenty of these 25 patients were successfully weaned from the intra-aortic balloon pump; yet six died within 3 months, five within the first 10 days of balloon weaning. Of the 14 patients who survived for more than 3 months, 13 were still alive at the time of the report, and 12 of the 13 were functional class II. Six have resumed full activity. This report indicates that the early application of intra-aortic balloon pumping during cardiogenic shock associated with acute myocardial infarction may improve patient survival. In addition, it is generally thought that enhanced coronary blood flow reduces the propensity for new clot formation and increases exposure of disrupted plaque to antiplatelet agents. Intra-aortic balloon pumping, by improving diastolic flow, may prove 'protective' in the setting of preventing reocclusion of an infarct related artery after a patient has received either percutaneous transluminal coronary angioplasty or thrombolytic therapy.

An overall survival rate of 30–85% has been reported (Bourdarias, Gourgon and Bardet, 1978) for patients in cardiogenic shock secondary to either a mechanical defect complicating acute myocardial infarction, or in patients with cardiogenic shock treated by the combination of intra-aortic balloon pumping and surgery.

In a recent report of intra-aortic balloon use in 728 patients (Mueller *et al.*, 1972), the rate of intra-aortic balloon pump-related mortality was only 0.8%, and the survival of a large number of patients with acute myocardial ischaemia was attributed to the use of the intra-aortic balloon pump. The success of this treatment modality, coupled with its low mortality rate, has encouraged many authors (Weintraub *et al.*, 1974; Scully *et al.*, 1976; Bardet *et al.*, 1977; Bahn, 1978; Bregman, 1978; Cohn *et al.*, 1978; Kuhn, 1978; Leinbach *et al.*, 1978; McEnany *et al.*, 1978; Roberts *et al.*, 1978) to advocate the earlier institution of intra-aortic balloon counterpulsation support for cardiogenic shock.

Still unresolved completely, is the question of how to proceed after the institution of the counterpulsation. If the patients is completely stable on the intra-aortic balloon pump, it has been suggested that the maximal benefit from intra-aortic balloon counterpulsation will be achieved with 5 days of support, and accordingly, attempt should be made to wean the patient from balloon support at this time. If the catheterization studies then indicate that the patient should undergo either coronary bypass surgery (CABG) or percutaneous transluminal coronary angioplasty (PTCA), the definitive procedure should be performed within the same hospitalization.

The patients who may best profit from this therapeutic route seem to be those who respond most promptly to the intra-aortic balloon, and those who have major ischaemic changes on their electrocardiogram which return to normal with the onset of intra-aortic balloon pumping.

At present, for the patient with cardiogenic shock requiring intra-aortic balloon support and ultimately coronary revascularization surgery, the overall survival, as mentioned, is now being reported in excess of 50% (Berger *et al.*, 1973). However, if the patient becomes dependent on intra-aortic balloon support and can not be successfully weaned with the addition of pharmacologic manoeuvres (i.e. inotropic support), this situation has uniformly led to a nearly 100% mortality, even when surgical intervention is attempted.

Myocardial infarction without shock

Much evidence suggests that support with the intra-aortic balloon pump can limit infarct size, thereby preserving myocardium. For over a decade, investigators (Mueller *et al.*, 1972; Scheidt *et al.*, 1973; Willerson *et al.*, 1975; Bardet *et al.*, 1977; Hagemeijer *et al.*, 1977; Bahn, 1978; Bourdarias, Gourgon and Bardet, 1978; Bregman, 1978; Cohn *et al.*, 1978; Kuhn, 1978) have supported using the intra-aortic balloon pump in the setting of acute myocardial infarction in patients without shock. Leinbach *et al.* (1978) studied the reversibility of myocardial ischaemia through the use of the intra-aortic balloon pump in patients with acute myocardial infarction who were not in clinical shock. Their criteria for selection was that the patients be under the age of 65 with continued chest pain unrelieved by standard medical therapy, including morphine, oxygen, and intravenous nitrates; and anterior ST-segment elevation on the surface electrocardiogram. Continuous electrocardiographic monitoring was used, and as soon as current therapy failure was observed, prompt institution of the intra-aortic balloon pump was initiated. Five of the 11 patients studied responded with an 84% fall in ST-segment elevation in 1 h, while maintaining precordial R-waves and good ventricular function. The other six patients responded poorly, with a 40% fall in the ST-segment elevation in 1 h, Q-wave development and poorer residual left ventricular function. Patient response correlated well with the presence and absence of complete left anterior descending coronary artery occlusion as demonstrated by coronary angiography.

Thus, experimental documentation supports aggressive therapy with the intra-aortic balloon pump in the setting of acute myocardial infarction, specifically, anterior wall infarctions. This adjunct will be of particular use and benefit for those patients in whom thrombolysis would be contraindicated (i.e. those patients above 70 years of age, or with recent history of cerebral vascular events, surgery, or severe hypertension).

Safety with thrombolytic therapy

As alluded to above, the safety record of the intra-aortic balloon pump when used in patients receiving thrombolytic therapy is encouraging. Goodwin *et al.* (1989) retrospectively reviewed patients given streptokinase and intra-aortic balloon counterpulsation between 1985 and 1987. They found no statistically significant differences among three groups: (1) those treated with streptokinase during acute myocardial infarction; (2) those with acute myocardial infarction or unstable angina treated with intra-aortic balloon counterpulsation without thrombolysis; and (3) those treated with streptokinase followed by intra-aortic balloon counterpulsation, with regard to requirement of surgical repair of the femoral artery, percent of patients requiring transfusion, and number of units of packed red blood cells transfused (*see* Figure 18.21a and b). They suggest that intra-aortic balloon pumping may be used safely and early in patients with acute myocardial infarction who receive thrombolytic therapy. Of note is the fact that the complication rate of patients treated with thrombolysis and intra-aortic balloon pumping compared with patients who were treated with heparin alone was no greater.

High-risk patients requiring cardiac catheterization and percutaneous transluminal coronary angioplasty

At present there is little doubt that a patient who has evidence of either a significant degree of left ventricular failure, ventricular tachyarrhythmia, or one of the acute mechanical complications of myocardial infarction can be safely carried through cardiac catheterization without significant risk using the intra-aortic balloon pump (Webb *et al.*, 1974; Goldman *et al.*, 1976; Gunstensen *et al.*, 1976; Mundth, 1976; Lappas, Powell and Daggett, 1977). During the catheterization procedure, the intra-aortic balloon is momentarily switched off as the guidewire passes the balloon into the thoracic aorta. As soon as the catheter and/or guidewire is positioned in the ascending aorta, the intra-aortic balloon pump is turned on again, and the cardiac catheterization procedure can proceed. Clearly, the intra-aortic balloon pump has significantly reduced the potential complications of cardiac catheterization in these critically ill patients.

As the levels of technology and skill improve in the area of non-surgical revascularization, more and more patients originally considered purely surgical

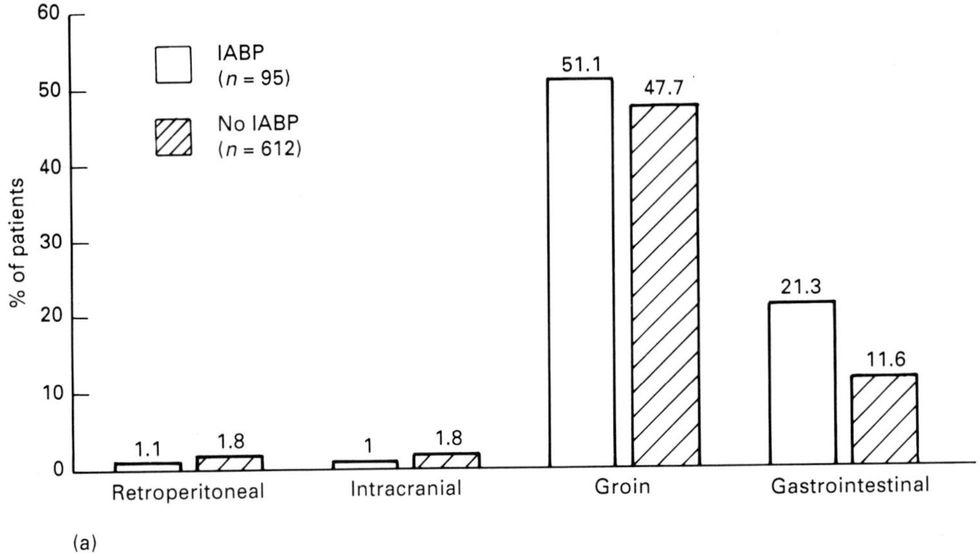

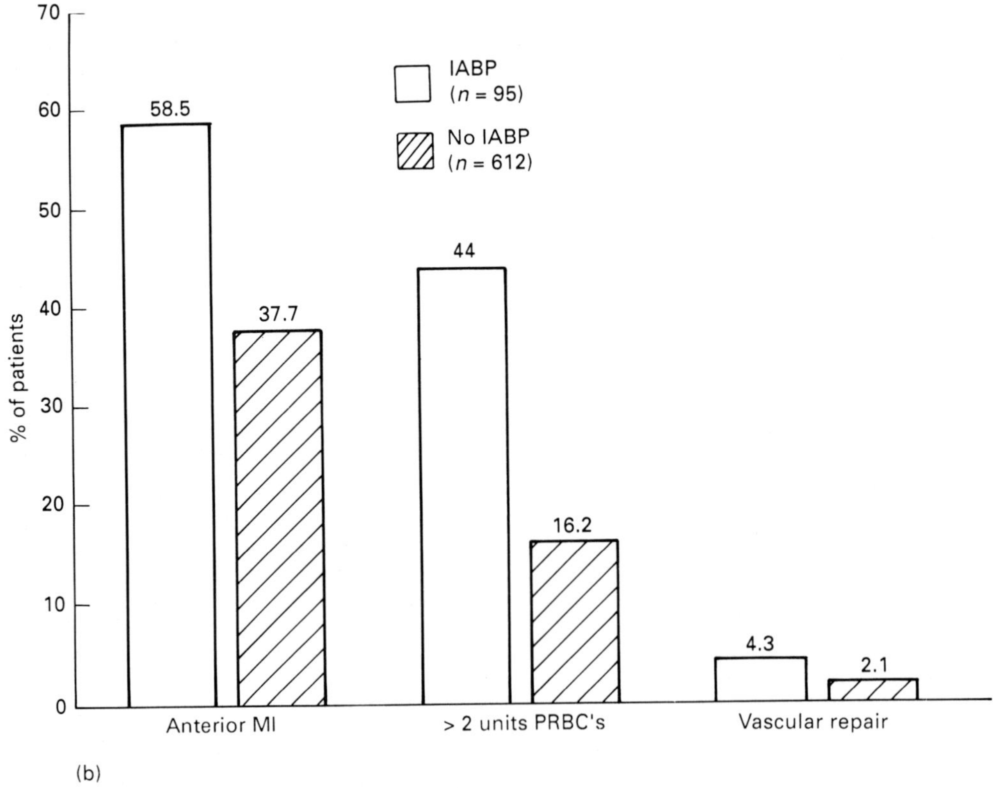

Figure 18.21a and b Intra-aortic pump use during the TAMI trials. (a) There was no greater incidence of bleeding complications in the group that received treatment with intra-aortic balloon pumping as compared with the group that did not. (b) Although the intra-aortic balloon pump patients required more than two units of PRBCs more often than the non-intra-aortic balloon pump patients, the difference between the two groups was not statistically significant

candidates are now being offered PTCA. Intra-aortic balloon pump support during these procedures is proving to be very effective. The latest information demonstrates that intra-aortic balloon pumping can be carried out in 'high–risk' PTCA as an adjunctive and relatively benign procedure. Kahn *et al.* (1990) performed PTCA on 28 'high-risk' patients. Mean ejection fraction was 24%. Ninety-three percent had three-vessel disease, with significant left main disease in 25%. They successfully dilated 90 of 94 lesions (96%), including multi-vessel dilatation in 75% and five left main coronary artery dilatations. They reported no deaths or myocardial infarctions in any patient at 3 days post-procedure. None of the patients required emergency coronary artery bypass surgery.

In examining the TAMI I data, Califf and Phman (1990) discovered that only 7% of 85 patients who had undergone PTCA while on the intra-aortic balloon pump had reocclusion. More importantly, however, none of the reocclusion occurred while the intra-aortic balloon pump was in place. They go on to propose the mechanism of prevention of reocclusion; as alluded to previously, improved diastolic blood pressures translates into improved coronary blood flow. This may reduce the propensity for clot formation, while increasing the delivery time of antiplatelet agents and anticoagulants. In addition, improved coronary filling pressure may prevent closure of the initial flap made during PTCA against the opposing wall of the vessel.

Preoperative intra-aortic balloon pumping in high-risk cardiac patients

The risks of early infarction and death in patients with acute coronary insufficiency undergoing cardiac surgery are generally considered greater than in patients with stable angina pectoris. The most appropriate therapy, however, and the timing of that therapy, are points of controversy. Cooper *et al.* (1977) reported on 63 high-risk myocardial revascularization patients who had preoperative intra-aortic balloon pumping. Only six patients required rapid institution of cardiopulmonary bypass after anaesthetic induction despite a marked drop in blood pressure in 50% of the patients. There were two instances of post-pump power failure, with two deaths in this series. The author concluded from this experience that preoperative intra-aortic balloon pumping in a valid method of limiting morbidity associated with coronary surgery in high risk patients.

Scully *et al.* (1976) have recently studied the effects of preoperative intra-aortic balloon pumping in 42 patients with acute coronary insufficiency complicated by abnormal left ventricular haemodynamics and refractory chest pain. Aggressive medical therapy had previously failed in all cases.

The perioperative mortality rate, when compared with that of similar patients treated before and after the use of the intra-aortic balloon pump, was lowered from 25% to 8%. Similar results have been achieved by Weintraub *et al.* (1978), Langon *et al.* (1978), and McEnany *et al.* (1978). In addition, inotropic support and duration of stay, both in the intensive care unit and in the hospital, were significantly decreased in the patients treated preoperatively with the intra-aortic balloon pump. Bolooki *et al.* (1976) also reported a shorter time on cardiopulmonary bypass, and Feola *et al.* (1977) have noted an improvement in metabolic status as measured by decreased cardiac lactate production.

Others (Sammel, O'Rouke and Chang, 1976; Lefemine *et al.*, 1977; Lamberti and Resnekov, 1978) have applied the intra-aortic balloon pump preoperatively in cases of decreased left ventricular function, but the interpretation of the data is not as clear-cut as in the case of acute coronary insufficiency.

Use in non-cardiac surgery

An indication which ultimately may prove to be very practical is the prophylactic use of intra-aortic balloon counterpulsation in major non-cardiac surgery. Perloth and Haltgren (1975) reported a 6% to 7% risk of perioperative myocardial infarction in patients with prior myocardial infarction. That number may be as high as 37% in patients undergoing major non-cardiac surgery within 3 months of a previous infarction with an associated mortality of 54% (Tarhan *et al.*, 1972). Grotz and Yeston (1989) recently presented three case reports supporting the thinking that prophylactic intra-aortic balloon pumping in high-risk patients may improve myocardial perfusion and overall haemodynamics, thereby reducing the risk of perioperative myocardial infarction and mortality.

Tachyarrhythmia and ventricular irritability

The increase in coronary blood flow associated with the use of the intra-aortic balloon pump as well as the decrease in myocardial wall tension as a result of the acute reduction in left ventricular afterload is ideally suited for the treatment of refractory ventricular tachyarrhythmia, both in the setting of the coronary care unit and in the postoperative surgical patient (Bregman, 1976). Unfortunately, while the treatment of tachyarrhythmia after open-heart surgery with the intra-aortic balloon pump can frequently be definitive (Willerson *et al.*, 1975), it is underutilized in this setting. Likewise, in the coronary care unit, many patients with ventricular irritability can be stabilized, and the frequency of their arrhythmias decreased significantly. It is the policy of these authors to catheterize every medical patient on an intra-aortic balloon pump whose indication for insertion has been ventricular tachyarrhythmia so that the patient's anatomy can be defined; and surgical intervention can proceed if indicated.

Mundth *et al.* (Mundth *et al.*, 1975; Mundth, 1976) have indicated that in the medical setting life-threatening, recurrent ventricular tachyarrhythmia in the acute postinfarction phase and in chronic coronary disease can be controlled initially with intra-aortic balloon pumping as a prelude to cardiac catheterization and cardiac surgery. Ten patients with recurrent ventricular tachyarrhythmia underwent cardiac surgery, and seven of those patients survived.

Williams *et al.* (1975) have reported success with intra-aortic balloon pumping therapy even when no surgically correctable lesion is present, and recommend the use of the intra-aortic balloon pump for all patients who develop ventricular arrhythmias and low nodal bradyarrhythmia, which are refractory to standard medical therapy.

Septic shock

Sepsis is usually responded to by an increase in cardiac output, the limitation of which is posed by both Starling's law and the functional cardiac reserve of the individual patient. Ultimately, the patient in septic shock will develop a low cardiac output state mediated by 'myocardial depressant factors' and, if the appropriate medical therapy fails, death will ensue. Berger *et al.* (1973) reported on the fortuitous use of the intra-aortic balloon pump in a patient with septic shock, who was initially thought to have a myocardial infarction with low-output state. The distinct improvement in this patient prompted the authors to use the intra-aortic balloon pump in another patient with septic shock. In both of these patients, cardiac output could be maintained while the appropriate treatment, including antibiotics and steroids, could be administered. Our experience has also justified the concept of intra-aortic balloon pumping in septic shock patients with low cardiac output syndrome. Indeed, Berger's two initial patients were ultimately discharged from the hospital. Since then, other investigators (O'Rouke, 1977; McEnany *et al.*, 1978) have considered septic shock an indication for use of the intra-aortic balloon pump.

Myocardial contusion

Myocardial contusion complicates approximately 20% of cases of blunt anterior thoracic chest wall trauma (Saunders and Doty, 1978). Steering wheel injuries are the most prevalent cause of myocardial contusion. Unfortunately the diagnosis is frequently delayed or missed, complicating the treatment of myocardial contusion, which in turn may affect the treatment of associated injuries.

One of the most important physiological consequences of myocardial contusion, which is always associated with severe blunt chest wall trauma, is decreased cardiac output. Proper treatment may be a major determinant of survival in some cases of myocardial contusion. While clinical intra-aortic balloon pumping therapy for myocardial contusion has yet to be reported in the literature, Saunders and Doty have applied this technique in dogs with experimentally induced myocardial contusion. The results of their study show that intra-aortic balloon pumping does, in fact, improve left ventricular performance following myocardial contusion, especially when applied early after injury.

Cardiac arrest

Another role for the intra-aortic balloon pump made possible by the rapidity of the percutaneous approach is mechanical support during cardiac resuscitation. Conventional balloon insertion is not feasible during resuscitation because of the time required for surgical insertion. Because percutaneous insertion can be instituted in several minutes without interfering with resuscitative efforts or closed chest massage, this approach can be used to provide mechanical circulatory support during resuscitation.

Lane *et al.* in 1987, reported on the successful resuscitation of a patient with massive propanolol overdose and cardiac arrest with the use of the intra-aortic balloon pump.

Time and scientific inquiry yield a more complete understanding of both the indications and contraindications for use of the intra-aortic balloon pump in this setting. Since it is simple in both theory and practice (Igo *et al.*, 1978), intra-aortic balloon pump insertion may be accomplished rapidly and efficiently, and thus, appears ideal for the emergency situation. The haemodynamic effects of intra-aortic balloon pump actuation on left and right ventricular performance are immediate and can not be duplicated by pharmacological agents. These unique effects decrease right and left ventricular myocardial oxygen requirements (systolic unloading), increase biventricular indices of myocardial oxygen supply (diastolic augmentation), and increase right and left ventricular external performance (stroke volume) by conservation of less efficient pressure work to more efficient volume work.

Long-term survival of IABP patients

The ability of the intra-aortic balloon pump to haemodynamically support and stabilize the failing circulation is well established. However, does the short-term stabilization of patients by IABP result in improved long-term survival for any group of patients? Because most of the patients requiring intra-aortic balloon counterpulsation would have otherwise succumbed in the short-term, intuitively, the intra-aortic balloon pump has improved their long-term outlook. For these patients most certainly would not have survived to hospital discharge had it not been for intra-aortic balloon pump support. One must consider this fact when reviewing the literature concerning long-term survival of intra-aortic balloon pump patients. Several investigators have looked at this issue.

The first study on the long-term effect of balloon pumping was initiated by Bolooki *et al.* (1976) in their review of 43 patients who required intra-aortic balloon pump support to be weaned off the cardiopulmonary bypass circuit. Twenty-three patients (53%) were discharged from the hospital and were living 4 months or longer. Golding *et al.* (1980) at the Cleveland Clinic, studied 197 patients who underwent intra-aortic balloon pumping, pre-, peri-, or postoperatively. Of the 197 patients, 143 (72.6%) were discharged from the hospital. The 2 year cardiac actuarial survival for the hospital survivors was 134 (96%). Eighty-five per cent of the surviving patients remained asymptomatic during the follow-up period. Golding also reported that the survival statistics for patients who required intra-aortic balloon pumping in conjunction with myocardial revascularization were similar to the patients who did not require intra-aortic balloon pump assistance. This becomes even more significant assuming that the patients requiring support, in general, are a sicker group of patients.

Sanfelippo *et al.* (1986) reported their experiences with 283 patients discharged from the hospital following cardiac surgery and IAB support. Of these 283 patients, 181 (64%) survived 3 years or more. Kuchner *et al.* (1987) studied 225 patients with left ventricular failure refractory to medical management after myocardial infarction and cardiac surgery. All patients had undergone intra-aortic balloon counterpulsation; 43% were discharged from the hospital with an average follow-up of 5.8 years.

Long-term support by IABP

There have been several instances where patients have remained on the intra-aortic balloon pump for an extended period of time (greater than 3–5 days). Except for patient discomfort associated with a lengthy immobilization of the limb with the catheter, no toxicity has been associated with long-term balloon pumping (Madras *et al.*, 1969). Brantigan, Grow and Schoonmaker (1976) have reported on a woman with peripartum cardiomyopathy who was balloon dependent for 7 weeks and improved during this period; she subsequently expired 3 weeks after balloon removal.

The majority of cases on long-term balloon support can not be weaned off, and are in fact balloon dependent. Most often these are patients with end-stage coronary artery disease and cardiomyopathy, although several instances of septicemia with cardiogenic shock have been reported (Frazier *et al.*, 1986).

In 1978, Reemtsma *et al.* reported the successful heart transplantation in two patients maintained on the IAB. Both patients were discharged and survived over one year. Subsequent to this, Reemtsma and associates (Bregman *et al.*, 1982) reported another four cardiac transplantations performed on balloon maintained patients. These four patients survived the operation, with one living 12 months; the other three patients expired within a month from acute transplant rejection. Cooley reported a successful cardiac transplant in a woman with septicaemia who required IAB support.

IABP at the community hospital

With the advent of coronary care units, many patients with acute coronary insufficiency or mechanical complications of acute myocardial infarction are being cared for in community hospitals. The ability to insert the intra-aortic balloon rapidly through the percutaneous technique has made it possible for the IAB to be inserted and maintained in the community hospitals setting. Many primary and community hospital with staff members trained in cardiac catheterization techniques find themselves now able to take advantage of counterpulsation. For the patient with unstable haemodynamics and surgically correctable lesions, the intra-aortic balloon pump can serve as life support during transfer to a cardiac surgery centre. For years, several community hospitals have purchased intra-aortic balloon pump apparatus, and have inserted intra-aortic balloons in selected patients in their coronary care units (Bass, Katzman and Pois, 1978; Bolooki, 1984). McEnany *et al.* (1978) have reported that 32 of their 747 intra-aortic balloon pumps were started at peripheral community hospitals and the patients were then transported to the Massachusetts General Hospital while receiving diastolic augmentation support.

Several investigators have reported their experience in transporting IAB dependent patients from community hospitals to major cardiac centres. Hines *et al.* (1982) describe a mobile cardiac shock van that contains a portable balloon pump. The van transports patients in need of counterpulsation to a hospital equipped with these facilities. The balloon is inserted by the mobile team on arrival at the community hospital. Once the patient is stabilized with IABP support, he can be safely transported. In the first 16 patients, 14 had the balloon successfully inserted, one was unable to be inserted, and one could not have intra-aortic balloon pumping performed for administrative reasons. All 16 arrived at the destination safely although one patient required en route defibrillation. Kramer (1988) describes his experience with the use of the intra-aortic balloon during helicopter transport of 32 patients since 1984. The system was easily adapted for airborne use.

Singh and associates (1981) have reported their experience with the intra-aortic balloon pump at the community hospital level. Insertions were performed in the intensive care unit at the bedside by the thoracic surgeons. Patients requiring cardiac surgery were transported on the intra-aortic balloon pump using a specially equipped ambulance. In a group of 22 patients with unstable angina, 16 were considered operable and were transported to another institution for cardiac surgery. In a 15-month follow-up, all 16 were doing well. LoCicero and colleagues (1985) had similar experiences with 50 patients who after being placed on intra-aortic balloon pump, were transferred on the IAB pump to a regional medical centre. All patients were transported without incident and then underwent myocardial revascularization. Three (5%) patients expired postoperatively, and nine (20%) had complications directly related to the IAB catheter. Finally, Gottlieb *et al.* (1986) report similar results in 11 patients, who after undergoing intra-aortic balloon pump insertion and stabilization at the community hospital level were then transferred to a tertiary centre for cardiac surgery.

IABP in the paediatric population

Not long after the introduction of the intra-aortic balloon in clinical use, Pollock *et al.* (1982), in 1979, reported on the use of the intra-aortic balloon pump in a series of infants and children undergoing open-heart surgery. The patients ranged in age from 1 1/2 years to 18 years. There were six long-term survivors, however, all the patients under 5 years of age died. Insertion was via the common femoral artery using a side arm Dacron graft. Adult balloons, 8 mm and 10 mm, were inserted through the graft up into the thoracic aorta. It was noted that effective augmentation was difficult to achieve. This was felt to be related to the relatively compliant aortic walls in children. Although no bleeding or thrombocytopenia was seen, there were several serious complications noted, including superior mesenteric artery occlusion, renal artery occlusion, and severe limb ischaemia. The use of adult size balloons allowed a large segment of the pumping chamber to lie below the level of the diaphragm, thereby accounting for most of the ischaemic related complications.

In an effort to overcome these problems, Veasy *et al.* (1981) have sought to adapt the intra-aortic balloon pump for use in the paediatric population. The major obstacles, however, are balloon and catheter size. Unlike with adults, there is much concern over varying aortic diameters and length, as well as femoral artery length. Veasy developed balloons ranging from 0.75 ml to 5 ml attached to Nos 4.0 Fr and 5.0 Fr catheters. These were then tested *in vitro* in animal models using the Utah heart driver and three other pumping systems. All the balloons were introduced percutaneously. In small animals with reduced cardiac output from acutely produced mitral regurgitation, the newly developed intra-aortic balloons effectively reduced aortic peak systolic pressure (afterload), lowered aortic end-diastolic pressure and reduced left atrial pressure. In addition, the Datascope 80 system most effectively augmented diastolic pressure and increased aortic forward and negative flow as compared with the AVCO^{R} and UHS^{R} systems.

A balloon catheter should be selected with a volume equal to at least 50% of the stroke volume. The following formula has been suggested (Veasy and Webster, 1985):

$$\frac{2000 \times (\text{cardiac index}) \times (\text{body surface area})}{\text{Heart rate}} \times 0.5 = \text{Balloon volume}$$

with a larger size balloon being employed should the calculation fall between available sizes.

One concern with the use of intra-aortic balloon pumping in paediatric patients is poor augmentation. This is due to several reasons: (1) the paediatric aortic wall displays increased elasticity and compliance compared with the adult aorta. Since the balloon inflates against a relatively distensible lumen, the degree of augmentation seen in children may not match that of adults; (2) the increased heart rates seen in the paediatric population at any given level of cardiac output, can present a timing challenge even to the experienced operator. Therefore, it has been recommended (Dunn, 1988 unpublished data) that larger balloons than expected be used to overcome the distensibility problem, and that at heart rates greater than 160, 1:2 intra-aortic balloon assistance may afford better diastolic augmentation than at every beat assistance. Other difficulties include designing catheters capable of permitting rapid exchange of gas to match the faster heart rates of infants and children.

Through 1985, clinical experience of Veasy *et al.* included patients from age 5 days to 12 years, with weights ranging from 3.2 kg to 33.2 kg. Of their first 18 patients, nine survived over the short term, tolerating weaning from the intra-aortic balloon pump; and, of these, five left the hospital and were surviving 6 months after discharge. The inherent complications were few. Only one patient required discontinuation because of lower limb ischaemic injury.

Del Nido, in 1988, reported the successful circulatory support of a low cardiac output state in a 2 kg, 3-week-old infant.

As with adults, diligent monitoring of balloon position, respiratory support, inotropic support, renal function, infection control, anticoagulation, and more specifically for this population, of abdominal girths and gastrointestinal function is paramount.

Conclusion

Since the intra-aortic balloon pump was first introduced in the early 1960s, there has been a dramatic increase in its use. Currently more than half a million have been inserted world wide. Since the transition to the percutaneous method of insertion, it is now relatively easy to initiate intra-aortic balloon pumping in patients who require its use. No longer is the only indication cardiogenic shock. Recently, its applications have been substantially broadened; the intra-aortic balloon pump is used not only as an aid to the failing heart and as a last resort anti-arrhythmic device but during thrombolytic therapy, and as an adjunct to percutaneous transluminal angioplasty in patients with marginal haemodynamics to salvage ischaemic myocardium. The intra-aortic balloon pump is now used easily during transportation of patients, and in smaller community hospitals with relative safety. The intra-aortic balloon has been adapted efficiently for use in infants and small children. Further advances in hardware and software will no doubt continue to maintain the intra-aortic balloon pump as the most widely used temporary circulatory assist device.

References

Alcan, K.E., Stertzer, S.H., Wallsh, E., *et al.* (1984) Current status of intra-aortic balloon counterpulsation in critical care cardiology. *Critical Care Medicine*, **12**, 489

American Heart Association (1981) *Heart Facts*. American Heart Asssociation, New York

Bahn, C.H. (1978) Cardiac catheterization and intra-aortic balloon counterpulsation. (Letters to the editor). *American Journal of Cardiology*, **42**, 873

Bardet, J., Masquet, C., Kahn, J.C., *et al.* (1977a) Clinical and haemodynamic results of intra-aortic balloon counterpulsation and surgery for cardiogenic shock. *American Heart Journal*, **63**, 280

Bardet, J., Rigaud, M., Kahn, J.C., *et al.* (1977b) Treatment of post-myocardial infarction angina by intra-aortic balloon pumping and emergency revascularization. *Journal of Thoracic and Cardiovascular Surgery*, **74**, 299

Baron, D.W. and O'Rouke, M.F. (1976) Long-term results of arterial counterpulsation in acute severe cardiac failure complicating myocardial infarction. *British Heart Journal*, **38**, 285

Bass, J., Jr., Katzman, L. and Pois, A.J. (1978) Experience with intra-aortic balloon counterpulsation in a community hospital. *American Surgeon*, **44**, 324

Bedderman, C., McGee, M.G., Turner, S.A., *et al.* (1985) Intra-aortic balloon pumping in women: effects of balloon size on survival. *Journal of Thoracic and Cardiovascular Surgery*, **28**, 428

Berger, R.L., Saini, V.K., Long, W., *et al.* (1973) The use of diastolic augmentation with the intra-aortic balloon pump in human septic shock with associated coronary artery disease. *Surgery*, **74**, 601

Bernstein, E.F. and Murphy, A.E. (1973) The importance of pulsation in preventing thrombosis from intra-aortic balloons. A note of caution. *Journal of Thoracic and Cardiovascular Surgery*, **62**, 906

Bolooki, H. (1984) *Clinical Application of Intra-aortic Balloon Pump*, Futura Publishing Co, New York

Bolooki, H., Williams, W., Thurer, R.J., *et al.* (1976) Clinical and hemodynamic criteria for the use of the intra-aortic balloon pump in patients requiring cardiac surgery. *Journal of Thoracic and Cardiovascular Surgery*, **72**, 756

Bourdarias, J.P., Gourgon, R. and Bardet, J. (1978) Mechanical circulatory assistance by intra-aortic balloon pumping for the treatment of cardiogenic shock. *Intensive Care Medicine*, **4**, 29

Brantigan, C.O., Grow, J.B., Sr. and Schoonmaker, F.W. (1976) Extended use of intra-aortic balloon pumping in peripartum cardiomyopathy. *Annals of Surgery*, **183**, 1

Braunwald, E., Covell, J.W., Maroko, D.R. and Ross, J.R., Jr. (1969) Effects of drugs and of counterpulsation on myocardial oxygen consumption. *Circulation*, **38** and **40 (Suppl. IV)**, 220

Bregman, D. (1971) Intra-aortic balloon in open-heart surgery. *New England Journal of Medicine*, **284**, 393

Bregman, D. (1974) Management of patients undergoing intra-aortic balloon pumping. *Heart and Lung*, **3**, 916

Bregman, D. (1976) Mechanical support of the failing heart. In *Current Problems in Surgery* (ed. M.M. Ravitch), Year Book Medical Publishers, Chicago

Bregman, D. (1978) Cardiac assist devices. In *Blades Surgical Diseases of the Chest*, 4th edn, (ed. D.B. Effler), C.V. Mosby Co, St. Louis

Bregman, D. (1980a) A new percutaneous intra-aortic balloon. *Transactions of the American Society for Artificial Internal Organs*, **26**, 8

Bregman, D. (1980b) Intra-aortic balloon counterpulsation. In *Circulatory Assistance and the Artificial Heart* (ed. W.S. Pierce), USA–USSR Joint Symposium. Tibilsi, USSR, Sept. 20–22, 1979, U.S. Dept of Health and Human Services, PHS, NIH, pp. 155–165

Bregman, D. (1982) Percutaneous intra-aortic balloon pumping: a time for reflection. *Chest*, 82, 397

Bregman, D. and Casarella, W.J. (1979) Percutaneous intra-aortic balloon pumping: initial clinical experience. *Annals of Thoracic Surgery*, **29**, 153

Bregman, D., Bailin, M., Bowman, F.O., Jr., *et al.* (1977) A pulsatile assist device (PAD) for improved myocardial protection during cardiopulmonary bypass. *Annals of Thoracic Surgery*, **24**, 574

Bregman, D., Bolooki, H. and Malm, J.R. (1973) A simple method to facilitate difficult intra-aortic balloon insertions. *Annals of Thoracic and Cardiovascular Surgery*, **15**, 636

Bregman, D., Grusin, R., Lamb, J., *et al.* (1982) Heart transplantation in patients requiring mechanical circulatory support. *Heart Transplantation*, **1**, 154

Bregman, D., Nicols, A.B., Weiss, M.B., *et al.* (1980) Percutaneous intra-aortic balloon insertion. *American Journal of Cardiology*, **46**, 261

Brown, B.G., Gundel, W.D., Gott, V.L. and Covell, J.W. (1972) Hemodynamic determinants of retrograde arterial coronary flow following acute coronary occlusion. (Abstract). *Circulation*, **45** and **46** (**Suppl II**), 100

Busch, H.N., Jr., Cogbill, T.H. and Gunderson, A.E. (1985) Splenic infarction: complications of intra-aortic balloon counterpulsation. *American Heart Journal*, **109**, 383–385

Califf, R.M. and Phman, E.M. (1990) Reocclusion after thrombolytic therapy and percutaneous transluminal coronary angioplasty. *Cardiac Assists*, **5**, 1

Caulfield, J.B., Dunkman, W.B. and Leinhbach, R.C. (1972) Cardiogenic shock. Myocardial morphology with and without artificial left ventricular counterpulsation. *Archives of Pathology*, **93**, 532

Clayman, R.V., DeLaria, G.A., Johansen, K.H. and Berstein, E.F. (1973) The hypertensive balloon: a beneficial synergism for salvage of ischemic myocardium. *Surgical Forum*, **24**, 152

Cohn, L.H. (1975) Intra-aortic balloon counterpulsation in low cardiac output states. *Surgical Clinics of North America*, **55**, 545

Cohn, L.H., Alpert, J., Koster, J.K., Jr., *et al.* (1978) Changing indications for the surgical treatment of unstable angina. *Archives of Surgery*, **113**, 1312

Collier, P.E., Liebler, G.A., Park, S.B., *et al.* (1986) Is percutaneous insertion of the intra-aortic balloon pump through the femoral artery the safest technique? *Journal of Vascular Surgery*, **3**, 629

Cooper, G.N., Jr., Singh, A.K., Vargas, L.L. and Karlson, K.E. (1977) Preoperative intra-aortic balloon assist in high risk revascularization patients. *American Journal of Surgery*, **133**, 463

Corday, E., Swan, J.C., Lang, T.W., *et al.* (1970) Physiologic principles in the application of circulatory assist for the failing heart. *American Journal of Cardiology*, **26**, 595

Cox, J.L., McLaughlin, V.W., Flowers, N.C. *et al.* (1968) The ischemic zone surrounding acute myocardial infarction. Its morphology as detected by dehydrogenase staining. *American Heart Journal*, **76**, 650

Del Nido, P.J. (1988) Successful use of intra-aortic balloon pumping in a 2-kilogram infant. *Annals of Thoracic Surgery*, **46**, 574

Dormandy, J.A., Goetz, R.H. and Kripke, D.C. (1965) Hemodynamics and coronary blood flow with counterpulsation. *Surgery*, **65**, 311

Ehrich, D.A., Biddle, T.L., Kronenburg, M.S. and Yu, P.N. (1977) The hemodynamic response to intra-aortic balloon counterpulsation in patients with cardiogenic shock complicating acute myocardial infarction. *American Heart Journal*, **93**, 274

Feola, M., Limet, R.R. and Glick, G. (1971) Direct and reflex vascular effects of intra-aortic balloon counterpulsation in dogs at four levels of aortic pressure. *Clinical Research*, **19**, 313

Feola, M., Wiener, L., Walinsky, P., *et al.* (1977) Improved survival after coronary bypass surgery in patients with poor left ventricular function: role of intra-aortic balloon counterpulsation. *American Journal of Cardiology*, **39**, 1021

Frazier, O.H., Cooley, D.A., Okereke, O.J., *et al.* (1986) Cardiac transplantation in a patient with septicemia after prolonged intra-aortic pump support: implications for staged transplantation. *Texas Heart Journal*, **13**, 13

Furman, S., Vijaynagar, R., Rosenbaum, R., *et al.* (1971) Lethal sequelae of intra-aortic balloon rupture. *Surgery*, **69**, 121

George, B.S. (1988) Thrombolysis and intra-aortic balloon pumping following acute myocardial infarction–experience in four TAMI studies. *Cardiac Assists*, **4**, 3

Gill, C.C., Weschler, A.S., Newman, G.E. and Oldham, H.N., Jr. (1973) Augmentation and redistribution of myocardial blood flow during acute ischemia by intra-aortic balloon pumping. *Annals of Thoracic Surgery*, **16**, 445

Gold, H.K., Leinbach, R.C., Buckley, M.J., *et al.* (1976) Refractory angina pectoris: follow-up after intra-aortic balloon pumping and surgery. *Circulation*, **54**, 41 (**Suppl III**)

Golding, L.A., Loop, F.D., Peter, M., *et al.* (1980) Late survival following use of intra-aortic balloon pump in revascularization operations. *Annals of Thoracic Surgery*, **30**, 48

Goldman, B.S., Gunstensen, J., Gilbert, B.W., *et al.* (1976) Increasing operability and survival intra-aortic balloon pumping assist. *Canadian Journal of Surgery*, **19**, 69

Goodwin, M. (1989) Saefty of intra-aortic balloon counterpulsation in patients with acute myocardial infarction receiving streptokinase intravenously. *American Journal of Cardiology*, **64**, 937

Gottlieb, S.O., Chew, P.H., Chandra, N., *et al.* (1986) Portable intra-aortic balloon counterpulsation. *Catheterization and Cardiovascular Diagnosis*, **12**, 18

Grotz, R.L. and Yeston, N.S. (1989) Intra-aortic balloon counterpulsation in high-risk cardiac patients undergoing non-cardiac surgery. *Surgery*, **106**, 1

Gueldner, T.L. and Lawrence, G.H. (1975) Intra-aortic balloon assist through cannulation of the asecnding aorta. *Annals of Thoracic Surgery*, **19**, 88

Gunstensen, J., Goldman, B.S., Scully, H.S., *et al.* (1976) Evolving indications for preoperative intra-aortic balloon pump assistance. *Annals of Thoracic Surgery*, **22**, 535

Hagemeijer, F., Laird, J.D., Haalebos, M.P. and Hugenholtz, P.G. (1977) Effectiveness of intra-aortic balloon pumping without cardiac surgery for patients with severe heart failure secondary to a recent myocardial infarction. *American Journal of Cardiology*, **40**, 951

Harken, D.E. (1958) *Presentation at the International College of Cardiology Meeting*, Brussels, Belgium

Hines, G.L., Mehbe, U., Chang, P., *et al.* (1982) Mobile cardiac shock van: An 18 month experience. *New York State Journal of Medicine*, **82**, 725

Igo, S.R., Hibbs, C.W., Trono, R., *et al.* (1978) Intra-aortic balloon pumping: Theory and practice–experience with 325 patients. *Artificial Organs*, **2**, 249

Inverson, L.I., Herfindahl, G., Ecker, R., *et al.* (1987) Vascular complications of intra-aortic balloon counterpulsation. *American Journal of Surgery*, **154**, 99–103

Isner, J.M., Cohen, S.R., Virmani, R., *et al.* (1980) Complications of the intra-aortic balloon counterpulsation device: clinical and morphologic observations in 45 necropsy patients. *American Journal of Cardiology*, **45**, 260

Jackson, G., Cullum, P., Pastellopoulos, A., *et al.* (1977) Intra-aortic balloon assistance in cardiogenic shock after acute myocardial infarction or cardiac surgery. *British Heart Journal*, **39**, 598

Jacoby, J.A., Craddock, L.D., Wolf, P.S. and Beckwitt, H.J. (1968) Clinical experience with counterpulsation in coronary artery disease. *Journal of Thoracic and Cardiovascular Surgery*, **56**, 846

Jacoby, J.A., Taylor, W.J., Smith, G.T., *et al.* (1963) A new therapeutic approach to acute coronary occlusion. II. Opening dormant coronary collateral channels by counterpulsation. *American Journal of Cardiology*, **11**, 218

Johnson, M.D., Holub, D.A., Winston, D.S., *et al.* (1977a) Retrospective analysis of 286 patients requiring circulatory support with the intra-aortic balloon pump. *Cardiovascular Diseases. Bulletin of the Texas Heart Institute*, **4**, 428

Johnson, S.A., Scanlon, P.J., Loeb, H.S., *et al.* (1977b) Treatment of cardiogenic shock in myocardial infarction by intra-aortic balloon counterpulsation and surgery. *American Journal of Medicine*, **62**, 687

Kahn, J.K., Rutherford, B.D., McConahay, D.R., *et al.* (1990) Supported high-risk coronary angioplasty using intra-aortic balloon counterpulsation. *Journal of the American College of Cardiology*, **15**, 1151

Kantrowitz, A. (1969) Experimental augmentation of coronary flow by retardation of the arterial pressure pulse. *Surgery*, **34**, 678

Kantrowitz, A., Tjonneland, S., Freed, P.S., *et al.* (1968) Initial clinical experience with intra-aortic balloon pumping in cardiogenic shock. *Journal of the American Medical Association*, **203**, 113

Kantrowitz, A. and McKinnon, W.M. (1958) The experimental use of the diaphragm as an auxiliary myocardium. *Surgical Forum*, **9**, 266

Karlson, S.B., Martin, E.C., Bregman, D., *et al.* (1981) Superior mesenteric artery obstruction by intra-aortic balloon simulating embolism. *Cardiovascular Interventional Radiology*, **4**, 236–238

Kralios, A.C., Zwart, H.H.J., Yenching, W., *et al.* (1972) Coronary flow supplementation in experimental myocardial infarction with shock. *Chest*, **61**, 365

Kramer, R.P. (1988) Helicopter-transported intra-aortic balloon pumping: advanced technology made airborne. *Cardiac Assists*, **4**, 2

Kucher, D.L., Campell, W. and O'Rouke, M.F. (1987) Long-term survival after counterpulsation for medically refractory heart failure complicating myocardial infarction and cardiac surgery. *European Heart Journal*, **8**, 490

Kuhn, L.A. (1970) Shock in myocardial infarction-medical treatment. *American Journal of Cardiology*, **26**, 578

Kuhn, L.A. (1978) Management of shock following acute myocardial infarction part II. Mechanical circulatory assistance. *American Heart Journal*, **95**, 789

Kuhn, L.A., Unger, A.H., Novick, S.A., *et al.* (1970) Hemodynamics and cardiac metabolic effects of diastolic intra-aortic balloon obstruction combined with distal aortic 'booster' occlusion in experimental acute myocardial infarction. *American Journal of Cardiology*, **25**, 111

Kveim, M., Cappelen, C., Jr., Froysaker, T. and Hall, D.V. (1976) Intra-aortic balloon pumping in the treatment of cardiogenic shock follow-up in open-heart surgery. *Scandinavian Journal of Thoracic and Cardiovascular Surgery*, **10**, 231

Lamberti, J.J., Cohen, L.W. and Collins, J.J., Jr. (1974) Iliac artery cannulation for intra-aortic balloon counterpulsation. *Journal of Thoracic and Cardiovascular Surgery*, **67**, 976

Lamberti, J.J. and Resnekov, L. (1978) Cardiac assist devices. *Annual Review of Medicine*, **29**, 571

Lane, A.S., Woodward, A.C. and Goldman, M.R. (1987) Massive propanolol overdose poorly responsive to pharmacologic therapy: Use of intra-aortic balloon pump. *Annals of Emergency Medicine*, **16**, 1381

Langon, R.A., Geha, A.S., Hammond, G.L and Cohen, L.S. (1978) Surgical approach for patients with unstable angina pectoris: role of the response to initial medical therapy and intra-aortic balloon pumping in perioperative complications after aortocoronary bypass grafting. *American Journal of Cardiology*, **42**, 629

Lappas, D.G., Powell, W.M., Jr., and Daggett, W.M. (1977) Cardiac dysfunction in the perioperative period. *Anesthesiology*, **47**, 117

Lefemine, A.A., Kosowsky, B., Madoff, I., *et al.* (1977) Results and complications of intra-aortic balloon pumping in surgical and medical patients. *American Journal of Cardiology*, **40**, 416

Leinbach, R.C., Gold, H.K., Harber, R.W., *et al.* (1978) Early intra-aortic balloon pumping for anterior myocardial infarction without shock. *Circulation*, **58**, 204

Leinbach, R.C., Goldstein, J., Gold, H.K., *et al.* (1982) Percutaneous wire-guided balloon pumping. *American Journal of Cardiology*, **49**, 1707

LoCicero, J., III., Hartz, R.S., Sanders, J.H., Jr., *et al.* (1985) Interhospital transport of patients with ongoing intra-aortic balloon pumping. *American Journal of Cardiology*, **56**, 59

McEnany, M.T., Kay, H.R., Buckley, M.J., *et al.* (1978) Clinical experience with intra-aortic balloon pump support in 728 patients. *Circulation*, **58** (**Suppl. I**), 124

Madras, P.N., Laird, J.D., Iatridis, E., *et al.* (1969) Effects of prolonged intra-aortic balloon pumping. *Transactions of the American Society for Artificial Internal Organs*, **15**, 400

Maroko, P.N., Bernstein, E.F., Lippy, P., *et al.* (1972) Effects of intra-aortic balloon counterpulsation on the severity of myocardial ischemic injury following acute coronary occlusion. *Circulation*, **45**, 1150

Martin, R.S., III., Moncure, A.C., Buckley, M.J., *et al.* (1983) Complications of percutaneous intra-aortic balloon insertion. *Journal of Thoracic and Cardiovascular Surgery*, **85**, 186

Merav, A.D., Solomon, N., Montefusco, C.M. and Bregman, D. (1981) A new guidable double-lumen percutaneous intra-aortic balloon. *Transactions of the American Society for Artificial Internal Organs*, **27**, 593

Moulopoulos, S.D., Topaz, S. and Kolff, W.J. (1962a) Diastolic balloon pumping (with carbon dioxide) in the aorta: A mechanical assistance to the failing circulation. *American Heart Journal*, **63**, 669

Moulopoulos, S.D., Topaz, S. and Kolff, W.J. (1962b) Extracorporeal assistance to the circulation and intra-aortic balloon pumping. *Transactions of the American Society for Artificial Internal Organs*, **8**, 85

Mueller, H., Ayres, S.M., Mazzara, J.T., *et al.* (1970) Responses of hemodynamics and myocardial energetics to intra-aortic phase shift balloon pumping in acute coronary shock (Abstract). *Circulation*, **41** and **42** (**Suppl. III**), 81

Mueller, H., Ayres, S.M., Conklin, E.F., *et al.* (1971) The effects of intra-aortic balloon counterpulsation on cardiac performance and metabolism in shock associated with acute myocardial infarction. *Journal of Clinical Investigation*, **50**, 1885

Mueller, H., Ayres, S.M., Gianelli, S., Jr., *et al.* (1972) Effect of isoproterenol, 1-norepinephrine and intra-aortic balloon counterpulsation on hemodynamics and myocardial metabolism in shock following acute myocardial infarction. *Circulation*, **45**, 335

Mundth, E.D. (1976a) Perioperative intra-aortic balloon pump assistance. *Annals of Thoracic Surgery*, **22**, 603

Mundth, E.D. (1976b) Mechanical and surgical interventions for the reduction of myocardial ischemia. *Circulation*, **53** (**Suppl. I**), 176

Mundth, E.D., Buckley, M.J., Daggett, W.M., *et al.* (1975) Intra-aortic balloon pump assistance and early surgery in cardiogenic shock. Integrated medical-surgical care in acute coronary artery disease. *Advances in Cardiology*, **15**, 159

Nachlas, H.M. and Sieband, M.P. (1967) The influence of diastolic augmentation on infarct size following coronary artery ligation. *Journal of Thoracic and Cardiovascular Surgery*, **53**, 698

Nicols, A.B., Weiss, M.B. and Bregman, D. (1981) Percutaneous intra-aortic balloon insertion in patients with aorto-iliac disease. *Catheterization and Cardiovascular Diagnosis*, **7**, 443

Norman, N.A. and Kennedy, J.H. (1971) Arterial baroreceptor responses to intra-aortic balloon assistance. *Journal of Surgical Research*, **11**, 396

O'Rouke, M.F. (1977) Arterial counterpulsation in the management of ischemic heart disease. *Australian and New Zealand Journal of Surgery*, **47**, 1

Pappas, G. (1974) Intrathoracic intra-aortic balloon insertion for pulsatile cardiopulmonary bypass. *Archives of Surgery*, **109**, 842

Perloth, M.G. and Huftgren, H.N. (1975) The cardiac patient and general surgery. *Journal of the American Medical Association*, **232**, 1279

Pollock, J.C., Charlton, M.C., Williams, W.G., *et al.* (1980) Intra-aortic balloon pumping in children. *Annals of Thoracic Surgery*, **29**, 6

Reemtsma, K., Drusin, R., Edie, R., *et al.* (1978) Cardiac transplantation for patients requiring mechanical circulatory support. *New England Journal of Medicine*, **298**, 670

Reemtsma, K., Parodi, E.N., Bregman, D., *et al.* (1974) Clinical intraoperative coronary artery saphenous vein bypass graft pressure-flow relationship. In *Coronary Artery Medicine and Surgery: Concepts and Controversies* (ed. J.C. Norman), Appleton-Century-Crofts, New York

Roberts, A.J., Alonso, D.R., Combes, J.R., *et al.* (1978) Role of delayed intra-aortic balloon pumping in the treatment of experimental myocardial infarction. *American Journal of Cardiology*, **41**, 1202

Rodigas, P.C. and Bridges, K.G. (1986) Occlusion of the left internal mammary artery with intra-aortic balloon: clinical implications. *Journal of Thoracic and Cardiovascular Surgery*, **91**, 142–143

Rodigas, P.C. and Finnegan, J.O. (1985) Technique for removal of percutaneously placed intra-aortic balloons. *Annals of Thoracic Surgery*, **40**, 80

Rosenweig, J., Chatterjee, S. and Merino, F. (1970) Treatment of acute myocardial infarction by counterpulsation. Experimental rationale and clinical experience. *Journal of Thoracic and Cardiovascular Surgery*, **69**, 243

Sammel, N., O'Rouke, M.F. and Chang, V. (1976) Arterial counterpulsation: review of the first 100 patients. *Medical Journal of Australia*, **2**, 802

Sanfelippo, P.M., Baker, N.H., Ewy, H.G., *et al.* (1986) Experience with intra-aortic counterpulsation. *Annals of Thoracic Surgery*, **41**, 36

Saunders, C.R. and Doty, D.B. (1978) Myocardial contusion: effect of intra-aortic balloon pumping on cardiac output. *Journal of Trauma*, **18**, 706

Scheidt, S., Wilner, G., Mueller, H., *et al.* (1973) Intra-aortic balloon counterpulsation in cardiogenic shock. Report of a co-operative clinical trial. *New England Journal of Medicine*, **288**, 979

Scully, H.E., Gunstansen, J., Williams, W.G., *et al.* (1976) Surgical management of complicated acute coronary insufficiency. *Surgery*, **80**, 437

Seldinger, S.L. (1953) Catheter replacement of the needle in percutaneous arteriography: a new technique. *Acta Radiologica*, **39**, 368

Shirley, A.L., Loughridge, B.P. and Lain, K.C. (1976) Insertion of the intra-aortic balloon through the aortic arch. *Annals of Thoracic Surgery*, **21**, 560

Singh, J.B., Connelly, P., Kocat, S., *et al.* (1981) Intra-aortic balloon counterpulsation in a community hospital. *Chest*, **79**, 58

Snow, N. and Horrigan, T.P. (1986) Intra-aortic balloon counterpulsation via the ascending aorta. *Journal of Cardiovascular Surgery*, **27**, 337

Spotnitz, H.M., Covel, J., Ross, J.,Jr., and Braunwald, E. (1969) Left ventricular mechanics and oxygen consumption during artrial counterpulsation. *American Journal of Physiology*, **217**, 1352

Sugg, W.L., Rea, M.J., Webb and Ecker, R.R. (1970) Cardiac assistance (counterpulsation) in ten patients. *Annals of Thoracic Surgery*, **9**, 1

Sugg, W.L., Webb, W.R. and Ecker, R.R. (1969) Reduction of extent of myocardial infarction by counterpulsation. *Annals of Thoracic Surgery*, **7**, 311

Summers, D.N., Kaplitt, M., Morris, J., *et al.* (1969) Intra-aortic balloon pumping. Hemodynamic and metabolic effects during cardiogenic shock in patients with triple coronary artery obstructive disease. *Archives of Surgery*, **99**, 733

Talpins, N.L., Kripke, D.C. and Goetz, R.H. (1968) Counterpulsation and intra-aortic balloon pumping in cardiogenic shock. Circulatory dynamics. *Archives of Surgery*, **97**, 991

Tarhan, S., Moffitt, E.A., Taylor, W.F. and Guiliani, E.R. (1972) Myocardial infarction after general anesthesia. *Journal of the American Medical Association*, **220**, 1451

Todd, G.L., Bregman, D., Voorhees, A.B. and Reemtsma, K. (1983) Vascular complications associated with percutaneous intra-aortic balloon pumping. *Archives of Surgery*, **93**, 280

Ugogi, C.C., Turner, S.A. and McGee, M.D. (1980) Transcending aortic intra-aortic balloon insertion with delayed sternal closure: A retrospective analysis. *Cardiovascular Diseases*, **7**, 307

Veasy, L.G., Blaybock, N., Fukumasu, H. and Orth, J.L. (1981) Preclinical evaluation of intra-aortic balloon pumping for pediatric use. *Transactions of the American Society for Artificial Internal Organs*, **27**, 490

Veasy, L.G. and Webster, H. (1985) Intra-aortic balloon pumping in infants and children. *Cardiac Assists*, **2**, 1

Vignola, P.A., Swaye, P.S. and Gosselin, A.J. (1981) Guidelines for effective and safe percutaneous intra-aortic balloon pump insertion and removal. *American Journal of Cardiology*, **48**, 660

Watson, J.T., Willerson, J.T., Fixler, D.E., *et al.* (1973) Changes in collateral coronary blood flow (CCBF) distal to a coronary occlusion during intra-aortic balloon pumping (IABP). *Transaction of the American Society for Artificial Internal Organs*, **19**, 402

Webb, W.R., Parker, F.B., Jr., Neville, J.F., Jr. and Hanson, E.L. (1974) Acute mechanical complications of coronary arterial disease. *Archives of Surgery*, **109**, 251

Weber, K.T. and Janicki, J.S. (1973) Coronary collateral flow and intra-aortic balloon counterpulsation. *Transactions of the American Society for Artificial Internal Organs*, **19**, 402

Weber, K.T. and Janicki, J.S. (1974) Intra-aortic balloon counterpulsation: a review of physiological principles, clinical results, and device safety. *Annals of Thoracic Surgery*, **17**, 602

Weber, K.T., Janicki, J.S. and Walker, A.A. (1972) An assessment of intra-aortic balloon pumping in hypovolemic and ischemic heart preparations. *Journal of Thoracic and Cardiovascular Surgery*, **64**, 869

Weintraub, R.M., Voukydis, P.C., Aroesty, J.M., (1974) Treatment of preinfarction angina with intra-aortic balloon counterpulsation and surgery. *American Journal of Cardiology*, **34**, 809

Willerson, J.T., Curry, G.C., Watson, J.T., *et al.* (1975) Intra-aortic balloon counterpulsation in patients with cardiogenic shock, medically refractory left ventricular failure and/or recurrent ventricular tachycardias. *American Journal of Medicine*, **58**, 183

Williams, E.H., Tyers, G.F., Carter, S.L and Williams, D.R. (1975) Ventricular arrhythmias following mitral valve replacement: control with intra-aortic balloon counterpulsation. *Chest*, **68**, 641

Wolvek, S. (1989) The evolution of the intra-aortic balloon: The Datascope contribution. *Journal of Biomedical Applications*, **3**, 527

Yellin, E., Levy, L. and Bregman, D. (1973) Hemodynamic effects of intra-aortic balloon pumping in dogs with aortic incompetence. *Transactions of the American Society for Artificial Internal Organs*, **19**, 389

19

Ventricular assist devices

Timothy Locke and Christopher McGregor

Mechanical support of the circulation became a reality in the late 1960s when Spencer (Spencer *et al.*, 1965) successfully used a perfusion circuit for left heart assistance and DeBakey (1971) used a left ventricular assist device (LVAD) to treat postcardiotomy shock. A variety of systems is now available for support or replacement of the failing heart, including counterpulsation catheters, roller pumps, centrifugal pumps, pneumatically or electrically driven artificial ventricles, total artificial hearts, skeletal muscle ventricles, and extracorporeal membrane oxygenation.

The need for mechanical circulatory support was underlined by the report of the Working Group of the National Heart, Lung and Blood Institute (1985) which estimated that 17 000 to 35 000 patients would be candidates for long-term circulatory support each year in the United States. At present, cardiac transplantation represents the only form of long-term palliation available for such patients, but there is a serious shortage of cardiac donors. In 1987 only 1512 suitable cardiac donors became available for transplantation in the USA (Report to the Chairman, Subcommittee on Health, Committee on Ways and Means, House of Representatives, 1989). The current technology of mechanical circulatory support does not yet allow for permanent artificial hearts, but the use of such support allows transplantation in candidates with terminal heart failure who would die while waiting for an organ to become available.

A second group of patients who may require mechanical circulatory support are those who develop postcardiotomy shock. The syndrome may develop in as many as 4% of all patients undergoing cardiac surgery (McEnany *et al.*, 1978), although the need may have decreased with more recent improvements in methods of myocardial preservation. As many as 70% of these patients can be weaned from cardiopulmonary bypass with a combination of volume loading, inotropic agents and vasodilator therapy, but in the other 30% of patients in whom early recovery of left ventricular function may be expected, death will result if a more radical form of support is not available.

In this chapter we will discuss the development and application of currently available devices for mechanical circulatory support.

Historical notes

A workable heart–lung machine was developed by Gibbon (1954), built by the IBM Corporation, and successfully applied by him for the clinical repair of an atrial septal defect under direct vision. Thereafter, Gibbon became disillusioned and discontinued his participation in open cardiac surgery but this contribution introduced the modern era of cardiac surgery. The Gibbon machine was modified by Kirklin and associates at the Mayo Clinic and, after a period of intense, careful experimentation, a series of eight clinical open heart operations was performed beginning in March 1955 with four survivors (Kirklin, 1989). As knowledge of the early Mayo experience spread in the subsequent years, the application of this technology became worldwide. The occurrence of postcardiotomy shock preventing weaning from cardiopulmonary bypass and the potential for recovery of such patients prompted the development of circulatory assist systems in the early 1960s. Early experience with venoarterial bypass and extracorporeal oxygenation in two patients was unsuccessful (Spencer *et al.*, 1965). The same group went on to describe the successful application of left atriofemoral bypass in a patient with left ventricular failure after aortic and mitral valve repairs. A second patient, supported by the same technique after aortic and mitral replacement, died of right ventricular failure, a problem that continues to occur during left heart assist alone. The need for a temporary mechanical device to support the circulation of a patient dying of cardiac decompensation stimulated Cooley *et al.* (1969) to implant a total artificial heart as a bridge to transplantation. Support for 64 h was followed by orthotopic cardiac transplantation but the patient later died of *Pseudomonas* pneumonia. The first successful use of a pulsatile left ventricular assist device to treat postcardiotomy shock was reported by DeBakey in 1971 who defined the problem of the interface between the blood and the synthetic surfaces of these devices that remains the subject of much research today.

Until the early 1980s the major thrust in the development of circulatory support was in the field of intra-aortic balloon pumping. Kantrowitz and Kantrowitz proposed the concept of phase shift diastolic augmentation in 1953 and showed experimentally that perfusion of the coronary arteries during diastole with peak systolic pressures increases coronary blood flow by 26–53%. In combination with Sarnoff's demonstration of the proportional relationship between myocardial oxygen uptake and tension-time index the feasibility of intra-aortic balloon pumping became a reality (Welch *et al.*, 1958). Clinical use of the intra-aortic balloon pump began in the late 60s (Leinbach *et al.*, 1971) and the device has become the most widely used form of mechanical support for postcardiotomy shock. The intra-aortic balloon pump has also been used as a bridge to transplantation (Reemtsma *et al.*, 1978; Hardesty *et al.*, 1986) and in the treatment of primary graft failure.

In the early 80s the application of several devices (roller pumps (Rose *et al.*, 1985), centrifugal pumps (Park *et al.*, 1986), and pneumatic ventricles (Gaines *et al.*, 1985)) to the treatment of refractory postcardiotomy shock resulted in many successes. The mid-1980s saw a rapid expansion in the number and applications of mechanical support devices. The first permanent total artificial heart was inserted in 1982 (DeVries, 1984) and the patient survived 112 days. The device worked well in maintaining a cardiac output of more than 6 l min^{-1} but the patient died of multiple organ failure. The first successful bridge to transplantation with a totally implantable artificial ventricle was performed at Stanford in 1984 (Portner *et al.*, 1985). The device worked well for 9 days before successful cardiac transplantation was performed and this patient remained alive 5 years later. At about the same time the first successful bridge using the external Pierce–Donachy pump was performed (Hill *et al.*, 1986). The initial use of a Jarvik-7 total artificial heart as a bridge to transplantation occurred in 1985 (Levinson *et al.*, 1986). The patient was supported for 9 days before transplantation was performed.

Pathophysiology of myocardial ischaemia

A review of the pathophysiology of myocardial ischaemia is necessary for an understanding of the way in which the intra-aortic balloon pump and ventricular assist devices are effective. Myocardial ischaemia occurs when there is an imbalance of oxygen supply and demand. Myocardial oxygen supply is closely related to blood flow, which is in turn dependent on the degree of coronary artery obstruction, on the duration of diastole, and on diastolic perfusion pressure. This is especially true for the left ventricle whose subendocardial blood flow is almost exclusively diastolic. Oxygen demand is dependent upon heart rate, inotropic state, and wall tension. The common factor present in all types of myocardial work is the area under the left ventricular pressure curve, the tension-time index (Figure 19.1). Wall tension is related to left ventricular volume and afterload by the law of Laplace. This relationship allows calculation of the effective coronary perfusion pressure by subtraction of the left ventricular end-diastolic pressure (or pulmonary capillary wedge pressure) from the aortic diastolic pressure.

When 40% or more of the left ventricular wall is ischaemic, cardiac output falls, activating the renin–angiotensin system and causing the release of

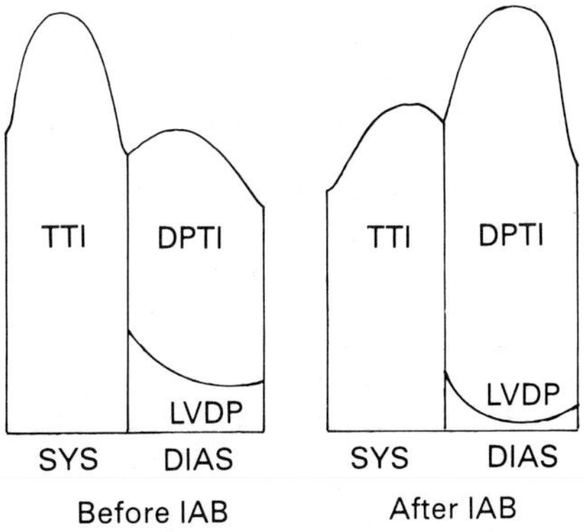

Figure 19.1 The tension-time index (TTI, derived from the area under the aortic pressure curve in systole) exceeds the diastolic pressure-time index (DPTI, which determines coronary blood flow). During intra-aortic balloon pumping, TTI is reduced by rapid deflation of the balloon just before systole and DPTI is increased by the counterpulse and the consequent decrease in left ventricular diastolic pressure (LVDP)

catecholamines, which elevate systemic vascular resistance. The work load of the heart increases and the oxygen demand of marginal areas of myocardium is increased. A vicious circle of decreasing tissue perfusion follows.

Principles of mechanical circulatory support

Mechanical circulatory support should simultaneously increase systemic and coronary perfusion, and decrease myocardial work load and oxygen consumption. The degree of improvement in systemic perfusion should be sufficient to prevent deterioration in the function of other organs. In milder degrees of heart failure, the intra-aortic balloon pump will suffice but if the cardiac output is severely depressed, use of a left ventricular assist device is required.

Adequate monitoring is necessary to determine the need for and timing of support, and to assess the resultant haemodynamic benefits. The use of a Swan–Ganz catheter allows the simultaneous measurement of right atrial pressure, pulmonary capillary wedge pressure, pulmonary artery pressures, and cardiac output.

The physiological criteria for the use of ventricular assist devices are fairly well defined. In general, less invasive measures should be tried before resorting to artificial ventricles, i.e. volume loading, inotropic therapy, vasodilator therapy, and the intra-aortic balloon pump. However, if undue delay occurs before mechanical circulatory support is instituted, the eventual outcome is compromised. The use of a left ventricular assist device is indicated in patients with non-surgically correctable left ventricular dysfunction, a systolic blood pressure of <90 mmHg, a left atrial or pulmonary wedge pressure of >25 mmHg in the absence of mitral valve disease, and a cardiac index of $<1.8\ l\ min^{-1}$. The use of pulmonary artery oximetry may aid decision making. In 1965, Spencer described the relationship between pulmonary artery oxygen saturation and cardiac output, noting that saturations of 30–40% are soon followed by progressive circulatory collapse and death, and persistent saturations of less than 30% are almost always fatal.

Candidates for right ventricular support should have had a technically satisfactory surgical repair, a cardiac index of $<1.8\ l\ min^{-1}$, a right atrial pressure of >20 mmHg in the absence of tricuspid valve disease, and a systolic blood pressure of <12 mmHg, and a left atrial pressure of <90 mmHg. At least 25% of patients with left ventricular failure can develop right ventricular failure (Farrar *et al.*, 1985), indeed in one series the incidence of right ventricular failure was 80% (Pennington *et al.*, 1988b). The pathophysiology of right ventricular failure in this context may be the same as for the left ventricle, but mechanical support of the left ventricle can contribute by reducing the septal contribution to right ventricular contraction (Farrar *et al.*, 1984). Farrar concluded that right ventricular performance can be optimized by avoidance of volume overloading and adjusting the decrease in left ventricular afterload so that the septum can contribute to right ventricular contraction.

The place of mechanical circulatory support after cardiotomy is uncertain. In the operating theatre, it is often difficult to determine the extent of cardiac injury or other organ failure that would preclude survival. It has been shown that perioperative myocardial infarction has a strong negative effect on survival but does not rule out myocardial recovery (Pennington *et al.*, 1988a). In an otherwise viable patient, the use of ventricular assistance is the next logical step in the treatment of cardiac failure after cardiotomy not amenable to balloon counterpulsation.

The surgical principles of mechanical circulatory support reflect those of general cardiac surgery and, as always, attention to detail can prevent complications. Device implantation techniques are specific to each pump. In general when the myocardium is expected to recover, it is preferable to avoid cannulation of the left ventricular apex. At device removal it is important to remove all prosthetic material. The small atrial cuffs left after excision of a Jarvik-7 have not caused major problems (Griffith, 1989). The posterior rectus sheath pocket left after removal of the Novacor left ventricular assist device must be inspected for haemostasis and drained into a closed system (Pennington, 1989).

Thromboembolism remains the major complication of artificial ventricles and total artificial hearts, and continues to occur despite all forms of therapy. Thrombus develops in up to 30% of ventricular assist devices (Hill, 1989) and most total artificial hearts (DeVries, 1988; Didisheim *et al.*, 1989). Embolization occurs less frequently than thrombus formation (Didisheim *et al.*, 1989); blood clots on almost all foreign surfaces. The rate of thrombus formation depends on factors including surface texture and chemistry, wettability, surface charge, turbulence of blood flow, blood rheology, shear stresses, and pump chamber design. Surface imperfections and crevices between connectors and valve housings are common sources of thrombus formation. Device infection and thromboembolism may be causally related (Didisheim *et al.*, 1989). Thromboembolism may be less common with electrical ventricular assist devices than with pneumatic devices, and the risk appears to increase with time, especially beyond 30 days of implantation

(Didisheim *et al.*, 1989). Multiple therapies including full anticoagulation to prevent thromboembolism have been tried but have not been successful in eradicating this complication.

Haemorrhage is another significant problem and is multifactorial in origin. The high shear forces generated at the suture lines by pneumatic devices often necessitate reinforcement with pledgetted sutures. Full reversal of heparin, meticulous suture technique, primary wound closure, and the use of topical thrombin on a collagen matrix are beneficial. Coagulopathy is treated by transfusion of fresh frozen plasma, cryoprecipitate, and platelets. When bridging to transplantation, reduced blood loss and transfusion decreases the risk of developing preformed antibodies.

A significant number of patients die of infectious complications of mechanical circulatory support despite maintenance of an adequate cardiac output (McBride *et al.*, 1987a). Most infections are nosocomial bacterial pneumonias and the rate of infection increases with duration of support. Local device-related sepsis and percutaneous line infection may be reduced by wound closure (Griffith, 1989), the use of prophylactic antibiotics until the chest drains are removed (Pennington, 1989), and meticulous local care of drive lines. The immunosuppressive effects of mechanical circulatory support *per se* may predispose to fungal infections but are minimized by adequate tissue perfusion (McBride *et al.*, 1987b).

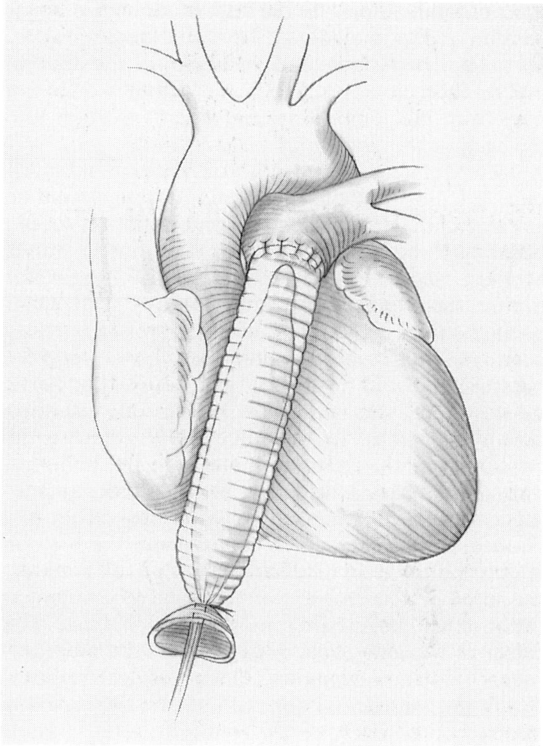

Figure 19.2 Pulmonary artery balloon counterpulsation. The end-to-side conduit and balloon position are shown

Intra-aortic balloon counterpulsation

The early balloon catheters used in the 1970s were large, bulky devices that required a cutdown on the femoral artery for insertion and the construction of an end-to-side Dacron graft as a conduit. Modern devices can be inserted percutaneously by Seldinger technique, allowing more rapid institution of counterpulsation in critically ill patients (Bregman and Caserella, 1980).

Intra-aortic balloon pumping acts on both sides of the myocardial oxygen supply–demand equation. Inflation of the balloon in diastole increases diastolic perfusion pressure, increasing blood flow to the myocardium. Deflation of the balloon at the beginning of systole rapidly reduces the afterload on the left ventricle (see Figure 19.1).

The indications for use of the intra-aortic balloon pump include cardiogenic shock due to myocardial infarction, shock following postinfarction ventricular septal defect or mitral regurgitation, medically uncontrollable angina pectoris, and the inability to wean from cardiopulmonary bypass. In the initial experience in this latter group, 42% survived to hospital discharge (Buckley *et al.*, 1973). Early application of the intra-aortic balloon pump can increase hospital survival of postcardiotomy shock to 70% and success is more likely if revascularization was complete. The intra-aortic balloon pump has also been used as a right ventricular assist after insertion through a Dacron end-to-side graft (Figure 19.2). Results have not been encouraging (Miller *et al.*, 1980; Moran *et al.*, 1984), though isolated successes have been reported (Flege, Wright and Reisenger, 1984).

As a bridge to transplantation, the intra-aortic balloon pump should be the first line therapy in patients with unstable haemodynamics refractory to inotropic support. Hardesty (1986) reported an experience of cardiac transplantation in 33 mortally ill patients, which included 14 patients supported to transplantation with intra-aortic balloon pump for a mean of 10 days (range 2 days to 3 weeks), but the survival rate of this subgroup was not given. Oaks *et al.* (1989) reported the use of the intra-aortic balloon pump as a bridge to transplantation in eight patients, of whom seven were transplanted with four discharged from hospital. As a bridge to transplantation, the intra-aortic balloon pump has the disadvantage of confining the patient to bed if the femoral artery is used for cannulation.

Contraindications to the use of the intra-aortic balloon pump include aortic valve regurgitation, aortoiliac obstruction, and aneurysm of the abdominal or thoracic aorta. When the catheter does not pass from the femoral artery, direct insertion into the arch of the aorta may be indicated.

Two elements of intra-aortic balloon management are essential: the timing of inflation should be as early in diastole as possible and deflation should occur just before opening of the aortic valve. Modern pumps use several forms of trigger for timing; the R-wave, atrioventricular or ventricular pacing spikes, and the arterial pressure trace. Timing of deflation is optimal if the aortic root pressure is about 50 mmHg just before the aortic valve opens. During support careful attention should be paid to the distal circulation and to the possibility of thrombus formation on the balloons, particularly during weaning. Some authors recommend anticoagulation after blood loss from the chest drains has ceased. Weaning from the balloon is accomplished by reducing the rate of counterpulsation or reducing the level of diastolic augmentation, the latter being more physiological. The effect of weaning is checked by repeated measurements of haemodynamics. Open surgical removal of the intra-aortic balloon catheter to allow confirmation of patency of the femoral artery seems prudent.

Complications represent the major limitation to the use of the intra-aortic balloon pump and occur in about 10% of patients (McEnany *et al.*, 1978; Amsterdam *et al.*, 1981). The incidence of complications however is probably reduced by the advent of smaller catheters and the use of percutaneous insertion techniques (Martin *et al.*, 1983). Limb ischaemia and arterial trauma are the most common complications and can be lessened by strict attention to insertion procedure. Thrombosis, aortic perforation, and gas embolism are rarer complications. Late complications in the bridge to transplant experience have been femoral seromas and false aneurysms (Hardesty *et al.*, 1986).

The Hemopump

A promising new device that fills the intermediate position between the intra-aortic balloon pump and the more invasive ventricular assist devices is the Hemopump, a percutaneous, miniature, cable-driven axial blood pump (Wampler *et al.*, 1988) (Figure 19.3). The device is implantable through the femoral artery and consists of a 20 cm inlet cannula that is positioned in the left ventricle. Blood is drawn into the cannula by the effect of the high speed rotor and is propelled into the aorta. In animal studies there was good circulatory support even during periods of ventricular fibrillation, with

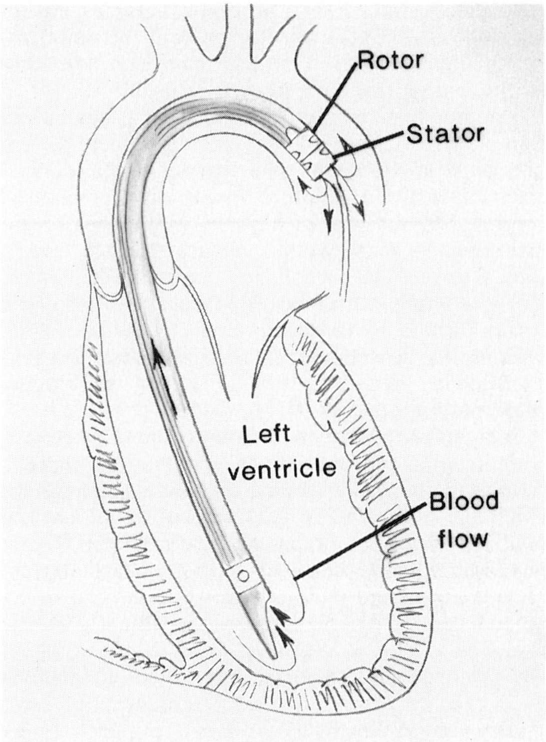

Figure 19.3 The Nimbus Hemopump

little haemolysis, but there were problems with renal infarction despite the absence of thrombus in the device and with migration of the device out of the left ventricle. Preliminary clinical results are available from 22 patients with cardiogenic shock supported with the Hemopump for 1–8 days. Survival in the treatment group was 41% against 0% in the non-treatment group (Wampler *et al.*, 1989) with an increase in cardiac index from 1.58 to 2.13 l min^{-1} m^{-2} and an associated reduction in pulmonary capillary wedge pressure to 7 cmH_2O.

Roller and centrifugal pumps

These pumps constitute the simplest and least expensive form of ventricular assist device. The basic circuit used for left heart assist consists of a venous drainage cannula in the left atrium, a pump, and an arterial return catheter; no reservoir is required (Rose *et al.*, 1989). Results with occlusive roller pumps are less impressive than with centrifugal devices. The centrifugal pumps (examples include the Biomedicus and Centrimed devices) are non-occlusive and use a rotating cone to generate energy recoverable as flow/pressure work. The drive is transmitted to the pump head by a

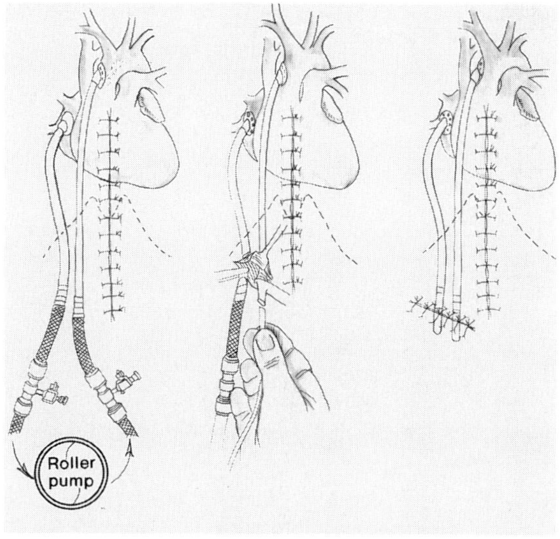

Figure 19.4 Discontinuation of left heart support without repeat sternotomy. After enlarging the skin incisions, the cannula tips are exposed, clamped and permanently occluded leaving two lengths of tube within the chest

magnetic coupling. At a given speed, the pump generates constant pressure over a range of flow rates. Specific cannulae for these pumps are currently being tested but, at the present time, most users have adapted standard cardiopulmonary bypass cannulae. Cannulation is straightforward; pursestring sutures are placed in the ascending aorta (after sternotomy in the case of bridge to transplantation) and in the roof of the left atrium or right superior pulmonary vein. For right heart support the right atrial appendage and pulmonary outflow tract are cannulated. Percutaneous trans-septal left atrial cannulation has been used for emergency resuscitation in patients with profound cardiogenic shock or cardiac arrest (Rose *et al.*, 1989). Litwak *et al.* (1985) further simplified separation from the pump by devising a cannulation system that does not require a second sternotomy for discontinuation of support (Figure 19.4). The use of a step motor in conjunction with a roller pump allows pulsatile flow; an intra-aortic balloon pump is required to produce a pulse when centrifugal pumps are used. The minimum flow required for good organ perfusion and a successful outcome is about 2.5 l min^{-1} m^{-2}, but higher flows are desirable if the patient's heart is not ejecting (Litwak *et al.*, 1985; Magovern, Sang and Maher, 1985; Rose *et al.*, 1989).

Clinical experience with roller pumps after open heart surgery has demonstrated the limitations of these devices. Of 72 patients undergoing left heart assist with a roller pump, 30% were discharged from hospital (Rose *et al.*, 1989). Causes of death included coagulopathy, biventricular failure, stroke, and arrhythmias. Later in the postoperative period, sepsis, multisystem failure, and pulmonary embolism became problems. None of the recipients of right heart or of percutaneous left heart assist survived hospitalization.

Centrifugal pumps have been used successfully for short term support after cardiotomy. In a review of 21 patients of whom five were long-term survivors, Magovern (Magovern, Sang and Maher, 1985) suggested that a fatal outcome was associated with increasing age, cardiogenic shock before surgery, and complex surgery. A feature of this clinical experience was the use of limited anticoagulation with maintenance of the activated clotting time of around 140 s. Centrifugal pumps should not be run at flows below 0.5 l min^{-1} without increasing heparinization to prevent thrombus formation in the pump head. Survivors of ventricular assist after cardiotomy tend to have had short-term support (less than 75 h), absent or mild right ventricular failure, some recovery of left ventricular function within 24 h, and no evidence of perioperative myocardial infarction (Magovern, 1989). With recent improvements in management, long-term survival rates of 44% can be achieved after left ventricular assist, and 33% after biventricular support (Magovern, Sang and Maher, 1985; Magovern, 1989).

Bridging to transplantation with centrifugal pumps has produced encouraging results (Golding *et al.*, 1988; Bolman *et al.*, 1989; Hill, 1989; Pennington, 1989). In one report, nine patients were supported for 0.5 to 4 days using centrifugal pumps. Six required mechanical support of the left ventricle, two required biventricular support, and one was supported by extracorporeal membrane oxygenation due to right ventricular decompensation. Seven patients underwent successful cardiac transplantation with six long-term survivors (Bolman *et al.*, 1989). A slightly higher rate of infection was seen in the first 3 months after transplantation (Bolman *et al.*, 1989). Pennington reviewed the experience of several centres (1989) using centrifugal pumps as a bridge to transplantation. Twenty patients were supported for a mean of 3.4 days, 15 were transplanted and 10 (67%) were discharged from hospital. In Hill's multicentre review of 25 bridge to transplantation procedures with centrifugal pumps 16 patients underwent transplantation and 10 were long-term survivors (40%). Serious complications included renal failure, bleeding, cerebrovascular accidents, and sepsis.

The limitation of centrifugal pumps remains the frequent formation of fibrin and, to a lesser extent, thrombus in the pumping chamber. The upper limit of duration of support appears generally to be 5–7 days.

Extracorporeal membrane oxygenation

Extracorporeal membrane oxygenation (ECMO) was developed in the 1970s as a treatment for fulminant lung pathology unresponsive to maximal mechanical ventilation. After the initial application in adults (Hill *et al.*, 1972) and children (Kolobow *et al.*, 1975), considerable experience with ECMO in respiratory failure was accumulated in the late 1970s. More recently ECMO has been used to support patients with cardiogenic shock (Pennington *et al.*, 1984).

In practice, ECMO uses venoarterial or venovenous bypass. In the former, blood is drained from a femoral vein and returned to a femoral artery; in neonates, the right internal jugular vein and the right carotid artery are used because of size considerations. T-shaped arterial cannulae may prevent the disastrous complication of distal limb ischaemia. For support of postcardiotomy patients, standard cardiopulmonary bypass cannulae can be used. The disadvantages of venoarterial extracorporeal membrane oxygenation include the risks of systemic embolization, arterial injury, and cerebral damage following carotid occlusion. Recently developed percutaneous systems allow rapid resuscitation of critically ill patients. Venovenous ECMO requires good underlying cardiac function and is not relevant to the field of cardiac support.

The circuit in general use (Kanter *et al.*, 1987; Pennington, 1989) comprises a membrane oxygenator, a heat exchanger, and either a centrifugal or simple roller pump (Figure 19.5). Continuous heparinization, to maintain an activated clotting time of about 150 s, is initiated after postoperative bleeding has ceased. Flow is not pulsatile but an intra-aortic balloon pump may be inserted to provide a pulsatile element.

Profound cardiogenic shock after cardiac surgery in children has been successfully managed with ECMO with a duration of support of 9–50 h (Kanter *et al.*, 1987). Five of 13 children supported with ECMO survived 7 months to 4.3 years. Seven required re-exploration for bleeding, five developed renal failure of whom four required dialysis or ultrafiltration, and three failed to wean from the oxygenator due to neurologic problems. Of the seven patients who were successfully separated from the pump, three developed mediastinitis. The treatment of postcardiotomy shock in adults has met with inferior results (Pennington *et al.*, 1983; 1984). Of 12 adults supported for a mean of 57.6 h, three survived and the spectrum of complications was similar to the paediatric experience. This experience included three patients supported as a bridge to transplantation, all of whom died. The only two reported successful uses of ECMO as a

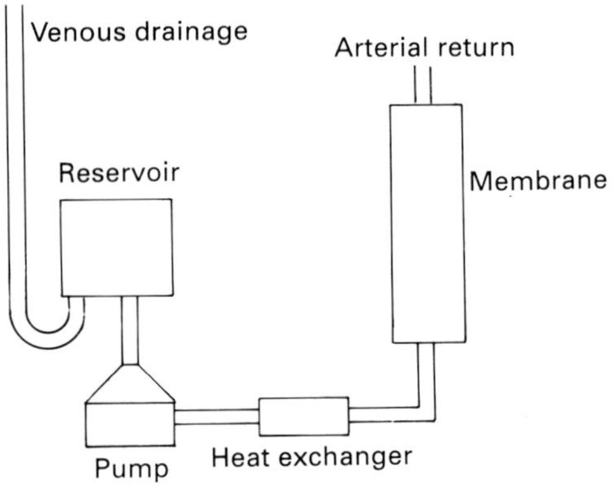

Figure 19.5 The circuit for extracorporeal membrane oxygenation

bridge to transplantation were performed for 4.2 days at Cambridge (Gifford *et al.*, 1986) and 2 days at St. Louis (Bolman *et al.*, 1987).

Extracorporeal membrane oxygenation is not suitable for long-term support of the failing heart due to the problems of anticoagulation, lack of patient mobility, bleeding and sepsis. Its role appears to be in the rapid resuscitation of acutely ill patients who may then be considered for a more sophisticated form of support if permanent organ damage has not occurred. The recent development of heparin-bonded tubing may obviate the need for anticoagulation, reducing bleeding and damage to platelets and red cells. Bindslev *et al.* (1986) successfully supported six dogs with ECMO using a surface heparinized venovenous bypass system for 30 h without systemic heparinization. The same group (Bindslev *et al.*, 1987) have successfully used a surface heparinized artificial lung for 9 days to support a 44-year-old woman with viral pneumonia. Low dose heparin was administered to maintain an activated partial thromboplastin time of 40–50 s.

Artificial ventricles (ventricular assist devices)

Used singly, these devices work in parallel with the patient's own heart. Pneumatic powered devices were introduced first, latterly electrically powered pumps have become available.

Most air-powered devices have a similar design. They consist of a rigid metal casing that encloses a seamless polyurethane sac. Compressed air is pulsed from an external drive console through percutaneous drive lines to the space between the blood sac and the rigid housing to produce pulsatile expulsion of blood. Inlet and outlet valves direct flow. These pumps can be used to support both sides of the heart individually or together to provide biventricular assistance. Currently available devices are the Pierce–Donachy, the Thermedics, Nimbus, Liotta, and Abiomed pumps.

The Pierce–Donachy VAD has a stroke volume of 65 ml with an ejection fraction of 75%, and uses Bjork–Shiley inlet and outlet valves. Postcardiotomy patients are cannulated via the left atrium with return to the aorta (Figure 19.6) whereas patients undergoing bridge to transplantation can be cannulated through the left ventricular apex. The pump can operate in three modes; manual set-rate mode, synchronized to the R-wave of the ECG, or in a fill-to-empty mode in which a Hall effect switch is activated when the sac is full and initiates the pump cycle. Usually the Pierce–Donachy pump is set in the fill-to-empty mode, but the device can be used in the ECG-synchronized mode as a counterpulsator in patients whose myocardium is expected to recover (Pennington, 1989). The fill-to-empty mode provides optimal washout of blood and may reduce thrombus formation. If the flow through the device is greater than 3 l min^{-1} heparinization is not necessary but anticoagulation should be introduced during weaning (Pennington *et al.*, 1988a). An alternative design is incorporated in the Thermedics device (Bernhard *et al.*, 1985). This pneumatic pump uses an axisymmetric blood sac. Blood is drained from the left ventricular apex and returned to the aorta.

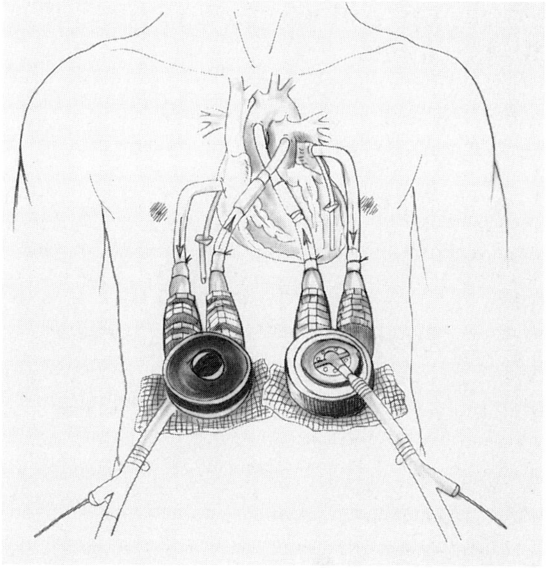

Figure 19.6 Biventricular support with Pierce–Donachy devices

The Pierce–Donachy device has been used most often in clinical practice (Pae *et al.*, 1987; Pennington, 1989; Pennington *et al.*, 1988a). Pae reported 25 patients requiring temporary support for 72–288 h after cardiotomy of whom nine were long-term survivors. One-third of the 18 patients, who had a left ventricular assist device only, died of right ventricular failure and there were no survivors of biventricular support. A similar pattern of problems was seen in the St. Louis experience; of 30 patients, 24 had biventricular failure. Fifty-three per cent of these patients required biventricular support, nine with biventricular assist devices and seven with right ventricular assist devices plus intra-aortic balloon pumps. The rate of weaning and survival was significantly better in the group with biventricular support than the remaining patients with biventricular failure treated with a left ventricular assist device only. Overall survival for the whole series was 37%.

The strongest determinants of survival appeared to be perioperative myocardial infarction and renal failure. Complications that may limit the duration of support such as the development of thrombus within the blood sac or percutaneous line-related sepsis were not common; two patients developed mediastinitis, and thrombus formation occurred in three ventricular assist device sacs. Two patients who had strokes did not have any ventricular assist device sac thrombus.

The Pierce–Donachy pump has produced rather better results when used as a bridge to transplantation (Farrar *et al.*, 1988; Pennington *et al.*, 1988a; Gray *et al.*, 1989; Hill, 1989). At least 57 patients have been treated for terminal heart failure with Pierce–Donachy pumps; 80% of these patients required biventricular support. Of these patients supported for a mean of 8.5 days, 46 were transplanted and 38 were discharged from hospital (67%). The most frequent medical reasons for patients on support not qualifying for transplantation were multiorgan failure, and haemorrhage. Device-related complications were uncommon, with three transient ischaemic attacks and two console dysfunctions. The Pierce–Donachy device has been used to support four patients who developed refractory cardiogenic shock after cardiac transplantation (Pennington *et al.*, 1988), but all patients died of renal failure and/or infection.

The Thermedics device has been used for postcardiotomy support in 22 patients, of whom eight were weaned from the device (Bernhard *et al.*, 1985). Only three patients left hospital. The report was interesting in that Bernhard experimentally seeded the textured lining of the electrically powered left ventricular assist device with fetal fibroblasts to accelerate the development of a collagenous sac lining which may inhibit the growth of calcium deposits on the polyurethane and ultimately prevent sac rupture. The Thermedics

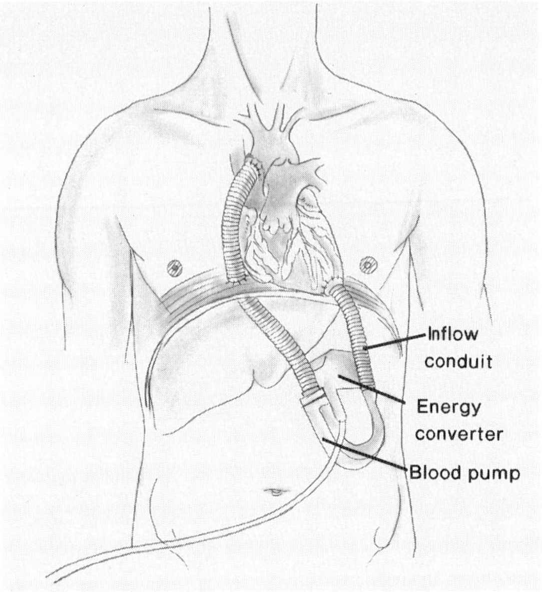

Figure 19.7 The Novacor left ventricular assist system configured for bridging to transplantation

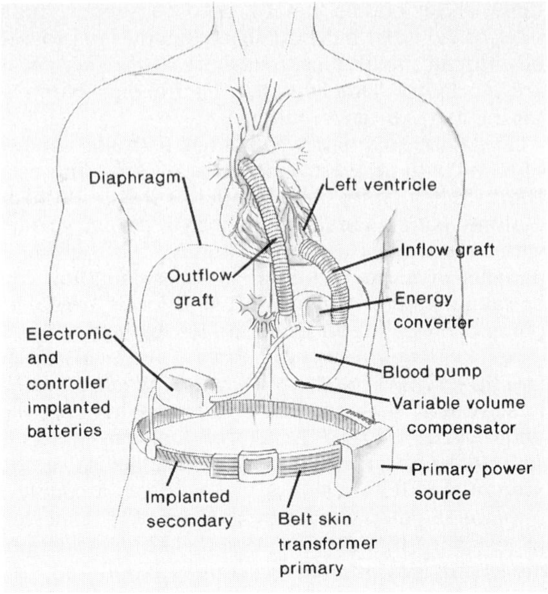

Figure 19.8 The totally implantable Novacor LVAS

pump has been used as a bridge to transplantation in four patients (Hill, 1989), and only one of three transplanted patients survived.

Electrically powered ventricular assist devices are designed to be totally implantable for permanent implantation in patients who do not meet the criteria for heart transplantation. The first of the second generation, and the only one currently available, is the Novacor ventricular assist system which employs a highly efficient electrical solenoid drive coupled by spring arms to dual pusher plates. The seamless, polyurethane blood sac is integral with the pusher plates, a design that reduces stress on the sac and allows continuous flow over the whole sac minimizing the risk of thrombus formation. Pericardial valves fitted to the Dacron inflow and outflow conduits provide unidirectional flow and the use of such tissue valves may reduce the incidence of thromboembolism. Most authors have heparinized recipients of this device beyond 4 days of support, although Warfarin and antiplatelet agents may be preferable (Starnes *et al.*, 1988). The pump has a maximum stroke volume of 67 ml. Cannulation of the apex of the left ventricle is achieved through a Teflon washer and blood is returned to the ascending aorta (Figure 19.7). The device itself sits in a posterior rectus sheath pocket. Three modes of operation are available: normal operation is synchronous counterpulsation based on internal sensors responsive to pump filling, but triggering from the R-wave and a fixed-rate are available. The Novacor device has an adjustable ejection fraction allowing progressive weaning in recovering hearts. Optimal effects of the Novacor pump are assessed by measurement of left ventricular pressures with a Millar transducer tipped catheter. Ultimately the complete system will incorporate an internal control box, an internal back up battery pack with a capacity of greater than 45 min, and a subcutaneous electrical coil for transcutaneous induction of power. The external coil will be connected to a rechargeable 10–12 h battery pack (Figure 19.8).

At least 20 patients have been supported using the Novacor device (Portner, 1989) for up to 90 days (mean 22.7). Ten of these patients received orthotopic heart transplants, eight of whom were discharged from hospital and there have been no late deaths. The most frequent reasons for not performing transplantation in patients supported with the Novacor device were multiorgan failure, stroke and haemorrhage. Device-related complications were uncommon, but did include two episodes of stroke. The single, small percutaneous control line may reduce the incidence of infection (Starnes *et al.*, 1988). Other electrically powered pumps are under development but no clinical results are available.

The total artificial heart

The aim of research into total artificial hearts (TAH) is to develop a readily available cardiac

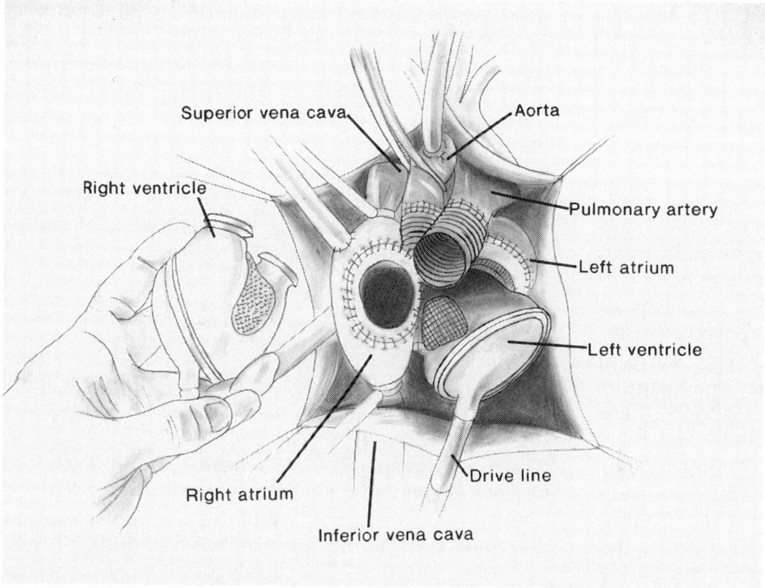

Figure 19.9 Implantation of the Jarvik-7 total artificial heart showing the 'quick' connect cuffs

replacement for patients with end-stage heart failure. The power requirements of a totally implantable system have, however, proved a major stumbling block. Current devices are pneumatic with transcutaneous drive lines which have increased potential for infection. Nuclear powered hearts have been designed but the use of plutonium-238 as a power source has, for the time being at least, proved societally unacceptable. Electrically powered total artificial hearts are under development but no clinical trials are yet reported although animal experiments have been conducted at Penn State (Davis *et al.*, 1989). The Penn State device consists of two blood pumps, one electrical roller-screw motor that converts rotational energy to linear force, and has Bjork–Shiley monostrut valves to ensure unidirectional flow. As with the Novacor left ventricular assist device, the absence of percutaneous power lines would allow permanent implantation in patients with severe biventricular failure who would not meet the criteria for heart transplantation.

Most TAHs consist of two pumps similar to the pneumatic ventricular assist devices, each with a rigid housing containing a seamless polyurethane blood sac. Expulsion of blood is achieved by pulsion of air between the sac and its casing. 'Quick' connect cuffs are used to attach the prosthesis to the atria and great vessels (Figure 19.9) and prosthetic valves direct the flow of blood. Two percutaneous drive lines connect the pumps to the console. At least eight different types of total artificial heart exist and 116 implants have been reported, the majority as a bridge to transplantation. The best known and most commonly used device is the Jarvik-7 which has been used as a permanent cardiac replacement in five patients and as a bridge to transplantation in 92 patients (Joyce, 1988). Some of the latter group received the smaller Jarvik-7/70 which has a stroke volume of 70 ml instead of the 100 ml of the standard model. Sixty-two of the 92 recipients of Jarvik devices were successfully bridged to transplantation, and of these 34 were overall survivors. Thirty patients developed complications and died during the period of support and a further 28 patients died after transplantation: the commonest causes were again multiorgan failure and sepsis. Support times were as long as 42 days. Thromboembolism was a major problem with clot found in most explanted devices and cerebral embolism affecting up to 10% of patients (Joyce *et al.*, 1988). Infection was the major cause of death after transplantation.

Major limitations to the use of TAHs are the blood rheologic abnormalities (increased viscosity and fibrinogen concentration) (Kormos *et al.*, 1987) that coupled with reduced microcirculatory perfusion results in cerebral injury and multiorgan failure, and the strikingly high incidence of mediastinitis, which may be due to the inability of the pericardial sac to fill the dead space around the device (Griffith *et al.*, 1988). Patients who would benefit from temporary support with a TAH are those with severe biventricular failure and complete absence of cardiac rhythm or uncontrollable arrhythmias, whereas patients with some remaining left ventricular function might be better supported with a left ventricular assist device alone.

The first permanent implant of a Jarvik-7 TAH was performed in 1982 (DeVries *et al.*, 1986) and the patient survived 112 days but died of multiorgan failure. The longest period of support has been 620 days (DeVries, 1988). Three of five recipients of total artificial hearts have had cerebral thromboembolism (Joyce *et al.*, 1988). The surgical complications including re-sternotomy for haemorrhage, and end-organ failure predispose these patients to infection (Kunin *et al.*, 1988) and have made the use of this device as a permanent cardiac replacement unacceptable to many. A further disadvantage to the long-term application of the TAH is the loss of normal cardiovascular regulation by the autonomic nervous system and circulating catecholamines after excision of the heart. The computerized control of the total artificial heart by microchips programmed with Starling's law may not provide sufficient fine tuning for optimal end-organ perfusion.

Skeletal muscle ventricular assist

The concept of electrical conditioning of skeletal muscle to generate fatigue-resistant muscle grafts for augmentation of cardiac contraction is attractive as living, autologous tissue is used. The latissimus dorsi muscle lends itself to the purpose due to its neurovascular anatomy and its ability to reach the heart. Skeletal muscle can be used to wrap the heart as a cylinder or as a spiral cone, or can be used to provide counterpulsation when interposed into the descending thoracic aorta. A number of investigators have investigated the technique experimentally (Chachques *et al.*, 1953; Macoviak *et al.*, 1981). At least 19 patients have been treated with latissimus dorsi cardiomyoplasty for left ventricular augmentation following resections for aneurysms (Magovern *et al.*, 1988), and fibroma (Carpentier and Chachques, 1985), as well as for treatment for cardiomyopathy (Hagege *et al.*, 1988; Molteni *et al.*, 1989). In most cases electrical conditioning of the myograft was begun after implantation. Improvements in resting left ventricular ejection fraction ranged from 0% to 13% at 10–17 months after cardiomyoplasty (Hagege *et al.*, 1988; Magovern *et al.*, 1988; Molteni *et al.*, 1989). In some patients with dilated cardiomyopathy and increased left ventricular end-diastolic volumes, small increases in ejection fraction may result in significant improvements in cardiac output (Hill and Chiu, 1989).

Selected patients may benefit from functional muscle grafts, particularly for augmentation of the right ventricle. There are, however, major limitations to this technique; a significant muscle mass is required that carries its endogenous neurovascular bundle without tethering, skeletal muscle is thrombogenic (this complication can be avoided if the endocardium is intact (Magovern *et al.*, 1986)), and the long-term performance characteristics of conditioned myografts are unknown.

Conclusions

Mechanical support of the circulation in patients with cardiogenic shock has become a reality. For the treatment of postcardiotomy shock and as a bridge to transplantation, a variety of sophisticated devices is available. In both sets of circumstances, conventional means of circulatory support, such as inotropes and the intra-aortic balloon pump should be tried initially. The application of centrifugal pumps and artificial ventricles to postcardiotomy shock should be confined to those patients with a reasonable chance of myocardial recovery. Patients with cardiogenic shock who are potential transplant candidates are suitable candidates for insertion of a mechanical support device. The decision to support such patients must be taken before end-organ failure, particularly renal failure, has developed. The use of mechanical support devices before transplantation should be confined to transplant centres and should not give the patient priority over other transplant candidates. It must also be remembered that the use of such devices reduces the cost-effectiveness of a transplant programme, by increasing cost but not improving overall survival. No series has shown an improvement in survival after mechanical support and cardiac transplantation. The relative merits of short term support with electrical versus pneumatic devices and left ventricular assist versus total artificial heart remain to be resolved. With optimal haemodynamic and pharmacological management, however, many patients can be maintained with a left ventricular assist device only, even in the presence of right ventricular dysfunction. At the present time, the marginal improvement in quality and duration of life resulting from the long-term use of pneumatic devices is not sufficient to justify their widespread application. Totally implantable electrically powered total artificial hearts are unlikely to be available for 10 years. The implantable electrical left ventricular assist system (Novacor) will be available for long-term implantation within 1–2 years. Improvements in biomaterials, biocompatible surfaces, system integration, and power sources are required for the use of permanent systems to become a routine part of cardiovascular practice, but these developments will surely occur, making permanent artificial cardiac support or replacement a reality in the forseeable future.

References

Amsterdam, E.Z., Awan, N.A., Lee, G., *et al.* (1981) Intraaortic balloon counterpulsation; rationale, application and results. *Cardiovascular Clinics*, **11**, 79–96

Bernhard, W.F., Clay, W., Gernes, D., *et al.* (1985) Temporary and permanent left ventricular bypass: laboratory and editorial investigations. *World Journal of Surgery*, **9**, 54–64

Bindslev, L., Gouda, I., Inacio, J., *et al.* (1986) Extracorporeal elimination of carbon dioxide using a surface heparinised veno-venous bypass system. *Transactions of the American Society of Artificial Internal Organs*, **32**, 530–534

Bindslev, L., Eklund, J., Norlander, O., *et al.* (1987) Treatment of acute respiratory failure by extracorporeal carbon dioxide elimination performed with a surface heparinised artificial lung. *Anaesthesiology*, **67**, 117–120

Bolman, R.M.III, Cox, J.L., Marshall, W., *et al.* (1989) Circulatory support with a centrifugal pump as a bridge to cardiac transplantation. *Annals of Thoracic Surgery*, **47**, 108–112

Bolman, R.M., Spray, T.L., Cance, C., *et al.* (1987) Heart transplantation in patients requiring preoperative mechanical support. *Heart Transplantation*, **5**, 374 (Abstract)

Bregman, D. and Casserella, W.J. (1980) Percutaneous intraoartic balloon pumping; initial clinical experience. *Annals of Thoracic Surgery*, **29**, 153–155

Buckley, M.J., Craver, J.M., Gold, H.K., *et al.* (1973) Intraaortic balloon pump assist for cardiogenic shock after cardiopulmonary bypass. *Circulation*, **48** (**Suppl III**), 90–94

Carpentier, A. and Chachques, J.G. (1985) Myocardial substitution with a stimulated skeletal muscle: first successful clinical use. *Lancet*, **i**, 1267

Chachques, J.C., Mitz, V., Hero, M., *et al.* (1985) Experimental cardioplasty using latissimus dorsi muscle. *Journal of Cardiovascular Surgery*, **26**, 457

Cooley, D.A., Liotta, D., Hallman, G.L., *et al.* (1969) Orthotopic cardiac prosthesis for two-staged cardiac replacement. *American Journal of Cardiology*, **24**, 723–730

Davis, P.K., Rosenberg, G., Snyder, A.J. and Pierce, W.S. (1989) Current status of permanent artificial hearts. *Annals of Thoracic Surgery*, **47**, 172–178

DeBakey, M.E. (1971) Left ventricular bypass pump for cardiac assistance: clinical experience. *American Journal of Cardiology*, **27**, 3–11

DeVries, W.C., Anderson, J.L., Joyce, L.D., *et al.* (1984) Clinical use of the artificial heart. *New England Journal of Medicine*, **310**, 273–278

DeVries, W.C. (1988) The permanent artificial heart: four case reports. *Journal of the American Medical Association*, **259**, 849–859

Didisheim, P., Olsen, D.B., Farrar, D.J., *et al.* (1989) Infections and thromboembolism with implantable cardiovascular devices. *Transactions of the American Society of Artificial Internal Organs*, **35**, 54–70

Farrar, D.J., Compton, P.G., Dajee, H., *et al.* (1984) Right heart function during left heart assist and the effects of volume loading in a canine preparation. *Circulation*, **70**, 708–716

Farrar, D.J., Compton, P.G., Hershon, J.J., Hill, J.D. (1985) Right ventricular function in an operating room model of mechanical left ventricular assistance and its effect in patients with depressed left ventricular function. *Circulation*, **72**, 1279–1285

Farrar, D.J., Hill, J.D., Gray, L.A., *et al.* (1988) Heterotopic prosthetic ventricles as a bridge to cardiac transplantation. *New England Journal of Medicine*, **318**, 333–340

Flege, J.B., Jr., Wright, C.B. and Reisenger, T.J. (1984) Successful balloon counterpulsation for right ventricular failure. *Annals of Thoracic Surgery*, **37**, 167–168

Gaines, W.E., Pierce, W.S., Donachy, J.H., *et al.* (1985) The Pennsylvania State University paracorporeal ventricular assist pump: optimal methods of use. *World Journal of Surgery*, **9**, 11–17

Gibbon, J.H. Jr (1954) Application of a mechanical heart and lung apparatus to cardiac surgery. *Minnesota Medicine*, **37**, 171–180

Gifford, D., Wheeldon, D., Wallwork, J. and Spratt, P. (1986) Balloon counterpulsation together with Bio-Medicus pump closed circuit membrane oxygenation for left ventricular assist: a case report. *Journal of Extracorporeal Technology*, **18**, 29–33

Golding, L.A.R., Stewart, R.W., Sinkewich, M., *et al.* (1988) Nonpulsatile ventricular assist bridging to transplantation. *Transactions of the American Society of Artificial Internal Organs*, **34**, 476–479

Gray, L.A., Ganzel, B.L., Mavroudis, C. and Slater, A.D. (1989) The Pierce–Donachy ventricular assist device as a bridge to cardiac transplantation. *Annals of Thoracic Surgery*, **48**, 222–227

Griffith, B.P. (1989) Interim use of the Jarvik-7 artificial heart: lessons learned at the Presbyterian–University Hospital of Pittsburgh. *Annals of Thoracic Surgery*, **47**, 158–166

Griffith, B.P., Kormos, R.L., Hardesty, R.L., *et al.* (1988) The artificial heart: infection related morbidity and its effect on transplantation. *Annals of Thoracic Surgery*, **45**, 409–414

Hagege, A.A., Fernandez, F., Desnos, M., *et al.* (1988) Hemodynamic study of the long-term efficiency of dynamic cardiomyoplasty. *Circulation*, **78** (**Suppl II**), 345

Hardesty, R.L., Griffith, B.P., Trento, A., *et al.* (1986) Mortally ill patients and excellent survival following cardiac transplantation. *Annals of Thoracic Surgery*, **41**, 126–129

Hill, A.B. and Chiu, R.C-J. (1989) Dynamic cardiomyoplasty for treatment of heart failure. *Clinical Cardiology*, **12**, 681–688

Hill, J.D., Farrar, D.J., Hirshon, J.J., *et al.* (1986) Use of a prosthetic ventricle as a bridge to cardiac transplantation for post infarction cardiogenic shock. *New England Journal of Medicine*, **314**, 626–628

Hill, J.D., O'Brien, T.G., Murray, J.J., *et al.* (1972) Prolonged extracorporeal oxygenation for post-traumatic respiratory failure (shock lung syndrome). *New England Journal of Medicine*, **286**, 629–634

Hill, J.D. (1989) Bridging to cardiac transplantation. *Annals of Thoracic Surgery*, **47**, 167–171

Joyce, L.D., Johnson, K.E., Cabrol, C., *et al.* (1988) Nine year experience with the clinical use of total artificial hearts as cardiac support devices. *Transactions of the American Society of Artificial Internal Organs*, **34**, 703–707

Kanter, K., Pennington, D.G., Weber, T.R., *et al.* (1987) Extracorporeal membrane oxygenation for postoperative cardiac support in children. *Journal of Thoracic and Cardiovascular Surgery*, **93**, 27–35

Kantrowitz, A. and Kantrowitz, A. (1953) Experimental augmentation of coronary flow by retardation of arterial pressure pulse. *Surgery*, **34**, 678–687

Kirklin, J.W. (1989) The middle 1950s and C. Walton Lillehei. *Journal of Thoracic and Cardiovascular Surgery*, **98**, 822–824

Kolobow, T., Stool, E.W., Sacks, K.L. and Vurek, G.G. (1975) Acute respiratory failure: survival following ten days support with a membrane lung. *Journal of Thoracic and Cardiovascular Surgery*, **69**, 947–953

Kormos, R.L., Borovetz, H.S., Griffith, B.P., *et al.* (1987) Rheologic abnormalities in patients with the Jarvik-7 total artificial heart. *Transactions of the American Society of Artificial Internal Organs*, **33**, 413–417

Kunin, C.M., Dobbins, J.J., Melo, J.C., *et al.* (1988) Infectious complications in four long-term recipients of the Jarvik-7 artificial heart. *Journal of the American Medical Association*, **259**, 860–864

Leinbach, R.C., Buckley, M.J., Austen, W.G., *et al.* (1971) Effects of intraaortic balloon pump on coronary flow and metabolism in man. *Circulation*, **44 (Suppl I)**, 77–81

Levinson, M.M., Smith, R.G., Cork, R., *et al.* (1986) Three recent cases of the total artificial heart before transplantation. *Journal of Heart Transplantation*, **5**, 215–228

Litwak, R.S., Koffsky, R.M., Jurado, R.A., *et al.* (1985) A decade of experience with a left heart assist device in patients undergoing intracardiac operation. *World Journal of Surgery*, **9**, 18–24

McBride, L.R., Pennington, D.G. and Tsai, C.C., *et al.* (1987b) Influence of ventricular assist devices on lymphocytes. *Heart Transplantation*, **5**, 379

McBride, L.R., Ruzevich, S.A., Pennington, D.G., *et al.* (1987a) Infectious complications asssociated with ventricular assist device support. *Transactions of the American Society of Artificial Internal Organs*, **33**, 201–202

McEnany, M.T., Kay, H.R., Buckley, M.R., *et al.* (1978) Clinical experience with intra-aortic balloon pump support in 728 patients. *Circulation*, **58 (Suppl I)**, 124

Macoviak, J.A., Stephenson, L.W., Alavi, A., *et al.* (1981) Effect of electrical stimulation on diaphragmatic muscle used to enlarge right ventricle. *Surgery*, **90**, 271–277

Magovern, G.J. (1989) Panel 5. Weaning and bridging. *Annals of Thoracic Surgery*, **47**, 102–107

Magovern, G.J., Park, S.B., Magovern, G.J.. Jr *et al.* (1986) Latissimus dorsi as a functioning synchronously paced muscle component in the repair of a left ventricular aneurysm. *Annals of Thoracic Surgery*, **41**, 116

Magovern, G.J., Heckler, F.R., Park, S.B., *et al.* (1988) Paced skeletal muscle for dynamic cardiomyoplasty. *Annals of Thoracic Surgery*, **45**, 614–619

Magovern, G.J., Sang, B.P. and Maher, T.D. (1985) Use of a centrifugal pump without anticoagulants for postoperative left ventricular assist. *World Journal of Surgery*, **9**, 25–36

Martin, R.S., Moncure, A.C., Buckley, M.J., *et al.* (1983) Complications of percutaneous intra-aortic balloon insertion. *Journal of Thoracic and Cardiovascular Surgery*, **85**, 186–190

Miller, D.C., Moreno-Cabral, R.J., Stinson, E.B. *et al.* (1980) Pulmonary artery balloon counterpulsation for acute right ventricular failure. *Journal of Thoracic and Cardiovascular Surgery*, **80**, 760–763

Molteni, L., Almada, H.E., de Palma, C. and Ferriera. R. (1989) Dynamic cardiomyoplasty: clinical experience. In *Transformed Muscle in Cardiac Assist and Repair* (eds R.C.J. Chiu and I. Bourgeois), Futura Publishing Company Inc., Mount Kisco, New York

Moran, J.M., Opravil, M., Gorman, A.J., *et al.* (1984) Pulmonary artery balloon counterpulsation for right ventricular failure: II. Clinical experience. *Annals of Thoracic Surgery*, **38**, 254–259

Muneretto, C., Solis, E., Pavie, A., *et al.* (1989) Total artificial heart: survival and complications. *Annals of Thoracic Surgery*, **47**, 151–157

Oaks, T.E., Wisnan, C.B., Pae, W.E., *et al.* (1989) Results of mechanical assistance before heart transplantation. *Journal of Heart Transplantation*, **8**, 113–115

Pae, W.E., Pierce, W.S., Pennock, J.L., *et al.* (1987) Long-term results of ventricular assist pumping in post-cardiotomy cardiogenic shock. *Journal of Thoracic and Cardiovascular Surgery*, **93**, 434–441

Park, S.B., Liebler, G.A., Burkholder, J.A., *et al.* (1986) Mechanical support of the failing heart. *Annals of Thoracic Surgery*, **42**, 627–631

Pennington, D.G. (1989) Circulatory support before transplantation. In *Heart and Heart–lung Transplantation* (ed J. Wallwork), WB Saunders, Philadelphia, pp. 41–86

Pennington, D.G., Cood, J.E., Merjavy, J.P., *et al.* (1983) The expanded use of ventricular bypass system for severe cardiac failure and as a bridge to tranplantation. *Heart Transplantation*, **3**, 38–46

Pennington, D.G., Merjavy, Codd, J.R., *et al.* (1984) Extracorporeal membrane oxygenation for patients with cardiogenic shock. *Circulation*, **70 (Suppl 1)**, 130–137

Pennington, D.G., Kanter, K.R., McBride, L.R., *et al.* (1988a) Seven years' experience with the Pierce–Donachy ventricular assist device. *Journal of Thoracic and Cardiovascular Surgery*, **96**, 901–911

Pennington, D.G., McBride, L.R., Kanter, K.R., *et al.* (1988b) Effect of perioperative myocardial infarction on survival of post cardiotomy patients supported with ventricular-assist devices. *Circulation*, **78**, (**Suppl 3**), 110-115

Portner, P.M., Oyer, P.E., McGregor, C.G.A., *et al.* (1985) First human use of an electrically powered implantable ventricular assist system. *Artificial Organs*, **9**, 36

Portner, P.M., Oyer, P.E., Pennington, D.G., *et al.* (1989) Implantable electrical left ventricular assist system: bridge to transplantation and the future. *Annals of Thoracic Surgery*, **47**, 142–150

Reemtsma, K., Krusin, R., Edie, R., *et al.* (1978) Cardiac transplantation in patients requiring mechanical circulatory support. *New England Journal of Medicine*, **298**, 670–671

Report to the Chairman, Subcommittee on Health, Committee on Ways and Means, House of Representatives (1989) *Heart Transplants: concerns abouts costs, access, and availability of donor organs.* United States General Accounting Office, Washington DC

Rose, D.M., Connolly, M., Cunningham, J.N.Jr and Spencer, F.C. (1989) Technique and results with a roller pump left and right heart assist device. *Annals of Thoracic Surgery*, **47**, 124–129

Rose, D.M., Laschinger, J., Grossi, E., *et al.* (1985) Experimental and clinical results with a simplified left heart assist device for treatment of profound left ventricular dysfunction. *World Journal of Surgery*, **9**, 11–17

Spencer, F.C., Eiseman, B., Trinkle, J.K., Rossi, N.P. (1965) Assisted circulation for cardiac failure following intracardiac surgery with cardiopulmonary bypass. *Journal of Thoracic and Cardiovascular Surgery*, **49**, 56–73

Starnes, V.A., Oyer, P.E., Portner, P.M., *et al.* (1988) Isolated left ventricular assist as a bridge to cardiac transplantation. *Journal of Thoracic and Cardiovascular Surgery*, **96**, 62–71

The Working Group on Mechanical Circulatory Support of the National Heart, Lung, and Blood Institute (1985) *Artificial heart and assist devices: Directions, needs, costs, societal, and ethical issues.* US Dept of Health and Human Services, Public Health Service, Publication No. (NIH)85-2723. Washington, DC

Wampler, R.K., Johnson, D.V., Rutan, P.M. and Riehle, R.A. (1989) Multicenter study of the Hemopump in the treatment of cardiogenic shock. *Circulation*, **80** (**Suppl II**), 670

Wampler, R.K., Moise, J.C., Frazier, O.H. and Olsen, D.B. (1988) In vivo evaluation of a peripheral vascular access axial flow blood pump. *Transactions of the American Society of Artificial Internal Organs*, **34**, 450–454

Welch, G.H.,Jr., Sarnoff, S., Braunwald, E., *et al.* (1958) The influence of cardiac output, aortic pressure, and heart rate on myocardial oxygen utilization. *Surgical Forum*, **8**, 294–298

20

Artificial hearts–present and future

W.J. Kolff and Jack Kolff

At present artificial hearts are used exclusively as a bridge to transplantation. Indeed, during 1987, 46 artificial hearts were implanted in patients waiting for a donor heart, and 36 of these patients left hospital with a functioning donor heart. This is a remarkable success considering the preoperative status of the patients.

However, before the cyclosporin-A era in heart transplantation the Food and Drug Administration (FDA) permitted the use of an artificial heart only in those patients who were not candidates for cardiac transplantation. Indeed in the first protocol used in Salt Lake City we were specifically forbidden to use an artificial heart in a patient who could be a candidate for cardiac transplantation.

The first artificial heart was implanted in December 1982. The recipient was Dr Barney Clark (Figure 20.1). He was 61 years old, and at that time fell outside the age range for heart transplantation. During the first few days postimplantation of the artificial heart, Dr Clark made a dramatic improvement. Later he suffered a number of complications, most of which were unrelated to the artificial heart (Joyce *et al.*, 1983; Kolff *et al.*, 1983).

This remarkable improvement following successful implantation of an artificial heart has been seen by many surgeons. In these failing patients it may be impossible to ascertain whether pulmonary failure, hepatic failure and nutritional disturbances are irreversible disease entities rather than being secondary to the heart failure. We know of many cases where successful implantation of an artificial heart has resulted in patients putting out large volumes of urine causing a resolution of pulmonary oedema and bronchopneumonia, and a rise to haematocrit. Furthermore their liver function would improve with activation of clotting factors necessitating the use of anticoagulation to prevent strokes (Levinson *et al.*, 1986).

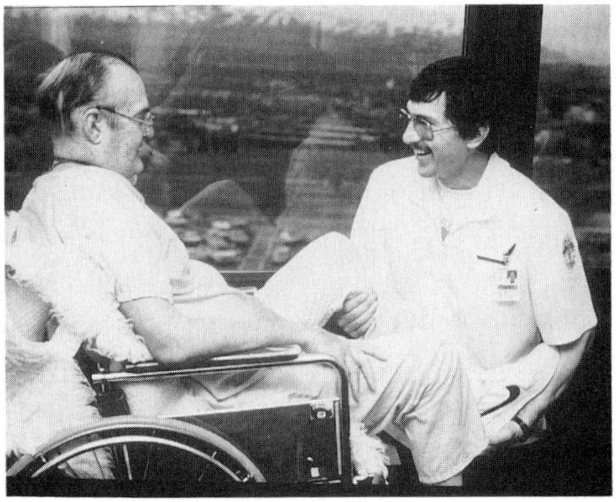

Figure 20.1 Barney Clark – A photograph of Barney Clark who was the first recipient of a 'permanent' artificial heart in December 1982. We learned from Dr Clark that (1) the artificial heart causes no pain or discomfort in the chest, (2) that the noise of the drive system did not bother him, (3) that he did not lose his sense of humour, (4) that he still loved his family, (5) and that he still wanted to help and serve his fellow men, so that all essential functions of the human mind were preserved

Thrombosis was a major problem with the initial artificial heart. Of the first six patients who received artificial hearts with the intention that these would be a permanent device five have thrown emboli to their brain which have ruined their lives (DeVries *et al.*, 1988a). This experience caused considerable worry for surgeons who then implanted artificial hearts for as short a time as possible until a donor heart was available. Thus the artificial heart would be inside the chest for only a few days. This seems illogical. It would be much more appropriate if the patient were allowed to recover fully from the secondary sequela of his heart failure before organ transplantation.

Levinson *et al.* (1986) described the occurrence of thrombosis in recipients in the Symbion type of artificial heart. They found that in many instances the thrombus originated either on the connecting system (the so called 'quick connects') or on the valves or valve rings of the artificial heart. To overcome this main source of thromboemboli the Utah-100 artificial heart with a different connecting system was developed. Alternatively, Kolff in Philadelphia encouraged the development of the Philadelphia-type heart where all connectors have been avoided.

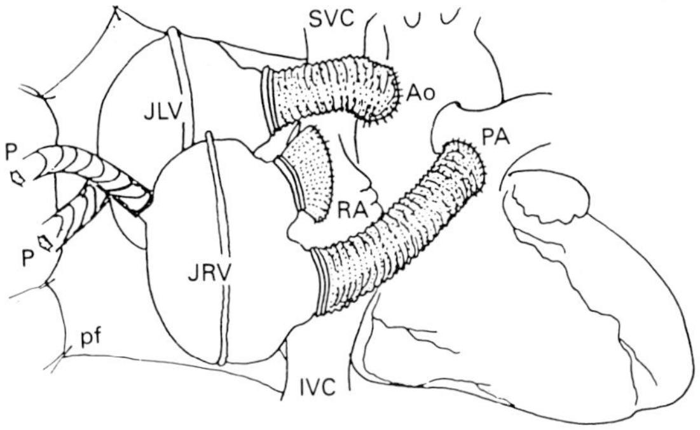

Figure 20.2 Arrangement suggested by Dr Jacques G. Losman with the LVAD and an RVAD both located in the right side of the chest. When the heart recovered, they could be removed

Intrathoracic LVAD–RVAD or total artificial heart

Of the 130 patients who received Thoratec Left Ventricular Assist Device (LVAD) (unmodified extracorporeal Pierce-Donachy Heart) until September 1987, 50% needed a biventricular assist. Of the 45 patients who received the LVAD as a bridge to transplantation 28 have done well after heart transplantation. Of the 85 patients in which the LVAD was applied in the hope that the natural heart would improve only 15 have been discharged from hospital.

There is no scientific evidence for the assumption that the intrathoracic LVAD is an easier and potentially more reliable device than the total artificial heart. Of course whenever there is the possibility of the natural heart recovering the LVAD plus RVAD would be preferable to a total artificial heart. Barnard's patients in South Africa whose natural hearts recovered after heterotopic transplantations of donor hearts proved that such recovery can occur, particularly in cases of viral myocarditis. It is also true that an ailing natural heart might still be able to sustain life if the LVAD and RVAD failed. There is no doubt that decisions regarding implantation of an artificial heart or ventricular assist device must be made promptly. The sooner use of the 'device' is begun the better chance the patient has of survival. Our maxim has become LVAD plus RVAD is a total artificial heart. We suggest the following therapeutic regime. The natural heart can be left in place and LVAD put on the left side and an RVAD on the right, or both on the right (Losman, Replogle and Kolff, 1982) (Figure 20.2). If the natural heart recovers then the LVAD and RVAD can be removed. If it does not recover the natural heart can be removed and a donor heart put in its place. The LVAD-RVAD can then be removed when the donor heart has taken over the circulation.

This argument only applies to intrathoracic LVAD and RVADs. With the exception of axial flow pump developed by Nimbus, which fits between the left ventricle and the aorta, most of the presently used L-RVADs are extracorporeal.

Surgical implantation of the artificial heart

Kwan-Gett and co-workers (1971) demonstrated that it was possible to implant an artificial heart without the use of a pump oxygenator. He first implanted the left ventricle and then the right ventricle. Then he took out the natural heart and joined the two artificial ventricles together. However it is more usual to use a membrane oxygenator and a pump combined with moderate hypothermia. The surgical techniques have been described and revised recently (Rieben *et al.*, 1986; DeVries, 1988b). In animals that lie on their sternum such as the calf or the sheep the chest is opened by removal of the fifth rib on the right side. In human patients as a rule a sternal split is performed.

Postoperative management

Heparin is neutralized with protamine sulfate as soon as the heart–lung machine is stopped. Anticoagulation therapy is started on the following day when there is no bleeding from the chest tubes. Dextran may be started earlier. The following drugs are considered: Heparin, warfarin, dextran, dipyridamole and aspirin. In experimental animals we often give nothing as we wish to determine if and where the thrombosis develops. Warfarin treatment in calves is difficult. Aspirin is broken down in the four stomachs of the ruminant and we give it rectally. Dr Fazal Mohammad and co-workers

(Swier *et al.*, 1989) have recently shown that aspirin has little effect in bovine platelets, contrary to its marked effect on human platelets. The aspirin inhibition of platelet function lasts as long as the life of the platelets, which is about ten days. In case of bleeding a transfusion of fresh platelets is required.

We use cephalosporin prophylaxis in calves for a period of 5 days and amikacin when infection with *Pseudomonas* is suspected.

Air-driven artificial hearts

Most artificial hearts are driven by compressed air. This method has the advantage that the intrathoracic pumps are light; there is no hardware and there is no need for electronics inside the chest. The drive system can be repaired or replaced on the outside reducing the demand on its durability and greatly reducing the cost. Certainly if the artificial heart is meant only as a bridge to transplantation and there is no justification for putting the hardware inside the chest.

There has been a great deal of discussion about the bulkiness of the presently used drive systems. These systems are necessarily bulky because the FDA requires two heart drivers on the console. In many instances an extra compressor or large tanks with compressed air are incorporated as a safeguard in the event of failure of the electricity supply.

There are several drive systems available for air driven artificial hearts. The Utah Heart Driver using a solenoid valve is a further development of the Detroit Coil Heart Driver and the Kwan-Gett Driver. The Philadriver uses a pneumatic logic and is therefore independent of electric power and uses electronics only for recording. It has a gentle dp/dt since a small air valve opens first (Kolff, 1988) (Figures 20.3 and 20.4).

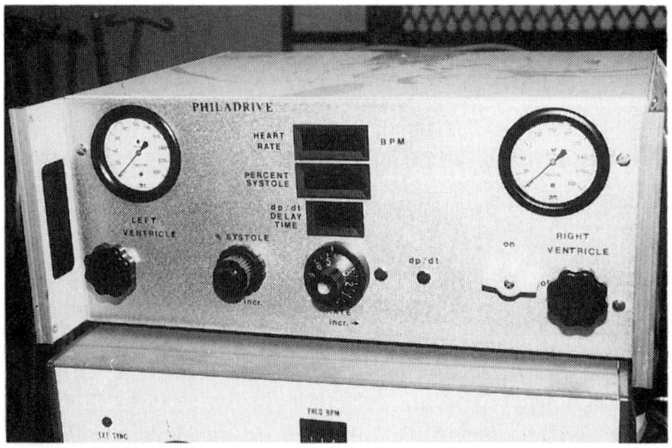

Figure 20.3 The Philadriver is a pneumatic system that operates without electricity. The air pressure required is low so that smaller compressors can be used. Electricity from a battery is used for the readouts

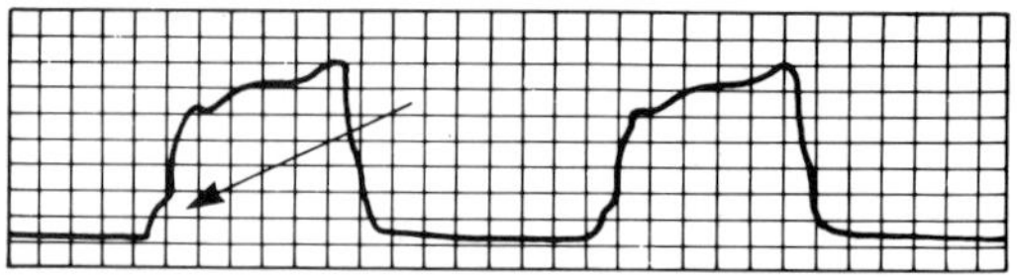

Figure 20.4 Drive pressure of the left ventricle in a calf. The Philadriver has a gentler onset of dp/dt than the Utah heart driver. This is accomplished by a small valve that opens first, hopefully long enough to close the mitral valve gently with 30 mmHg pressure indicated by the arrow. Thereafter, the full pressure comes on

There are also portable drive systems. The most sophisticated one that we are familiar with is the Heimes Drive System (Heimes and Klasen, 1982). Whalen is developing a simple pneumatic heart driver whose power is provided by a high force (178 N) electromagnetic linear activator (Whalen and Briskman, 1988).

Reciprocating mechanical pumps

These pumps are the simplest of all. A two cylinder gasoline engine can be converted, driven with an electric motor, putting the air hose in the spark plug opening and changing the camshaft that lifts the valves (Figure 20.5). A very simple design is shown in Figure 20.6.

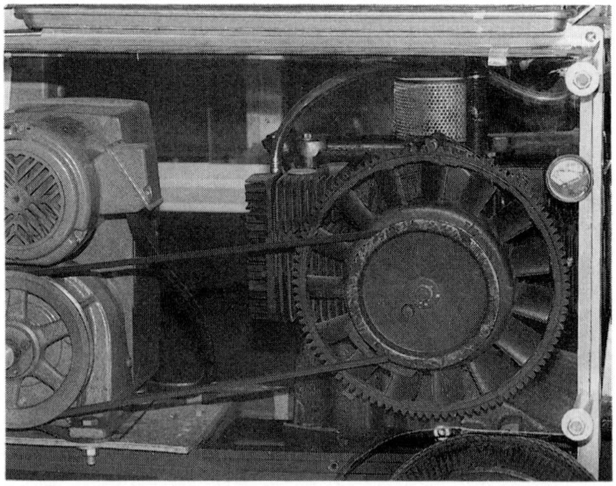

Figure 20.5 A two-cylinder gasoline engine energized by an electromotor can be used to drive an artificial heart. The driveline to the artificial heart comes from the hole for the spark plug. The shaft that lifts the valves has been changed: outflow (systole) 1/4 of cycle, inflow 3/4 of cycle

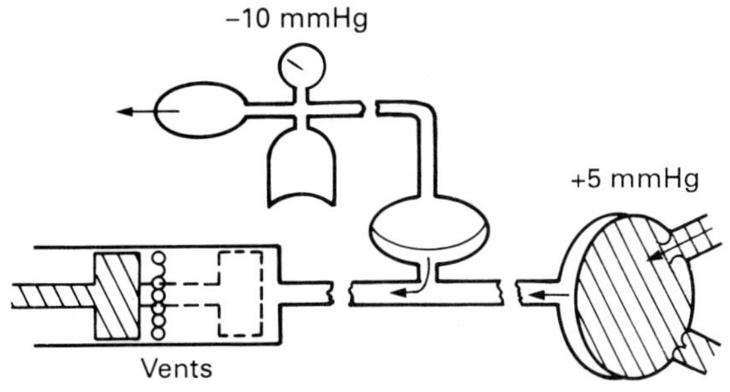

Figure 20.6 A very simple reciprocating drive pump. The position of the holes in the cylinder determines the ratio between systole and diastole. If desired, an extra ventricle connected to a bottle with subatmospheric pressure can regulate the maximum suction

Postoperative management

It is imperative that the postoperative management teams understand the action of the artificial heart. For example endotracheal suction may stop left ventricular output because it may reduce intrathoracic pressure and the filling pressure of the left ventricle. Positive pressure ventilation also has an effect. These effects must be studied in a mock circulation (Pantalos and Kolff, 1984).

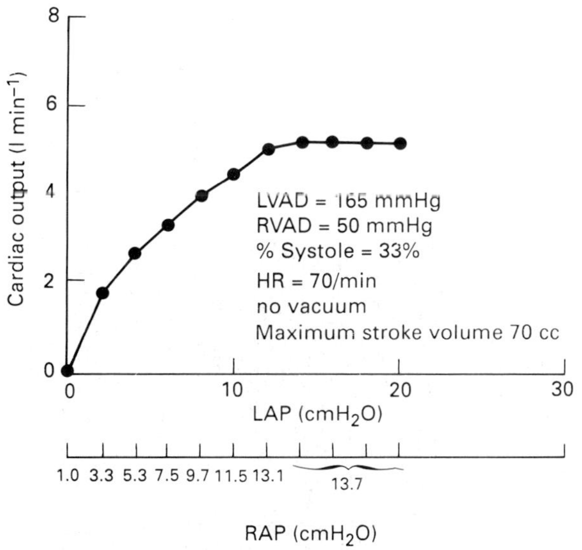

Figure 20.7 Starling's law. Curve plots the cardiac output versus the filling pressures of the left atrium (LAP) and of the right atrium (RAP). This curve is made in a cascade-type mock circulation for right and left sides, when a plateau of cardiac output is reached. Further addition of water does not increases the cardiac output. In this case, the left atrial pressure rises more than the right

Control of artificial hearts – Starling's law

Though there are many sophisticated controls we believe that Starling's law is of the utmost importance in the control of the artificial hearts. Approximately 87% of all cardiac output is governed by Starling's law. Thus if the venous supply to either right or left heart increases and the pressure rises then that ventricle will pump out more automatically (Figure 20.7). Starling's law can easily be demonstrated in mock circulation. All one does is to alter the total blood volume. The blood volume is increased in a mock circulation then venous pressure rises and the cardiac output goes up. Starling's law also provides for balance between right and left ventricles. Starling's law can be obtained by:

1. Variable rate fixed stroke volume – usually a full-fill, full-empty mode.
2. Fixed rate with variable stroke volume but the rate can be manually changed if desired. When the venous or filling pressure is higher a larger volume in the ventricle will be pumped out during the next stroke.
3. A combination of the above.

Artificial hearts developed in Utah mostly use the manually set rate and a variable stroke volume.

Artificial hearts that have soft and flexible pumping membranes, and have inflow valves with low resistance respond well to Starling's law. We know of no artificial heart that can equal the rapidity of response of the natural heart but the heart with antisuction balloon has come close (Norton, Akutsu and Kolff, 1962).

Starling's law develops a plateau when the maximum output has been reached (Figure 20.7).

A condition for the proper functioning of Starling's law in an artificial heart is that the ventricles are driven by sufficient pressure to empty the ventricle. We know examples of clinical cases where the surgeon was afraid of overloading the lungs and therefore drove the right ventricle with an insufficient pressure for emptying that ventricle. In that case the response to Starling's law is lost. (See below: Learning how to drive the artificial heart.)

Shift of Starling's curve to left by diastolic suction

Our aim is to build ventricles that have so little resistance to inflow and have diaphragms that move so easily, that the variable volume ventricle will respond to Starling's law. However, if we have not reached that ideal, or if there is some impediment to these functions, the Starling's curves can be

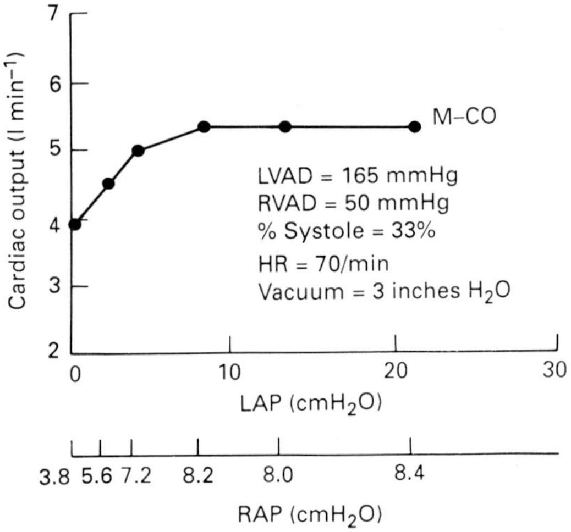

Figure 20.8 Starling's curve shifts to the left when suction is applied during diastole to the drivelines. The higher the suction, the more the curve shifts to the left and the sooner a plateau of cardiac output is reached. Of course, this abolishes Starling's response.

shifted to the left by applying extra suction during diastole to the outflow of the drive line of artificial heart (Figure 20.8). Modest suction does not interfere with the function of the Cardiac Output Monitor and Diagnostic Unit (COMDU) which measures cardiac output. This can be accomplished by a simple pump, remembering that one needs a relatively large volume, and if the pump does not work, it should not impede the outflow to the atmosphere. The suction that we use with pumps does not exceed 15 cmH_2O. It can also be accomplished by a Venturi device, if it is combined with a simple flap valve to release the first gust of air. It should be remembered that excessive suction by the artificial ventricles runs the risk of aspirating the atrial wall into the inflow valve.

Other controls of cardiac output

The belief that Starling's law was insufficient to regulate cardiac output during exercise led other groups to develop other automatic control systems. The system developed at the Pennsylvania State University (Magovern, Rosenberg and Pierce, 1986) employs a negative feedback loop to control the output of each ventricle. On the left side, the pump is set to maintain a desired aortic pressure range. If aortic pressure falls, due to a drop in peripheral resistance as occurs during exercises, the pump rate increases. On the right side, the system is designed to maintain a defined left atrial pressure. If the left atrial pressure increases beyond a certain range, the right pump rate decreases, pumping less blood through the pulmonary circulation and reducing the left atrial pressure.

Both the aortic and left atrial pressures are derived from the pneumatic power unit driveline pressures, eliminating the need for implanted transducers.

Control mechanisms have also been designed by two European groups. The Berlin group employs a system where changes in right atrial pressure are used as the input to a negative feedback loop that changes the output of both pumps. The Vienna group employs a hot-wire thermistor probe anemometer in the pneumatic power line to detect complete filling and complete emptying, and uses these signals to initiate the systole and diastole.

The COMDU or the Heimes Driver gives us the cardiac output every third beat (Willshaw *et al.*, 1984).

Driving mode

The dp/dt of the various drive systems is different. The Philadriver has a small air valve which opens first, just long enough to close the mitral valve gently, followed by a large air valve to bring in full pressure. Stress on the mitral valve at the incident of closure is thus reduced (Figure 20.4). The aortic valves will close immediately after the ending of the blood ejection from the ventricle.

In the natural tricusp semilunar valves, the leaflets will close like the rolling out of a carpet starting at the periphery, so that little stress occurs on the commissures (Figure 20.9). However, this is difficult to accomplish with elastomer valves. If there is a pause after ventricular ejection, the valve may open again and regurgitation will occur.

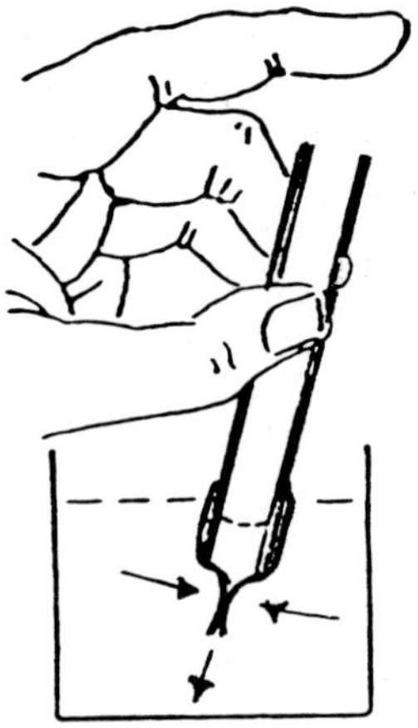

Figure 20.9 Henderson and Johnson showed this figure in 1912–when the flow suddenly stops, the valve closes. Henderson, Y., Johnson, F.E. (1912) Two modes of closure of heart valves. *Heart–A Journal of Circulation*, **4**, 69

For the artificial heart, this means that the percentage of systole should be adjusted so that a pause after ejection is avoided.

Measuring the cardiac output

Analysis of the drive pressure curve indicates whether there is complete emptying of the ventricle. If that is the case, there is a small peak at the end of systole (see Figure 20.4).

Using exhausted air, the measuring of the cardiac output in air driven artificial hearts is simple. It can be done with a non-invasive technique using the drive lines that are already going through a chest wall. If a pneumotoachograph or other flow meter is put into the exhaust port of the air coming out of the drive lines to the artificial heart, one can very easily measure the amount of air that is expelled.

The COMDU does this with every third beat (Willshaw *et al.*, 1984). The amount of air expelled during diastole is equal to the amount of blood entering the ventricle. With the next stroke, this volume of blood is expelled.

Thus, with every third beat we see on the diagram not only the volume at blood that entered each ventricle but also the rate of which it entered. From this, one can estimate the venous pressure in the left and right atrium. One can then make a diagnosis of the things that can go wrong with either the patient or the artificial heart (Figure 20.10).

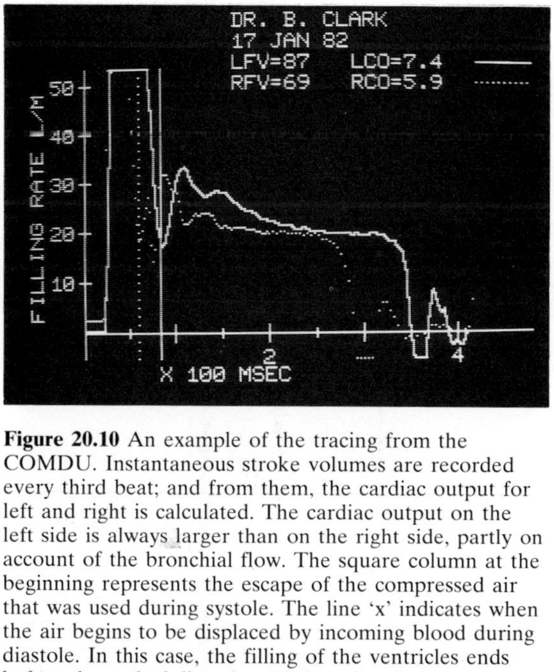

Figure 20.10 An example of the tracing from the COMDU. Instantaneous stroke volumes are recorded every third beat; and from them, the cardiac output for left and right is calculated. The cardiac output on the left side is always larger than on the right side, partly on account of the bronchial flow. The square column at the beginning represents the escape of the compressed air that was used during systole. The line 'x' indicates when the air begins to be displaced by incoming blood during diastole. In this case, the filling of the ventricles ends before the end of diastole and there is a little extra flow near the end

The pneumotachograph is basically a multiple tube resistance in the air line. One measures the pressure on either side of this resistance, and from this, one can calculate the flow.

Earlier, the air flow was measured by using thermistors (Kless *et al.*, 1974). Abiomed uses this system.

It should be understood that although the COMDU measures the volume of blood that enters the heart and one assumes that under normal conditions the same volume is pumped out with the next stroke, the calculation by the COMDU does not differentiate how the blood enters or leaves the ventricle. In other words, if there is a leaking aortic valve or a mitral valve, the COMDU calculates a large stroke, but it is not 100% effective. Fortunately the shape of the filling curve can often make the diagnosis.

Learning how to drive the artificial heart

Someone on the surgical team should understand the mechanics of the circulation and the mechanics of the artificial heart and how it is driven. The personnel responsible for the postoperative care should be allowed to practice with an artificial heart connected to a mock circulation.

W.J. Kolff prefers the cascade mock circulation because it not only allows testing of the heart and flow measurements, but it also demonstrates changes in the blood volume between the lesser and greater circulation (Pantalos and Kolff, 1984) (Figure 20.11).

To give an example, sometimes patients with an air driven artificial heart have mucus in their bronchi or have aspirated vomitus. The physician or the nurse then decides that it has to be sucked out with an endotracheal tube. This may cause a subatmospheric pressure inside the chest. The cascade mock circulation shows convincingly that when an subatmospheric pressure is induced in the thoracic cavity or in the mock circulation over the pulmonary artery and over the pulmonary veins, suddenly all cardiac output on the left side stops. Since the artificial heart is dependent on Starling's law, the venous pressure determines the filling of the heart, and this determines the cardiac output. If subatmospheric pressure prevents the filling of the ventricle, the cardiac output on the left side becomes zero.

An immediate shift of the blood occurs from the vena cavae and the greater circulation with its larger volume of blood to the lung veins and the lesser circulation where the capacity is much smaller. This produces a shift in blood volume and pulmonary oedema.

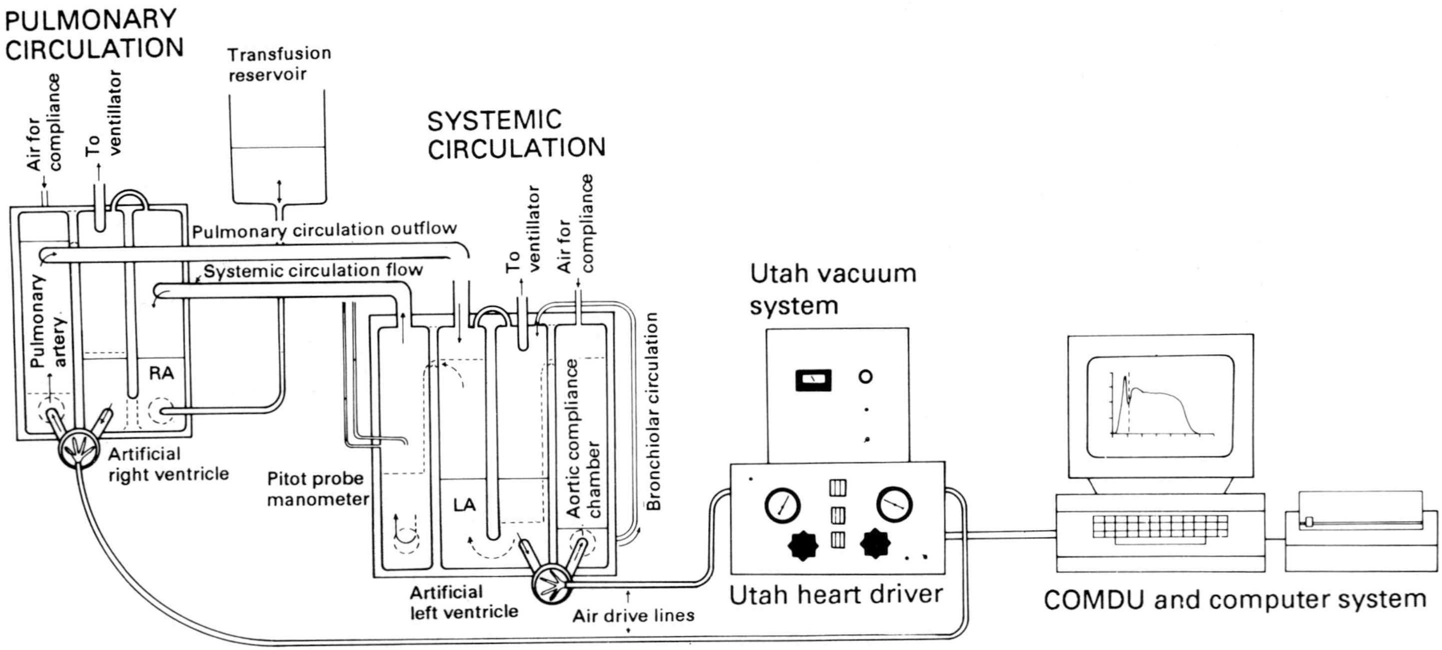

Figure 20.11 The Mock Circulatory System has two series of water cascades to represent the systemic and pulmonary circulations. They provide the typical physiological afterload pressures to the ejecting artificial ventricles. Air chambers in the cascade provide compliance. With its transparent walls, the mock circulatory system vividly displays the flow movement and balance of fluid volume between the lesser (pulmonary) and greater (systemic) circulation. Many of the circumstances that arose with the first human recipient, can be demonstrated with this system. Other pathologic states can also be created for the education of the physicians

The cardiac output in the left side is always later than the right side due to the bronchial circulation which returns to the left side. In calves this may be 3–15% of the stroke volume. In addition the COMDU records as a cardiac output, the amounts that leak through the valves. The loss due to distension is mainly accounted for during the square column before the counting of the displaced volume begins.

The onset of drive pressure (measured at the machine), ventricular pressure and aortic pressure do not start at the same time due to physical delays. The aortic pressure will obviously start much later than the driveline pressure.

When the drive system indicates '33% systole', this means the systolic air inlet valve is open 33% of the cycle, but since it takes some time for the high air pressure to leave the heart, systole may actually be longer and diastole is not 100% – 33% = 67%. To understand this, look at the COMDU tracings (Figure 20.10). A large square column precedes the curve that indicates diastolic filling. The square column represents decompression of the air that was under pressure during systole. Diastole cannot begin before this high pressure air has escaped. It may take 7% of the cycle time, leaving only 60% for diastole.

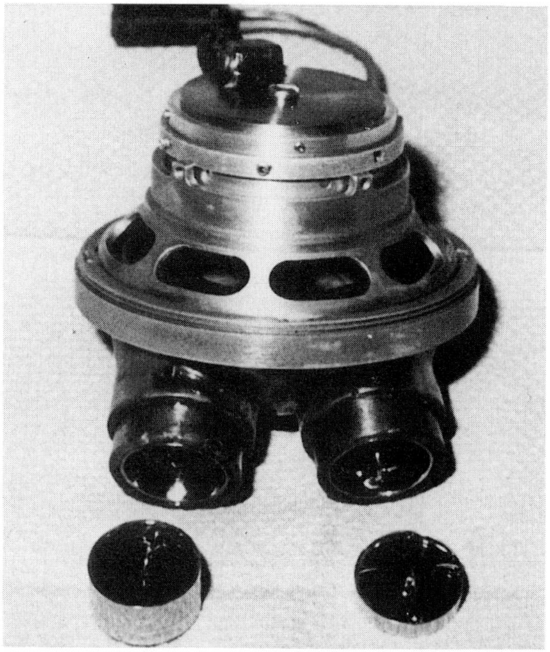

Figure 20.12 A magnetically driven left assist pump developed in 1988 by Dr Stephen G. Kovacs. It is the simplest design available

Drive systems for implantation inside the chest

Electromechanical drive systems

These drive systems are being developed by contracts with the National Institutes of Health (NIH). Some have also been developed for use with LVADs (Portner *et al.*, 1988). Electromechanical devices will be developed, but they will be heavy. The simplest device familiar to us is the magnetically powered device developed by Kovacs (Yarnoz and Kovacs, 1983) (Figure 20.12). He has managed to direct and control the magnetic flux in such a way that a large stroke volume is possible.

Electrohydraulic drive systems

The smallest and lightest system is probably the electrohydraulic system. It uses a small electric motor directly connected to an axial flow pump. This pump can be reversed in 0.012 s, so that the hydraulic fluid is pumped from left to right and right to left (Jarvik, 1981).

One of the problems is that normally the left ventricle displaces more blood than the right for the following two reasons:

1. The bronchial circulation receives its blood from the aorta and returns via the pulmonary veins to the left side of the heart. This can be large; it may amount to 15% of the cardiac output even in patients without congenital heart disease. Sometimes we have observed a bronchial circulation in normal calves of 1–2 l min^{-1}.
2. Since the left side is the highest pressure side, all losses on the left side are more severe than on the right side. Valves leak more on the left side than the right. Distension of the left ventricle is more.

How to cope with the differences? One solution might be to produce a leaking pulmonary valve on the right side. Thus, high cardiac stroke volume on the right side is frustrated by the leak. In case this is not quite adequate, Jack Kolff has proved that a hole in the intra-atrial septum would equilibrate pressures between the two sides. Thereby, increased pressure in the left atrium would be eliminated since the blood will go to the right side through the foramen ovale. It increases the pulmonary circulation without doing any damage (Brownstein, Clancy and Kolff, 1983). In an individual with a natural heart, this might lead to hypertrophy of the right ventricle and finally to its insufficiency. However, this would not be a problem in the mechanical heart.

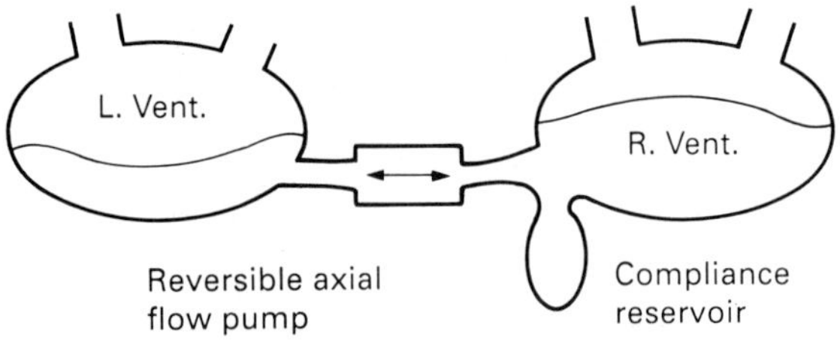

Figure 20.13 A diagram of the electrohydraulic heart. This system has only one moving mechanical part, the axial flow pump directly connected to a motor which is reversed 160 times per minute to propel the hydraulic fluid from left to right and them from right to left. The great simplicity of the electrohydraulic heart is its main advantage, and it can use the ventricles otherwise driven by compressed air with which we have had years of experience. The difference in stroke volume between the left ventricle (which is larger on account of the bronchial circulation) and the right ventricle must be compensated for one way or another. A small compliance sac on the right side is suggested in the diagram

To reduce the cardiac output in the right side of the electrohydraulic heart, W.J. Kolff prefers to provide an extra sac in the hydraulic fluid line that leads to the right ventricle, thereby, some of the hydraulic fluid can be diverted into this hydraulic sac, and the volume of this hydraulic sac can be varied according to the need (Figure 20.13).

The advantage of the Utah-type electrohydraulic heart is that the drive system has only one motor with one axial flow pump, only two bearings and otherwise, no moving parts, no valves, no switching mechanisms, except the reversing of the electric motor. This can be done electronically very safely and very quickly.

Another advantage of this system is that the same type of artificial hearts with which we have years of experience while they were driven with compressed air, can now simply be adapted to the use of a hydraulic fluid. Perhaps an advantage of the hydraulically driven diaphragm is that since there is little difference between the specific gravity of the blood and the specific gravity of the hydraulic fluid, gravity has no influence on the flexing of the diaphragm when the heart's position changes.

Valves for the artificial heart

When the artificial heart is used as a bridge to transplantation, it makes no sense to put in four valves costing between $2000 and $4000 each. Since the average time the artificial heart served as a bridge to transplantation was only 14 days, the FDA decided the durability of these artificial hearts should be 35 days. Our polyurethane tricusp semilunar valves will last much longer.

The Philadelphia-type artificial heart (22)

Since connectors and valve rings have been a major source of thrombosis in patients with artificial hearts and since donor hearts are implanted without connectors, Jack Kolff decided to eliminate all connectors.

Indeed, the Philadelphia-type artificial heart without quick connects, which has a direct connection of the atria to the ventricles and of the aorta and the pulmonary artery to the ventricles, has now been implanted in a number of calves with sufficient results.

There are two types of the Philadelphia heart:

Philadelphia heart, Type 1

Using this type of artificial heart, at the time of surgery, the surgeon can implant the valves of his choice (Figures 20.14 and 20.15). (The first FDA approval will be for the St. Jude Valves only.) Tissue valves could be implanted. They have no shelf life in an artificial heart, but they could be implanted in the operating room and if this is done, the valves would almost certainly by free of thrombosis. The trouble is that the valves are so expensive (Figure 20.16).

Therefore, we have started using polyurethane valves made in our own laboratory. These valves are made either by solution casting or vacuum forming. They are presently being made of Biomer or of Pellethane (2363-75AE) or 2363-80AE (Figure 20.17).

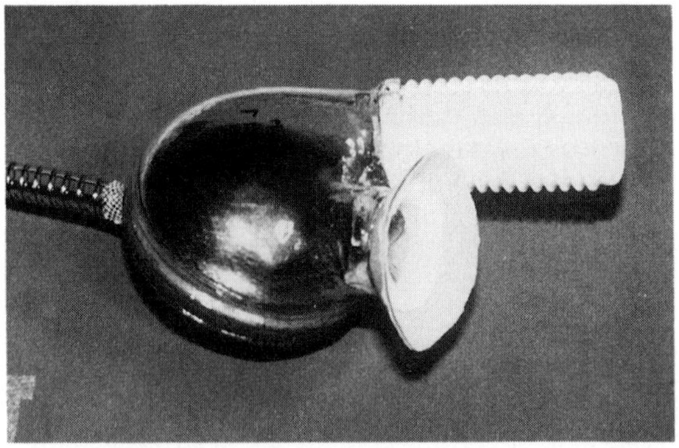

Figure 20.14 The Philadelphia Type-I artificial heart (left ventricle). The quick connects were eliminated to help avoid the occurrence of thromboembolism. In the Philadelphia Type-I model, the aorta and the atrium are directly connected to the ventricle and the surgeon can, on the operating table, sew in the valve of his choice, even if he wants to use a tissue valve. However, the FDA did not approve of this and required Cardiac System to insert the valves before the artificial hearts are delivered

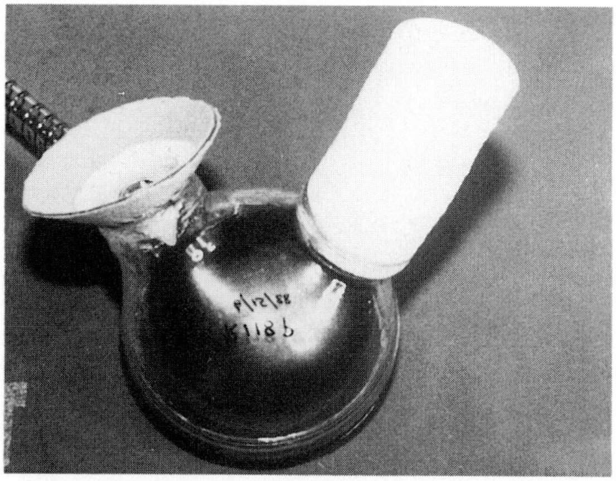

Figure 20.15 The Philadelphia Type-I artificial heart (right ventricle). This photograph shows the artificial heart without quick connects developed by Cardiac Systems and the University of Utah

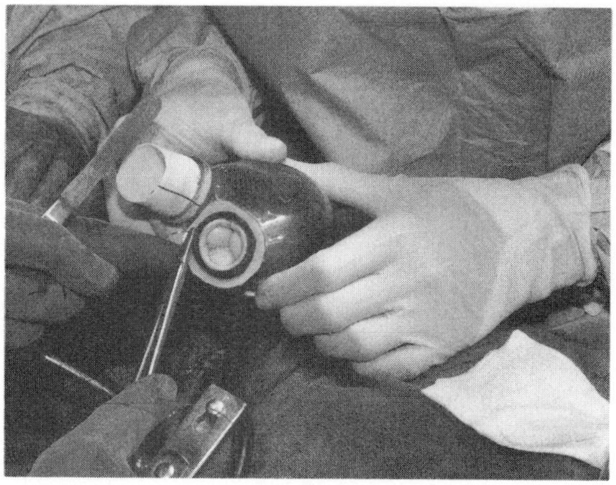

Figure 20.16 A tissue valve, which was in the inflow port of an artificial heart, shown here from the left atrium, 3 days after insertion. It is free of thrombosis. This valve was made by Sorin Biomedica in Italy

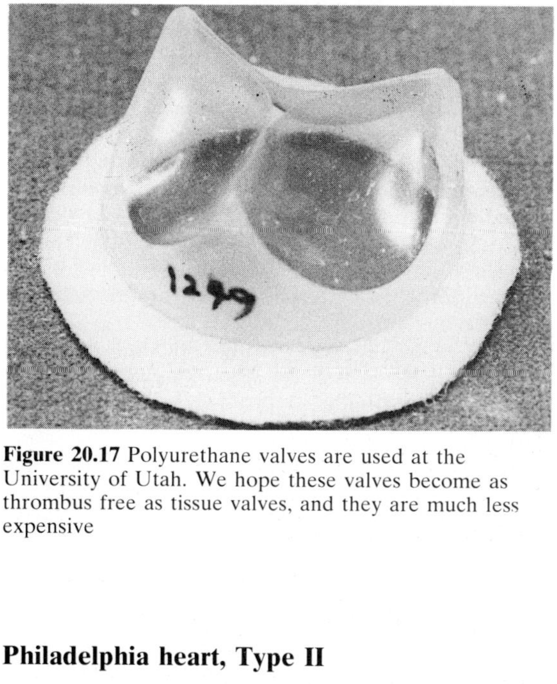

Figure 20.17 Polyurethane valves are used at the University of Utah. We hope these valves become as thrombus free as tissue valves, and they are much less expensive

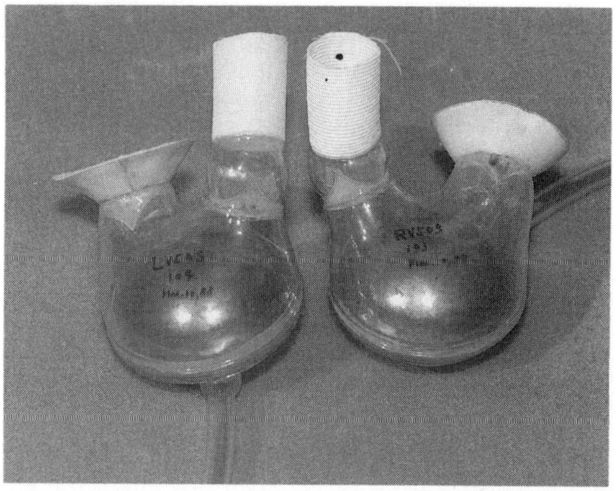

Figure 20.18 The Philadelphia Type-II artificial hearts do not have quick connects either. They contain tricusp semilunar valves which are fixed into the inflow and outflow ports at the factory. Note that these ports are provided with sinus valsalvae. These half circular cavities on the outflow side of each cusp make a revolving blood flow possible to wash the back side of the valve

Philadelphia heart, Type II

The Philadelphia Type II artificial hearts are provided with sinus valsalva in the outflow tract of the ventricles and in the roots of the aorta and the pulmonary artery (Figure 20.18).

The sinus, if properly constructed, helps the washout with blood behind the leaflets. The roots of the aorta and pulmonary artery should be as straight as they are in all mammals.

We now have a series of animals that have had a 50 ml vacuum-formed Philadelphia type artificial heart implanted with our own polyurethane tricusp valves with or without sinus valsalvae. There has been remarkably little thrombosis.

Clamshell artificial heart

It became apparent that if we could give the surgeon a ventricle that would be entirely soft and

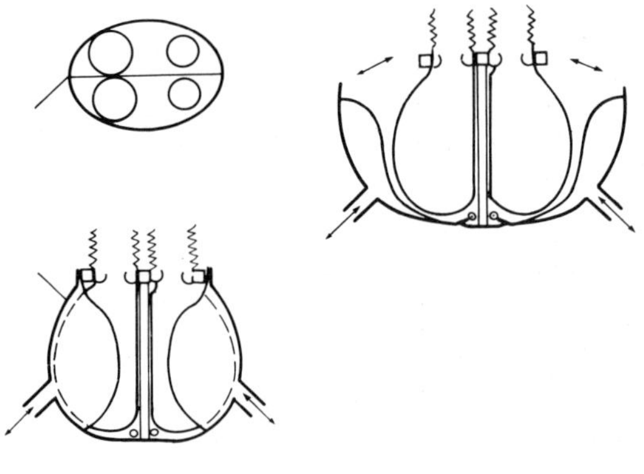

Figure 20.19 A sketch of the clamshell artificial heart. It has a very soft left ventricle connected with its atrium and aorta and can be easily implanted by a surgeon, as can the right ventricle. After implantation, checking of the suture lines and removal of air, both ventricles are enclosed in a clamshell. The driving mechanism (air or mechanical) is also inside the clamshell

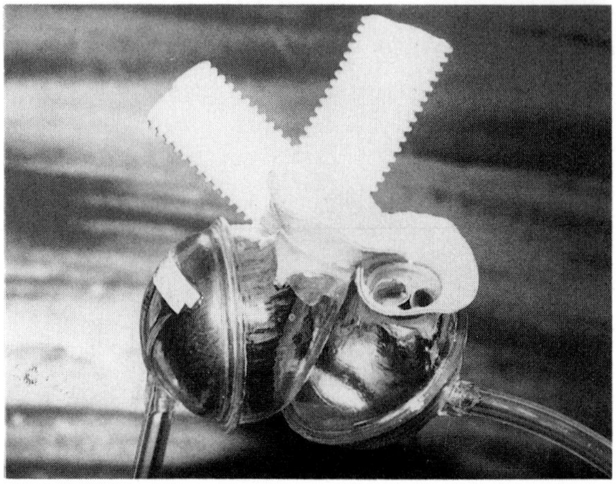

Figure 20.20 The soft heart with a stroke volume of 65 ml has a very soft body and polyurethane valves. At the time of writing, March 1989, we have a calf implanted with this type of artificial heart that has lived for 42 days. Patent applications for the clamshell heart and the soft heart are being submitted

could be rolled or folded up, that the implantation would become very convenient. The left ventricle has the artificial atrium and artificial aorta connected. The right ventricle has a similar arrangement. After the ventricle has been implanted, we have two shells (like a clam) which close over the ventricle. The drive system is in one side of the shell. It can be an air sac like we presently use or it can be mechanical. The first tests with this type of heart are under way (Figure 20.19).

Soft artificial heart

It would be even simpler to make an artificial heart that would be entirely flexible. It will not be as flexible as the blood sac of the clamshell heart, but still very flexible. With the use of the newer polyurethanes and the vacuum forming technique, it is now possible to make very inexpensive artificial hearts with the valves already incorporated in them.

Long Sheng Yu, using a radiofrequency (RF) welding technique, suggested earlier by Dan Bishop, has made such ventricles (Figure 20.20).

In March 1989, we had three calves with artificial heart implantations in the Experimental Heart Research Laboratory at the University of Utah living for up to 35 days with these new soft hearts.

Soft shell hearts can be driven by simple reciprocating piston pumps.

W.J. Kolff has a patent which has almost expired, describing the soft shell mushroom heart (Patent 3,641,591). At the time, we worked with silicone. The advantage of a soft shell heart is that it can be driven by a simple reciprocating pump. You never want to create excessive suction by any artificial ventricle. This cannot happen because as soon as you apply excessive suction, the soft shell of the heart collapses inwards (Figure 20.21).

However, we must be certain that during systole, the heart does not distend. This was accomplished in the heart to be driven by atomic energy by incorporating a Dacron mesh in the thin, flexible silicone (Smith *et al.*, 1975).

The newer polyurethanes are very flexible but distensible only under higher pressure. Dacron support is not needed. All soft, flexible ventricles can be driven either by the conventional drive systems or by simple reciprocating pumps.

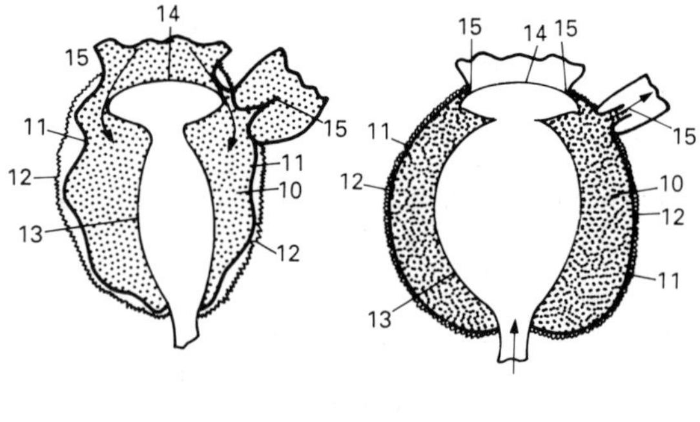

Figure 20.21 Drawing of the mushroom heart. The soft shell mushroom heart had an actively opening and closing inflow valve. During suction, the head of the mushroom collapses much further down than is shown in the picture (patent #3,641,591)

Starling's curves of the soft UVAD 60 show their excellent performance (refer to Figure 20.7).

Silicones

All polyurethanes change with age. Therefore, we have started producing valves and artificial hearts of Silastic.

Silastic HP-100 is said to be 100 times stronger than the old Silastic and has a remarkable resistance to the propagation of a tear. If the silicone is at the inner surface of the ventricles, it should be very blood compatible. There is hope that if it is formed by injection or transfer moulding, that during the flow along a smooth surface, the silica (which is a filler) will remain inside, and the silicone will be at the surface. If not, the surface can be treated by plasma polymerization of either silicone or Teflon.

Complications of artificial hearts

Fortunately there is no problem with immune rejection, which is the main disadvantage of heart transplantation. Although there is no rejection, there seems to be some activation of the complement. This forms the subject of a study being done by Burns at the University of Utah (Burns, Lamb and Olsen, 1989). Multipara women may reject a donor heart if the donor HL-A resembles that of the husband. There is at least one example that showed how the immune bodies decreased while the woman was maintained with an artificial heart.

Poor fit inside the chest

Perhaps the least recognized but most important difficulty for artificial hearts is their poor fit inside the chest.

For an artificial heart, the natural atrium should be left in, and not removed as is done for heart transplantation. A famous heart transplant surgeon removed the atria from a patient to receive an artificial heart. Consequently the patient's chest could not be closed, and it was left open, painted with betadine, and covered with plastic. Even then, the venous return from the left lung became obstructed so that the patient also needed an oxygenator.

The early 'pancake heart' was located against the ribs and left the entire section between the sternum and the vertebral column free for the connection to the blood vessels (Jarvik *et al.*, 1974) (Figure 20.22).

A kink in the pulmonary artery or in the aorta may not be very serious since these are high pressure sides. However, if there is a kink or fold in the atria or vena cava, or if the location of the inflow port is such that the opposite side of the atrium is sucked into the port, there is serious trouble.

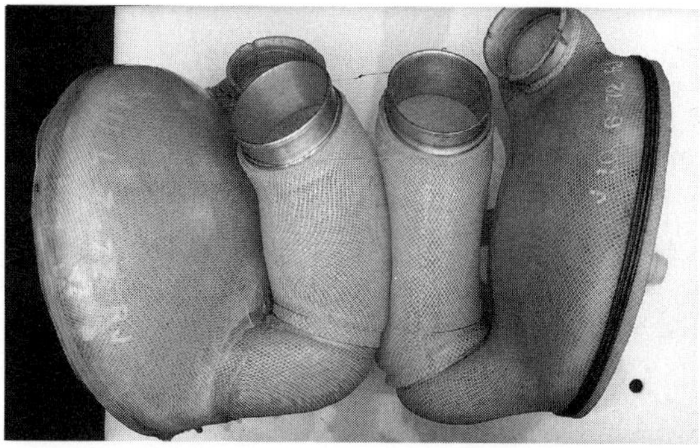

Figure 20.22 The pancake artificial heart has the ventricles against the ribcage and leaves the entire area between the sternum and the vertebral column open for the connections to the atria, the aorta and the pulmonary artery. A calf with this kind of artificial heart did not have the rise in venous pressures that we saw in previous calves. The rise in venous pressure was blamed on an obstruction in the venous return

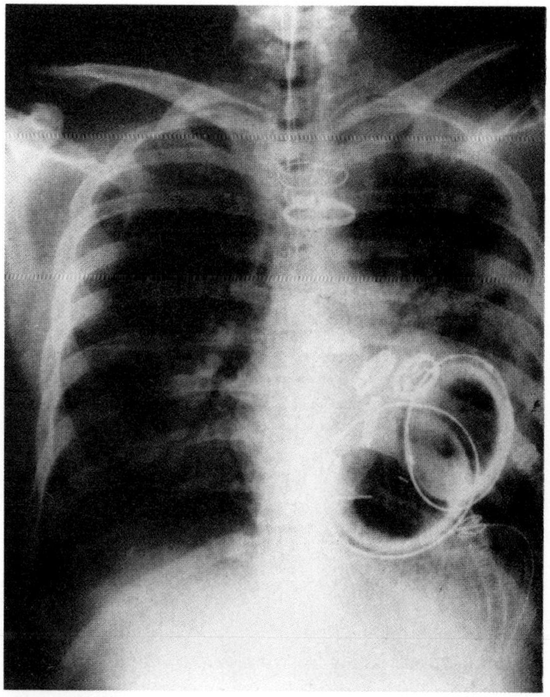

Figure 20.23 Dr Jack Kolff in Philadelphia explored implantation of artificial hearts in brain-dead cadavers. For relatively large artificial hearts, one should move the ventricles either to the left, as is the case here, or to the right. One should not try to put them between the sternum and the vertebral column. This will lead to an obstruction of the venous return

The space between the sternum and vertebral column is small. During experiments of implantations in human, brain-dead cadavers, Jack Kolff, Temple University, Philadelphia, proved that space can be gained by moving either the right ventricle more to the right or the left ventricle more to the left. During the first artificial heart implantation at the University of Utah in Dr Barney Clark, the heart did not fit properly, the pericardium was split and the left ventricle was placed more to the left (Kolff *et al.*, 1984) (Figure 20.23).

It may be remembered that in small patients receiving a larger donor heart the posterior left side of the pericardium can be split to provide more space. The same can be done for an artificial heart.

Presently, we provide the surgeons with a 'dummy' right and left ventricle. The atria, the aorta or the pulmonary artery are attached, but the driveline is not, because the ventricles cannot be fitted easily when the long driveline is attached to it.

Using the 'dummy' heart, the proper location for the heart is determined, then the surgeon can indicate where he wants to make the incision for the drivelines. For the real ventricles, he can then insert the drivelines through the incision and when they are pulled through, the artificial ventricles will fall into proper place.

Most of the surgeons who presently implant artificial hearts clinically, have been trained by Olsen at the University of Utah. Dr Olsen now heads the Institute for Biomedical Engineering, and continues to train surgeons. Kolff's laboratory will make artificial hearts available without cost, if the surgeon to be trained is willing to pay for the expense of the calf and the operation.

Infection

Endocarditis of the valves

Since it is well known that mechanical artificial heart valves are prone to attract endocarditis, it is not surprising that the artificial heart which has four heart valves, is also prone to infection. Wurzel of Cardiac Systems, Inc. was able to show a relation between infection in general and vegetative endocarditis in calves with artificial hearts in an application for an Investigational Device Exemption (IDE) to the FDA in 1988.

Our hope is that the polyurethane valves will be less infected than the mechanical valves, since they are apparently less prone to the formation of thrombosis. This still has to be proven. Riebman *et al.* (1987) and Gristina *et al.* (1988) have pointed out that in many cases, more than one micro-organism is found. Originally this was dismissed as contamination of the sample, but that is probably not so. Gristina also pointed out that specific inserts or elastomers attract specific bacteria.

Infection around the driveline

Infection can occur along the pathway of the drivelines of air-driven artificial hearts by bringing bacteria inside the body. Yet with appropriate skin buttons provided with velour, infection can usually be avoided.

However if infection does occur, it can usually be contained. A better surgical technique with a skin flap that avoids necrosis, was described in a paper by Holmberg *et al.* (1987).

The newest skin button designed by Topaz and a device to pull the driveline through the button are shown in Figure 20.24

Pierce in Hershey, Pennsylvania, has covered his artificial hearts with Dacron velour. Since infection can spread easily along the smooth surface of a ventricle, this is probably a wise move. However, it can be a disadvantage if the surgeon cannot see through the crystal clear ventricular wall to detect and remove air during implantation.

We plan to cover most of our ventricles with velour, but will leave a small area clear which will be located at the highest spot where the air bubbles usually accumulate. We are also working on an artificial heart that has no space between the two ventricles, since that space is where bacteria can flourish.

In calves and other ruminants, neomycin is used before surgery to restrict gas formation in the rumen. Details of antibiotics in postoperative management are given on p.284.

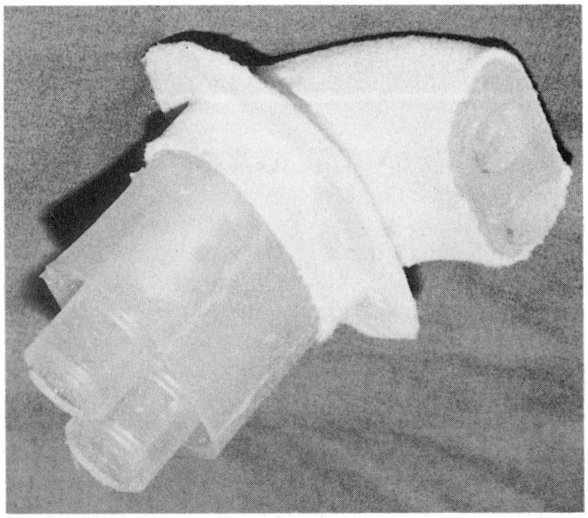

Figure 20.24 Proper skin buttons reduce the risk of infection along the drive lines. A velour-covered flange under the skin allows sealing with connective tissue. A loose outer tube prevents disruption of the skin wound when the tubes move. This is a double skin button made by Steve Topaz at the University of Utah

Transcutaneous energy

In the future, drivelines and percutaneous wires can be avoided. Transmission of energy through the intact skin is possible for artificial hearts with power converters inside. The primary coil is a belt or a cone and a secondary coil picks up the alternating current.

Power source inside the body

The only way in which this can really be obtained would be with an atomically-powered artificial heart.

Indeed, the Atomic Energy Commission, which later became known as the Energy Resource and Development Administration (ERDA), and then later evolved into the Department of Energy, financed the development of artificial hearts driven by atomic power. In 1977, at the University of Utah, a calf survived for 37 days with a prototype of such an artificial heart (Smith *et al.*, 1975).

In this case, the artificial heart was not driven by an atomic hot finger, but by an electric motor (Figure 20.25). Many years later, that record for a mechanically driven heart was broken in the laboratory of Pierce at Hershey, Pennsylvania.

The NIH has continued the development of the Sterling Engine, which is a hot-air engine to power artificial hearts that ultimately should be powered by an atomic hot finger.

These thermal engines have become very small and reliable and can be linked hydraulically or mechanically to the blood sacs that pump the blood. It should ideally power axial flow pumps suspended in the blood stream by magnetic force, for which Olsen has a patent (Figure 20.26) (also see Figure 20.13).

Thrombosis and anticoagulation

During the use of the heart–lung machine, heparinization is used, although it is not started before the operating field is dry. When the connection with the artificial heart is completed, the heparin is neutralized with protamine sulfate. The first 24 h are the most likely that thrombosis will occur. From this point of view, the inside coating of artificial hearts with either heparin or prostaglandin might be advantageous even if it does not last very long (Heyman *et al.*, 1985).

DeFeo and co-workers (1988) showed that there is little difference between the pictures made by the electronic microscope when they look at thrombocytes adhering to the surface at various times after implantation of an artificial heart, which suggests constant formation and removal.

Renal complications

Complications in the form of uraemia are extremely rare in experimental animals (Westenfelder *et al.*, 1985). However, the kidneys of the calf and the sheep write a very reliable history about the occurrence of infarctions. Old and young infarctions can often be seen in the kidneys, and to our great relief, we see them far less in the first animals which have received the Philadelphia-type heart with polyurethane valves. The pre-existing uraemia due to heart failure of the patient is often reversible, and as long as it is not proven otherwise, this should be the assumption.

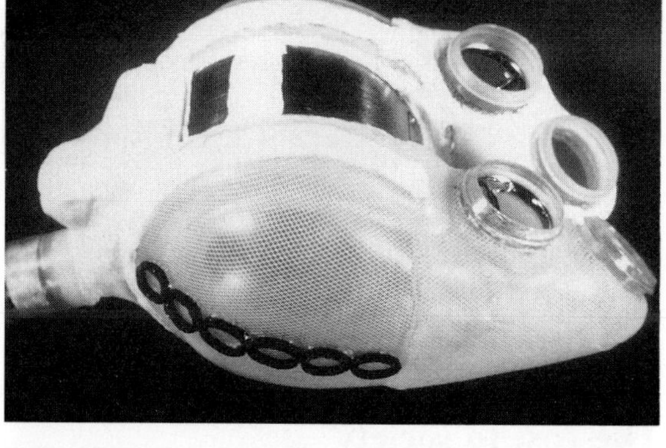

Figure 20.25 A photograph of the ERDA heart, which was the first heart designed to be powered by atomic energy. Driven by an electromotor, it sustained a calf for 37 days. The soft ventricular wall made it respond to Starling's law

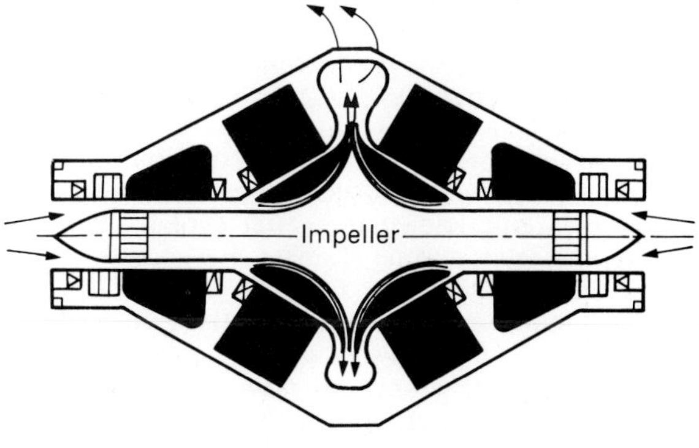

Figure 20.26 A diagram of an axial flow pump, magnetically suspended in the bloodstream, no axles, no bearings. The impeller is provided with permanent magnets that follow the rotation of a magnetic flux induced by solenoids outside

Haematological consequences

It is customary to see the haematocrit of the experimental animal drop severely at first, probably as a consequence of the blood damage done by the heart–lung machine, then to regenerate, but never to regain the normal value. We believe part of the haemolysis is caused by the four mechanical valves used in most artificial hearts, no matter what kind of mechanical valves are tried.

We were very encouraged that the calf Chivas Regal had a gradual increase of his haematocrit during the 62 days of his experiment. Chivas Regal had tricusp semilunar valves.

We do not see demonstrable haemolysis. Free plasma Hb is usually less than 5%.

If we do not see overt signs of coagulopathy, that does not mean that there is none. There is a compensated coagulopathy. The survival time of the thrombocytes appears to be less than normal, but it is compensated. The survival time of red blood cells is also less. White blood cells seem to be impaired, but so little that it is hard to prove. All this should improve with better designs of the hearts, less 'residence time of blood' in the ventricle, (Shettigar *et al.*, 1989), avoidance of shear stress, better valves, and better intima (inside surface of the heart).

We all know that rough intimas give more haemolysis until they are coated with a smooth fibrin surface. Personally, we prefer smooth intimas, and they can always be improved.

Avoid drugs

If the heart is properly implanted and if it functions well, the physician should learn to use a minimum of drugs and adapt the control of the artificial heart to the patient's need. The accumulation of fluid, both in patients and animals with the artificial heart, may be improved by diurectics.

Atrial function

Oedema has been blamed on reduction of the natriuretic hormone produced in the natural atrium, which is lacking immediately after cardiac implantation and later returns (Kablitz, Baranowski and Westenfelder, 1986).

The natural atria are usually left in place, but their blood supply is always severely compromised. The tissue in the atrial wall may regenerate to a certain extent as is evident by the persistence of P wave and even of some atrial contractions.

In the beginning, these atrial contractions are usually very rapid, but later they slow down. It does not seem to be practical to use them as a pacemaker for the artificial heart, as we have tried.

Although this article is about artificial hearts, we may be allowed a remark about LVADs supported by our own experience in animals. We do not believe that the synchronizing of the LVAD with the natural heart beat has a considerable advantage. To the contrary, it may be better to not synchronize it, since the natural heart is allowed to make a decent beat from time to time, and this may prevent atrophy of the muscle.

Future needs

We mentioned in the introduction of this chapter that the artificial heart is presently used only as a bridge to transplantation. In 1988, there were 115 surgical institutes in the United States which were doing heart transplantations. There are 35 000 patients per year who need a replacement of their irreparably sick heart; 2000 donor hearts are all that will be available. It is likely that we will not even reach that number per year. Heterotransplantation of hearts from pigs will not be possible in the near future. Moreover the life of a pig's heart is short because the pig's life is short.

This means that 33 000 patients per year in the United States will either die or will need an artificial heart. No one really wants an artificial heart, but when the time comes to make that choice, the alternative is death.

Since most people do not want to die, the future for the artificial heart seems to be assured, particularly when it can be made more efficiently and less expensively than the present hearts.

A totally implantable artificial heart would be preferable, but since they are not available yet, they offer no help to patients who are going to die shortly. During the time that air-driven artificial hearts are being applied, we can gain important information which can be used in future applications.

As far as the patient's happiness is concerned, we include the photograph of Leif Stenberg taken as he was leaving a restaurant near Stockholm, Sweden. Mr Stenberg was carrying the Heimes Drive System on a strap over his shoulder. None of the waiters or other patrons of the restaurant even noticed that this was a man with an artificial heart. Stenberg sent a telegram to the United States reading, 'I am the happiest man in Europe' (Figure 20.27).

The cost to society

We will not accept the notion that the USA is unwilling to spend money to save its fellow citizens in need. We simply have to redefine our priorities.

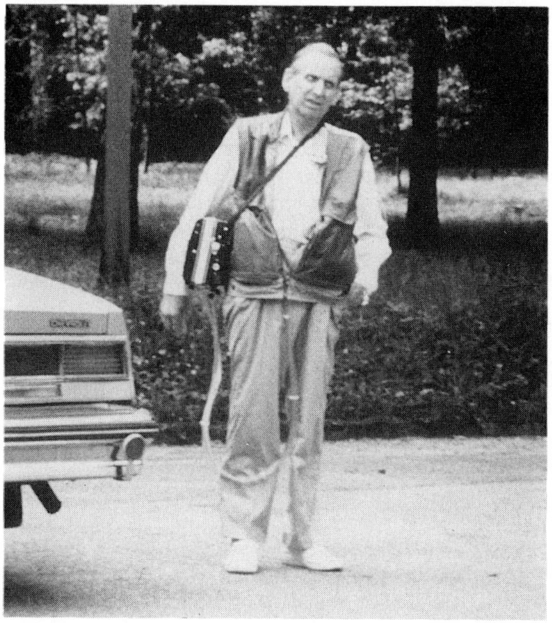

Figure 20.27 Leif Stenberg, wearing the portable drive system which drives his artificial heart, returns from a restaurant where he had just served himself four times from a smorgasbord. He sent a telegram to the United States, stating 'I am the happiest man in Europe!'

The cost of a permanent artificial heart is the same as for a heart transplant operation, approximately $120 000. That cost should be compared with the cost of dying slowly and miserably in an intensive care unit.

We believe that an artificial heart can restore the recipient to a worthwhile and happy existence, even with a portable drive system outside the chest.

Acknowledgements

The artificial heart has been supported in the past by multiple grants from the National Heart, Lung and Blood Institute and by the Development Fund of the Division of Artificial Organs to which contributions have been made by many including: Coronary Heart Disease Research, a programme of the American Health Assistance Foundation, Rockville, Maryland; Beatrice Foods; Burroughs–Wellcome Fund; Digital Equipment Corp.; General Instruments Corp.; Mr Ernest W. Hahn; Mr Lawrence Harvey; Mrs Iris Margolis; Mr Ben Matthews; Albert Penick Fund; Lionel I. Pincus Foundation, Inc.; Square D Foundation; Mr Wallace Rasmussen; Rothschild Fund; Mr Charles E. Spahr; The Stichting Alfred Heineken Funds, etc.

References

Brownstein, L., Clancy, M. and Kolff, J. (1983) Operation of cardiopulmonary bypass versus an intracorporeal total artificial heart. *Transactions of American Society for Artificial Internal Organs*, **29**, 110–115

Burns, G.L., Lamb, J. and Olsen, D. (1989) Immune response to blood pump use in calves. *Abstracts for American Society for Artificial Internal Organs*, **18**, 11

DeFeo, P.A., Wurzel, D., Wildevuur, W., *et al.* (1988) Deposition of blood elements on vacuum-formed ventricles in calves. *Transactions of the American Society for Artificial Internal Organs*, **34**, 550–556

DeVries, W.C. (1988a) The permanent artificial heart: four case reports. *Journal of American Medical Association*, **259**, 849–859

DeVries, W.C. (1988b) Surgical technique for implantation of the Jarvik-7-100 total artificial heart. *Journal of American Medical Association*, **259**, 875–889

Gristina, A.G., Dobbins, J.J., Giammara, B., *et al.* (1988) Biomaterial-centered sepsis and the total artificial heart. *Journal of American Medical Association*, **259**, 870–874

Heimes, H.P. and Klasen, F. (1982) Completely integrated wearable TAH-drive unit. *Journal of Artificial Organs*, **5**, 157–159

Heyman, P.W., Cho, C.S., McRea, J.C., *et al.* (1985) Heparinized polyurethanes: in vitro and in vivo studies. *Journal of Biomedical Materials Research*, **19**, 419–436

Holmberg, D.L., Dew, P., Crump, C., *et al.* (1987) Percutaneous access devices in calves receiving an artificial heart. *Journal of Artificial Organs*, **12**, 34–39

Jarvik, R.K. (1981) The total artificial heart. *Scientific American*, **244**, 74–80

Jarvik, R., Volder, J., Olsen, D., *et al.* (1974) Venous return of an artificial heart designed to prevent right heart syndrome. *Annals of Biomedical Engineering*, **2**, 335–342

Joyce, L.D., DeVries, W.C., Hastings, W.L., *et al.* (1983) Response of the human body to the first permanent implant of the Jarvik-7 total artificial heart. *Transactions of the American Society for Artificial Internal Organs*, **29**, 81–87

Kablitz, D., Baranowski, R.L. and Westenfelder, C. (1986) Atrial natriuretic peptide levels in a patient prior to and following implantation of an artificial heart. *Kidney International*, **29**, 192A

Kless, H., Blumenthal, N.V., Mohnhaupt, R., *et al.* (1974) Extracorporeal measurement of haemodynamic parameters of the artificial heart. *Proceedings of the European Society of Artificial Organs*, **1**, 166–169

Kolff, W.J. (1988) Tenth Hastings Lecture: experiences and practical considerations for the future of artificial hearts and of mankind. *Journal of Artificial Organs*, **12**, 89–111

Kolff, W.J., DeVries, W.C., Joyce, L.D., *et al.* (1984) Lessons learned from Dr Barney Clark, the first patient with an artificial heart. *Progress in Artificial Organs–1983*. International Society Artificial Organs, ISAO Press No. 204, Cleveland, Vol. **2**, 165–174

Kolff, J., Deeb, G.M., Cavarocchi, N.C., *et al.* (1984) The artificial heart in human subjects. *Journal of Thoracic and Cardiovascular Surgery*, **87**, 825–831

Kwan-Gett, C., Backman, D.K., Donovan, F.M., *et al.* (1971) Artificial heart with hemispherical ventricles II and disseminated intravascular coagulation. *Transactions of the American Society for Artificial Internal Organs*, **17**, 474–481

Levinson, M.M., Smith, R.G., Cork, R.C., *et al.* (1986) Thromboembolic complications of the Jarvik-7 artificial heart: case report. *Journal of Artificial Organs*, **10**, 236–244

Losman, J.G., Replogle, R.L. and Kolff, W.J. (1982) An alternative to the orthotopic artificial heart: a point of view. *Journal of Artificial Organs*, **6**, 319–324

Magovern, J.A., Rosenberg, G. and Pierce, W.S. (1986) Development and current status of a total artificial heart. *Journal of Artificial Organs*, **10**, 357–363

Norton, S.H., Akutsu, T. and Kolff, W.J. (1962) Artificial heart with antivacuum bellows. *Transactions of the American Society for Artificial Internal Organs*, **8**, 131–134

Pantalos, G.M. and Kolff, W.J. (1984) An improved mock circulation for total artificial heart instruction and performance analysis. *VIth International Conference and Workshop on Cardiovascular System Dynamics Society*, University of Pennsylvania.

Portner, P.M., Jassawalla, J.S., Oyer, P.E., *et al.* (1988) A totally implantable ventricular assist system for terminal heart failure. *American Society for Internal Organs Primers*, **3**, Ch. VII, 57–76

Riebman, J.M., Liotta, D., Cabrol, C., *et al.* (1986) Orthotopic univentricular artificial heart. *Life Support Systems, The Journal of the European Society of Artificial Organs*, **4**, (**Suppl 2**), 47–49

Riebman, J.B., Liotta, D., Navia, J.A., *et al.* (1987) Orthotopic univentricular artificial heart. In *Artificial Organs: Proceedings of the International Symposium on Artificial Organs, Biomedical Engineering and Transplantation* (eds J.D. Andrade, J.J. Brophy, D.E. Detmer *et al.*), VCH Publishers, Inc., New York, pp. 73–81

Shettigar, U.R., Dropmann, M., Christian, P. and Kolff, W.J. (1989) Residence time distributions in artificial ventricles. *Abstract for American Society for Artificial Internal Organs*, **14**

Smith, L., Sandquist, G., Olsen, D.B., *et al.* (1975) Power requirements for the A.E.C. artificial heart. *Transactions of the American Society for Artificial Internal Organs*, **21**, 540–543

Swier, P., Mohammad, S.F., Olsen, D.B. and Kolff, W.J. (1989) Comparison of antiplatelets effect of aspirin on human and bovine platelets. *Abstracts for American Society for Artificial Internal Organs*, **18**, 74

Westenfelder, C., Englard, T., Holmberg, D.L., *et al.* (1985) Renal function in calves with total artificial hearts. *Transactions of the American Society for Artificial Internal Organs*, **31**, 383–387

Whalen, R.L. and Briskman, R.N. (1988) An electromagnetic pneumatic blood pump driver. *Transactions of American Society for Artificial Internal Organs*, **34**, 721–725

Willshaw, P., Nielsen, S.D., Nanas, J., *et al.* (1984) A cardiac output monitor and diagnostic unit (COMDU) for pneumatically driven artificial hearts. *Journal of Artificial Organs*, **8**, 215–219

Wurzel, D., Kolff, J., Missfeldt, W., *et al.* (1988) Development of the Philadelphia heart system. *Journal of Artificial Organs*, **12**, 410–422

Yarnoz, M.D. and Kovacs, S.G. (1983) Magnetically actuated LVAD. *Transactions of the American Society for Artificial Internal Organs*, **29**, 574–579

21

Heart and heart–lung transplantation

G. Fradet, J.P. Scott, T.R. Graham, R.L. Smyth, E. Solis and J. Wallwork

Since Christian Barnard's impressive clinical experiment (Barnard, 1967), now over 20 years ago, cardiac transplantation has become an accepted form of treatment for many patients with end-stage cardiac failure. Much of this expansion has taken place since 1980 following the pioneering work of Shumway in Stanford (Shumway and Lower, 1964; Shumway, Dong and Stinson, 1969; Stinson *et al.*, 1970; Stinson *et al.*, 1972; Watson *et al.*, 1979). The demand for cardiac transplantation world-wide has increased rapidly as results have shown it to be an effective form of therapy. Improved survival has been largely, although not exclusively, due to the impact of the introduction of cyclosporin A into immunosuppressive regimes. There are now about 150 centres in the United States and more than 50 in Europe. The world-wide activity for heart transplantation as recorded in the International Society for Heart Transplantation Register is shown in Figure 21.1. Combined heart and lung transplantation is, by contrast, still in its developmental period, but over the last 5 years there has been a rapid increase in the number of heart–lung transplants performed (Figure 21.2).

In this chapter we will outline the current experience of heart and heart–lung transplantation with special emphasis on perioperative management and results as illustrated by the activities of the transplant programme at Papworth Hospital. Beginning in 1979, there has been a steady increase in the number of transplantations performed annually, the heart–lung transplant programme being initiated in 1984 (Figure 21.3). The number of heart transplantations had reached a plateau in 1987 and the continued increase in the total number of transplants performed is largely due to the heart–lung transplantation programme activities. The planned performance of 100 transplants for the year 1988

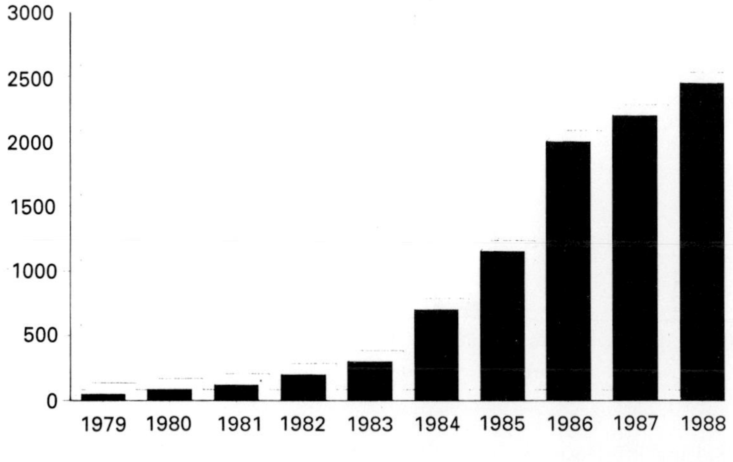

Figure 21.1 Number of heart transplants: registry of the International Society for Heart Transplantation

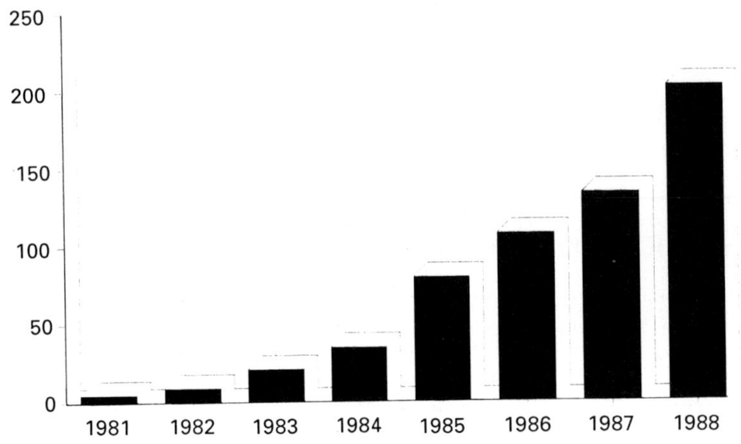

Figure 21.2 Number of heart–lung transplants: registry of the International Society for Heart Transplantation

was not fulfilled due to limitations of suitable donor organs. As transplantation becomes more successful, both for heart and heart–lung recipients, the demands on the service outgrow our ability to provide for them and approximately 20–25% of patients can be expected to die while on the waiting list. This stresses the importance of careful selection of potential recipients for heart and heart–lung transplantation in order to make the best use of the available but limited resources.

As the long-term survival of transplanted adult patients improved, heart and heart–lung transplantation for the paediatric population became a more attractive proposition. As a result, we have now begun to expand transplantation into the paediatric field in association with the Hospital for Sick Children at Great Ormond Street. A total of 12 paediatric heart (n = 4) and heart–lung (n = 8) transplants have now been performed from 1988 to July 1989.

Heart transplantation

Patients

Between November 1977 and June 1989, 1169 patients have been referred for transplantation. Of these, 680 have been assessed in hospital as being potentially suitable candidates and 516 were accepted for transplantation. A subgroup of patients (40) were offered conventional cardiac surgery for whom various procedures were performed, and of those assessed for transplanta-

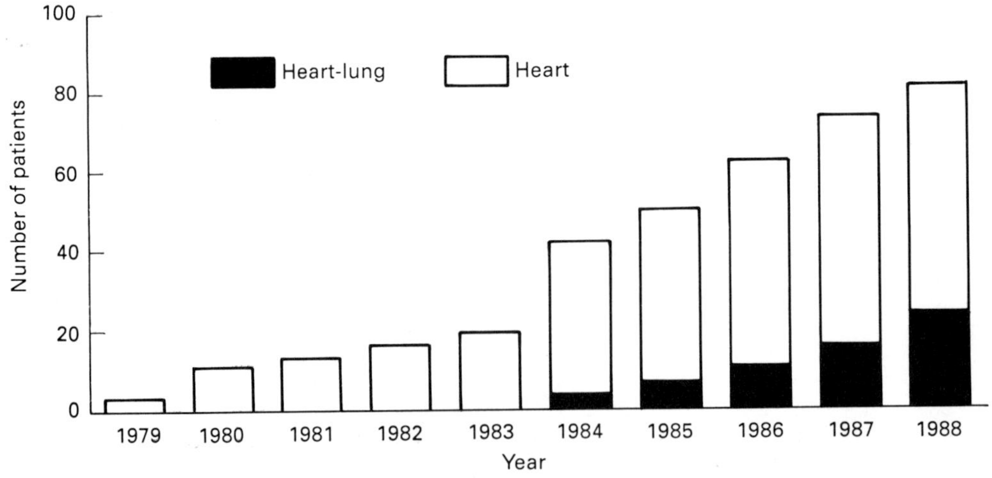

Figure 21.3 Transplant operations 1978–1988: Papworth Hospital

Table 21.1 Cardiac transplantation: recipient selection

Indications	*Contraindications*
Terminal disease (prognosis 6–12 months)	Infection
Age: 6–65 years	Malignancy
Positive attitude	Raised pulmonary vascular resistance (PVR) (>7 woods units)
Good family support	Recent pulmonary infarction
	Primary renal failure
	Primary hepatic failure
	Extensive vascular disease
	Active peptic ulceration

Table 21.2 Cardiac transplantation: patients accepted, description

	Transplanted	*Died waiting*
Patients	331	116
Mean age (range)	43(6–63)	43(15–63)
Diagnosis		
Ischaemic heart disease	176	69
Cardiomyopathy	144	39
Other	11	8
Waiting period mean (days)	110	52

Table 21.3 Multi-organ retrieval

Donor organ	
Heart	341
Heart and lung	66
Kidney	789
Cornea	206
Liver	181
Pancreas	29
Lung	3

tion , 113 were rejected for not meeting the criteria for acceptance.

As with all centres, these criteria have been liberalized as results improved. In particular, age limits have been relaxed so that patients are now accepted with an upper age limit of approximately 65 years. Many of the patients in their sixth decade have terminal cardiac failure as a result of severe coronary artery disease and this is now the single largest indication for heart transplantation. Patients with primary cardiomyopathy are the next largest group. Our actual criteria of acceptance are represented in Table 21.1. Of the 516 patients accepted for transplantation, 331 were transplanted. All received an orthotopic heart. Nine patients have undergone 10 retransplants, one patient having been retransplanted after 3 years for coronary occlusive disease and again after another 3 years for the same condition. The age, diagnosis and mean waiting time before transplantation of the 331 transplanted patients are shown in Table 21.2.

The donor

The principle factor limiting cardiac transplant activity remains the supply of donor organs, and although access to suitable donor organs is increasing, the demand for cardiac transplantation is even greater. For this reason we have not felt it appropriate to accept patients from abroad for transplantation. Criteria for donor selection have also been relaxed as a result of demand and donors up to the age of 45 will be considered for heart transplantation. Over 50% of the donors in the UK are multiorgan donors and the other organ usage for donors for heart and heart–lung transplantation is shown in Table 21.3. There is much current research directed towards better donor care. The recognition that major hormonal imbalances may occur along with massive fluid shifts following brain death is leading towards improved donor management and the prospects of salvaging more hearts for transplantation.

Nevertheless, despite improvements in preservation techniques over the years, for practical purposes, the upper limit for the ischaemic time of the heart is still only 4 h; early survival of patients receiving hearts with greater than 4 h ischaemic time is less good.

Some hearts are now becoming available for transplantation from patients receiving heart–lung transplantation, the so-called 'domino' procedure. This both increases the general organ pool and negates any criticism that heart–lung transplantation is denying patient access to the more established technique of heart transplantation. We have now performed two domino heart transplants and retrieved five hearts for similar procedures at other centres from our heart–lung recipients. This technique, originally described by the Harefield Group (Yacoub *et al.*, 1988), was introduced at our institution in early 1989.

Postoperative management and immunosuppression

The cardiac transplant operation itself has changed little in the last decade and what used to be a service provided exclusively by consultants is now well within the capability of a trained senior registrar or chief resident. The procedure is well described elsewhere (Cabrol *et al.*, 1989). Postoperative management has been simplified and the need for barrier nursing in intensive care curtailed. At the beginning of the programme, 10 years ago, patients were expected to be barrier nursed in the intensive care unit for some 4 weeks; this has now been reduced to 3 days. The majority of patients are able to leave hospital for intermediate care in about 2–3 weeks following cardiac transplantation.

Table 21.4 Cardiac transplantation: immunosuppression protocols (summary)

Patients (n)	*Protocol*
1–29	Azathioprine and steroids
30–89	Cyclosporin A and low dose steroids
90–150	Cyclosporin A and steroids or Cyclosporin A and azathioprine
151+	Triple therapy (Table 21.5)

Table 21.5 Cardiac transplantation: current immunosuppression protocol

Steroids
- Methylprednisolone 500 mg i.v. on induction
- Methylprednisolone 500 mg i.v. at reperfusion
- Methylprednisolone 125 mg i.v. at 8/16/24 h post CPB
- Prednisolone 1 mg kg^{-1} day^{-1} down to 0.2 mg kg^{-1} day^{-1} p.o. (decreasing 5 mg day^{-1})

RATG-Merieux (POD 0,1,2)
- 0.5–1.5 mg kg^{-1} i.v. infusion over 10 h started on CPB
- Day 1,2:dose adjusted to T cells (<10%, <100 per mm^2)

Cyclosporin
- Introduced on POD 1 and gradually increased up to 10 mg kg^{-1} day^{-1} in two doses, adjusted to renal function (creatinine <200 μm/l) and whole blood trough level (wbt) (200–500 ng ml^{-1})

Azathioprine
- 2–3 mg kg^{-1} i.v./p.o. pre-op
- 2 mg kg^{-1} p.o. daily post-op (WBC>5000 cells ml^{-1})

CPB Cardiopulmonary bypass
RATG Rabbit anti-thymocytic globulin
POD Postoperative day

There have been 4 distinct immunosuppressive protocols for cardiac transplantation since the programme began and these are shown in Table 21.4. The results have improved with each successive protocol and the current expected 1 year survival is 85% (Figure 21.4). Most cardiac transplant centres are adopting a protocol of triple therapy in an attempt to ameliorate the nephrotoxic effects of cyclosporin A. All these protocols have included a prophylactic course of anti-thymoctic globulin (ATG), originally for 28 days but now for only 3 days. Our actual immunosuppression protocol is summarized in Table 21.5.

Rejection

The detection of rejection following cardiac transplantation relies on the histological appearances of endomyocardial biopsies. This technique introduced by Caves in 1973 (Caves, 1974) has not been superseded by any reliable non-invasive methods. The use of echocardiography, sophisticated ECG measurements and cytoimmunological monitoring have all been used as adjuncts, but biopsies performed at decreasing frequency following transplantation remain the gold standard for the detection of rejection. Episodes of moderate or more severe rejection at biopsy are treated with pulse doses of steroids.

Infection

Infection episodes are a common feature of the postoperative care of the immunosuppressed host. The transplanted patient is particularly susceptible to usual nosocomial pathogens in the initial perioperative period where easy access is provided through the different angio access lines, ventilation system and drainage catheters. It is for this reason that we feel it is of the utmost importance to

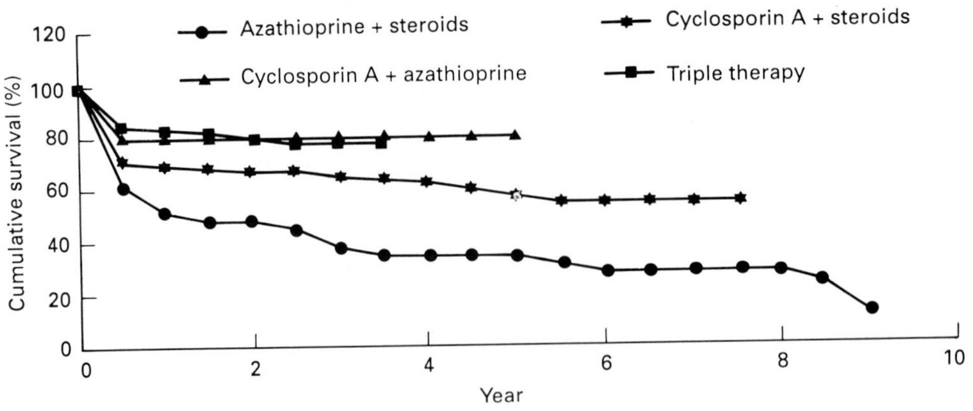

Figure 21.4 Heart transplant patient survival by immunosuppression protocol

encourage early extubation and mobilization. We also give prophylactic antibiotherapy consisting of flucloxacillin or erythromycin if penicillin allergy, and a third generation cephalosporin. This prophylaxis is continued until the lines and catheters are removed, usually on the second or third postoperative day, at which time the patient is transferred to the ward.

Opportunistic infections are rare in the early postoperative period, but more frequent after the first postoperative month and a variety of opportunistic pathogens can be involved (McGiffin *et al.*, 1989). In our initial experience, we have encountered a number of *Pneumocystis carinii* pneumonia (PCP) with its associated morbidity and mortality in one case. Since then, we have been giving cotrimoxazole (480 mg twice daily) prophylaxis to patients receiving steroids (usually first 3 months). This protocol has proven to be successful.

Of interest also within the first 6 months after transplantation are infections acquired from the donor organs (cytomegalovirus and *Toxoplasma*) and viral reactivations (*Herpes simplex* virus (HSV) and cytomegalovirus (CMV)). We do give prophylaxis for *Toxoplasma* recipient–donor mismatch (pyrimethamine 25 mg daily along with folinic acid 15 mg three times a day for 6 weeks). Because of the increased morbidity and mortality associated with cytomegalovirus infection, we now avoid mismatch by prospectively matching recipient and donor before surgery. After the initial 6 months post-transplantation, the incidence of infection decreases, but patients remain at risk, this being particularly true when their immunosuppression is increased during rejection episodes.

Results

The overall survival for heart transplantation in our series is shown in Figure 21.5. Since the introduction of cyclosporin A, survival has improved as shown in Figure 21.6. As previously seen in Figure

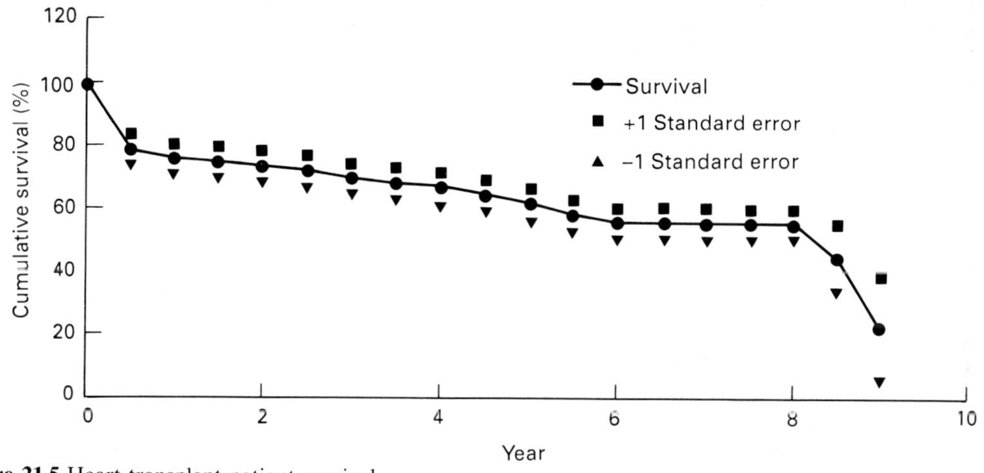

Figure 21.5 Heart transplant patient survival

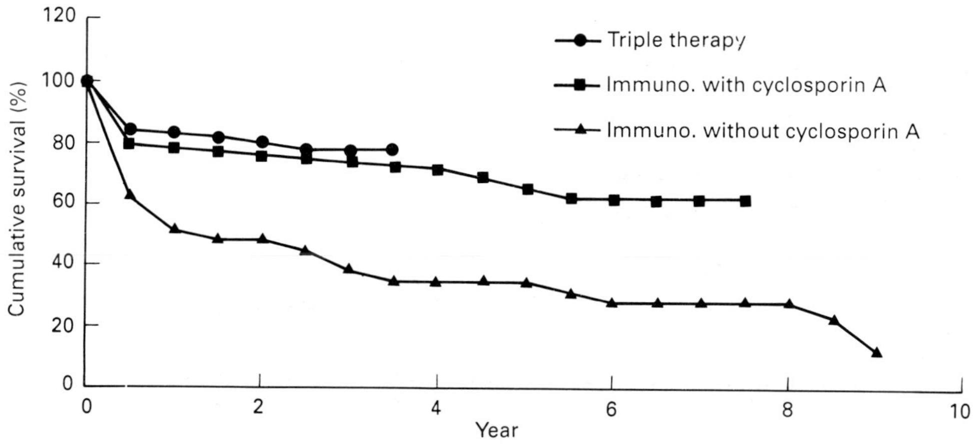

Figure 21.6 Heart transplant patient survival by immunosuppression therapy

Table 21.6 Cardiac transplantation: causes of death

	0–90 Days	*90 Days–1 year*	*>1 Year*
Rejection	25	9	–
Infection	17	5	3
Coronary occlusive disease	–	1	16
Donor heart failure	5	–	–
Multifactorial	4	–	–
Lymphoma	1	–	1
Non-lymphoma	–	–	3
Cerebrovascular	4	1	–
Raised PVR	3	–	–
Intestinal infarct	2	–	–
Operative haemorrhage	1	–	–
Total	62	16	23

21.4, subgroups of patients treated with different cyclosporin A based regimes have shown an incremental improvement in survival with each regime.

The causes of death are shown in Table 21.6. As might be anticipated, rejection and infection have been the principal causes of death during the first 3 months; indeed, it is during this period that most of the deaths occur. Both remain important causes of mortality during the remainder of the first year, but thereafter, accelerated coronary occlusive disease in the allografted heart becomes the most important determinant of survival. It is the incidence of this disease which will determine the long-term outlook for cardiac transplantation. Analysis of angiograms performed on an annual basis following transplantation showed that the prevalence of significant angiographic coronary disease was 18% at 2 years and 25% at 5 years. Progressive coronary occlusion may be an indication for retransplantation in appropriate patients. The aetiology of this condition is complex, but undoubtedly immunologically based; the incidence, time of onset, severity and rate of progress are variable and unpredictable.

Heart–lung transplantation

Transplantation of the heart and lungs is progressing rapidly through its developmental phase, following the first successful operation in 1981 (Reitz *et al.*, 1982). Since then there have been developments in distant procurement using both a simple pulmonary artery flush technique (Hakim *et al.*, 1988) or cardiopulmonary bypass (Yacoub *et al.*, 1989). In the last 2 years the development of an early, precise histological diagnosis of rejection using transbronchial biopsies has enabled patients to be better managed and has contributed to good survival.

Patients

There are three main groups of diseases for which heart–lung transplantation is appropriate:

1. Parenchymal lung disease, with or without secondary cardiac disease
2. Primary cardiac disease associated with pulmonary hypertension (Eisenmenger's syndrome)
3. Pulmonary vascular disease

The criteria for patient acceptability have changed over the years, for instance patients with cystic fibrosis are now accepted as candidates for heart–lung transplantation and may well form the single largest group of patients suitable for this surgery. The demand for heart–lung transplantation is large and increasing and thus recipients are selected carefully; moribund patients, or patients with pulmonary aspergillosis or multi-system disease are not considered to be suitable candidates. In addition, because of the scarcity of suitable donor organs, emergency heart–lung transplantation is normally not available.

Since November 1982, 581 patients have been referred for heart–lung transplantation. Of these 228 patients were admitted for a period of assessment and 150 were accepted as potential recipients. The demographic data and diagnoses of the 66 patients who have been given transplants are shown in Table 21.7; in one of these cases a liver was trans-

Table 21.7 Heart–lung transplantation: population (April 1984–June 1989)

Patients transplanted		66
Age	Mean	30
	Range	11–53
Sex	Male	32
	Female	34
Diagnosis		
Eisenmenger syndrome		18
Cystic fibrosis		16
Primary pulmonary hypertension		7
Thromboembolic pulmonary hypertension		2
Emphysema		4
Sarcoidosis		3
Fibrosing alveolitis		3
Histiocytosis X		2
Bronchiectasis		3
Alpha 1 antitrypsin deficiency		3
Pulmonary fibrosis		1
Systemic lupus erythematosus + pulmonary hypertension		1
Cardiomyopathy + pulmonary hypertension		1
Pulmonary artery sarcoma		1
Primary biliary cirrhosis + pulmonary hypertension		1
Survival	alive	44

Table 21.8 Heart–lung transplantation: donor criteria

Age ideally <40 years
ABO compatibility
Normal gas exchange
Good pulmonary compliance
Low ventilation pressures
Clear chest X-ray
No infections
Short ventilation period
Appropriate size matching donor/recipient
CMV serology compatibility

planted simultaneously. Of the accepted patients, 25% have died awaiting a suitable organ. The upper age limit for acceptability for heart–lung transplantation has been arbitrarily set at 50, but even with this age limit, the waiting list continues to lengthen.

Donors

Donors for heart–lung transplantation are even less available than donors for heart transplantation. Probably some 15–20% of donors who would be suitable for heart transplantation would be suitable for heart–lung transplantation. The donor criteria for heart and lung donation are shown in Table 21.8. Rapid deterioration of the lungs can result from inadequate monitoring of the donor and great care needs to be taken to avoid oedematous organs. The quality of the donor lungs is extremely important in determining the ease of care in the immediate postoperative period and subsequently the patient's chances of survival.

The sizes of the donor and recipient are matched according to the total lung capacity of the recipient, measured at the time of assessment, and predicted values for the donor, based largely on the donor's height (Otulana *et al.*, 1989). The final comparison of chest X-rays is made at the donor hospital. A latex agglutination test for CMV is now used prospectively at the donor hospital to avoid primary CMV infection in the CMV negative recipient by transplanting organs from a CMV positive donor. As primary CMV disease has been a major determinant of death in the early postoperative period, we regard this as an important aspect of donor selection.

Until 1985 all donors for heart–lung transplantation were transported to the recipient hospital. Since that date all donors in the UK have been obtained by long distance procurement. We have used a single flush technique (Wallwork *et al.*, 1987), but others (Yacoub *et al.*, 1989) have used cardiopulmonary bypass and total body cooling for the donor. Using a single flush technique of extra cellular fluid combined with perioperative prostacyclin infusion, donor organ preservation has been satisfactory for up to 4 h of ischaemia time. There have been no primary organ failures and early lung function has been poor in only two patients who received transplants from donors with oedematous lungs.

Postoperative management and immunosuppression

The operative technique for heart–lung transplantation has been well described and although this

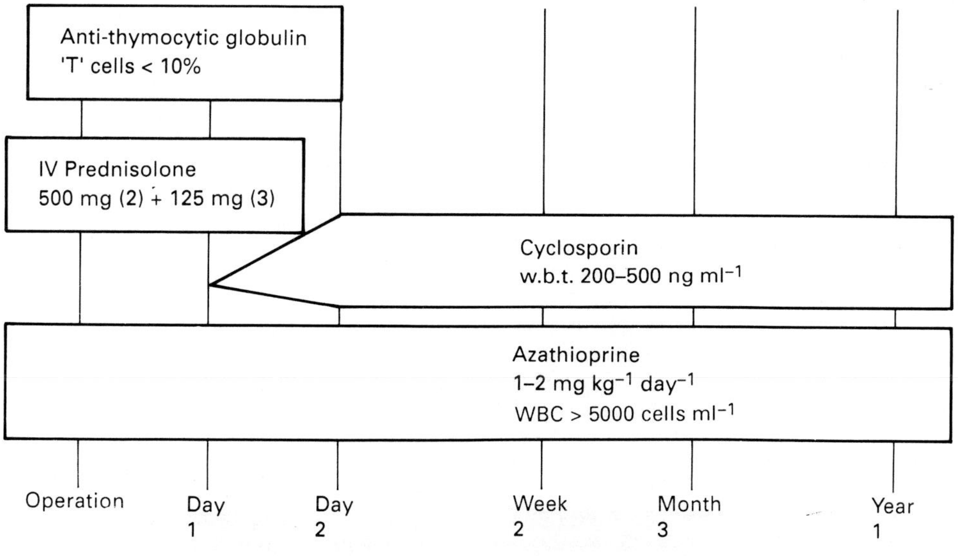

Figure 21.7 Immunosuppression protocol for heart–lung transplantation

procedure is not yet as standard as heart transplantation and by its very nature more complex, the necessary stages of surgery are well worked out (Jamieson and Kaye, 1989).

The majority of patients are extubated within 24 h following transplantation and a regime similar to that described for heart transplantation is followed. The patients are barrier nursed in the intensive care unit for 3 days and are often transferred to the ward before the end of the first week where they will stay until their discharge at 3–4 weeks. Immunosuppression for heart–lung transplantation is based on cyclosporin A and azathioprine with steroids being reserved for rejection episodes. In addition, perioperative methylprednisolone and a short 3 day course of rabbit ATG is given (Figure 21.7).

Diagnosis of rejection

When clinical heart–lung transplantation began there was no reliable or accurate method of detecting lung rejection. This is no longer the case due to developments at Papworth Hospital. Rejection is now diagnosed by biopsies (Higenbottam *et al.*, 1987): the indications for biopsy include new clinical symptoms and signs, alterations in chest X-ray or lung function changes (fall in FEV1 (forced expiratory volume in one second) >10% on 3 occasions over a 24 h period). Transbronchial biopsies are also of use in distinguishing infection from rejection and in defining their coexistence. The routine use of endomyocardial biopsy has been shown to be of no value in the detection of rejection in heart–lung transplantation (Cooper *et al.*, 1986; McGregor *et al.*, 1985). It is likely that lung biopsy will be established as the gold standard against which less invasive methods of detecting rejection can be compared as they develop.

Infection

Most considerations of infection addressed in the previous section on heart transplantation remain pertinent for the heart–lung transplant patients. However, for these patients the general issue of infection is compounded by the similar clinical presentation of both rejection and infection in the transplanted lungs and moreover by the frequent coexistence of both situations (Higenbottam and Wallwork, 1988). Indeed, in our group of heart–lung transplanted patients documented to have rejection at transbronchial biopsy, 29% also had coexistence of an infective process requiring therapy (Igboaka *et al.*, 1989). More so, while sputum culture and viral serology are a useful guide to pulmonary infection, either can be misleading in the immunosuppressed host. Bronchoscopy in order to perform bronchoalveolar lavage (BAL) and to perform transbronchial biopsy allows us to obtain viral culture of both BAL and lung tissue and to seek any histological evidence of infection. This makes bronchoscopy an invaluable tool in the postoperative management of these patients.

Of special interest in the heart–lung transplanted patients are the cystic fibrosis (CF) patients whose airways have been chronically infected with pathogens, mostly *Pseudomonas* species. In these particular patients, our antibiotic prophylaxis is guided by the antibiogram of the last sputum obtained before surgery. The antibiotherapy is then modified if necessary according to the culture and antibiogram of the specimen obtained at surgery from the recipient and donor trachea. The antibiotics are continued for 7–10 days. For the other groups of patients our prophylactic antibiotherapy is similar to the one used for heart transplantation.

All patients CMV and/or HSV seropositive are given acyclovir 400 mg three times daily prophylactically. This is commenced after extubation and continued for the following 3 months. Thereafter, acyclovir prophylaxis will be resumed in seropositive CMV patients when they receive steroids or they have their immunosuppression increased because of rejection. Primary CMV infections are treated with intravenous Ganciclovir (10 mg/kg/day in two doses) with or without hyperimmune globulin (Cytotec) depending on the severity of their clinical presentation. A similar protocol is used for the treatment of symptomatic CMV reactivation. Finally, HSV seropositive patients developing evidence of orofacial lesions or HSV pneumonia are treated with intravenous acyclovir (5 mg/kg tds) until improvement and then kept on oral acyclovir prophylactically. Similar to the heart transplant protocol, *Toxoplasma* mismatch patients are given a prophylactic 6-week course of pyrimethamine 25 mg daily along with folinic acid 15 mg three times daily. Also, patients receiving steroids are given cotrimoxazole (480 mg twice daily) for *Pneumocystis carinii* pneumonia prophylaxis.

Past the perioperative period and later in the first year post-transplantation is the time of the emergence of invasive aspergillosis. We have five such cases where in four the problem developed in patients who have had recurrent CMV reactivation or primary CMV infection. In all cases patients had a positive sputum culture of *Aspergillus fumigatus* previously. In all our cases the diagnosis was established histologically on tissue obtained at transbronchial biopsy using the Grocott's methamine silver stain and the treatment was with amphotericin B. One of these patients died of progressive respiratory failure and chronic rejection. In our experience few of these infections occurred in the absence of rejection.

In summary, we consider any patient with an FEV1 less than 70% of predicted at 3 months after

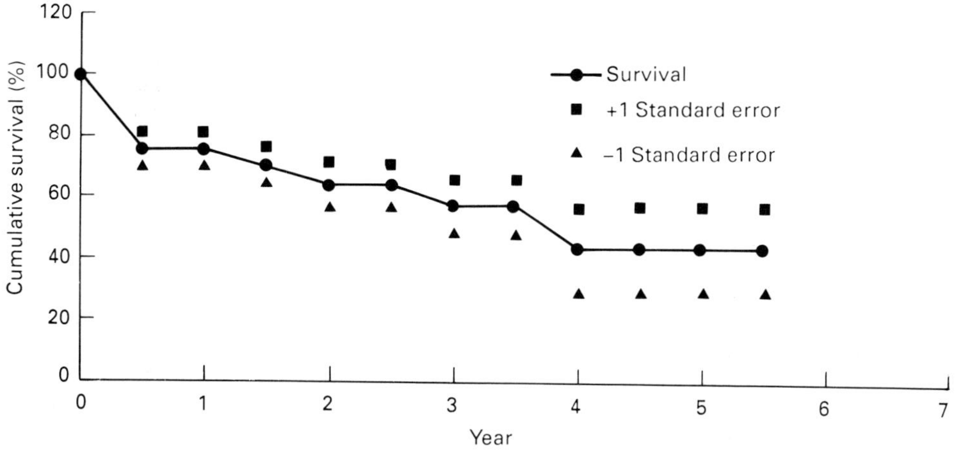

Figure 21.8 Heart–lung transplantation: actuarial survival analysis

transplantation to be at high risk and to require intensive monitoring through serial clinical assessments at short intervals along with continuous daily monitoring of FEV1 and repeated bronchoscopy for BAL and transbronchial biopsies. We expect an FEV1 of 100% of predicted at 6 months post-transplantation.

Results

A total of 66 patients have undergone heart–lung transplantation at Papworth Hospital and 44 are alive and well between 1 week and 66 months after surgery. The actuarial survival curve in Figure 21.8 shows a 1 year survival figure of 75.8%. The causes of death are shown in Table 21.9. The quality of life of these patients is good and comparable to patients having had heart transplants. The long-term complication of obliterative bronchiolitis, which is analogous to coronary occlusive disease in the donor heart in heart transplantation is a continuing concern and will probably be the most important determinant of long-term survival. We believe that this condition is a result of persistent or missed rejection episodes and there are some indications that patients at risk can be diagnosed early in their postoperative period and have their immunosuppression enhanced accordingly. Nevertheless, the long-term results of heart–lung transplantation are as yet unknown.

Table 21.9 Heart–lung transplantation: causes of death (June 1989)

Infection	
CMV	4
Others	8
Obliterative bronchiolitis	3
Cerebrovascular event	2
Donor heart failure/infection	1
Infection/liver failure	1
Tracheal dehiscence	1
Infection/ruptured aorta	1
Small bowel infarction/systemic lupus erythematosus	1
Total	22

References

Barnard, C.N. (1967) A human cardiac transplant: an interim report of a successful operation performed at Groote Schuur Hospital, Capetown. *South African Medical Journal*, **41**, 1271–1274

Cabrol, C., Gandjbakhch, I., Pavie, A., *et al.* (1989) Surgical procedure. In *Heart and Heart–Lung Transplantation* (ed. J. Wallwork), W.B. Saunders & Co., Philadelphia, USA, pp. 119–143

Caves, P.K., Schulz, W.P., Dong, E., Jr, *et al.* (1974) A new instrument for transvenous cardiac biopsy. *American Journal of Cardiology*, **33**, 264–267

Cooper, D.A.C., Novitzky, D., Rose, A.G. and Reichart, B.A. (1986) Acute pulmonary rejection precedes cardiac rejection following heart–lung transplantation in a primate model. *Journal of Heart Transplantation*, **5**, 129–131

Hakim, M., Higenbottam, T., Bethune, D., *et al.* (1988) Selection and procurement of combined heart and lung grafts for transplantation. *Journal of Thoracic and Cardiovascular Surgery*, **95**, 474–479

Higenbottam, T.W. and Wallwork, J. (1988) Transplantation of lungs. *Postgraduate Medical Journal*, **64**, (Suppl. 4), 120–124

Higenbottam, T.W., Stewart, S., Penketh, A.R.L. and Wallwork, J. (1987) The diagnosis of lung rejection and opportunistic infection by transbronchial lung biopsy. *Transplantation Proceedings*, **19**, 3777–3778

Igboaka, G.U.A., Higenbottam, T.W., Scott, J.P., *et al.* (1989) The distribution of lung rejection and infection in heart–lung transplantation. *American Review of Respiratory Disease*, **139**, A242 (Abstract)

Jamieson, S.W. and Kaye, M.P. (1989) Operative procedure and postoperative management. In *Heart and Heart–Lung Transplantation* (ed. J. Wallwork), W.B. Saunders & Co., Philadelphia, USA, pp. 481–490

McGregor, C.G.A., Baldwin, J.C., Jamieson, S.W., *et al.* (1985) Isolated pulmonary rejection after combined heart–lung transplantation. *Journal of Thoracic and Cardiovascular Surgery*, **90**, 623–626

McGiffin, D.C., Bonner, J.R., Kirklin, J.K. and Naftel, D.C. (1989) Patterns of infection and management in cardiac transplantation. In *Heart and Heart–Lung Transplantation* (ed. J.Wallwork), W.B. Saunders & Co., Philadelphia, USA, pp. 251–298

Otulana, B.A., Mist, B.A., Scott, J.P., *et al.* (1989) The effect of recipient lung size on lung physiology after heart–lung transplantation. *Transplantation*, **48**, 625–629

Reitz, B.A., Wallwork, J., Hunt, S.A., *et al.* (1982) Heart–lung transplantation: successful therapy for patients with pulmonary vascular disease. *New England Journal of Medicine*, **306**, 557–564

Shumway, N.E. and Lower, R.R. (1964) Special problems in transplantation of the heart. *Annals of the New York Academy of Science*, **120**, 773–777

Shumway, N.E., Dong, E. and Stinson, B. (1969) Surgical aspects of cardiac transplantation in man. *Bulletin of the New York Academy of Medicine*, **45**, 387–393

Stinson, E.B., Griepp, R.B., Clark, D.A., *et al.* (1970) Cardiac transplantation in man. VIII. Survival and function. *Journal of Thoracic and Cardiovascular Surgery*, **60**, 303–321

Stinson, E.B., Griepp, R.B., Schroeder, J.S., *et al.* (1972) Hemodynamic observations one and two years after cardiac transplantation in man. *Circulation*, **45**, 1183–1193

Wallwork, J., Jones, K., Cavarocchi, N., *et al.* (1987) Distant procurement of organs for clinical heart–lung transplantation using a single-flush technique. *Transplantation*, **44**, 654–658

Watson, D.C., Reitz, B.A., Baumgartner, W.A., *et al.* (1979) Distant heart procurement for transplantation. *Surgery*, **86**, 56–59

Yacoub, M., Khaghani, A., Aravot, D., *et al.* (1988) Cardiac transplantation from live donors. *Journal of the American College of Cardiology*, **11**, 102A

Yacoub, M., Khaghani, A., Banner, N., *et al.* (1989) Distant organ procurement for heart–lung transplantation. *Transplantation Proceedings*, **21**, 2548–2550

22

Extracorporeal respiratory support

John H. Dark

Historical background

The first membrane oxygenator was introduced into clinical use as early as 1964 (Bramson *et al.*, 1965) and successful long-term perfusion was described in 1972 (Hill, O'Brien and Murray, 1972). Techniques were refined during the 1970s, but a review of published results in 1976 suggested a survival rate of only 15% (Gille and Bagnewsky). To test what was an expensive technique of questionable worth, the National Institutes of Health in the USA sponsored a randomized trial of venoarterial ECMO (Extracorporeal Membrane Oxygenation) from 1975 to 1977. Nine centres took part, and entry criteria were so strict that only 10% of patients managed conservatively survived. Unfortunately for the technique, there were only the same number of survivors in the ECMO group (Zapol *et al.*, 1979). Although venoarterial bypass improved gas exchange, it did not effect survival. Ten years ago this approach to treatment had largely been abandoned.

There have been three lines of development during the 1980s. The most important is that of neonatal and paediatric ECMO. The initial reports of Bartlett and colleagues (1976) have been supported by many other groups. Success in neonates with persistent fetal circulation due to meconium aspiration and diaphragmatic hernia has been extended to infants with other aetiologies of respiratory failure, and to older patients with cardiac and respiratory failure after cardiopulmonary bypass. By 1990 there had been over 3500 paediatric perfusions in the USA (ELSO Registry, 1990). Experience in Europe remains much more limited, and there have been suggestions that current enthusiasm is not justified in the absence of any controlled trials (Meinert, 1990; Sosnowski *et al.*, 1990; Elliot, 1991).

In adults, progress has mainly revolved around the work of Gattinoni and Kolobow, with their techniques of extracorporeal carbon dioxide removal ($ECCO_2R$) (Gattinoni *et al.*, 1980; Gattinoni, 1989). They argue that the approaches employed during the NIH trial, which aimed only at normal oxygenation, did nothing to help recovery of the original lung pathology. $ECCO_2R$ specifically tries to spare the lung from the potentially damaging high pressure, high volume ventilation of traditional IPPV (intermittent positive pressure ventilation) with PEEP (positive end expiratory pressure). Exciting results are reported by a small group of enthusiasts, but widespread acceptance is still lacking.

During this ten-year period a number of groups have continued 'traditional' ECMO on a small scale, hoping particularly for success in patients with very easily reversible lung pathology. A number of technical advances have made the application of ECMO in adults more straightforward.

Percutaneous cannulation obviates the need for extensive surgical procedures and probably reduces local bleeding problems so support can be established rapidly and almost at the bedside (Harwood, 1986). Equally important has been the widespread use of centrifugal pumps, which do away with the need for venous reservoirs and complex safety switches. They can be run in very simple circuits with minimal supervision. This is particularly important if the cost of prolonged extracorporeal perfusion is to be reduced as the constant presence of experienced perfusionists is not required. Finally the use of heparin bonded oxygenators has been described both experimentally and now clinically (Bindslev, 1988). As bleeding with systemic anticoagulation remains the greatest source of morbidity this advance may have a very real place in making the whole technique more acceptable.

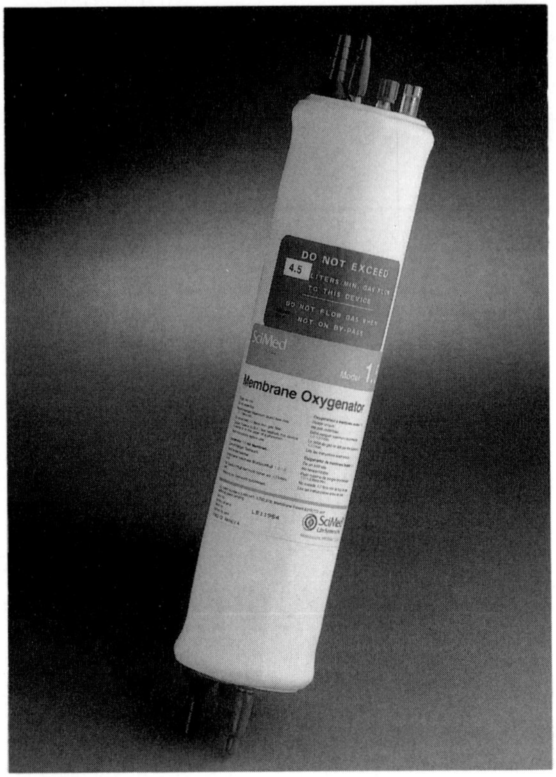

Figure 22.1 The Sci-Med hollow fibre membrane oxygenator

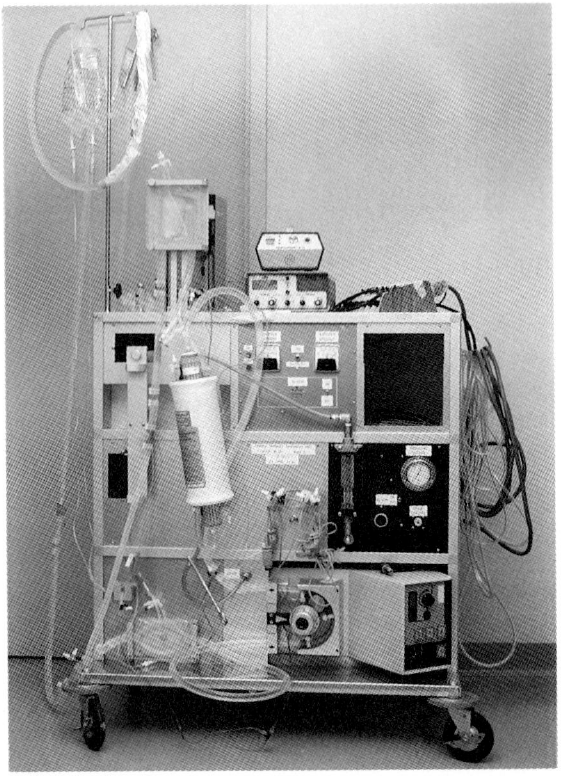

Figure 22.2 A self-contained 'ECMO cart'. The venous reservoir, roller pump and bubble trap can be clearly seen in the circuit. Also visible are pressure transducers, built-in oximeters and the Haemochron machine for measurement of the ACT..(Illustration from Toronto General Hospital, with the permission of Dr J.D. Cooper)

Adult ECRS

The techniques of oxygenator support in children and infants have evolved along different lines from those in adults. They will be described in a completely separate section (see below).

Notes on nomenclature

The emphasis in the early (1970s) application of these techniques was on oxygenation. The crucial advance, at least in the minds of the pioneers, was the development of a reliable membrane oxygenator. The term extracorporeal membrane oxygenation (ECMO) was obvious and easily understood. It did not define methods of access or routes of perfusion, but did however emphasize complete replacement of pulmonary gas exchange. In this sense it was really a form of long-term cardiopulmonary bypass, and the perfusion route was venoarterial (VA) – see below. High flow venovenous perfusion, as for instance practised by the Toronto group in the 1970s and 1980s, comes into this category, and is also usually termed 'ECMO'.

Gattinoni introduced the term $ECCO_2R$ (extracorporeal CO_2 removal), but this and its variant 'low flow $ECCO_2R$' (Pesenti, Kolobow and Gattinoni, 1988) are also forms of venovenous perfusion. Although based on a different philosophy they present the same technical problems and require the same solutions to those problems.

All of these concepts can be united under the term 'extracorporeal respiratory support' – ECRS. This should supplant the former 'ECMO', which should be reserved for the perfusion techniques developed in the 1970s – high flow venovenous or venoarterial – and paediatric support.

The 'Hardware' is common to all these techniques, and will be discussed before a description of the individual perfusion methods.

Oxygenators

Nearly all clinical experience has been obtained with Kolobow spiral coil silicone rubber

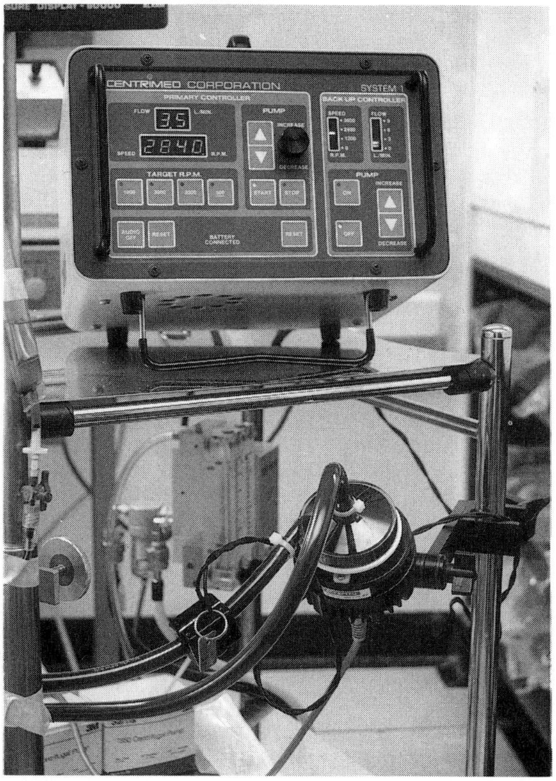

Figure 22.3 Centrifugal pump (Centrimed) with associated flow probe (see Figure 22.4). Illustration reproduced with the permission of the Audio Visual Service Department, University of Newcastle upon Tyne

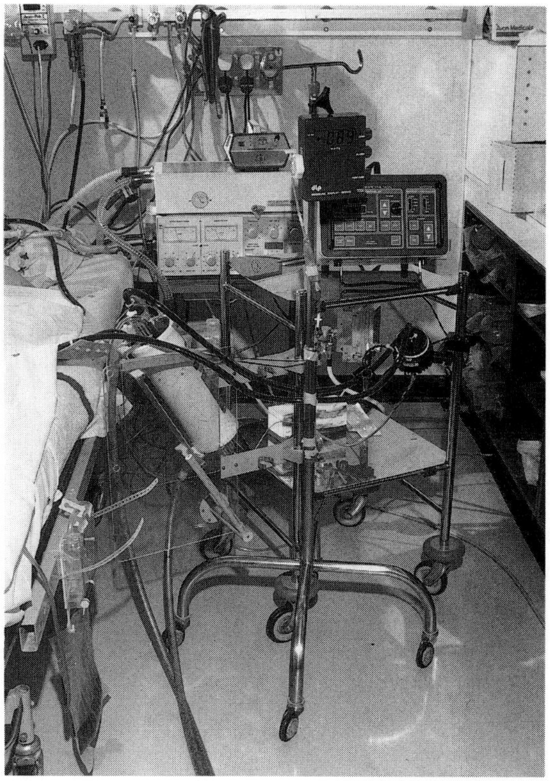

Figure 22.4 Bedside ECRS, rapidly established with standard centrifugal pump and oxygenator. Illustration reproduced with the permission of the Audio Visual Service Department, University of Newcastle upon Tyne

membrane lung (Sci Med, Minneapolis) (Figure 22.1). These oxygenators are available in a variety of sizes with up to 4.5 m^2 surface area. For complete respiratory support 1 m^2 of oxygenator surface is required per 10 kg. For maximum CO_2 removal, Gattinoni uses two oxygenators in series, whereas others have put them in parallel, to minimize pressure drop. The pressure gradient across the oxygenator is 75–150 mmHg at a typical flow rate. Even for venoarterial perfusion, only a single pump is required, as long as the return cannula is of a reasonable size.

These oxygenators are exceedingly reliable, and continuous perfusion for up to 19 days is recorded (Egan *et al*., 1988). Although failure is uncommon, the perfusion circuit should contain appropriately sited Y connectors to permit rapid attachment of a second device. Plastic outflow surface should be examined hourly and if clot appears, or if the oxygen saturation of the blood leaving the membrane falls below 90%, it should be exchanged for a new oxygenator.

Pumps and associated apparatus

A number of groups experienced in ECRS have described purpose-built apparatus to gather together the various components required into a compact mobile form (Figure 22.2). In the past, a standard roller pump has been used by all groups. The only required modification is to replace the ordinary silicone rubber blood tubing with a segment of hard wearing polyurethane tubing (Tygothane) in the pump head itself (Egan *et al*., 1988).

With a roller pump system, blood is drained into a reservoir bag containing a servo switch which can slow or stop the pump as the reservoir empties. In addition a bubble trap is required at the highest point of the outlet tubing to guard against accidentally entrained air. This arrangement can be considerably simplified by the use of a centrifugal pump (Figure 22.3). Although not demonstrably less traumatic to the blood, the non-occlusive centrifugal pump does not require a drainage reservoir, and will not pump large boluses of air. This pump is particularly safe with the particular problem of obstructed drainage in that, unlike the roller pump, the continuous presence of a perfusionist is not required.

The ease with which perfusion can be performed with a centrifugal pump has rendered the so-called 'ECMO cart' obsolete. The whole system can be established at the bedside (Figure 22.4) using readily available component parts.

In addition to provision for a spare or additional oxygenator, the perfusion tubing should incorporate blood sampling and venous access sites for heparin infusions, blood transfusion and parenteral nutrition. Many patients will have a degree of renal impairment, and a haemofilter can easily be connected into the circuit, in parallel with the oxygenator. This may be used for removal of excess fluid or converted to a full dialysis system. The degree of anticoagulation required for the oxygenator is perfectly adequate for the haemofiltration device. In a recent report from Gattinoni's group, 15 out of 68 patients required formal dialysis (1989). In addition, the role of haemofiltration to remove fluid should not be underestimated in the management of, for instance, lung contusion.

Monitoring

Regardless of the perfusion technique being used, these critically ill patients require very intensive monitoring. On the perfusion system itself, it is usual to measure flow either with a calibrated pump head or an electromagnetic flow probe on a standard segment of tubing. The pressure gradient across the oxygenator is routinely observed, and in more sophisticated systems, oximeters can be placed in the drainage in the outflow lines for continuous oxygen saturation readings. To this can be added pulse oximetry on the patient and continuous monitoring of mixed venous oxygen saturation with a fibre optic pulmonary artery catheter (Oximetrix).

Anti-coagulation and bleeding

Only the perfection of heparin bonded tubing and oxygenators will permit ECRS without some form of anti-coagulation. Precise regimens will vary, but with almost all, bleeding remains a major source of morbidity, and the risk of bleeding, e.g. head injury or major trauma, remains a contra-indication.

All current techniques achieve anticoagulation with heparin infusions, and control this with the automated instruments to measure activated clotting time (ACT) such as the Haemochron. Gattinoni recommends 'full' anticoagulation with an ACT of 'two to three times' control values. At these levels, oozing from cannulation sites is inevitable and the average blood loss was quoted at 1.3 l day^{-1} (Gattinoni, 1989). Surgical interventions were often followed by significant blood loss. Other centres are less cautious, aiming for an ACT of 160–240 s (Snider *et al.*, 1988) or even 150–180 s (Egan *et al.*, 1988). This last group initiate perfusion with very low heparin loading doses (1 mg kg^{-1}); with this regime minor surgical procedures such as open lung biopsy could easily be achieved. The ACT should be checked hourly and heparin infusion rates are typically 3–800 units h^{-1} although there may be considerable variation. Falls in platelet count are inevitable and daily transfusions are usually required, to maintain a count greater than 50 000 mm^{-3}. Fibrin split products and fibrinogen should be measured at least once daily to detect occult intravascular coagulation.

If bleeding becomes a problem the ACT can be returned to normal for several hours; the spiral coil membrane oxygenator will not clot as long as flow rates are kept high.

Routes of perfusion and cannulation

Venoarterial perfusion

This technique was used in the early days of ECMO and in the subsequent NIH trial of the mid 1970s. Since then it has only been used in respiratory failure when venovenous ECRS was not possible. Thus indications include heart failure, particularly right heart failure, and high pulmonary artery pressures. More recently the technique has been used in a transplant setting, either as a bridge to keep the patient alive until an organ becomes available (Pennington *et al.*, 1989; Delius *et al.*, 1990), or during severe episodes of donor heart dysfunction. In this application it reverts to its original role of providing long-term cardiopulmonary bypass.

The advantages of VA perfusion are obvious. Oxygenated blood is presented at physiological pressures to the systemic circulation (Figure 22.5). In practice arterial return is usually to the femoral artery and for perfusion for more than a few hours the distal vessel should also be cannulated to provide a blood supply to the leg. The relatively large access site requires formal vascular repair at the discontinuation of perfusion.

A major flaw of VA perfusion is the poor distribution of oxygenated blood. While there may be excellent perfusion of organs below the diaphragm, the mesenteric and renal beds in particular, if the heart continues to eject blood from functionless lungs, the brain and myocardium may remain hypoxic. Even sampling of specimens from the left radial artery may not detect significant desaturation in other aortic arch branches. A number of groups have sought to overcome this problem with arch perfusion using long thin-walled cannulae inserted

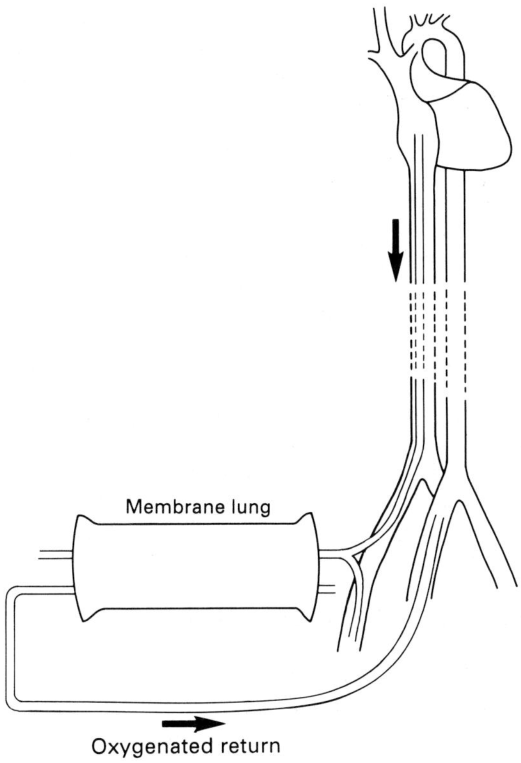

Figure 22.5 Venoarterial perfusion

at the femoral site (Cooper *et al.*, 1976). While the physiological situation is improved, there is a considerable price in surgical complications.

Return of oxygenated blood to the arterial side of the circulation obviously brings with it potential problems from gaseous and articular microemboli which do not exist with the venovenous techniques (see below).

A possible advantage of VA perfusion is the potential reduction in pulmonary artery pressure and the clearing of lung water resultant in reduction of transcapillary filtration pressure. In practice little change in pulmonary pressure is seen, and there may be an elevation of left arterial pressure consequent on inadequate cardiac decompression. A lack of oxygenated blood flowing into the lungs is likely to compromise repair of the original pulmonary lesion. This is particularly so at alveolar level, where the blood supply is almost entirely derived from the pulmonary artery.

Results of venoarterial perfusion

Until recently the only prospective trial of ECRS in adults was that sponsored by the Division of Lung Diseases of the National Heart Lung and Blood Institute in 1974. Ninety patients were recruited and the common entry criterion was arterial hypoxia (Pa_{O_2} less than 50 mmHg at Fi_{O_2} greater than 0.6, PEEP greater than or equal to 5 cmH_2O). Forty-eight patients were randomized to conventional mechanical ventilation with PEEP, and 42 received partial venoarterial bypass at nine separate centres in the United States. Four patients in each group survived. Perfusion improved arterial oxygenation but did not effect long-term outcome and most patients died with progressive lung damage. In the face of these unpromising results, and the technical difficulties described above, the technique was largely abandoned.

Even in recent reports from enthusiastic centres, such as that of Egan *et al.* (1988) from the Toronto group. the VA perfusions were in the very early part of the series. The one success for VA perfusion in that report was in the setting on multiple pulmonary emboli, (Cooper *et al.*, 1976) and obviously predates thrombolytic therapy.

More recently there have been reports of VA perfusion used as an extension of cardiopulmonary bypass to support the failing heart, either before or after transplantation. Application has been largely restricted to children and adolescents, for whom more conventional forms of mechanical support (ventricular assist devices and the total artificial heart) are not available. Results are disappointing, for instance two out of six survivors in the report of Delius and colleagues (1990). Their survivors were in the two youngest patients, a group for whom VA perfusion has very high success rates (see paediatric section). Results are similarly poor in adults bridged to heart transplant (Pennington *et al.*, 1989), and the technique has been superseded by mechanical ventricular assist devices.

High flow venovenous perfusion

While conventional VA ECMO provides physiological blood and gases in the systemic circulation, it was realized that simple improvement of oxygenation in the pulmonary artery could provide adequate support to many patients. Although a degree of arterial desaturation persists, many of the objections to VA perfusion are overcome.

In essence the technique involves draining venous blood from below the diaphragm, using wide bore cannulae, passing it through a membrane oxygenator, and returning it via the jugular vein into the right atrium (Figure 22.6). The pulmonary artery saturation is considerably improved, and this blood then passes through the damaged lungs where it might theoretically be expected to enhance recovery. This oxygenated blood is then pumped in a pulsatile fashion with physiological distribution round the systemic circulation by the patient's own left ventricle.

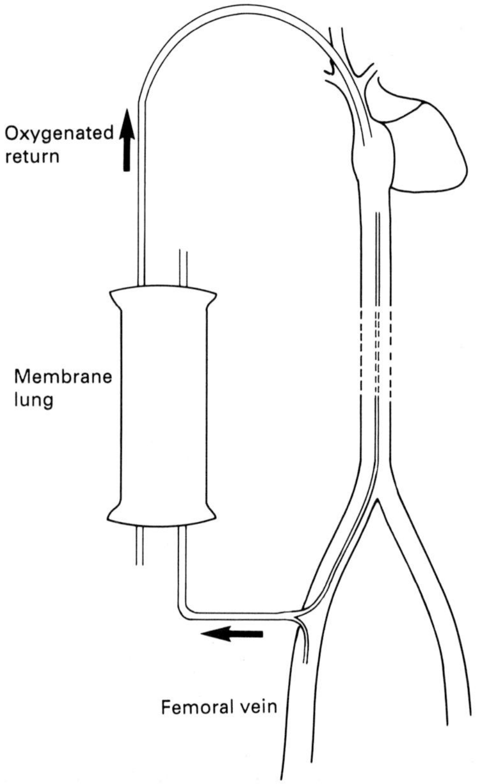

Figure 22.6 High flow venovenous perfusion

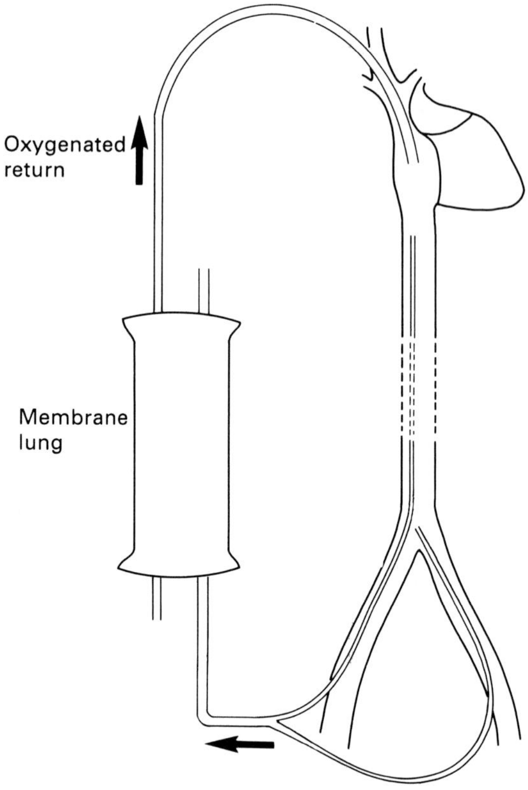

Figure 22.7 Percutaneous venovenous perfusion

In its conventional form, thin-walled cannulae are placed by an open approach into the common femoral vein and the internal jugular vein. The cannulation can be performed under local anaesthetic but haemostasis should be meticulous. An additional side limb on the drainage cannula should decompress the distal femoral vein. It is important to position the drainage cannula well below the diaphragm. It may be equipped with appropriately placed side holes to improve flow from the hepatic and renal beds. The return cannula is advanced into the right atrium and is ideally directed towards the tricuspid valve. Improvement in oxygenation is limited by mixing between the two cannulae. 'Mixed venous' saturation may be as high as 80% but will be a good deal lower in high cardiac output states. With severe lung damage there is often no step up in oxygen saturation across the pulmonary bed, but the $Pa\text{O}_2$ will obviously be improved compared with the preperfusion figure. Large air bubbles entrained into the perfusion circuit will not reach the systemic circulation, though the effect of microemboli being filtered by the lungs for several days must not be underestimated.

Results of high flow venovenous perfusion

This technique should be regarded as an intermediary between attempts with VA perfusion in the 1970s, and the more aggressive approach of Gattinoni and Kolobow with their rather different underlying philosophy. Thus it has been used on a sporadic basis for the rescue of profoundly hypoxic patients who seemed to have easily reversible lung pathology.

The Toronto group described 12 patients over a 10-year period, with two long-term survivors and one other patient who was successfully bridged to a lung transplant, although he subsequently died (Egan *et al.*, 1988). Similarly Snider and colleagues (1988) from Pennsylvania report three surviving patients out of six collected over a 5-year period. No particular ventilatory regime was followed in these patients, once they were established on perfusion. Most of the deaths were due to sepsis, or to progressive deterioration of the underlying lung condition with eventual organization and fibrosis and no recovery of alveolar damage.

Percutaneous venovenous perfusion

A further subgroup of patients has arisen more recently. The development of percutaneous bypass cannulae, now fairly widely available for partial bypass during coronary angioplasty, and the widespread familiarity with the centrifugal pump, have led to the possibility of 'bedside ECRS'. Perfusion can be readily established in the setting of rapidly worsening hypoxia of recent onset (Harwood, 1986). A flow of 3–5 l min^{-1} can easily be established using these cannulae using two in the inferior vena cava for drainage, and one placed via the internal jugular vein into the right atrium for return (Figure 22.7). Non-cardiogenic pulmonary oedema after bypass surgery has been an indication in several case reports (e.g. Katz *et al.*, 1988) and emergency perfusion has even been used for status asthmaticus (Tajimi *et al.*, 1988).

Extracorporeal CO_2 removal ($ECCO_2R$)

Underlying philosophy

It is well established that a high inspired oxygen and high ventilation pressure are deleterious even to healthy lungs, and certainly to injured lung (Kolobow, 1988). In the adult respiratory distress syndrome (ARDS) the lungs are poorly compliant and require high inflation pressures to maintain reasonable gas exchange.

The Milan group suggest that the apparent poor compliance is due to small but relatively normal areas of lung performing most of the gas exchange, while much larger areas are atelectatic and make no contribution. They have recently demonstrated this lack of homogeneity with a series of beautiful CT scans (Gattinoni, 1987). The assumption is made that aggressive ventilation of the healthy areas causes further damage and contributes to the very high mortality of ARDS. Gattinoni and colleagues suggest that $ECCO_2R$ is successful because it allows gentle ventilation of the healthy areas of lung and encourages recovery. Perfusion of the lung with oxygenated blood is an important part of the process, so the route of choice is venovenous.

Specific technical aspects

The hardware required for $ECCO_2R$ is largely as for other forms of ECRS. Two hollow fibre oxygenators are used in series (Gattinoni *et al.*, 1980) to allow almost complete clearance of CO_2 from the blood passing through the circuit. Because of this, relatively low flow rates, typically 20% of cardiac output, and rarely more than 2.5 l min^{-1} (Gattinoni, 1989). The Milan group favour cannulation via a superficial cutdown on to the saphenous veins. The distal vein is not obstructed and bleeding problems are largely eliminated.

The patients are kept sedated and paralysed, and the lungs kept inflated with PEEP of 15–25 cmH_2O (Pesenti *et al.*, 1988). Mechanically delivered 'sighs' are delivered 3–5 times per minute, and oxygen instilled by a catheter in the trachea during the prolonged inspiratory phase.

Results of $ECCO_2R$

In 1989, Gattinoni reported 68 patients, with 35 surviving. All had fulfilled the entry criteria for the NIH ECMO study, and only 10% might have been expected to survive if managed conventionally. Similar results are reported from Germany, although with smaller numbers (Knoch *et al.*, 1987). These results, while very exciting, remain uncontrolled. A prospective, randomized study has been commenced in the USA (Morris *et al.*, 1988), and the result of this trial will decide the future of $ECCO_2R$.

Future prospects in adult ECRS

Intravascular oxygenation–IVOX

No speculation about future applications would be complete without mention of the intravascular oxygenator (the IVOX device) (Vaslef *et al.*, 1989). This oxygenator, which unfolds in the inferior vena cava, remains connected to external gas exchange and exhaust connections (Figure 22.8). Up to 150 ml min^{-1} of oxygen can be exchanged, and although anticoagulation to an ACT of 200 s is required, no major surgery is involved in insertion. The device is currently undergoing trials in both the United States and Europe. If it fulfils its albeit very early promise (e.g. Kallis *et al.*, 1991) it will have a major role in pulmonary support in the future.

Low-flow venovenous perfusion

Percutaneous cannulation and simplified perfusion circuits open up the prospect of 'bedside ECRS', established as easily as dialysis or parenteral nutrition. The aim would be to remove, perhaps, enough CO_2 to prevent the need for intubation in a precariously balanced patient. Blood flows of 500–1000 ml min^{-1} will clear 25–30% of CO_2 production. Pesenti, Kolobow and Gattinoni (1988) have already described a patient with multiple air leaks in whom low flow perfusion was able to obviate the need for mechanical ventilation.

Heparin-free perfusion

Surface-heparinized pump tubing has long been available, but this process can now be applied to whole oxygenators. Bindslev (1988) described four patients in whom such a system had been used clini-

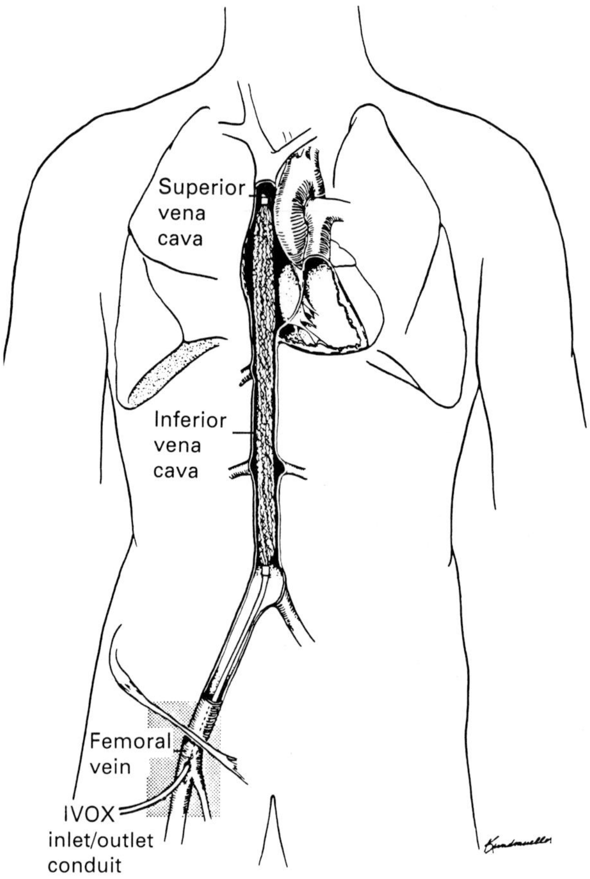

Figure 22.8 General concept of the IVOX intra-vascular oxygenator

cally. All patients received some systemic heparin, and three survived to leave hospital. The non-survivor developed DIC (disseminated intravascular coagulation) and an uncontrollable coagulopathy, clearly indicating that some problems remain. In the laboratory, animals have been perfused for up to 24 h without any additional heparin (Pesenti, Kolobow and Gattinoni, 1988).

It is likely that all three of these technical advances will be coupled with the concepts proposed by Gattinoni and his colleagues. If extracorporeal support can be established quickly, with minimal morbidity, and if it can be run inexpensively (without labour-intensive supervision) then we may see its application earlier in the progress of lung disease rather than waiting until the patient is actually dying from hypoxia (which was the case in the NIH trial). The patient will be supported before lung damage is irreversible, in the hope that such damage can be prevented by modification of mechanical ventilation.

Paediatric extracorporeal membrane oxygenation

In parallel with the early attempts at venoarterial perfusion in adults, a number of centres applied these techniques in children, and particularly in neonates. The leader in this field was Bartlett, first reporting encouraging results in 1976. After a slow early growth, confined to a handful of centres, there was an explosion of activity in the late 1980s. By the end of that decade, over 1000 patients were being treated per year in the USA and the neonatal registry held at Ann Arbor contained details of over 3500 patients (ELSO neonatal registry, 1990).

The best early results were achieved in conditions where there was pulmonary hypertension, usually due to the meconium aspiration syndrome or due to persistent fetal circulation (Bartlett, 1976). Survivors were achieved here, in contrast to the situation in adults, because the underlying problem was reversible. Perfusion broke the circle of hypoxia, acidosis and further shunting away from a constricted pulmonary circulation, both keeping the patient oxygenated and encouraging the pulmonary hypertension to subside.

Subsequently, ECMO was also offered to neonates with congenital diaphragmatic hernia. Although results were less good mortality was halved in some groups of patients (Heiss *et al.*, 1989). In a different age group there has been tentative exploration in other types of respiratory failure, such as viral bronchiolitis (Steinhorn and Green, 1990).

Finally ECMO has been used as a form of extended cardiopulmonary bypass to support older children who cannot be weaned and bypass in the course of cardiac surgery. There are no alternative mechanical support devices for this patient group, some of whom require to be bridged to heart transplantation.

Technical aspects of paediatric ECMO

The basic circuit now used by most centres is that developed by Bartlett from the adult veno-arterial perfusion experience. (Figure 22.9). With the infant inevitably ventilated and paralysed, a cut down is made over the right hand side of the neck to expose the internal jugular and internal carotid arteries. After systemic heparinization (1–200 unit kg^{-1} to give an ACT of 300–500 s) cannulae are passed into the right atrium and aortic arch. The length of these cannulae is critical and should be measured against an appropriate X-ray. In early series, paediatric chest tubes were used, but special cannulae (Elecath) are now available – 12 or 14 Fr for venous drainage, 8–10 or 12 Fr for arterial return (Moront *et al.*, 1989). The cannulae are connected by quarter

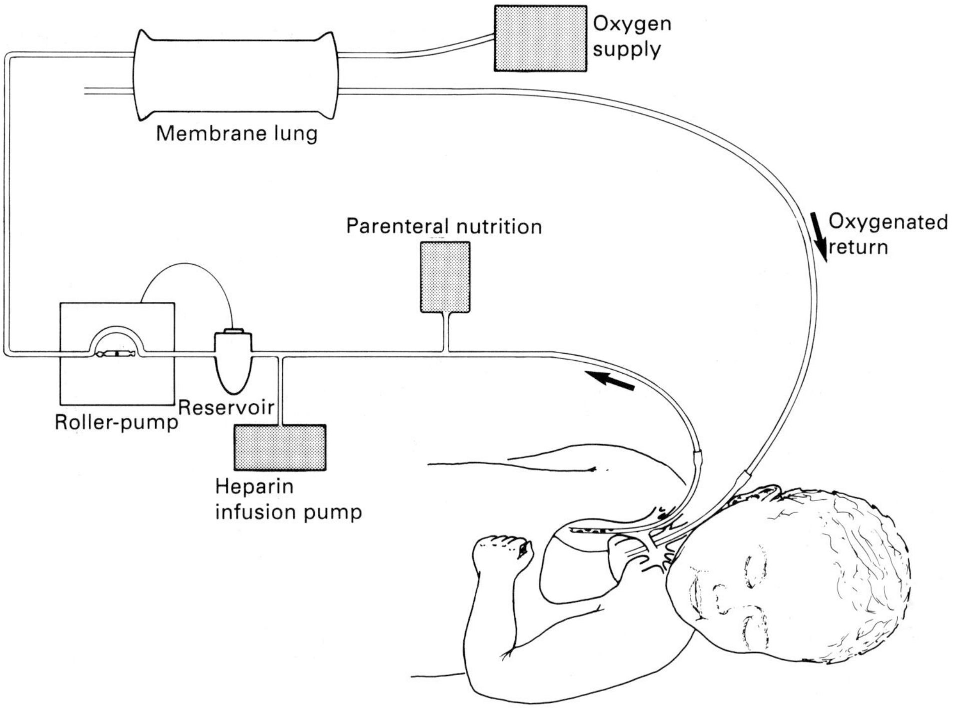

Figure 22.9 Basic circuit for paediatric venoarterial ECMO

inch tubing to a 50 ml reservoir bag with a servo switch to cut off the pump if venous drainage fails. Roller pumps have been used invariably: the centrifugal pump cannot be precisely controlled at low flow rates (Lillehei *et al.*, 1989).

Typically 80% of venous return, amounting to 100–150 ml kg^{-1} min^{-1} is drained from the right atrium to provide adequate oxygenation. As in adults, bleeding remains a serious problem. The ACT should be maintained at 200–250 s by heparin infusion. Platelet transfusions should be given if the platelet count falls below 100 000 mm^{-3}. Oozing from cannulation sites can be dealt with by direct application of fibrin glue (Moront *et al.*, 1989). Parenteral nutrition should be added to the circuit as a routine, and haemofiltration used without hesitation in renal impairment.

Ventilator settings should be adjusted to achieve lung rest. These include low $F\text{IO}_2$ (21 or 30%), relatively slow ventilation, 10–15 breaths min^{-1}, and low peak pressures, 20–25 cmH_2O. PEEP of around 10 cmH_2O is important to prevent a white lung appearance on chest X-ray.

Indications for weaning are a clearing chest X-ray and improving arterial blood gases, on a low inspired oxygen. Echocardiography may reveal increasing left to right shunting, indicating a fall in pulmonary vascular resistance (Foglia, 1990). The inspired oxygen concentration is increased up to 50% and pump flow is gradually reduced until it can be stopped and the patient decannulated. The circuit should be left heparinized for a further 12 h in case of an urgent return to ECMO.

A major disadvantage of this perfusion technique is the subsequent ligation of the carotid artery and internal jugular vein. Venovenous perfusion has been used in neonates, with some success (Klein *et al.*, 1985) but ligation of the femoral vein is not without problems, and many of these patients have cardiac decompensation. Anderson and colleagues (1989) have also described a double lumen catheter placed in the internal jugular vein which shows considerable promise.

Criteria for neonatal ECMO

Most centres with a significant experience have evolved rigid thresholds below which ECMO is indicated. In general these are based on retrospective analysis demonstrating high (greater than 80%) mortality if conventional therapy alone is continued. Thus it is suggested that an inability to raise

$Pa\text{O}_2$ above 8 kPa for greater than 8 h predicts a poor outcome (Foglia, 1990). In practice many patients require ECMO much more urgently for so-called failure of conventional medical therapy, with a $Pa\text{O}_2$ less than 5.5 kPa for more than 2 h (Klein, 1988).

Lillehei and colleagues (1989) put forward the Oxygenation Index:

$$\frac{F\text{iO}_2 \times \text{mean airway pressure}}{Pa\text{O}_2 \text{ in mmHg}}$$

and suggest that ECMO is indicated if this index is less than 0.4.

As might be expected, a number of contraindications have evolved. The commonest cause of death in Bartlett's review of his first 100 patients (Bartlett *et al.*, 1986) was intracranial haemorrhage. It occurred in 89% of infants less than 35 weeks gestation, and most of these weighed less than 2000 g. Small size and immaturity are accepted as contraindications and the others are set out in Table 22.1. Echocardiography should be used to exclude an intracardiac cause of arterial hypoxia.

Table 22.1 Contraindications to neonatal ECMO

<35 weeks gestational age
<2000 g weight at birth
Intracranial haemorrhage
Coagulopathy
>10 days mechanical ventilation
Structural cardiac disease

Indications and results for neonatal ECMO

As mentioned above, the best indication is persistent pulmonary hypertension, sometimes occurring alone, but usually the result of the meconium aspiration syndrome. Survival rates of greater than 90% can be achieved in the best centres (Moront *et al.*, 1989). Other insults – blood aspiration, congenital pneumonia, have a similar effect in terms of pulmonary hypertension and shunting. Another area where ECMO has made a major impact is congenital diaphragmatic hernia. A 50% mortality for those presenting in the 24 h can be halved (Heiss *et al.*, 1986), leaving the residuum who have lungs too hypoplastic for survival. Overall survival in this group, from the neonatal ECMO registry (ELSO registry, 1990) is 62% compared with a figure greater than 90% for the meconium aspiration syndrome.

Long-term follow up data is scanty, but now beginning to appear. The Ann Arbor group (Andrews *et al.*, 1986) report that 64% of patients followed 1–3 years after perfusion had normal motor development. Moderate to severe neurological deficit was present in 13% but whether this is a result of perfusion or occurred before ECMO was instituted is impossible to tell. Chronic lung problems are remarkably absent. Towne *et al.* (1985) report similar results from a different centre, but again the numbers are small.

Morbidity of neonatal ECMO

The principle side-effects of intracranial haemorrhage and generalized coagulopathy have already been mentioned. Other complications related to the perfusion itself include haemolysis, vocal cord paralysis, leucopenia and sepsis. Mechanical failure is relatively rare, occurring in less than 10% of perfusions, and rarely contributing to a poor outcome. Ligation of the common carotid artery results in striking alternations of blood flow in the right cerebral hemisphere, with retrograde perfusion from the contralateral internal carotid system (Lott *et al.*, 1990). The clinical importance of these changes is not yet known.

The current place of neonatal ECMO

The superb early results were undoubtedly a considerable improvement over those achieved in historical controls (Bartlett *et al.*, 1986). However, one must beware of continuing to use the same controls. Dworetz *et al.* (1989) demonstrated an 80% mortality for patients who met ECMO criteria in 1980 and 1981, but only a 10% mortality for conventionally ventilated infants reaching the same criteria in 1988. Prospective trials have taken place (e.g. O'Rouke *et al.*, 1989) but were biased towards ECMO and have been extensively criticized (Meinert, 1990; Elliot, 1991). It has been suggested that even though neonatal ECMO is not of 'proven' benefit a properly constructed prospective trial is now impossible in the USA. A trial would be possible and has indeed been suggested (Sosnowski *et al.*, 1990) in the United Kingdom where neonatal ECMO is not yet established.

Use of ECMO for postoperative surgical cardiac failure

Mechanical assist devices are not applicable to the paediatric population. A number of reports describe ECMO in this setting, as a form of prolonged cardiopulmonary bypass (Kanter *et al.*, 1987; Trento *et al.*, 1988; Weinhaus *et al.*, 1989; Rogers *et al.*, 1989). In many cases, perfusion was initiated several hours after the original surgery. Survival is 30–50%, reflecting the severe insult before ECMO was initiated. Bleeding was the most important problem reflecting extensive surgery and often central cannulation. Survival is unlikely if the original defect is not corrected or is incorrectable. In these patients, bridging to transplant is occasionally possible.

References

Anderson, H.L., Otsu, T., Chapman, R.A. and Bartlett, R.H. (1989) Venovenous extracorporeal life support in neonates using a double lumen catheter. *Transactions of the American Society for Artificial Internal Organs*, **35**, 650–653

Andrews, A.F., Nosum, G.A., Lilley, R.E., *et al.* (1986) One to three year outcome for 14 neonatal survivors of extracorporeal membrane oxygenation. *Paediatrics*, **78**, 692–698

Bartlett, R.H., Gazzaniga, A.B., Jefferies, M.B., *et al.* (1976) Extracorporeal membrane oxygenation (ECMO) cardiopulmonary support in infancy. *Transactions of the American Society for Artificial Internal Organs*, **22**, 80–93

Bartlett, R.H., Toomasian, J., Raloff, D.W., *et al.* (1986) Extracorporeal membrane oxygenation (ECMO) in neonatal respiratory failure: 100 cases. *Annals of Surgery*, **204**, 236–245

Bindlsev, L. (1988) Adult ECMO performed with surface-heparinized equipment. *Transactions of the American Society for Artificial Internal Organs*, **34**, 1009–1013

Bramson, M.L., Osborn, J.J., Main, B.F., *et al.* (1965) A new disposable membrane oxygenation with integral heat exchanger. *Journal of Thoracic and Cardiovascular Surgery*, **50**, 391–396

Cooper, J.D., Teasdale, S., Nelems, J.M., *et al.* (1976) Cardiorespiratory failure secondary to peripheral pulmonary emboli: survival following a combination of prolonged extracorporeal membrane oxygenator support and pulmonary embolectomy. *Journal of Thoracic and Cardiovascular Surgery*, **71**, 871–877

Delius, R.E., Zurischenberger, J.B., Cilley, R., *et al.* (1990) Prolonged extracorporeal life support of paediatric and adolescent cardiac transplant patients. *Annals of Thoracic Surgery*, **50**, 791–795

Dworetz, A.R., Moya, F.R., Sabo, B., *et al.* (1989) Survival of infants with persistent pulmonary hypertension with extracorporeal membrane oxygenation. *Paediatrics*, **84**, 1–6

Elliot, S.J. (1991) Neonatal extracorporeal membrane oxygenation: how not to assess novel technologies. *Lancet*, **337**, 476–478

Egan, T.M., Duffin, J., Glynn, M.F.X., *et al.* (1988) Ten year experience with extracorporeal membrane oxygenation for severe respiratory failure. *Chest*, **94**, 681–687

ELSO Neonatal Registry. *Summary report*. (1990) University of Michigan, Ann Arbor, Michigan, July

Foglia, R. (1990) Extracorporeal membrane oxygenation. *Current Opinion in Cardiology*, **5**, 20–24

Gattinoni, L. (1989) The use of extracorporeal support for adult respiratory distress syndrome. *Annual of Cardiac Surgery* 1989, 56–61

Gattinoni, L., Pesenti, A., Rossi, F., *et al.* (1980) Treatment of acute respiratory failure with low frequency positive-pressure ventilation and extracorporeal CO_2 removal. *Lancet*, **ii**, 292–294

Gattinoni, L., Pesenti, A., Avalli, A., *et al.* (1987) Pressure–volume curve of total respiratory system in acute respiratory failure: a computed tomographic scan study. *American Review of Respiratory Disease*, **136**, 730–736

Gille, J.P., Bagnewsky, T.E. (1976) Worldwide results of extracorporeal membrane oxygenation performed between 1972 and 1976. *Transactions of the American Society for Artificial Internal Organs*, **22**, 102–105

Harwood, S.J. (1986) Veno-venous ECMO–a rapid percutaneous method for patients in severe respiratory distress. *Transplantation and Implantation Today*, **3**, 44–47

Heiss, K., Manning, P., Oldham, K.T., *et al.* (1989) Reversal of mortality for congenital diaphragmatic hernia with ECMO. *Annals of Surgery*, **209**, 225–230

Hill, J.D., O'Brien, T.G. and Murray, J.T. (1972) Prolonged extracorporeal oxygenation for acute post traumatic respiratory failure (shock lung syndrome). *New England Journal of Medicine*, **286**, 629–634

Kallis, P., Al-Soady, N.M., Bennett, D. and Treasure, T. (1991) Clinical use of intravascular oxygenation. *Lancet*, **337**, 549

Kanter, K.R., Pennington, D.G., Weber, T.R., *et al.* (1987). Extracorporeal membrane oxygenation for post-operative cardiac support in children. *Journal of Thoracic and Cardiovascular Surgery*, **93**, 27–35

Katz, N.M., Bachholz, B.J., Howard, E., *et al.* (1988) Venovenous extracorporeal membrane oxygenation for non-cardiogenic pulmonary edema after coronary bypass surgery. *Annals of Thoracic Surgery*, **46**, 462–464

Klein, M.D. (1988) Neonatal ECMO. *Transactions of the American Society for Artificial Internal Organs*, **34**, 39–42

Klein, M.D., Andrews, A.F., Wesley, J.R., *et al.* (1985) Venovenous extracorporeal membrane oxygenation in neonates with respiratory failure. *Annals of Surgery*, **201**, 520–526

Knoch, M., Muller, E.E., Holtermann, W., *et al.* (1987) Ventilation with extracorporeal CO_2 removal (in German). *Anaesthetist*, **36**, 210–216

Kolobow, T. (1988) Acute respiratory failure: or how to injure healthy lungs (and prevent sick lungs from recovering) *Transactions of the American Society for Artificial Internal Organs*, **34**, 31–34

Lillehei, C.W., O'Rouke, P.P., Vacanti, J.P. and Crone, R.K. (1989) Role of extracorporeal membrane oxygenation in selected paediatric respiratory problems. *Journal of Thoracic and Cardiovascular Surgery*, **98**, 968–971

Lott, I.T., McPherson, D., Towne, B., *et al.* (1990) Long-term neurophysiologic outcome after neonatal extracorporeal membrane oxygenation. *Journal of Paediatrics*, **116**, 343–349

Meinent, C.L. (1990) Extracorporeal membrane oxygenation trials. (Editorial). *Paediatrics*, **85**, 365–366

Moront, M.G., Katz, N.M., Keszler, M., *et al.* (1989) Extracorporeal membrane oxygenation for neonatal respiratory failure. *Journal of Thoracic and Cardiovascular Surgery*, **97**, 706–714

Morris, A.H., Menlove, R.L., Rollins, R.J., *et al.* (1988) A controlled clinical trial of a new 3-step therapy that includes extracorporeal CO_2 removal for ARDS. *Transactions of the American Society for Artificial Internal Organs*, **34**, 48–53

O'Rouke, P.P., Crane, R.K. and Vacanti, J.P. (1989) Extracorporeal membrane oxygenation and conventional medical therapy in neonates with persistent pulmonary hypertension of the newborn: a propspective randomised study. *Paediatrics*, **84**, 957–963

Pennington, D.G., McBride, L.R., Kanter, K.R., *et al.* (1989) Bridging to heart transplantation with circulatory support devices. *Journal of Heart Transplantation* **8**, 116–123

Pesenti, A., Kolobow, T. and Gattinoni, L. (1988) Extracorporeal respiratory support in the adult. *Transactions of the American Society for Artificial Internal Organs*, **34**, 1006–1008

Rogers, A.J., Trento, A., Siewers, R.D., *et al.* (1989) Extracorporeal membrane oxygenation for postcardiotomy cardiogenic shock in children. *Annals of Thoracic Surgery*, **47**, 903–906

Snider, M.T., Campbell, D.B., Kofke, W.A., *et al.* (1988) Venovenous perfusion of adults and children with severe adult respiratory sickness syndrome. *Transactions of the American Society for Artificial Internal Organs*, **34**, 1014–1020

Sosnowski, A.W., Bonser, S.J., Field, D.J., *et al.* (1990) Extracorporeal membrane oxygenation. (Editorial) *British Medical Journal*, **301**, 303–304

Steinhorn, R.H. and Green, T.P. (1990) Use of extracorporeal membrane oxygenation in the treatment of respiratory syncytial virus bronchiolitis: the national experience 1983 to 1988. *Journal of Paediatrics*, **116**, 338–342

Tajimi, K., Kasai, T., Nakatani, T. and Kobayashi, K. (1988) Extracorporeal lung assist for patient with hypercapnia due to status asthmaticus. *Intensive Care Medicine*, **14**, 588–589

Towne, B.H., Lott, I.T., Hicks, D.A. and Healy, T. (1985) Long term follow-up of infants and children treated with extracorporeal membrane oxygenation (ECMO): a preliminary report. *Journal of Paediatric Surgery*, **20**, 410–414

Trento, A., Thompson, A., Siewers, R.D., *et al.* (1988) Extracorporeal membrane oxygenation in children: new trends. *Journal of Thoracic and Cardiovascular Surgery*, **96**, 542–547

Vaslef, S.N., Mockros, L.F. and Anderson, R.W. (1989) Development of an intravascular lung assist device. *Transactions of the American Society for Artificial Internal Organs*, **15**, 660–664

Weinhaus, L., Kanter, C., Woetzel, M., *et al.* (1989) Extracorporeal membrane oxygenation for circulatory support after repair of congenital heart defects. *Annals of Thoracic Surgery*, **48**, 206–212

Zapol, W.M., Snider, M.T., Hill, J.D., *et al.* (1979) Extracorporeal membrane oxygenation in severe acute respiratory failure: a randomized prospective study. *Journal of the American Medical Association*, **242**, 2193–2196

23

Future developments and potential applications of extracorporeal circulation in medicine and surgery

Hans Zwart

Extracorporeal circulation has been under development for more than 170 years (Le Gallois, 1813). Around the middle of the nineteenth century, it was discovered that blood turned light red by mixing it with air and that organ function could be sustained better with bright blood (Brown-Seguard, 1858). In 1885, a detailed description appeared of an apparatus for isolated organ perfusion with oxygenated blood (von Frey and Gruber, 1885). This machine functioned much like a heart–lung machine although on a smaller scale. Great improvements were made possible in perfusion experiments by the discovery of heparin in 1916 (McLean, 1959) and by the development of blood transfusion, anaesthesia and antimicrobial techniques.

The adaption of laboratory perfusion techniques to clinical use must be credited to Gibbon (1937) for the heart–lung machine and to Kolff (Kolff and Berk, 1944) for the artificial kidney. Gibbon was inspired by the high mortality of pulmonary embolectomy. He envisaged that a heart–lung machine could be used for the treatment of massive pulmonary embolism or severe cardiac failure. He also suggested the possible use of the apparatus for surgery on the heart. It has been the latter application that greatly stimulated further development of the heart–lung machine. It was applied to a patient for the first time by Dennis *et al.* in 1951. Gibbon himself performed the first successful clinical open heart operation using his heart–lung machine in 1953 (Gibbon, Miller and Feinberg, 1953).

At present, cardiopulmonary bypass for open heart surgery is a commonly accepted and relatively safe procedure. For the treatment of cardiac failure, the bypass was initially only sporadically used. Extracorporeal blood handling and oxygenation caused too much damage to be tolerated for more than a few hours. To be beneficial for the treatment of cardiac failure, it was believed that the bypass would have to be applied for much longer periods, possibly days or even weeks. It was hoped that during the period of assistance, while the circulation was maintained by the heart–lung machine, the heart would rest and be given a chance to recover.

The frightful death toll from arteriosclerotic coronary artery disease has continued to stimulate researchers to further refine bypass techniques to enable such prolonged perfusion. A major achievement in decreasing blood damage during bypass was the introduction of membrane oxygenators. The early models were bulky, cumbersome and unreliable devices. However, performance was gradually improved and over the last 5 years practical disposable oxygenators have become available and are now actually used more commonly than bubble oxygenators even in everyday application for heart surgery. Simultaneously, interest in using the heart–lung machine for the treatment of cardiac failure revived. This trend was intensified even more because of developments in techniques to treat coronary artery disease not only in the operating rooms but also in the heart catheterization laboratory. The application of balloon dilatation of coronary arteries may necessitate the standby of powerful mechanical assist devices in case the heart should develop fatal arrhythmias or intractable failure.

Still another field of possible application emerged. Refractory pulmonary failure such as occurs during the course of hyaline membrane disease in children and in acute respiratory distress syndrome in adults was treated with artificial oxygenation. In fact, it has been the latter clinical conditions where most experience has been gained with cardiopulmonary bypass for periods beyond 1 week.

To enable even longer use of mechanical assist devices, parts of the equipment of certain bypass techniques were designed to be incorporated within the body. This has been especially true for left heart bypass and to a lesser extent for prolonged artificial oxygenation. A totally implantable left heart bypass pump employing transcutaneous transmission of energy to implanted batteries has reached a point of development where it can be safely applied in calves for months (Portner *et al.*, 1989). Intravascular oxygenators have been studied and seem to function quite well in animal experiments (Mortensen, 1987). The ultimate artificial bypass device that is to be implanted permanently within the body is the artificial heart. The initial clinical results have been disappointing (DeVries, Anderson and Zoyce, 1986). The patients were plagued by embolization and infection. However, refinements in the design of the inside of the artificial hearts and the use of different energy sources will further improve tolerance of the artificial heart and lead to meaningful prolonged application. For temporary use in patients awaiting heart surgery, the artificial heart has functioned well in over a hundred cases (Lammermeir *et al.*, 1988; Hill, 1989).

It follows that the term extracorporeal circulation has become a misnomer because some of the equipment is intracorporeal. The broader term, artificial circulation, is more appropriate. A bewildering number of applications of artificial circulation have appeared in the literature and many more will undoubtedly emerge in the future. The technology of the artificial kidney is as much a part of artificial circulation techniques as the ones that will be described here. Thus, it appears that a rather broad field of possible applications of artificial circulation techniques is at hand. This area is suited quite well for the emergence of a new medical specialty.

Heart–lung machine for surgery

The heart–lung machine as it is used daily in heart surgery is quite safe. Where in the past the mortality of using cardiopulmonary bypass was high, it has now dropped to less than 0.5%. However, if close attention is paid to the function of several of the vital organs after surgery, it is found that in a high percentage of the patients severe damage may be inflicted by the bypass. The pulmonary function is often compromised after the use of the heart–lung machine. At close inspection, minor damage to the brain is common as well. Blood damage is inevitable and can be quite serious. Clearly, further refinements of the heart–lung machine are welcome.

The roller pump has been difficult to improve over the years. It causes little damage to the blood, is extremely reliable and can easily be operated by hand in case of power failure. However, during circumstances of prolonged application, parts of the tubing contained within the housing of the pump degenerate and small particles embolize to the blood stream. This process, which is called spallation, becomes more harmful the longer the bypass is applied.

The centrifugal or impeller pump is not plagued by this complication. In careful studies it was also demonstrated that after operation for some 16 h, blood damage caused by the impeller pump was significantly less than in the case where a roller pump was employed (Hoerr *et al.*, 1987). Another advantage off the impeller pump is that pulsations can be generated in the bypass circuit more easily. Furthermore, the impeller pump is smaller and can be positioned closer to the patient, an important advantage for long-term bypass systems. Thus, it is predictable that the use of the impeller pump will overshadow that of the roller pump.

Another pump type that came into use recently is the Archimedean pump. Although applied during the early years of the development of the heart–lung machine, it has not been in use for many years. However, it has now been incorporated in an intracorporeal left heart bypass system that actually pumps the blood from the left ventricle into the aorta (Wampler *et al.*, 1988). It is capable of pumping flows of up to 4 l min^{-1} causing little blood damage. It may be adapted and used again for regular heart–lung machines. Electromagnetically powered flow would be the least traumatic. It has not been used in clinical extracorporeal circulation as yet but surely deserves attention.

Claims on the benefits of altering the commonly employed non-pulsatile flow of the roller pump and the impeller pump to pulsatile flow continue to cause much controversy. However, more evidence is accumulating that pulsations are of importance (Taylor, 1988). Thus, it seems reasonable to pursue the application of pulse generators during the use of cardiopulmonary bypass. Where this was rather difficult with the roller pumps, it is quite easy when an impeller pump is used. It is to be expected that in future developments the goal will not be just to generate pulsations but to imitate the natural pulse wave as closely as possible.

The bubble oxygenator, which until recently was used nearly universally for short-term cardiopulmonary bypasses, is gradually being replaced by membrane oxygenators. Much controversy was focused during the last decade on the need to pursue this replacement. In the early days, when membrane oxygenators were unreliable, expensive and bulky, there was ample ground for these discussions. However, since the membrane oxygenators have now reached a stage of development where they are small, reliable and relatively inexpensive and disposable, there is little reason to continue to use bubble oxygenators. Recent studies have clearly shown that the incidence of microembolism in membrane oxygenators is less than in bubble oxygenators (Blauth *et al.*, 1986). Further developments in membrane technology and the construction of the oxygenator will surely make these devices even better. One of the goals should be to decrease the priming volume.

The use of filters in the bypass circuit is commonly accepted. The need for filtering the cardiotomy suction blood and fluids transfused into the bypass circuit was never under discussion. However, the wisdom of filtering the arterial blood return line has been debated for many years. With the development of modern filters, it is now clear that they do decrease the embolus load on the patient rather than cause embolization like the older filter types did. Modern filters are also designed specifically to remove air bubbles even when they are of very small size. Future developments will probably focus on the automatic purging of air that is captured in these filters during cardiopulmonary bypass (Marshall, 1988). The application of electromagnetic forces for the removal of microemboli needs further investigation.

In modern bypass circuits, the heat exchanger is usually an integral part of the oxygenator. The devices function well and allow for rapid cooling. However, the re-warming period is still rather long and this can prove cumbersome in some heart operations. If deeper hypothermia will come into use in the future, the ability of heat exchangers to increase the blood temperature faster but without causing damage could become important. In this context, the application of microwave techniques to heat blood is promising (Gazzaniga *et al.*, 1988).

It has been recognized for some time that the major source of blood damage is the suctioning of spilled blood from the operative area back into the heart–lung machine. The mixture of air with blood in the suction line is the culprit. Rather intricate suction tips have been designed to decrease this air mixing as much as possible and indeed, if carefully applied, blood damage decreases. Further developments in material technology may lead to bypass circuits with inner surface characteristics that preclude the use of heparin. The volume of spilled blood will then decrease but will still be higher than blood loss observed in general surgery. Thus, more emphasis will be placed on cell saving techniques where blood is suctioned from the operative field but purified before returning it to the bypass circuit. This process is at present rather time consuming.

Cardiac preservation techniques during heart surgery have greatly improved over the last few years. Cooling of the heart is now generally preferred to decrease damage to the myocardium during clamping of the aorta. The equipment used to cool the heart has undergone extensive development and now apparatus is available where the blood can be cooled and re-warmed at will and where mixtures can be prepared with predetermined amounts of blood and non-blood primes. The cannulation technique on the operating table itself is usually for intra-aortic perfusion but recent development may lead to wider acceptance of coronary sinus retrograde perfusion. It is to be expected that a combination of cannulation systems will be developed where the myocardium can be cooled either via the coronary arteries or via the coronary veins or both. At present, most surgeons simply remove the aortic clamp to rewarm the heart and to initiate cardiac action again. In the future it may be found that more elaborate techniques to re-warm the heart are of benefit.

Cannulation techniques for modern heart surgery seem to have reached a stable point. During the early days of heart surgery, the femoral artery was used most commonly for blood return. Over the last 15–20 years, however, the aorta has been the preferred site for cannulation for blood return. As the circuit of the heart–lung machine has improved over the years, the incidence of neurological complications has decreased. If at present an unexpected neurological calamity does occur, postoperatively, it is believed to be due to dislodgement of embolic material either from the heart or from manipulation of the ascending aorta including insertion of the blood return cannula. In an effort to decrease neurological complications further, it is foreseeable that the blood return cannulation technique will be changed. Blood can be returned either into the femoral artery again, into a subclavian or axillary artery or into the descending aorta by using a longer cannula so that the tip resides beyond the aortic arch. The use of the femoral artery is not to be encouraged, because in present day patients, arteriosclerosis is usually advanced and the iliofemoral vascular system is commonly involved.

In-line laboratory equipment has been developed quite rapidly over the last few years. At present, apparatus is available that continuously measures the pH, $P\text{O}_2$, $P\text{CO}_2$, haematocrit, potassium and calcium levels (Parault, 1988). However, the equipment is expensive. Yet, it seems beyond doubt that in the future such in-line laboratory measurements will become routine. Obviously, better control can be exerted over the condition of the patient. By improving the quality of the cardiopulmonary bypass one foresees less complications in the postoperative period. Continued savings resulting from less incidence of complications will amply justify the increased cost of laboratory equipment.

Cardiopulmonary bypass continues to cause widespread alterations in the blood. Shortly after bypass is started, fibrinogen deposits on the artificial surfaces (Vroman, Adams and Klings, 1975). This layer of fibrinogen causes platelets and white cells to adhere and to clump together (Salzman,

Lindon and Brier, 1977). Free floating aggregates of platelets and white blood cells are found as well (Taylor, 1987). In the process, the cells seem to be activated and release possible harmful products. This in turn can lead to intravascular blood coagulation and vasospasm (Stenach, Cottrell and Fisher, 1987). The need to heparinize the patient during artificial circulation is a further burden on the organism. This is especially true in those cases where assisted circulation is applied for prolonged periods of time. Bleeding becomes an often intolerable complication (Pesenti, Kolobow and Gattinoni, 1988). Despite extensive research in developing a biocompatible surface for artificial circulation equipment, few changes have occurred since the early days of the use of cardiopulmonary bypass. This is certainly true for the routine equipment used during heart surgery. Several techniques have been developed to bond heparin to blood facing materials. Early experience was disappointing in that the anti-clotting characteristics of such materials were of only short duration. Recent improvements in heparin bonding techniques have resulted in more acceptable surfaces for prolonged bypass without heparin (Bindslev, 1988).

An alternative approach to decreasing the above described changes in the blood as it comes into contact with foreign surfaces is to provide pharmacological inhibition of pathological changes in the formed blood elements. Research so far has focused primarily on prostaglandins and their ability to preserve platelet function (Taylor, 1987). The prostaglandins themselves cause too much vasodilatation but new analogues are being developed that apparently do not carry this disadvantage. Further research will undoubtedly be directed towards development of other pharmacological products with similar actions. These medications will be supplied in the future as a routine prophylactic measure in patients undergoing cardiopulmonary bypass or other artificial bypass techniques in an effort to prevent or at least minimize activation of formed blood elements.

As the equipment for cardiopulmonary bypass undergoes further improvements, it is to be hoped that the priming volume of the blood circuit will decrease further. At present, there are still situations where the non-blood prime causes too much dilution so that the haemoglobin falls to dangerously low levels and the oxygen carrying capacity of the blood becomes insufficient. In this context, research to develop clinically acceptable artificial blood is important. Up until now, the concentration of the artificial haemoglobin in the fluid could not be raised high enough to obtain satisfactory oxygen carrying capacity because it increased the oncotic pressure too much. However, with recent efforts to encapsulate haemoglobin within artificial cells, this problem is closer to being resolved (Zheng *et al.*, 1988). If artificial blood could be used safely in routine heart surgery, it would further decrease the need for blood transfusions.

Up until now, the heart–lung machine system in most cases is open to air. Even with the introduction of the membrane oxygenator, cardiopulmonary bypass is often operated with an open blood to air level. It is hoped that in the future this will change and that a completely closed system will evolve. It can also be foreseen that the entire cardiopulmonary bypass system would be pre-assembled and primed by the manufacturer. This would further reduce the incidence of bacterial contamination of the heart–lung machine circuits.

In most cases, the body temperature of the patients is allowed to drop to around 30°C during cardiopulmonary bypass. At that point, cooling provides for excellent protection against temporary hypoperfusion of the organism. It is actually possible that too much perfusion is offered to the patient which is evident in the high oxygen saturation of the returning venous blood. In the future, it may be worthwhile to investigate the application of deeper hypothermia. Hypothermia was used extensively in the past. It was abandoned as the heart–lung machine became safer to use at higher flows. However, the higher the bypass flow is, the more blood will be exposed to foreign surfaces per unit of time. This leads to more blood damage and increases the embolus load. If hypothermia techniques could be improved and made practical, the resulting decrease of bypass flow would certainly be beneficial. Problems relating to the acid–base balance, microcirculation and tissue metabolism during deep hypothermia need to be resolved.

The safeguarding of vital organs should be another goal for further studies. Even though the incidence of gross neurological abnormalities is low, minor complications that can be attributed to brain damage are common. Detailed examination of the psychological status frequently indicates postoperative changes. The function of the lungs, if measured carefully, is nearly always impaired after the use of the heart–lung machine. Although the majority of these abnormalities disappear after several weeks, in some cases pulmonary changes escalate to culminate in acute respiratory distress syndrome, a condition carrying a high mortality. Mild changes in kidney function are common as well. Observation on the effect of bypass on other organs and organ systems such as the liver, the pancreas, the gastrointestinal tract and the peripheral nerves are sparse. Much effort should be directed towards studying more closely the changes caused by the heart–lung machine on separate organs. Once such changes are identified, efforts can be undertaken to prevent damage.

The one organ that stands out in particular is the lung. The lungs uniformly undergo damage as a result of the heart–lung machine. It is surprising to see the difference in the attention paid to trying to protect the heart from damage as opposed to measures taken to do the same for the lung. The lung circulation during heart surgery is altered significantly in that most of the blood flow through the lungs via the pulmonary artery is discontinued. Thus, during cardiopulmonary bypass, the lungs depend on the bronchial circulation which is variable. Whether the lungs derive nourishment from pulmonary arterial blood is not clearly known. It may well be that selective deep cooling of the lungs such as is done for the heart is of benefit. Also, perfusion via the pulmonary arteries may be effective in preventing pathological changes in the lungs during cardiopulmonary bypass. Further research in this area is indicated.

The blood circuit used for cardiopulmonary bypass could be simplified if the natural lungs were used as an oxygenator. In the early days of heart surgery, the lungs were successfully used to preclude artificial oxygenation. In those days, extracorporeal oxygenation caused excessive blood damage. As better oxygenators became available, the use of the natural lungs for oxygenation was abandoned. However, since heart surgery has now developed into a specialty where most of the operations do not require opening of the heart cavities, it seems attractive to once more consider using the natural lungs for oxygenation. Some efforts in this direction have proven to be successful (Berglin *et al.*, 1986).

A number of possible advantages of such a system are evident. The surface area of foreign material exposed to the blood would be greatly decreased. This could lead to less change in the formed elements of the blood which in turn would decrease the release of toxic products and result in less bleeding after surgery. It is easier to coat such a blood circuit with heparin making heparinization unnecessary. The number of gaseous microemboli would be less. The cost of the cardiopulmonary bypass system would be decreased. The tubing system is better suited to transform to a long-term assist system. The cannulation technique is somewhat more complicated but in practice, this does not seem to be much of a problem to those who have tried it (Berglin *et al.*, 1986).

Keeping the above considerations in mind, one envisions the heart–lung machine of the future (American Heart Association, 1981) to be coated on the inside with heparin (Anderson, O'Hare and Fritz, 1970), equipped with an impeller pump and a sophisticated pulsatile device to imitate the natural pulse closely (Berglin *et al.*, 1986), to come without an oxygenator and thus have a small priming volume (Bindslev, 1988), to have all the usual laboratory studies sampled from in line systems (Blauth *et al.*, 1986) and to have a low bypass flow because of deeper hypothermia. It is hoped that such a system will cause less damage to patients.

To closely supervise cardiopulmonary bypass computer application would be of great value. If one analyses the many life or death decisions that need to be made by perfusionists, surgeons, and anaesthetists, it is surprising indeed that computer use has not gained wider acceptance in this field. Especially if monitoring, including laboratory studies becomes more refined, these variables should all be fed into a computer. The computer can display the values continuously to all those who make decisions. It can correlate the relevant factors to reach decisions. Many of these could actually be made by the computer and only be supervised by the persons involved in the process. For instance, if a sensor were to identify an increase in the incidence of microbubbles in the arterial line, this signal would be sent to the computer and cause it to query the gas flow rate, the level of the blood in the oxygenator, the level of the blood in the cardiotomy reservoir and other related factors. The computer could then discover that one of these factors actually causes the increase of arterial air emboli. If all this were presented to the heart–lung machine operator, fine tuning cardiopulmonary bypass would be feasible to a much greater extent than is possible at present (Anderson, O'Hare and Fritz, 1970; Hayes, 1987). Therefore, it is expected that the use of computers in cardiopulmonary bypass will increase significantly.

The heart–lung machine as an assist device

During the early development it was recognized that the heart–lung machine could be used to treat intractable heart failure and cardiogenic shock. However, in this setting, the bypass needs to be applied for prolonged periods of time and the early heart–lung machines caused too much damage to tolerate prolonged bypass. With the improvement of the blood circuit and especially the oxygenator, such extended applications are now possible. Techniques to attach heparin to the inner surface of the bypass circuit would be of great advantage since excessive bleeding is one of the major problems of long-term bypass (Bindslev, 1988). Recently developed transcutaneous techniques of cannulation of both the arterial and venous system have also greatly advanced the emergency application of the heart–lung machine (Phillips *et al.*, 1989). The technology of cannula fabrication and design has improved significantly resulting in a decrease of the wall thickness of cannulas. Such seemingly minor developments, nevertheless, can have a great impact on the possible application of bypass techniques in a variety of pathological conditions.

One area where artificial circulation can be significant is in the treatment of myocardial infarction. The number of patients in possible life threatening situations is much larger than that encountered in heart surgery. It is estimated that more than half a million people die each year in the United States from myocardial infarction (American Heart Association, 1981). The mortality of cardiogenic shock, if treated by medical means alone, is in excess of 95% (Haddy, 1970). Significant change of attitude is evolving in the approach towards patients with acute myocardial infarction. It is now considered an emergency situation where the goal of the immediate management of the patient is an exact knowledge of the anatomy of the coronary arteries and a plan for treatment. Where these patients used to be given symptomatic treatment with the hope for recovery, nowaday, they are rushed to the heart catheterization laboratory, for a coronary angiography, to establish the cause of the myocardial infarction. Then they undergo either balloon dilatation or coronary bypass operations to restore the blood circulation to the heart. Simultaneously, the need for speedy diagnosis and transport to a major health centre is being stressed. If somewhere along this process the heart is incapable of maintaining the circulation adequately, the need arises for an emergency artificial bypass. With the above indicated improvements in bypass techniques, the interest in the use of standard cardiopulmonary bypass for this purpose has been revived. The major advantage of this type of bypass is the ease of cannulation. All that is needed is a blood outflow cannula within a major vein and a blood return cannula inserted into a major artery. These is no need for major surgery. In the past, extensive research was directed towards other bypass systems where artificial oxygenation was not needed. These efforts were needed because safe oxygenation was impossible for long-term applications. With better oxygenators, it is now believed that standard cardiopulmonary bypass will serve well in the treatment of cardiogenic shock.

An important factor in this context is often overlooked: the fate of the heart itself. Cardiopulmonary bypass through peripheral cannulation can undoubtedly improve the circulation. But as it does, the afterload on the left ventricle is increased. This in turn may aggravate the failure of the left ventricle to empty itself and cause damage to the heart and pulmonary oedema. The danger of left ventricular overdistension was well recognized in the early years of assisted circulation (Zwart *et al.*, 1973). Fortunately it is re-emphasized in more recent literature, with the more frequent use of transcutaneous cardiopulmonary bypass. To decompress the left ventricle under these circumstances one can apply external cardiac massage. Obviously, such cannot be done over long periods of time and not during heart catheterization or surgery. Other techniques include direct decompression of the left ventricle with cannulae (Dennis *et al.*, 1962; Zwart, 1966), or rendering the pulmonary artery valve incompetent with a spring-like device (Kolobow *et al.*, 1988). Another easily available technique to decompress the left ventricle is to use counterpulsation while the bypass is applied. This may have the additional advantage of increased blood flow to the coronary arteries (Phillips *et al.*, 1989).

Future application of transcutaneous cardiopulmonary bypass will most likely be studied as part of the treatment of myocardial infarction. Moreover, it begins to play a role in the heart catheterization laboratory as a standby technique, in cases of sudden cardiac deterioration. Some even start cardiopulmonary bypass before the heart catheterization to prevent cardiac catastrophies (Vogel, Lommaso and Gundry, 1988). The bypass can be used after heart surgery if the heart needs to be further resuscitated. Since with an open chest any kind of cannulation is possible, it is more likely that under these circumstances a combination of right and left heart bypass will be used. The bypass system also has been used to assist patients awaiting heart transplantation who develop intractable cardiac failure (Hill, 1989). Here, as in other prolonged applications of the cardiopulmonary bypass technique, complications such as bleeding, infection and blood damage continue to be a problem. With further improvements of equipment, many of these problems may be circumvented.

Another application of transcutaneous cardiopulmonary bypass it to treat severe pulmonary failure in those patients who are expected to recover. In newborn babies, the bypass can be effective in some 50–90% of the cases depending on the underlying disease process (Snider *et al.*, 1988). In adults, the bypass is applied to patients with acute respiratory distress syndrome. The mortality rate of this severe pulmonary dysfunction of unknown cause is 80–90% if treated medically. Transcutaneous cardiopulmonary bypass can be life saving in these patients. When used for assistance to the failing lung, the bypass is usually called ECMO, an acronym for extracorporeal membrane oxygenation. The name stems from the days when membrane oxygenators were used in exceptional circumstances only. The bypass circuit may be different from the usual cardiopulmonary bypass, it can be venoarterial, arteriovenous, or venoveno or arterial-arterial. Much lower bypass flows are also used (Pesenti, Kolobow and Gattinoni, 1988). It was recognized that the transfer of oxygen to the blood could still be effected by the patient's lungs but at much lower oxygen concentration and inflation pressures and with less breathing frequency. The CO_2 removal is carried out primarily by the artificial lung. Here, as in other long-term applications of bypass systems, the ability to attach heparin to the plastic surfaces would significantly decrease major complications such as profuse bleeding.

Other circulatory assist devices

The most widely accepted mechanical assist device is intra-aortic balloon counterpulsation. This assist method originated as an artificial circulation technique where blood was actually removed from the femoral artery during systole and pumped back during diastole. Therefore, and because it is such an intricate part of resuscitating the failing heart, it is included in this discussion. Counterpulsation has been proven effective for the failing heart. However, it should be realized that at all times, a minimum cardiac output of about 1–2 l min^{-1} should be present for effective counterpulsation technique. It is a true assist device, and it cannot substitute the failing heart. With this limitation in mind, it is clear that there is ample room for application of alternate artificial circulation techniques. The development of methods other than the cardiopulmonary bypass itself was greatly stimulated during the last 20 years because of unacceptable blood damage caused by prolonged use of the heart–lung machine. Additional advantages emerged as different bypass techniques were studied.

Left heart bypass has received most attention as a mechanical means to assist the failing heart. It has the advantage of decompressing the left ventricle while at the same time maintaining the circulation, if necessary, entirely artificially. In left heart bypass blood is removed from either the left atrium or the left ventricle or from both and it is returned to the arterial circulation. It is capable of maintaining the circulation even during ventricular fibrillation. Under these circumstances, the circulation is of poor quality. However, for short periods of time, the bypass can be life saving.

Since the early development of left heart bypass, the problem of how to reach the left side of the heart without major surgery posed a hurdle. Intricate techniques were designed to cannulate the left side of the heart without thoracotomy (Dennis *et al.*, 1962; Zwart, 1966). One such technique employed a large bore catheter that was inserted via a peripheral vein and advanced into the right atrium, manipulated past a perforation in the atrial septum and advanced into the left atrium (Dennis *et al.*, 1962). Extensive experimental studies were undertaken providing evidence of the usefulness of this method in assisting the failing heart. The obvious drawback is the difficult cannulation technique with the risk of perforating the heart itself and thereby causing tamponade. Another obvious disadvantage is that shunting may occur from the right to the left atrium around the cannula tip especially if suction is applied to the left atrium (Zwart, 1966). This desaturation renders the bypass impractical under circumstances of left heart failure.

An alternative technique to reach the left side of the heart employs a cannula that is inserted via a peripheral artery and advanced past the aortic valve into the left ventricle (Zwart, 1966). This left heart bypass technique proved to be easy to carry out. However, over the years it could not be applied clinically because of the lack of suitable cannulas. Since the arterial system is small bored, the outside diameter of a catheter inserted via a peripheral artery also has to be small. Thus, to obtain a reasonable outflow from such a cannula, the wall thickness must be, at most 0.3 mm. Companies were incapable of producing such cannulas and thus the technique did not become widely accepted. More recently, however, the left ventricular drainage cannulas are used more often, especially in combination with transcutaneous cardiopulmonary bypass (Rose *et al.*, 1989).

An even more recent addition to left heart bypass has been an intravascular pump that actually removes the blood directly from the left ventricle and deposits it into the descending aorta (Wampler *et al.*, 1988). This catheter mounted blood pump is of the Archimedean type. It is attached to the tip of the catheter and has an inlet that is to be positioned within the left ventricle by advancing it via a peripheral artery past the aortic valve. The outlet of the pump is in the descending aorta. The pump is powered by a wire contained in the catheter to position the pump in the left ventricle. The pump is so bulky that it has to be inserted via a cutdown on a femoral artery, a transcutaneous technique has not been developed yet. The pump is capable of delivering flows of up to 4 l min^{-1} for prolonged periods of time without causing undue blood damage. It is a near ideal assist device. The left ventricle is decompressed effectively. The blood flow passages are very short and entirely contained within the body. Thus, there is little chance of infection and bleeding is no major problem either. It is anticipated that this pumping device will be used widely for the treatment of cardiogenic shock, but it remains to be seen whether left heart bypass will improve the outcome.

Left heart bypass has been envisioned to treat heart failure on a permanent basis as well. As an alternative to a complete artificial heart or heart transplant, it certainly does have appeal. During heart failure, often only the left side is dysfunctioning while the right side continues to perform adequately. As more experience was gained with mechanical treatment of heart failure, it became apparent that this isolated failure of the left ventricle is not as common as it was thought to be. It is now estimated that in half the cases, the right ventricle fails as well (Pennington *et al.*, 1988).

However, for those patients where isolated left ventricular failure occurs, long-term application of the left heart bypass system seems a good alternative to complete replacement of the heart. Much research has been directed towards implantable, permanent left heart bypass. Recent reports indicate that such systems are now available. They are safe, effective and can be powered entirely by implanted batteries that are recharged with transcutaneous techniques (Portner *et al.*, 1989). The bypass pumps employed are much like those used for the artificial heart. They are powered by electrical current and use pusher plate arrangements to empty a ventricle type pump. The pumps need an inlet and an outlet valve.

If right ventricular failure occurs, an additional bypass has to be instituted to assist the right side. It is easy to insert a right ventricular bypass via peripheral cannulation. Blood is removed from the right ventricle and returned into the pulmonary artery (Zwart, Kralios and Kolff, 1972). An even simpler way to assist the right ventricle is to initiate transcutaneous cardiopulmonary bypass. This has become an option since the availability of better oxygenators that cause less blood damage. Several cases have been published where an implantable right heart bypass system was added to a previously implanted left bypass pump, thus, effectively creating a total artificial heart with the natural heart in place (Pennington *et al.*, 1988). In some cases it is indicated to use a right heart bypass pump by itself without the necessity to assist the left ventricle. During heart surgery, as the heart is weaned off the heart–lung machine, there are instances where the right ventricle fails more than the left ventricle. In those cases, a cannulation system from the right atrium to the pulmonary artery is the simplest solution.

As the different bypasses were developed it became apparent that rather than to champion one particular technique, it was better to have them all available and use proper combinations. The most frequent scenario calls for the use of intra-aortic balloon counterpulsation initially to be followed by a left heart bypass and eventually if need be, a right heart bypass. This is accepted treatment during heart surgery. The future will tell whether such is true for other indications such as resuscitation after myocardial infarction as well.

Artificial hearts

The artificial heart continues to be a worthwhile alternative to heart transplantation. The scarce supply of donor hearts necessitates further research in this field. If a safe artificial heart were available, it would also obviate many of the ethical problems surrounding transplantations. Much experience has been gained in the last few years with the artificial heart in humans. In those cases where the artificial heart was used as an intended permanent replacement, the early results were disappointing (Gazzaniga *et al.*, 1988). The major problems encountered were thrombosis within the artificial heart with resulting embolization causing severe neurological abnormalities and infection. The early artificial heart implantations generated intense reactions from the public. As is often the case, interest soon waned. The steady flow of implantations that have occurred since escaped publicity. More than 100 clinical implantations have been carried out where the artificial heart was used to maintain life while a patient awaited heart transplantation (Lammermeir *et al.*, 1988). In these short-term applications, the artificial heart functioned satisfactorily. It is to be envisioned that acceptable long-term artificial hearts will become available for use as an alternative to heart transplantation.

A few basic technical considerations have been learned from clinical experience with the artificial heart. Compressed gas driven devices seem to be impractical for long-term application. The constant movement that inevitably occurs in the drive line that transmits the high pressure pulses causes a pathway for infection. Electrical power is better for long-term application of the artificial heart. With existing technology, it is possible to transmit enough electrical energy transcutaneously to energize an artificial heart for normal use (Davis *et al.*, 1989). Transmission occurs via the intact skin by electrical coupling using coils that are embedded subcutaneously and placed over the skin in that same area. It is expected that patients will use implanted batteries to power the artificial heart during the daytime. While asleep, the batteries have to be recharged. When the patient wakes up, they are recharged and ready to power the artificial heart another day. A major source of infection would thereby be eliminated. By improving the design of the artificial heart blood handling areas, it is hoped that thrombosis will decrease and that thereby emboli damaging peripheral organs such as the brain, will occur infrequently. This search for a better design will be facilitated as better materials become available. Not only will this decrease the incidence of thrombosis, it will also improve durability.

Efforts to replace the functioning heart have so far inspired the fabrication of pumps that imitate the natural heart. However, all that is needed is a driving force that transports blood from the venous to the arterial site. A variety of pumps that are non-pulsatile and different in configuration from the natural heart could be tested out for this purpose. Apparently, long-term application of non-pulsatile flow can be tolerated (Nose, 1988). Impeller pumps, because of their simplicity, seem an attractive alternative for cardiac function. Such pumps are easier to build and will probably last longer. They are powered electrically and could be used with battery systems that are presently available. It can be envisioned that a set of impellers positioned within the aorta and the pulmonary artery could effectively substitute the pumping function of the entire heart. Insertion of such pump units would be relatively simple. The impeller could conceivably be kept in place within the major vessels by electromagnetic forces from coils placed around the arteries.

Exciting times are ahead of us. Artificial circulation first envisioned at the beginning of the nineteenth century seems to only just outgrow infancy near the end of the twentieth century. Much remains to be done.

References

American Heart Association (1981) *Heart Facts*, American Heart Association, Dallas

Anderson, R.M., O'Hare, J.E. and Fritz, J.M. (1970) Automatic demand pump for cardiopulmonary bypass. *Annals of Thoracic Surgery*, **10**, 424

Berglin, E., Sandin, O., Windstedt, P. and William-Olsson, G. (1986) Extracorporeal circulation without an oxygenator in coronary bypass surgery. *Journal of Thoracic and Cardiovascular Surgery*, **92**, 306

Bindslev, L. (1988) Adult ECMO performed with surface-heparinized equipment, *Transactions of the American Society for Artificial Internal Organs*, **34**, 1009

Blauth, C., Kohner, E.M., Arnold, J. and Taylor, K.M. (1986) Retinal microembolism during cardiopulmonary bypass demonstrated by fluorescein angiography. *Lancet*, **ii**, 837

Brown-Seguard, E. (1858) Recherches experimentales sur les proprietes physiologiques et les usages du sang rouge et du sand noir et leurs principaux elements gazeux: l'oxygene et l'oxide carbonique. *Journal de Physiologie de l'Homme (Paris)*, **1**, 95, 353, 729

Davis, P.K., Rosenberg, G., Snyder, A.J. and Pierce, W.S. (1989) Current status of permanent total artificial hearts. *Annals of Thoracic Surgery*, **47**, 172

Dennis, C., Hall, D.F., Moreno, J.R. and Sennino, A. (1962) Left atrial cannulation without thoracotomy for total left heart bypass. *Acta Chirurgica Scandinavica*, **123**, 267

Dennis, C., Spring, D.S., Nelson, G.E., *et al.* (1951) Development of pump oxyengator to replace the heart and the lungs, an apparatus applicable to human patients and application to one case. *Annals of Surgery*, **134**, 709

DeVries, W.C., Anderson, J.L. and Zoyce, L.D. (1986) Clinical use of the total artificial heart. *New England Journal of Medicine*, **310**, 273

Gazzaniga, A.B., Day, A., Weber, C., *et al.* (1988) The microwave oven as a safe and rapid blood warmer. *Transactions of the American Society for Artificial Internal Organs*, **76**, (Abstract)

Gibbon, J.H. (1937) Artificial maintenance of circulation during experimental occlusion of the pulmonary artery. *Archives of Surgery*, **34**, 1105

Gibbon, J.H., Miller, B.J. and Feinberg, C. (1953) An improved mechanical heart and lung apparatus. *Medical Clinics of North America*, **37**, 1603

Haddy, F.J. (1970) Pathophysiology and therapy of the shock of myocardial infarction. *Annals of Internal Medicine*, **73**, 809

Hayes, R.S. (1987) Computerized data acquisition and data management for the open heart patient. *Journal of Extracorporeal Technology*, **19**, 287

Hill, J.D. (1989) Bridging to cardiac transplantation. *Annals of Thoracic Surgery*, **47**, 167

Hoerr, H.R., Kraemer, M.F., Williams, J.L., *et al.* (1987) In vitro comparison of the blood handling by the constrained vortex and twin roller blood pumps. *Journal of Extracorporeal Technology*, **19**, 316

Kolff, W.J. and Berk, H.T.J. (1944) Artificial kidney: dializer with great area. *Acta Medica Scandinavica*, **117**, 121

Kolobow, T., Rossi, F., Borelli, M., and Foti, G. (1988) Long term closed chest partial and total cardiopulmonary bypass by peripheral cannulation. *Transactions of the American Society for Artificial Internal Organs*, Abstract I

Lammermeier, D., Frazier, O.H., Iso, S.R. and Cooley, D.A. (1988) Total artificial hearts and ventricular assist devices as bridges to heart transplantation. *Texas Medicine*, **84**, 56

Le Gallois, J.J.C. (1813) *Experiences sur le principe de la vie.* D'Hautel, Paris. (Experiments on the Principles of Life, Translation M.C. and J.C. Nancrede, Thomas, Philadelphia)

McLean, J. (1959) The discovery of heparin. *Circulation*, **19**, 75

Marshall, L. (1988) Filtration in cardiopulmonary bypass: past, present and future. *Perfusion*, **3**, 135

Mortensen, J.D. (1987) An intravenacaval blood gas exchange device. *Transactions of the American Society for Artificial Internal Organs*, **33**, 570

Nose, Y. (1988) The need for a non-pulsatile pumping system. *Artificial Organs*, **12**, 113

Parault, B. (1988) Technique for improved patient care: initial experience with the GEM-6. *Journal of Extracorporeal Technology*, **20**, 47

Pennington, D.G., Kanter, K.R., McBride, L.R. and Willman, V. (1988) Seven year experience with the Pierce–Donachy ventricle ventricular assist device. *Journal of Thoracic and Cardiovascular Surgery*, **96**, 901

Pesenti, A., Kolobow, T. and Gattinoni, L. (1988) Extracorporeal respiratory support in the adult. *Transactions of the American Society for Artificial Internal Organs*, **34**, 1006

Phillips, S.J., Zeff, R.H., Konstakworn, C., *et al.* (1989) Percutaneous cardiopulmonary bypass: application and indication for use. *Annals of Thoracic Surgery*, **47**, 121

Portner, P.M., Oyer, P.E., Pennington, D.G. and Zassawalla, J.S. (1989) Implantable electrical left ventricular assist system: bridge to transplantation and the future. *American Thoracic Surgery*, **47**, 142

Rose, D.M., Connolly, M., Cunningham, J.N. and Spencer, F.C. (1989) Technique and results with a roller pump left and right heart assist device. *Annals of Thoracic Surgery*, **47**, 124

Salzman, E.W., Lindon, J. and Brier, D. (1977) Surface induced platelet adhesion: aggregation and release. *Annals New York Academy of Science*, **283**, 114

Snider, M.T., Campbell, D.B., Kafke, W.A., *et al.* (1988) Venovenous perfusion of adults and children with severe acute respiratory distress syndrome. *Transactions of the American Society for Artificial Internal Organs*, **34**, 1014

Stenach, N., Cottrell, E.D. and Fisher, C.A. (1987) Preservation of canine platelets with iloprost during extracorporeal circulation. *Journal of Extracorporeal Technology*, **19**, 258

Taylor, K.M. (1987) Prostacyclin therapy during cardiopulmonary bypass – is it beneficial? *Perfusion*, **2**, 1

Taylor, K.M. (1988) Vasopressor release and multiple organ failure in cardiac surgery. *Perfusion*, **3**, 1

Vogel, R.A., Iommaso, C.L. and Gundry, S.R. (1988) Initial experience with coronary angioplasty and aortic valvuloplasty using elective semipercutaneous cardiopulmonary support. *American Journal of Cardiology*, **62**, 811

von Frey, M. and Gruber, M. (1885) Untersuchunsen über den Stoffwechsel isolierter Organe. Ein Respirations-Apparat fur isolierter Organe. *Virchow's Archives*, **9**, 519

Vroman, L., Adams, A.L. and Klings, M. (1975) Fibrinogen globulin, albumin and plasma at interfaces. *Advances in Chemistry*, **145**, 255

Wampler, R.K., Moise, J.C., Frasier, O.H. and Olsen, D.B. (1988) In vivo evaluation of a peripheral vascular access axial flow blood pump. *Transaction of the American Society for Artificial Internal Organs*, **34**, 450

Zhens, S., Borwankar, C., Beissinger, R. and Wassan, D. (1988) A multiple emulsion of hemoglobin-in-oil-in-water as a blood surrogate. *Transaction of the American Society for Artificial Internal Organs*, (Abstract)

Zwart, H.H.J. (1966) Complete left heart bypass without thoracotomy, an experimental study in dogs. *Thesis*, S.O.L. Offset, Amsterdam, The Netherlands

Zwart, H.H.J., Kralios, A.C. and Kolff, W.J. (1972) Effects of right heart bypass on acute ventricular failure with and without ventricular fibrillation. *Chest*, **61**, 159

Zwart, H.H.J., Kralios, A., Backman, D.K., *et al.* (1973) The effects of transarterial left ventricular bypass on hemodynamics of the failing left ventricle in sheep. *Annals of Surgery*, **178**, 710

Index

Acidosis, metabolic, 11, 12, 16, 40, 72, 89, 98, 216
ACTH (adrenocorticotropic hormone), 11, 218
Acyclovir, 197–198, 204, 306
Adenosine, 89, 93, 102
  in cardioplegia, 109
  and kidney, 179
  in reperfusion, 116
Adenosine triphosphate (ATP), 88, 89–90, 93, 102, 115
  in brain, 232
  in cardioplegia, 108–109
Adrenaline (epinephrine), 85, 218, 247
Adult respiratory distress syndrome, 162–163, 171, 315, 324, 326
Advancing front theory of oxygen transfer, 44–46
Aerobic metabolism, 88
Air embolism, 25, 186
Air venting, 60
Albumin, 74, 113, 170
Aldosterone, 10, 218
Alfentanil, 80, 140
Alkalosis, 40
Allopurinol, 91, 112
Alpha-adrenergic blockade, 10, 11, 12, 83, 84
Alpha-2-antiplasmin, 17
Aminoglycoside, 200
Amphotericin B, 306
Amylase, pancreatic, 220
Anaerobic metabolism, 11, 16, 88, 89, 98, 102, 115, 216
  neonatal, 118
Anaesthesia, 10, 78–86
  cerebral dysfunction and, 186, 189
  contamination of, 66
Anaphylotoxins, complement-derived, 150, 156, 159, 160, 163–165, 171
  in disease processes, 161–163
Angiotensin II, 10, 179, 180, 218
Antiarrhythmic drugs, 79
Antibiotic prophylaxis, pre-transplantation, 196, 197–198, 202, 303, 306
Anticoagulant agents, 79
  citrate toxicity, 151
  see also Heparin
Antidiuretic hormone, 218
Antifoam, 25
Antifungal prophylaxis, preoperative, 196, 202
Antiplatelet drugs, 79, 146
Antithrombin III, 17–18, 40
Aprotinin, 18, 147
Archimedean pump, 322, 327
Arterial line filtration, 61–63
  cerebral dysfunction and, 61, 62, 190
Arteriovenous difference, 13–14
Artificial blood, 324
Artificial heart, 269, 276–278, 282–297, 322, 328–329
Artificial ventricle, 269, 274–276, 283, 296, 327–328
Aspartate, 110, 115
Aspergillus infection, 202, 203, 306
Aspirin, 79, 146
Atrial natriuretic factor, 11, 180
Atrioventricular node, 102, 103–104
Atropine, 83
Autotransfusion, 23, 64, 150–151, 205–208
Azathioprine, 301, 306
Aztreonam, 201, 202
Azygos principle, 2

Bacteria
  filtration of, 57–58, 66
  see also Infection
Baroreceptors, 10, 12, 73, 217, 247
Benzalkonium chloride, 60
Benzodiazepines, 79, 80, 140
Beta-adrenergic blockade, 83
  pretreatment with, 92, 95
Bicarbonate buffer, 98
Blood, effects of cardiopulmonary bypass on, 16–20, 49–52, 145–147, 323–324
Blood banks, 205, 209
Blood cardioplegia, 100–101
  warm, 93, 116–117, 118
Blood filtration, 56–57, 61–64, 149–150
  autotransfusion and, 64, 207–208
Blood flow, 8–10, 214–215
  cerebral, 84, 187–189, 219, 230–231

Blood flow (*cont.*)
  mechanical limitations to, 11–13
  rates of, 40, 47, 216
  surface effects and, 18–19
Blood salvage, 23, 150–151, 205–208
Blood transfusion
  avoidance of, 23, 64, 150–151, 205–208
  infection *via*, 148–149, 150, 198
  massive, 144–145
  mismatched, 148–149
Blood volume, 10
  expansion, 208
Brain
  assessment of, 140
  blood flow in, 84, 187–189, 219, 230–231
  postoperative dysfunction of, 20–21, 61, 82, 149, 183–191, 232–233, 324
  pulsatile perfusion and, 219
Bronchial sepsis, chronic, 202
Bronchiolitis, obliterative, 307
Bronchoalveolar lavage, 194, 200, 202–203, 306
Bubble oxygenator, 14–15, 33–34, 322
  blood damage in, 49–52
  carbon dioxide transfer in, 49
  cerebral dysfunction and, 21, 190
  complement and, 164, 168–170
  development of, 3, 33, 42–43
  filters and, 19
  oxygen transfer in, 44–45
Bubble point pressure (BPP), 59, 60–61
'Bubble tube' system, 214
Buffering
  of cardioplegic solution, 98
  of reperfusate, 115
Bundle of His, 102

Calcium, 24, 89, 90, 91
  in cardioplegia, 96–97
  and citrate, 151
  paradox, 90, 96, 100
  in reperfusion, 113–114
Calcium-channel blockers
  and cardioplegia, 92–93, 95, 97, 111
  and cerebral dysfunction, 190
  and kidney, 180
Candida infection, 202, 203
Cannulation techniques, 5, 12, 82, 323, 325
Capillary permeability, 10
Carbon dioxide, 13, 48–49
  in brain, 187, 188, 231
  extracorporeal removal of, 309, 310, 315
  in intra-aortic balloon, 243
Cardiac arrest, 260
Cardiogenic shock, 326
  extracorporeal membrane oxygenation and, 274
  intra-aortic balloon pump and, 237, 245–247, 256–257, 271
  reperfusion and, 117–118
Cardiomyoplasty, 278
Cardioplegia, 95–113
  administration of, 104–108
  filtration and, 64–66, 106
  neonatal, 119
  reperfusion following, 113–118
  secondary, 117–118
Cardiopulmonary bypass, hypothermic, 93–94
Cardiotomy reservoir, 37
  autotransfusion and, 207–208, 209
  filtration and, 61, 64, 207–208
  venting to, 60
Catalase, 90, 91, 112, 116
Catecholamines, 10, 12, 73, 218
Catheterization, cardiac, 257, 326
Cell washing, 23, 207
Centrifugal (impeller) pump, 36–37, 272–273, 309, 311–312, 322, 325, 328–329
Cerebral dysfunction *see under* Brain
Cerebral function analysis monitor, 231
Cerebrospinal fluid, pulsation of, 219
Children
  circulatory arrest in, 231–233
  extracorporeal membrane oxygenation in, 274, 309, 316–318
  intra-aortic balloon pumping in, 262–263
  myocardial protection in, 118–119
  pulsatile perfusion in, 223–224
  transplantation in, 203–204, 300
Ciprofloxacin, 201
Circulatory arrest, total, 231–234
Citrate toxicity, 151
Clamshell artificial heart, 291–292
Cleaning of extracorporeal circuit, 24
Clear fluid filtration, 57–58, 64–66
Coagulation, 16–18, 20, 40, 146–147
  of salvaged blood, 206
Colloid primes, 23, 74–75
Community hospital, intra-aortic balloon pumping at, 261–262
Complement system, 10, 15, 19, 150, 156–171
Compressed air, contamination of, 66
Computers, 325
Cooling, cardiac, 103–104, 323
Coronary circulation, 88–89
  pulsatile flow and, 220–221
Coronary ostial perfusion, 94
Coronary sinus cardioplegia, 106–107
Coronary steal effect, 81
Corticosteroids, 113, 169
Cortisol, 11, 84, 218
Co-trimoxazole, 201, 202, 303, 306
Counterpulsation, 212, 236
  intra-aortic balloon, 236–263, 269, 271–272, 327
C-reactive protein
  complement and, 164, 166
  transplantation and, 200, 202
Creatine phosphate, 88, 89, 108
Crystalloid cardioplegic solutions, 96, 99, 101
  oxygenated, 99–100, 102
  with perfluorocarbons, 101–102
Crystalloid primes, 23, 73–74
Cyclosporin A, 200–201, 302, 303–304, 306
Cystic fibrosis, 202, 203, 304, 306
Cytomegalovirus (CMV), 64
  testing for, 196, 197, 305
  transplantation and, 198–199, 201, 203, 303, 306

Depth filtration, 57, 62
Desferrioxamine, 91, 112, 116, 180
Desmopressin, 17, 147, 206
Dextrans, 72, 74–75, 113

Dextrose 5% in water, 72, 73–74
Diaphragm pump, 4
Diaphragmatic hernia, congenital, 316, 318
Diazepam, 80, 189
Differential mass balance, 44
Dilazep, 93
Diltiazem, 111
Dipyridamole, 18, 79, 93, 146
Dobutamine, 85
Dopamine, 85, 180

Eisenmenger's syndrome, 304
Electrolytes, 23–24
  in cardioplegic solutions, 96–99
  in priming solutions, 74
see also individual electrolytes
Endothelial derived relaxing factor, 88, 179
Endothelium
  coronary, 88
    damage to, 102–103
  renal, 179
Endotoxins, 66
Enflurane, 80, 81, 189
Enoximone, 85
Epinephrine (adrenaline), 85, 218, 247
Epstein-Barr virus (EBV), 196, 197–198
Erythrocytes, damage to *see* Haemolysis
Ethylene oxide toxicity, 24
Etomidate, 80
Extracellular fluid, 10, 23–24
Extracorporeal carbon dioxide removal ($ECCO_2R$), 309, 310, 315
Extracorporeal membrane oxygenation (ECMO), 274, 309–314, 326
  paediatric, 274, 309, 316–318

Factors, clotting, 17–18, 146, 168, 206
Fentanyl, 80, 81, 84
Fever, postoperative, 200, 201
Fibrin/fibrinogen, 16–18, 146–147, 206, 323
Fibronectin depletion, 64
Film oxygenator, 3–4, 14–15, 42
Filtration/filters, 19, 56–57, 149–150, 323
  of autotransfused blood, 64, 207–208
  in cardioplegia, 64–66, 106
  and cerebral dysfunction, 61, 62, 190
  product details, 66–67
Flucloxacillin, 197, 202, 303
Fluid(s), 10, 23–24
  see also Oedema
Flumazenil, 140
Fluorocarbon emulsions, 23, 73, 101–102
Fluosol-DA, 23
Foam oxygenator, 3, 14–15
Folinic acid, 306
Free radicals, 90–91, 111–112, 115–116
  kidney and, 180
  scavengers of, 19, 91, 112, 116
Fresh frozen plasma, 149
Frusemide, 180
Fumarate, 110–111

Ganciclovir, 198–199, 306
Gas exchange process, 13–16, 43–49
Gas filtration, 58–59, 66
Gas microemboli, 61–62, 100, 313, 314
Gastrointestinal complications, 21
Gelatins, 75, 113
GIK (intravenous glucose-insulin-potassium), 92, 115
Glucocorticoids, 113, 169
Glucose, 11, 74, 110, 115
Glutamate, 110–111
  in brain, 191
  as buffer, 98
  in reperfusion, 115
Glycogen loading, 92
Gravity drainage, 5
Growth hormone, 11

Haemodialysis, 181
Haemodilution, 8–10, 17, 23, 73, 144
Haemofiltration, 56, 181, 312
Haemolysis, 19, 49, 145
  filtration and, 62–63
  kidney and, 21–22, 179
  pulsatile perfusion and, 217
Haemorrhage, postoperative, 144, 145, 146–147, 149
Halothane, 10, 81, 186
Hearing loss, postoperative, 184
Heart transplantation, 194–201, 299–304
  artificial heart and, 269, 277, 282, 296
  extracorporeal membrane oxygenation and, 274, 312
  intra-aortic balloon pump and, 261, 271
  shortage of donors for, 268, 296
  ventricular assist devices and, 269, 273, 275–276
Heart-lung transplantation, 201–203, 299–300, 304–307
Heat exchanger, 37–38, 43, 323
Hemopump, 272
Heparin, 16–18, 40
  artificial heart and, 295
  complement and, 165–168
  discovery of, 1, 33
  dosage of, 5, 147
  equipment coated with, 60, 274, 309, 312, 315–316, 324, 325
  extracorporeal respiratory support and, 312
  rebound of, 147–148
  reversal of, 20, 40, 85, 147, 166–168
Hepatitis B virus (HBV)
  blood transfusion and, 148–149, 150
  transplantation and, 196
Herpes simplex virus (HSV), 303, 306
Histamine, 8, 10
Histidine buffer, 98
Human immunodeficiency virus (HIV)
  blood transfusion and, 148–149, 150
  transplantation and, 196
Hydralazine, 83
Hydrogen peroxide, 90–91, 170
Hydroxyethyl starch, 75, 113
Hyperbilirubinaemia, 21
Hyperglycaemia, 11, 74
Hyperkalaemia, 145
Hypertension, 10, 40, 83
  postoperative, 208–209
  pulmonary, neonatal, 316, 318
Hypokalaemia, 24, 74
Hypotension, 8–10, 40
  cerebral dysfunction and, 186
  pre-operative, 83

Hypothermia (hypothermic), 10, 23, 40, 73, 84, 324, 325
cardioplegia, 95–113
cardiopulmonary bypass, 93–94
low flow, 230–231
circulatory arrest, 231–234
intermittent ischaemia, 94, 95
ventricular fibrillation, 94–95
Hypoxanthine, 89, 93, 102, 109
oxidation of, 90–91

Iloprost, 18
Imidazole, 180
as buffer, 98
Impeller pump *see* Centrifugal pump
Infection, 25
of artificial heart, 294
of mechanical circulatory support, 271
septic shock, 260
and transfusion, 148–149, 150, 198
and transplantation, 194–204, 302–303, 306–307
Inosine, 89, 93, 102, 109
Insulin, 11, 74, 115
Intellectual impairment, postoperative, 20–21, 183, 184–186
Intensive care unit, transfer to, 85–86, 138–139
Intermittent ischaemia, hypothermic, 94, 95
Intra-aortic balloon pump, 212, 236–263, 269, 271–272, 327
Intravascular oxygenation (IVOX), 315, 322
Intravenous therapy solutions, filtration of, 64–66
Ischaemia, myocardial, 89–90, 269–270
neonatal, 118–119
Isoflurane, 81, 84

Jaundice, postoperative, 21
Jugular vein cannulation, 82

Kallikrein, 168
Ketamine, 80
Kidney, 21–22, 40, 178–181, 324
artificial heart and, 295
cyclosporin A and, 200
non-pulsatile flow and, 12, 179, 219
pulsatile perfusion and, 219
K-score, 51

Labetalol, 83
Leukocytes, 19, 22, 145–146, 323–324
filtration of, 63, 64
reperfusion injury and, 63
Lidoflazine, 93, 95
Liquid filtration, 56–58
blood, 56–57, 61–64, 149–150, 207–208
bubble removal in, 59–60
clear fluid, 57–58, 64–66
Liver damage, 21
Low flow cardiopulmonary bypass, 230–231
Low molecular weight dextran (LMWD), 72, 74
Lungs
postoperative dysfunction of, 22, 63, 72, 140–141, 170–171, 220, 324–325
postoperative infection of, 194, 197, 201
pulsatile perfusion and, 219–220
transplantation of, 201–203, 299–300, 304–307

Magnesium, 24, 89
in cardioplegia, 97
Maintenance of extracorporeal circuit, 24
Malate, 110–111
Mannitol, 22, 74, 112, 115, 180
Meconium aspiration syndrome, 316, 318
Mediastinum, blood salvaged from, 206, 207
Membrane filtration, 57–58
Membrane oxygenator, 14–15, 34, 322–323
blood damage in, 49–52
carbon dioxide transfer in, 48–49
cerebral dysfunction and, 21, 190
complement and, 168–170
development of, 4, 33, 42–43
extracorporeal respiratory support with, 274, 309, 310–311, 315
microbubbles in, 61–62
oxygen transfer in, 45–48
Metaraminol, 83, 84
Methoxamine, 84
Methyl-prednisolone, 19, 113, 169, 302
Metronidazole, 202
Microemboli, 18, 61–64, 149–150, 220
cerebral, 21, 149, 186–187, 189, 190
gas, 61–62, 100, 313, 314
Midazolam, 140
Mioflazine, 93
Morphine, 140
Muscle *see* Myocardium; Skeletal muscle
Muscle relaxants, 80
Myocardium (myocardial), 22
contusion, 260
infarction, 326
intra-aortic balloon pump and, 257
see also Cardiogenic shock
ischaemia, 89–90, 118–119, 269–270
protection, intraoperative, 88–119
cardioplegic, 95–113
non-cardioplegic, 93–95
paediatric, 118–119
pulsatile perfusion and, 220–221
reperfusion injury, 63, 90–92, 119
suppression of, 113–117
stunning, 89, 91

Natamstat mesilate, 170
Nervous system, 10
damage to, 20–21, 56, 61, 62, 82, 149, 183–191, 323, 324
pulsatile perfusion and, 219
see also Brain
Neutrophils, 10, 19, 22
complement and, 10, 19, 162, 164, 170
kallikrein and, 168
reperfusion injury and, 91
Nifedipine, 111
Nimodipine, 190
Nitroglycerin, 83, 84, 85
Nitrous oxide, 80, 81, 186
NMDA (*N*-methyl-*D*-aspartate) antagonists, 191
Noradrenaline (norepinephrine), 85, 218, 247
Nucleoside(s), 88, 89–90, 93, 102
in cardioplegia, 109
transport inhibition, 93, 95, 109–110
see also Adenosine triphosphate

Nystatin, 196

Oedema
cardioplegia and, 112–113
pulsatile perfusion and, 217
reperfusion and, 114–115
Opiates, 80, 81, 84, 140
Oxygen
consumption, 15–16, 40, 47–48, 73
delivery, 13–14, 15–16, 44–48, 73
paradox, 90
Oxygenated cardioplegic solutions, 99–102
Oxygenator(s), 33–34, 42–52, 322, 325
blood damage in, 16–20, 49–52
cerebral dysfunction and, 21, 190
complement and, 168–170
gas transfer in, 13–16, 43–49
heparin-bonded, 309, 312, 315–316
history of, 3–4, 33, 42–43
intravascular, 315, 322
performance of, 13–14
types of, 3–4, 14–15
see also Bubble oxygenator; Membrane oxygenator

Paediatrics *see* Children
Pancreas, 220
Pancreatitis, postoperative, 21, 220
Pancuronium, 80
Parathyroid hormone, 24
Percutaneous transluminal coronary angioplasty (PICA), 257, 259
Perfusion, adequacy of, 38–40, 73, 230–231
pH
of blood, 40
of cardioplegic solution, 96, 98, 100
of myocardium, 104
of reperfusate, 115
of skeletal muscle surface, 11
Phentolamine, 83, 84, 231
Phenylephrine, 83, 84, 231
Philadelphia-type artificial heart, 290–291
Phosphodiesterase inhibitors, 85
Plasmin/plasminogen, 17–18
Platelet(s), 16, 18–19, 49–52, 146, 206, 323–324
concentrate, 149
defects, 20
filtration and, 62–63
oxygenator type and, 15
pulsatile perfusion and, 217
reticuloendothelial function and, 22
Pleural cavity, blood salvaged from, 206, 207
Pneumococcal lobar pneumonia, 201
Pneumocystis carinii, 201, 202, 303, 306
Poiseuille's Equation, 214
Polyvinyl chloride (PVC) tubing, 24–25, 38
spallated, 64, 65
Postoperative management/morbidity, 85–86, 138–142
blood conservation and, 208–209
complement and, 170–171
lung dysfunction, 22, 63, 72, 140–141, 170–171, 220, 324–325
neurological dysfunction, 20–21, 56, 61, 62, 82, 149, 183–191, 323, 324
renal failure, 180–181
in transplant patients, 194, 197, 200–201, 202–203, 204

Potassium, 23–24, 74, 89, 145
in cardioplegia, 96, 103
Prebypass fluid filtration, 64–66
Predeposit donations, 150, 205
Pressure-controlled intermittent coronary sinus occlusion, 108
Priming solutions, 23, 24, 72–75, 144, 324, 325
complement and, 169–170
Procaine, 97
Profentanyl, 189
Prophylaxis, pre-transplantation, 197–198, 202, 303, 306
Propofol, 80, 84, 140
Propranolol, 92, 180
Prostacyclin, 18, 89, 180
cerebral dysfunction and, 190–191
Prostaglandins, 18, 89, 180, 190–191, 324
Protamine sulphate, 20, 40, 85, 147
complement and, 166–168
Pulmonary artery catheterization, 82–83
Pulsatile assist device (PAD), 212–214, 221–225
Pulsatile perfusion, 12, 211–225, 322, 325
Pump(s), 4–5, 35–37, 41, 212–214
see also Centrifugal pump; Roller pump
Pyrimethamine, 306

Rated flow, 13–14
Renal function *see* Kidney
Renin, 10, 179, 218
Reperfusion, 113–118
Reperfusion injury, 90–92
filtration and, 63
neonatal, 119
Respiratory support, extracorporeal, 274, 309–318, 326
Respiratory syncytial virus, 204
Reticuloendothelial function changes, 22
Right atrial cardioplegia, 107–108
Rigid reservoir, 37
Ringer's lactate primes, 74
Roller pump, 4–5, 35, 212, 272–273, 311, 322
Rotavirus, 204

Screen filtration, 57, 62–63, 149–150
Sedation: during mechanical ventilation, 139–140
Septic shock, 260
Shear stress, 49, 145
Silicone
artificial hearts, 293
rubber tubing, 38, 65
Skeletal muscle
surface pH measurement, 11
ventricular assist, 278
Sodium, 23–24, 89
in cardioplegia, 97
Sodium metabisulphite, 197
Sodium nitroprusside, 83, 84, 208–209
Soft artificial heart, 292–293
Soft reservoir, 37
Soluflazine, 93
Sorenson autotransfusion system, 207
'Stepping' motor pump, 214
Stored blood, filtration of, 63–64
Streptokinase, 257
Stroke, 184, 186
Strome free haemoglobin solutions, 73
Succinate, 110–111

Suction drainage, 5
Sufentanial, 80
Superoxide dismutase, 91, 112, 116
Superoxide radical, 90–91
Systemic vascular resistance, 40, 73, 216

Tachyarrhythmias, ventricular, 259–260
Tension-time index, 269
Thromboxanes, 146, 167–168, 187
Thrombus formation, 18–19, 49
  artificial heart/ventricle and, 270–271, 282–283, 295
  balloon catheter and, 253
Total artificial heart, 269, 276–278, 283
Toxicity
  of circuit materials, 24
  of citrate, 151
Toxoplasma gondii, 199, 303, 306
  testing for, 196, 197
Tranexamic acid, 18, 147
Transbronchial lung biopsy, 194, 200, 202–203, 304, 306
Transplantation
  in children, 203–204, 300
  heart, 194–201, 299–304
    artificial heart and, 269, 277, 282, 296
    extracorporeal membrane oxygenation and, 274, 312
    intra-aortic balloon pump and, 261, 271
    shortage of donors for, 268, 296
    ventricular assist devices and, 269, 273, 275–276
  heart-lung, 201–203, 299–300, 304–307
  lung, 201–203
  microbiological aspects of, 194–204, 302–303, 306–307
Triiodothyronine (T_3), 115
Tubing, 24–25, 38
  filtration and, 64, 65
  heparin-bonded, 274, 312

Urine output, 11, 40, 223
  artificial heart and, 282

Valves, artificial heart, 290, 294
Varicella zoster, 203, 204
Vascular resistance, 40, 73, 216, 218, 220
  pulmonary, 141, 216, 219
Vasoconstrictor/vasodilator drugs, 83, 84–85
Vasopressin, 10, 218
Vecuronium, 80
Venous reservoir, 37
Ventilation, mechanical, 139
  weaning from, 141–142
  see also Respiratory support
Venting mechanisms, 60
Ventricular assist devices, 268, 269, 270, 274–276, 283, 296, 327–328
Ventricular fibrillation, hypothermic, 94–95
Ventricular tachyarrhythmias, 259–260
Verapamil, 111

Xanthine oxidase, 90–91

Yeast infection, 196